Essentials of Interventional Nephrology

Essentials of Interventional Nephrology

Editors

Vinant Bhargava
DNB (Med) DNB (Nephro) MNAMS FASN FRCP (Lon) FACP MBA (HCM)
Senior Consultant and Associate Professor
Ganga Ram Institute of Postgraduate Medical Education and Research (GRIPMER)
Department of Nephrology
Sir Ganga Ram Hospital
New Delhi, India

J Balasubramaniam
MBBS MD DM (Nephro) FRCP (Glas) FRCP (Lon) FASN (USA)
Transplant and Interventional Nephrologist
Department of Nephrology
Kidney Care Centre
Tirunelveli, Tamil Nadu, India

Prashant C Dheerendra
MD DM (Nephrology)
Senior Consultant
Department of Nephrology
Apollo Hospitals and Dharma Kidney Care
Bengaluru, Karnataka, India

Associate Editors

AK Bhalla
MD DM MNAMS FISN FASN (US) FRCP (Edinburgh) FISOT
Chairman and Head
Department of Nephrology
Sir Ganga Ram Hospital
New Delhi, India

Sanjiv Jasuja
MD DNB MNAMS FIMSA
Professor and Senior Consultant
Department of Nephrologist
Indraprastha Apollo Hospitals
New Delhi, India

Section Editors

Gireesh Reddy G
MD DM FASDIN
Assistant Professor
Interventional Nephrologist and Transplant Physician
Course In-charge, Fellowship in Interventional Nephrology
Department of Nephrology, Division of Interventional Nephrology, Institute of Nephro-Urology
Bengaluru, Karnataka, India

Lalathaksha Kumbar
MD MBA FASDIN
Clinical Associate Professor of Medicine
Michigan State University School of Medicine
Henry Ford Hospital
Detroit, MI, USA

Forewords

Padma Shree Professor DS Rana, Padma Shree Professor AK Bhalla, Mohan Rajapurkar

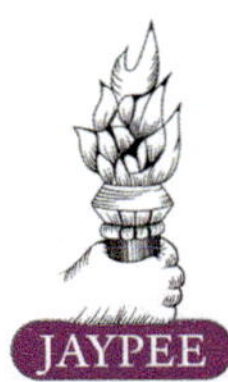

JAYPEE BROTHERS MEDICAL PUBLISHERS
The Health Sciences Publisher
New Delhi | London

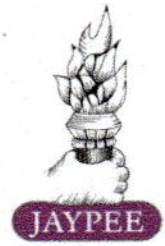

Jaypee Brothers Medical Publishers (P) Ltd

Headquarters
EMCA House, 23/23-B
Ansari Road, Daryaganj
New Delhi 110 002, India
Landline: +91-11-23272143, +91-11-23272703
+91-11-23282021, +91-11-23245672
e-mail: jaypee@jaypeebrothers.com

Corporate Office
4838/24, Ansari Road, Daryaganj
New Delhi 110 002, India
Phone: +91-11-43574357
Fax: +91-11-43574314
e-mail: jaypee@jaypeebrothers.com

Overseas Office
JP Medical Ltd.
83, Victoria Street, London
SW1H 0HW (UK)
Phone: +44-20 3170 8910
e-mail: info@jpmedpub.com

EU GPSR Authorised Representative
Logos Europe, 9 rue Nicolas Poussin
17000, La Rochelle, France
Phone: +33 (0) 6 67 93 73 78
e-mail: contact@logoseurope.eu

Website: www.jaypeebrothers.com
Website: www.jaypeedigital.com

Inquiries for bulk sales may be solicited at: jaypee@jaypeebrothers.com

Essentials of Interventional Nephrology

First Edition: **2026**

ISBN: 978-93-6616-143-8

Printed in India

Contributors

Aadil Beigh MD DNB
Director
Department of Nephrology
Paras Health
Srinagar, Jammu and Kashmir, India

Aakash Kirit Shingada
DNB DNB MRCP SCE FASN
Chief of Transplantation
Department of Nephrology
Namaha Specialised Healthcare
Mumbai, Maharashtra, India

Abhijit Madhav Konnur MD DNB
Senior Consultant
Department of Nephrology
Muljibhai Patel Urological Hospital
Nadiad, Gujarat, India

Abhilasha Soni MD DM
Associate Consultant Nephrologist
Department of Nephrology
Venkateshwar Hospital
New Delhi, India

Adrian P Sequeira
MD FACP FASN FASDIN
Professor of Clinical Medicine and
Director of Interventional Nephrology
Department of Nephrology
LSU Health Shreveport Academic
Medical Center
Shreveport, LA, USA

Ajit K Yadav DNB FVIR EBIR
Senior Consultant
Department of Interventional Radiology
Sir Ganga Ram Hospital
New Delhi, India

AK Bhalla
MD DM MNAMS FISN FASN (US) FRCP
(Edinburgh) FISOT
Chairman and Head
Department of Nephrology
Sir Ganga Ram Hospital
New Delhi, India

Ambarish Satwik MS DNB
Senior Consultant and Director
Vascular Cath Lab
Institute of Vascular and
Endovascular Sciences
Sir Ganga Ram Hospital
New Delhi, India
Professor of Vascular Surgery
Ganga Ram Institute of Postgraduate
Medical Education and Research
(GRIPMER), New Delhi, India

Amrita Dua MS DNB
Senior Resident
Department of Urology and
Renal Transplant
Sir Ganga Ram Hospital
New Delhi, India

Anantharam Jairam MD DNB DM
Professor
Department of Nephrology
St John's Medical College Hospital
Bengaluru, Karnataka, India

Anirudha Datta DNB DM
Clinical Associate
Department of Nephrology
Kolkata Kidney Institute
Kolkata, West Bengal, India

Anish Kumar Gupta
BPharm MPharm
Senior Research Officer
Department of Nephrology and
Renal Transplant Medicine
Max Super Speciality Hospital
New Delhi, India

Anurag Gupta MD DM FASN
Director Dialysis and Professor (GRIPMER)
Department of Nephrology
Sir Ganga Ram Hospital
New Delhi, India

Arushi Nautiyal DNB DrNB
Consultant
Department of Nephrology and
Kidney Transplantation
Jaipur Golden Hospital
New Delhi, India

Ashwani Gupta MD DM FISN FASN
Professor (GRIPMER) and Co-Director
Department of Nephology
Sir Ganga Ram Hospital
New Delhi, India

Ayush Thomas
US Doctor of Medicine Bachelor of Science
Resident, Post Graduate Year 2
Department of Radiology
Lahey Hospital and Medical Center
Burlington, Massachusetts, USA

Bharat Sachdeva MD
Professor of Clinical Medicine
Chief of Nephrology
Director of Dialysis
LSU Health Shreveport, LA, USA
President, American Society of
Diagnostic and Interventional
Nephrology (ASDIN)

Cherin Josi C DNB DrNB
Interventional Nephrologists Consultant
Department of Nephrology,
Division of Interventional Nephrology
Institute of Nephro-Urology
Bengaluru, Karnataka, India

Daniel Rubin DO
Fellowship
Department of Interventional Radiology
Cleveland Clinic
Cleveland, Ohio, USA

Darshan Thummar MD DNB DrNB
DrNB Registrar
Department of Interventional Radiology
Sir Ganga Ram Hospital
New Delhi, India

Denis Dawle Tirkey MD DrNB
Superspecialist
Department of Nephrology
ESIC Medical College and Hospital
Faridabad, Haryana, India

Dileep Kumar P MD DM
Interventional Nephrologists Consultant
Department of Nephrology
Division of Interventional Nephrology
Institute of Nephro-Urology
Bengaluru, Karnataka, India

Dinesh Khullar
DM MD FASN FISN FISOT FRCP (Edin) FACP
Chairman
Department of Nephrology and Renal Transplant Medicine
Max Super Speciality Hospital
New Delhi, India

Dwarak S MD DNB FIN
Assistant Professor
Department of Nephrology
Division of Interventional Nephrology
Institute of Nephro-Urology
Bengaluru, Karnataka, India

Edwin Mervin Fernando MD DM
Professor and Head
Department of Nephrology
Government Stanley Medical College
Chennai, Tamil Nadu, India

ET Arun Thomas
MD DNB DM DrNB MNAMS SCE (Nephro) RCP (UK)
Professor
Department of Nephrology
Believers Church Medical College Hospital
Thiruvalla, Kerala, India

Gireesh Reddy G MD DM FASDIN
Assistant Professor
Interventional Nephrologist and Transplant Physician
Course In-charge, Fellowship in Interventional Nephrology
Department of Nephrology
Division of Interventional Nephrology
Institute of Nephro-Urology
Bengaluru, Karnataka, India

Hardik B Patel MD DNB
Consultant
Department of Nephrology
Muljibhai Patel Urological Hospital
Nadiad, Gujarat, India

Hemant J Mehta
MD DM DNB FASDIN (USA) FISN (International) FISN (India)
Head
Department of Nephrology
Lilavati Hospital and Research Centre
Mumbai, Maharashtra, India

J Balasubramaniam
MBBS MD DM (Nephro) FRCP (Glas) FRCP (Lon) FASN (USA)
Transplant and Interventional Nephrologist
Department of Nephrology
Kidney Care Centre
Tirunelveli, Tamil Nadu, India

James Andrews
PGCert (Ultrasound) FRCP (Edin)
Consultant Interventional Nephrologist
Department of Renal Medicine
South Tyneside and Sunderland NHS Foundation Trust
and Newcastle University
Sunderland, Tyne and Wear, UK

Jia Shen-Goh MRCP (UK)
Trust Doctor
Department of Renal Medicine
South Tyneside and Sunderland NHS Foundation Trust
Sunderland, Tyne and Wear, UK

Jishnu Mohan MD DM
Consultant in Nephrology
Department of Nephrology
Ananthapuri Hospitals and Research Institute
Thiruvananthapuram, Kerala, India

Jitendra Kumar
MD DNB DM FISN
Chairman
Department of Renal Sciences and Transplant Medicine
Accord Hospital
Faridabad, Haryana, India

Kanav Anand MD FPN
Senior Consultant Pediatric Nephrologist
Division of Pediatric Nephrology and Renal Transplantation
Institute of Child Health
Sir Ganga Ram Hospital
New Delhi, India

Karthik Balasubramaniam MD DM
Consultant Nephrologist
Fellow in Interventional Nephrologist
Department of Nephrology
Kidney Care Centre
Tirunelveli, Tamil Nadu, India

Karthikeyan Balasubramanian
MD DM FASN
Senior Consultant
Department of Nephrology
Kauvery Hospital
Chennai, Tamil Nadu, India

Kasi Visweswaran R MD DM
Chief Consultant
Department of Nephrology
Ananthapuri Hospitals and Research Institute
Trivandrum, Kerala, India

Krishnaswamy Sampathkumar
MD DM FRCP (Glasgow) FASN FISN
Senior Consultant and Head
Department of Nephrology
Meenakshi Mission Hospital and Research Centre
Madurai, Tamil Nadu, India

Kristin George MD DM
Consultant Nephrologist and Renal Transplant Physician
Department of Nephrology
Aster Whitefield
Bengaluru, Karnataka, India

Kulwant Singh
MD DNB MNAMS FICP
Principal Consultant
Department of Nephrology
Max Super Specialty Hospital
New Delhi, India

Lalathaksha Kumbar MD MBA FASDIN
Clinical Associate Professor of Medicine
Michigan State University School of Medicine
Henry Ford Hospital
Detroit, MI, USA

Manish Lalwani MD DNB
Assistant Professor
Department of Nephrology
Christian Medical College
Vellore, Tamil Nadu, India

Manish Malik MD DNB MNAMS
Vice Chairman and Professor (GRIPMER)
Department of Nephrology
Institute of Renal Sciences
Sir Ganga Ram Hospital
New Delhi, India

Manish Rathi MD DM
Professor
Department of Nephrology
Postgraduate Institute of Medical Education and Research
Chandigarh, India

Manisha Sahay
MD DNB FAMS FRCP (Lon)
Professor and Head
Department of Nephrology
Osmania Medical College and General Hospital
Hyderabad, Telangana, India

Mehak Singla
MD DrNB (Nephrology)
Consultant Nephrologist
Department of Nephrology
Primus Super Speciality Hospital
New Delhi, India

Mrinal Pahwa MS DNB MNAMS
Director (Urology, Uro-Oncology and Kidney Transplant)
Max Super Speciality Hospital
New Delhi, India

Namrata S Rao MD DM
Additional Professor
Department of Nephrology
Dr Ram Manohar Lohia Institute of Medical Sciences
Lucknow, Uttar Pradesh, India

Narinder Pal Singh
MD FACP FRCP (Edin) FASN ISHF FISN FAMS FICP MBA
Consultant (Academic Programs in Nephrology)
Max Super Speciality Hospital, Saket
Dean Research, Eternal University
Baru Sahib, Himachal Pradesh
Advisor Research
Faculty of Medicine and Health Sciences
SGT Medical College Hospital and Research Institute, SGT University
Gurugram, Haryana, India

Neil Saldanha DNB DrNB ESENeph FASN
Consultant Nephrologist and Transplant Physician
Department of Nephrology
Namaha Hospital
Mumbai, Maharashtra, India

Nikhil Chaudhari MS DNB
Associate Consultant
Department of Vascular and Endovascular Surgery
Sir Ganga Ram Hospital
New Delhi, India

Nikhil Sharma MS DNB
Consultant
Institute of Vascular and Endovascular Sciences
Sir Ganga Ram Hospital
New Delhi, India

Oladunni O Akin-Akintayo MD MPH
Fellowship
Department of Interventional Radiology
Cleveland Clinic
Cleveland, Ohio, USA

Pavitra Manu Dogra
MD DM FISN FASN FRCP (Edin)
Consultant and Head
Department of Nephrology
Army Hospital (Research and Referral)
New Delhi, India

Prabhu Kumarappan Chidambaram
MS DrNB
Consultant
Department of Vascular Surgery
Meenakshi Mission Hospital and Research Centre
Madurai, Tamil Nadu, India

Pranay Pawar MS MCH FEBVS FACS
Associate Professor
Department of Vascular Surgery Unit
Christian Medical College and Hospital
Ludhiana, Punjab, India

Prashant C Dheerendra
MD DM (Nephrology)
Senior Consultant
Department of Nephrology
Apollo Hospitals and Dharma Kidney Care
Bengaluru, Karnataka, India

Pratik Das MD DNB DM
Chief Consultant
Department of Nephrology
Rabindranath Tagore International Institute of Cardiac Sciences
Kolkata, West Bengal, India

Prem P Varma
MD DM MNAMS FICP FACP FRCP (Edin) FISN FASN FAMS
Principal Director and Head
Department of Nephrology
Venkateshwar Hospital
New Delhi, India

Priti Meena MD DNB FASN FRCP
Assistant Professor
Department of Nephrology
All India Institute of Medical Sciences
Bhubaneswar, Odisha, India

Purva Suhas Bavikar MD DM
Consultant Nephrologist and Transplant Physician
Department of Nephrology
Kamalnayan Bajaj Hospital
Chhatrapati Sambhajinagar, Maharashtra, India

Raghav Seth MD DNB FVIR
Consultant
Department of Interventional Radiology
Sir Ganga Ram Hospital
New Delhi, India

Rajdeb Saha MD DM
Associate Consultant and Interventional Nephrologist
Department of Nephrology
Sir Ganga Ram Hospital
New Delhi, India

Rajendran Vilvendan MD
Staff Interventional Radiologist
Department of Radiology
Lahey Hospital and Medical Center
Burlington, Massachusetts, USA

Ram Kishore Gurajala
MRCSEd FRCR DABIR
Assistant Professor
Department of Radiology
The Lerner College of Medicine
Case Western Reserve University
Cleveland, Ohio, USA

Ranjan Shetty MD DM
Medical Director
Department of Interventional Cardiology
Sparsh Group of Hospital
Bengaluru, Karnataka, India

Rashid Sharaf MD FASDIN
Penal Associate
Department of Interventional Nephrology
Star Vascular Access Centre
San Antonio, Texas, USA

Rauri A Clerk FRCF (Edin)
Consultant Interventional Nephrologist and Clinical Director
Department of Renal Medicine
South Tyneside and Sunderland NHS Foundation Trust
and Newcastle University
Sunderland, UK

Rekulapally Praneetha
MD Fellowship in Pediatric Nephrology
Fellow in Pediatric Nephrology
Department of Pediatric Nephrology
Sir Ganga Ram Hospital
New Delhi, India

Rozil Jayesh Gandhi
MD DMRD DNB Fellowship in Interventional Radiology
Senior Consultant
Department of Interventional Radiology
Sushrut Hospital
Ahmedabad, Gujarat, India

Ruhani Sachdeva MD
Professor of Medicine
Department of Nephrology
Northwestern University
Chicago, IL, USA

Sachin S Soni MD DNB MNAMS DrNB
Associate Professor
Department of Nephrology
Ulhas Patil Medical College and Hospital
Nashik, Maharashtra, India

Saeed Ahmed FRCP (Lon)
Consultant Interventional Nephrologist
Department of Renal Medicine
South Tyneside and Sunderland NHS Foundation Trust and Newcastle University
Sunderland, UK

Sahil Arora
MD DM DrNB MNAMS ESENeph FISN
Interventional Nephrologists Consultant
Department of Nephrology, Division of Interventional Nephrology
Institute of Nephro-Urology
Bengaluru, Karnataka, India

Sandeep Mahajan
MD DM FASN FISN FRCP MNAMS FICP
Professor
Department of Nephrology
All India Institute of Medical Sciences
New Delhi, India

Sanjay Srinivas MD DNB
Associate Professor
Department of Nephrology
Sri Siddhartha Medical College, Tumkur
Medical Director
Dr Sanjay's Center for Kidney and Diabetes
Bengaluru, Karnataka, India

Sanjiv Jasuja MD DNB MNAMS FIMSA
Professor and Senior Consultant
Department of Nephrologist
Indraprastha Apollo Hospitals
New Delhi, India

Santosh Varughese
MD DN FICN FRCP MBA
Professor
Department of Nephrology
Christian Medical College
Vellore, Tamil Nadu, India

Sarah McCloskey FRCP (Edin)
Consultant Nephrologist and Clinical Lead for Nephrology Services
Department of Renal Medicine
South Tyneside and Sunderland NHS Foundation Trust
and Newcastle University
Sunderland, UK

Sarvanan Balamuthuswamy
MD MPH FASN FASDIN
Professor of Medicine
Anne Burnette School of Medicine
Texas Christian University
Texas, USA

Saurabh Maruti Thanekar MD DM
Consultant Nephrologist
Department of Nephrology
Sachin Multispeciality Hospital
Kolhapur, Maharashtra, India

Shahbaj Ahmad
MD DNB ISN Scholar ISN Fellow
Professor
Department of General Medicine
Himalayan Institute of Medical Sciences
Dehradun, Uttarakhand, India

Shalabh Srivastava
PhD FRC (Edin)
Consultant Interventional Nephrologist and Programme Director (Nephrology and Interventional Nephrology)
Department of Renal Medicine
South Tyneside and Sunderland NHS Foundation Trust
and Newcastle University
Sunderland, UK

Shalini Priya MD DNB
Consultant
Department of Nephrology
Orchid Medical Centre
Ranchi, Jharkhand, India

Shamnad P MD DrNB
Consultant
Department of Nephrology
Believers Church Medical College Hospital
Thiruvalla, Kerala, India

Shyam B Bansal MD DM FRCP
Chairman
Department of Nephrology
Medanta—The Medicity
Gurugram, Haryana, India

Sishir Dashrathmal Gang
MD DM DrNB
Chairman
Department of Nephrology
Muljibhai Patel Urological Hospital
Nadiad, Gujarat, India

Smriti Sinha MD DrNB FASN
Consultant
Department of Nephrology
NEO Hospital
Noida, Uttar Pradesh, India

Sneha Anna Joy MD DM
Consultant
Department of Nephrology
Believers Church Medical College Hospital
Thiruvalla, Kerala, India

Sowrabha Rajanna MD DNB DM DrNB
Associate Professor
Department of Nephrology
St John's Medical College Hospital
Bengaluru, Karnataka, India

Srinivasavaradan Govindarajan
MD DM (Pediatric Nephrology)
Assistant Professor
Department of Pediatrics
Vardhman Mahavir Medical College and Safdarjung Hospital
New Delhi, India

Sukanya Govindan
MD DM ISN (Fellow)
Senior Consultant
Department of Pediatric Nephrology
Dr Mehta's Hospitals
Chennai, Tamil Nadu, India

Sumiran Mahajan MD DM
Interventional Nephrologist and Consultant
Department of Nephrology
Division of Interventional Nephrology
Institute of Nephro-Urology
Bengaluru, Karnataka, India

Suresh Kumar Margassery
MD MRCP (UK) FASDIN
Interventional and Consultant Nephrology
Department of Vascular Centre
Advanced Surgical Centre, SCA Health and Dallas Vascular Centre
Dallas, Texas, USA

Tarun Kumar MD DNB
Consultant Nephrologist
Department of Nephrology
Sir Ganga Ram Hospital
New Delhi, India

Tauhidul Alam Choudhury
MD DM ISN_IN Scholar PGDM—Organ Transplant
Consultant Nephrologist
Department of Nephrology
Dispur Hospitals
Guwahati, Assam, India

Tushar J Vachharajani MD FASN MBA
Vice Chair
Department of Medicine
Wayne State University School of Medicine
Detroit, Michigan, USA

Umapati N Hegde MD DNB
Vice Chairman
Department of Nephrology
Muljibhai Patel Urological Hospital
Nadiad, Gujarat, India

Umesh B Khanna MD DNB
Founder Chairperson
Department of Nephrology
Kidney Associates Pvt Ltd
Mumbai, Maharashtra, India

Upal Sengupta MD DM
Senior Consultant and Director
Department of Nephrology
Fortis Hospital and Kidney Institute
Kolkata, West Bengal, India

Urmila Anandh
MD DNB DM DNB FRCP
Adjunct Professor
Department of Nephrology
Amrita Institute of Medical Sciences and Research Centre
Faridabad, Haryana, India

Vaibhav Tiwari
MD DM ESE (Neph) FISN FASN
Associate Consultant and Associate Professor (GRIPMER)
Department of Nephrology
Sir Ganga Ram Hospital
New Delhi, India

Valentine Lobo MD DNB
Senior Consultant
Department of Nephrology
King Edward Memorial Hospital
Pune, Maharashtra, India

Varinder Singh Bedi
MS Fellow Vascular Society of India
Chairman and Senior Consultant
Institute of Vascular and Endovascular Sciences
Sir Ganga Ram Hospital
New Delhi, India

Vel Arvind MD DM DNB
Director
Department of Nephrology Services
Pineapple Dialysis Care and Apollo Hospitals
Tiruchirappalli, Tamil Nadu, India

Venkatesh Rajkumar S
MD DM FISN
Consultant
Department of Nephrology
Apollo Hospitals
Chennai, Tamil Nadu, India

Vidhi Singla MD DrNB
Senior Resident
Department of Nephrology
Sir Ganga Ram Hospital
New Delhi, India

Vijayaprakash Sreenarasimhaiah
MD FASDN RPVI
Interventional Nephrologist
Department of Nephrology
Houston Nephrology Group
Houston, Texas, USA

(Gp Cpt) Vijoy Kumar Jha
MD DNB DM
Professor
Department of Nephrology
Army Base Hospital Delhi Cantt
New Delhi, India

Vinant Bhargava
DNB (Med) DNB (Nephro) MNAMS FASN FRCP (Lon) FACP MBA (HCM)
Senior Consultant and Associate Professor
Ganga Ram Institute of Postgraduate Medical Education and Research (GRIPMER)
Senior Consultant
Department of Nephrology
Sir Ganga Ram Hospital
New Delhi, India

Vineet Behera
MD DM FISN FASN FACP FRCP FICP FGD
Consultant Nephrologist and Professor Medicine
Department of Nephrology
Armed Forces Medical College
Pune, Maharashtra, India

Vineeth Kurki M MD DNB EBIR
DrNB Resident
Department of Interventional Radiology
Sir Ganga Ram Hospital
New Delhi, India

Vipul Prakash Sanghavi
MRCP (UK) DrNB Renal Transplant and Interventional Nephrology Fellow
Consultant Interventional Nephrologist and Renal Transplant Physician
Department of Nephrology
Sanghavi Multispeciality Hospital
Kolhapur, Maharashtra, India

Vivek Goel DrNB ESENeph (UK) MD
Consultant Nephrologist and Transplant Physician
Department of Nephrology
Apollo Multispecialty Hospital
Kolkata, West Bengal, India

Wasiyeeullah Z Shaikh
DNB (Med) DNB (Nephrology)
Consultant
Department of Nephrology
Lilavati Hospital and Research Centre
Mumbai, Maharashtra, India

Yimeng Zhang
BSc (Hons) MD MRCP (UK)
Renal Registrar
Department of Renal Medicine
University Hospitals Birmingham NHS Foundation Trust
Birmingham, West Midlands, England

Yogita Sharma MD DNB DrNB
Senior Resident
Department of Nephrology
Sir Ganga Ram Hospital
New Delhi, India

Foreword

Interventional nephrology stands at the crossroads of innovation and patient-centered care, offering transformative solutions for individuals living with kidney disease. As the field is evolving, so too has the need for a comprehensive, practical, and evidence-based resource to guide clinicians, trainees, and allied health professionals through its rapidly expanding landscape. This textbook fulfills that need with clarity, definition, and vision.

The present-day nephrologist is no longer confined to the realm of diagnosis and medical management alone. Today, he is called upon to master a suite of interventional procedures ranging from vascular access creation and maintenance, to peritoneal dialysis catheter placement, to advanced diagnostic and therapeutic interventions. These skills not only enhance patient outcomes but also empower nephrologists to deliver more holistic and timely care.

This textbook brings together the collective intelligentsia of leading experts in the field of interventional nephrology. It offers a meticulous review of foundational principles, step-by-step procedural guidance, and thoughtful discussions of complications and their management. Each chapter is crafted to bridge the gap between theory and practice, enriched by illustrative cases, high-quality images, and pearls gleaned from years of clinical experience.

As you embark on this journey through the pages ahead, you will find a resource that is practical and comprehensive. Whether you are a seasoned practitioner seeking to refine your skills, a trainee eager to build a strong foundation, or a member of the multidisciplinary team striving for excellence, this textbook will serve as your indispensable companion.

The future of nephrology is interventional. With this textbook in hand, you are well equipped to meet its challenges and embrace its opportunities, ultimately improving the lives of those we serve.

Padma Shree Professor DS Rana
MD MNAMS
Professor
Department of Nephrology
Chairman, Institute of Renal Sciences
Chairman
Sir Ganga Ram Trust Society
New Delhi, India
Dr BC Roy Awardee

Padma Shree Professor AK Bhalla
MD DM MNAMS FISN FASN (USA) FRCP (Edinburgh) FISOT
Professor and Chairman
Department of Nephrology
Sir Ganga Ram Hospital
New Delhi, India
Dr BC Roy Awardee

Foreword

It gives me immense pleasure to introduce the *Essentials of Interventional Nephrology* to you. This book has been the result of contributions by nearly 100 authors with 49 chapters.

The aim of the book is to provide a genuine source of authentic information regarding interventional nephrology for students as well as junior faculty interested in the practice of this emerging in nephrology services. It is designed to provide a thorough and practical guide to the principles, techniques, and evolving landscape of interventional nephrology.

Interventional nephrology by nephrologists may provide a shift in the care delivery paradigm to consolidate interventional nephrologist and the conventional nephrologist to provide comprehensive management of patients needing these lifesaving procedures. This is the field that is most in demand by young nephrologists over past five years. The text I believe will provide for the needs of these professionals.

Interventional nephrology is presently in the realm of innovation, bridging the gap between traditional nephrology and procedural medicine. Over the past two decades, this subspecialty has evolved tremendously, empowering nephrologists to directly deal with complex vascular and peritoneal access needs of patients with chronic kidney disease at all stages. With integration of diagnostic and therapeutic procedures, such as ultrasonography, renal biopsy, vascular access creation and maintenance, and peritoneal dialysis catheter placement, interventional nephrology has transformed patient outcomes through timely, individualized, and cost-effective care. In the past, these interventions were performed by surgeons or radiologists, often resulting in delays and fragmented care. The emergence of interventional nephrology has enabled nephrologists to deliver comprehensive and seamless management, reducing cost of creation, intervention, maintenance of access, and improving the overall quality of life for their patients.

This book will certainly benefit nephrology trainees, practicing nephrologists, and allied professionals who seek to enhance their procedural skills and deepen their understanding of this essential field. The contributors have used evidence-based insights and collective experience of leading experts to inspire a new generation of nephrologists.

I express my best wishes to my young friend and colleague Dr Vinant Bhargava and his team for the success of this book for achieving its' aims.

Mohan Rajapurkar
MD
Former Trustee, VT Desai Charity Trust
Former Member, Board of Governors
Muljibhai Patel Society for Research in Nephro-Urology
Director (Retired) Post-Graduate Studies and Research
Muljibhai Patel Urological Hospital
Dr VV Desai Road
Nadiad, Gujarat, India
Recipient, BC Roy National Award 2007
Past President Indian Society of Nephrology 2018
Recipient, Pioneer Award, South Asia ISN 2023

Preface

Interventional nephrology is presently in the realm of innovation, bridging the gap between traditional nephrology and procedural medicine. Over the past two decades, this subspecialty has evolved tremendously, empowering nephrologists to directly deal with complex vascular and peritoneal access needs of patients with chronic kidney disease and end-stage renal disease. With integration of diagnostic and therapeutic procedures, such as ultrasonography, renal biopsy, vascular access creation and maintenance, and peritoneal dialysis catheter placement, interventional nephrology has transformed patient outcomes through timely, individualized, and cost-effective care.

In the past, these interventions were performed by surgeons or radiologists, often resulting in delays and fragmented care. The emergence of interventional nephrology has enabled nephrologists to deliver comprehensive and seamless management, reducing cost of creation, intervention, maintenance of access, and improving the overall quality of life for their patients.

This book aims to provide a thorough and practical guide to the principles, techniques, and evolving landscape of interventional nephrology. It is designed keeping in mind problems faced by nephrology trainees, practicing nephrologists, and allied professionals who seek to enhance their procedural skills and deepen their understanding of this essential field. We have used evidence-based insights and collective experience of leading experts to inspire a new generation of nephrologists to embrace interventional practice and continue advancing the care of patients with vascular access problems.

Vinant Bhargava
J Balasubramaniam
Prashant C Dheerendra

Acknowledgments

To our mentors in nephrology

To our colleagues, well-wishers, and contributors whose work has paved the path forward for the future generations

To our parents, wives, and families who have endured with us with their patience and unfailing support during the preparation of this edition

To our God and our patients, without whom we would not have had the privilege to cure and care.

To the future glory of interventional nephrology.

Contents

SECTION 11: Ethical and Legal Considerations in Intervention for Nephrologist

SECTION 12: Peritoneal Dialysis

Video Archive

Chapter 5. Ultrasound/Doppler for Vein Mapping

Nikhil Chaudhari

Video 1 Ultrasound/Doppler for vein mapping

Chapter 6. Renal Ultrasound

Yimeng Zhang, Shalabh Srivastava, Sarah McCloskey, James Andrews

Video 1 Left forearm radiocephalic AVF. How to position the patient for fistula assessment using a high frequency linear probe.

Video 2 Left forearm radiocephalic AVF. Video showing how to assess the access. Ultrasound assessment starts with a transverse and then longitudinal assessment of the inflow artery and juxta-anastomotic segment. Ideally assess pre-anastomotic waveform using spectral Doppler looking for a characteristic monophasic antegrade low resistive waveform with spectral broadening.

Video 3 Left forearm radiocephalic AVF. Longitudinal and transverse assessment of juxta-anastomotic segment followed by a transverse assessment of the body of the fistula noting areas which will need further assessment in longitudinal orientation either in B-mode or using color Doppler.

Video 4 Left forearm radiocephalic AVF. Longitudinal assessment of the fistula outflow. In this case following initially the median cubital to basilic vein, followed by an assessment of the cephalic vein. In cases where outflow stenosis is suspected, follow the veins until they enter the deep venous system, making assessments of the vessels in transverse and longitudinal views with the addition of color Doppler where appropriate.

Chapter 8. Preoperative Evaluation of Arteriovenous Fistula

Shalini Priya, Vidhi Singla, Vinant Bhargava

Video 1 Preoperative assessment for arteriovenous fistula creation

Video 2 Preoperative evaluation for arteriovenous fistula by ultrasound

Chapter 10. Arteriovenous Fistula Creation

10.1 Surgical Arteriovenous Fistula

Yogita Sharma, AK Bhalla, Ashwani Gupta, Sanjiv Jasuja

Video 1 Incision, dissection and preparation of radial artery and cephalic vein for RC AV fistula creation.

Video 2 Incision, dissection and preparation of radial artery and cephalic vein for RC AV fistula creation.

Video 3 Incision, dissection and preparation of radial artery and cephalic vein for RC AV fistula creation.

10.2B Endovascular Arteriovenous Fistulas: Options, Maintenance, and Salvage

Sarvanan Balamuthuswamy, Vijayaprakash Sreenarasimhaiah

Video 4 Evaluation of an endovascular AV fistula

Chapter 11. Arteriovenous Graft Placement

Ambarish Satwik, Pranay Pawar

Video 1 Flushing the prosthetic graft with a feeding tube to remove clots and fibrin.

Video 2 De-airing the graft before commencing flow.

Chapter 12. Tunneled Cuffed Catheter Insertion

Prashant C Dheerendra, Karthikeyan Balasubramanian, Denis Dawle Tirkey

Video 1 Tunneled dialysis catheter (permcath) insertion

Video 2 Tunneled dialysis catheter removal.

Chapter 13. Vascular Access Creation for Hemodialysis by Nontunneled Catheters

Shahbaj Ahmad, Smriti Sinha

Video 1 Nontunneled catheter procedure

Chapter 15. Access Maintenance and Cannulation Techniques

Aakash Kirit Shingada, Vivek Goel, Neil Saldanha

Video 1 Steps of cannulation

Video 2 Steps of decannulation

Chapter 19. Hardware Requirements for Cath Laboratory Interventions by Nephrologists

J Balasubramaniam, Karthik Balasubramaniam

Video 1 Fluoroscopy guided fistuloplasty for RCF. Illustrative demo to show the hardwares required for juxta-anastomotic stenosis causing fistula dysfunction.

Video 2 Fluoroscopy guided angioplasty for central vein stenosis of left brachiocephalic vein in a patient with left BCF. Illustrative demo to show the hardwares required for central vein stenosis intervention by nephrologist.

Chapter 20. Angioplasty/Stenting

Rajendran Vilvendan, Ayush Thomas

Video 1 Purse-string technique for closure of access site

Chapter 21. Thrombolysis Techniques

Jia Shen-Goh, Rauri A Clerk, Saeed Ahmed, Shalabh Srivastava

Video 1 Initial fistulographic evaluation of the left brachiocephalic AV fistula revealed extensive thrombosis within the outflow vein.

Video 2 Fistuloplasty resulted in partial resolution of thrombotic occlusion with restoration of limited flow. Residual stenosis/thrombus remains evident.

Video 3 The Cleaner XT™ Rotational Thrombectomy System was utilized for mechanical maceration of residual thrombus within the thrombosed fistula, resulting in further clearance of the occlusion.

Video 4 Fistula patency was effectively restored using the Cleaner XT™ device, with good flow noted on final angiography.

Video 5 Another video illustrates enhanced restoration of flow in a previously thrombosed fistula, which had already been treated with AngioJet™ thrombectomy, balloon angioplasty, and catheter aspiration. This improvement was achieved using the Cleaner XT™ device under ultrasound guidance.

Chapter 26. Stenosis or Thrombosis of Vascular Access
26.2 Arteriovenous Fistula and Grafts
Venkatesh Rajkumar S, Nikhil Sharma, Varinder Singh Bedi

Video 1 JAS
Video 2 PTA
Video 3 Post-PTA

Chapter 28. Accessory Veins: Identification and Management
Arushi Nautiyal, J Balasubramaniam

Video 1 Accessory vein: AV fistula
Video 2 Accessory branches vis-à-vis maturation failure

Chapter 32. Vascular Access in Patients with Complex Anatomy
Sachin S Soni, Sanjay Srinivas, Umapati N Hegde

Video 1 Translumbar IVC permcath

Chapter 34. Kidney Biopsy
Vineet Behera, Tauhidul Alam Choudhury

Video 1 USG Doppler imaging of kidney for vascular supply

Chapter 37. Renal Denervation Techniques
Kristin George, Ranjan Shetty

Video 1 Selective renal angiography with Simplicity Spyral system—Part I
Video 2 Selective renal angiography with Simplicity Spyral system—Part II

Chapter 39. Renal Allograft Complications and Their Management
Vel Arvind, Karthik Balasubramaniam

Video 1 Biopsy bleed—Post-BX bleeding. Microcatheter localizes bleeding artery
Video 2 Biopsy bleed—Post-BX bleeding. Note extravasation by RA angio
Video 3 Biopsy bleed—Post-BX bleeding arrested by gel foam injection: no bleed now
Video 4 TRAS twisted—TRAS due to twisting/rotating of renal artery right internal iliac artery accessed through left femoral
Video 5 TRAS twisted—Stenting for twisted TX renal artery some residual wasting

Chapter 46. Percutaneous Insertion of Peritoneal Dialysis Catheter
Pavitra Manu Dogra, Purva Suhas Bavikar

Video 1 Percutaneous PD catheter insertion

Chapter 49. Peritoneal Dialysis Catheter Insertion in Pediatric Patients
Sowrabha Rajanna, Kanav Anand, Rekulapally Praneetha

Video 1 Acute PD catheter insertion technique in children

SECTION 1

Introduction to Intervention Nephrology

CHAPTER 1

Evolution of Interventional Nephrology in India

Kasi Visweswaran R, Jishnu Mohan

INTRODUCTION

Interventional nephrology is evolving as a specialty within nephrology. To ensure that a skilled nephrologist is qualified and competent to execute invasive procedures as part of diagnosis and treatment, other areas such as creating and preserving accesses should also fall under the purview of nephrology training. All nephrology interventions should ideally be carried out by nephrologists with the necessary training and authorization. One benefit is that the operator knows exactly what is expected of them while performing the specific procedure. Today, they are trained to undertake procedures related to routine dialysis therapy since a typical fellowship or specialty training equips them in that direction only. Free access to facilities such as ultrasound machine and cardiac catheterization laboratory/interventional radiology suite is one of the challenges experienced by many nephrologists working in smaller organizations. Nearly identical set of expensive equipment is required for the departments of cardiology, interventional radiology, and nephrology. There is a need for a balanced view in terms of equipment procurement and sharing so that nephrology training becomes all inclusive.

Dr Kripal Singh Chugh **(Fig. 1)**, who is widely regarded as the "Father of Nephrology" in India, made the first attempt to perform any kind of interventional procedure relating to nephrology in the 1950s while pursuing an MD (Medicine) at Panjab University. He made a concerted effort to secure permission from the university to conduct a kidney biopsy and conduct research on the subject as part of his MD thesis. As nephrology was not regarded as a specialty at the time, the institution strongly objected initially and finally permitted to undertake the study under "Genitourinary Medicine". After completing MD degree in medicine and training in nephrology at Hammersmith Hospital in London, he established the Department of Nephrology at PGI in Chandigarh. The first hemodialysis was initiated in the Department of Medicine, Christian Medical College (CMC), Vellore, by Dr P Koshy **(Fig. 2)**. Later, at KEM Hospital in Mumbai, Dr Vidya N Acharya **(Fig. 3)**, known as the "Mother of Nephrology" in India, was involved with

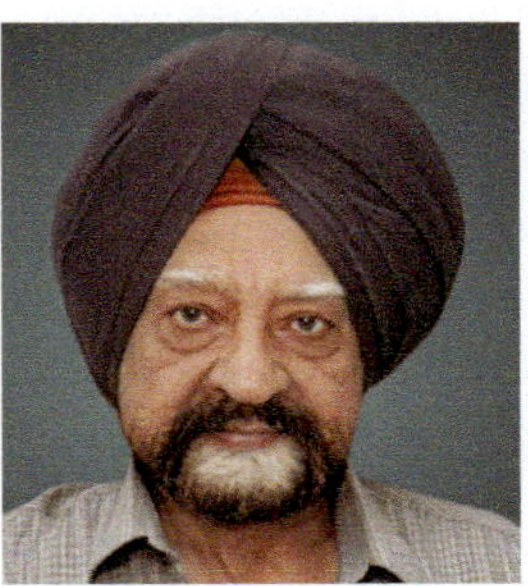

Fig. 1: (Late) Professor Kripal Singh Chugh, PGI, Chandigarh.

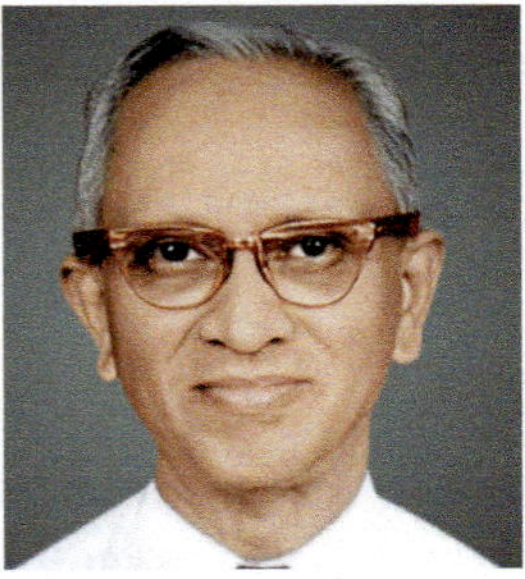

Fig. 2: (Late) Professor P Koshy, Christian Medical College, Vellore.

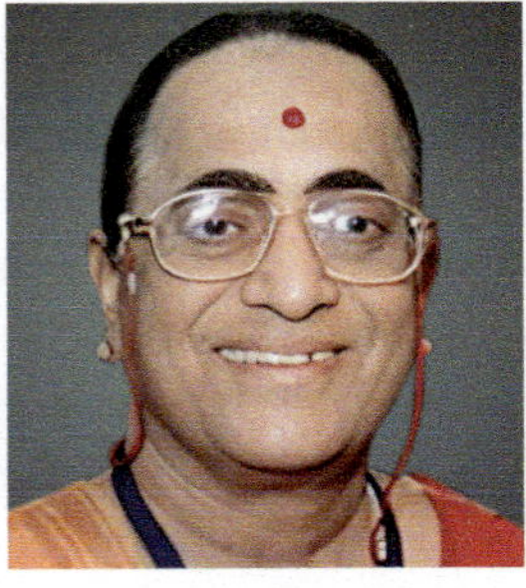

Fig. 3: (Late) Professor Vidya N Acharya, KEM Hospital, Mumbai.

Professor P Raghavan in performing the first hemodialysis in Mumbai in 1963. Later, she established a functioning department devoted to kidney disorders. By the 1970s, the nation had many more training and teaching facilities. In North India Sir Ganga Ram Hospital under the stewardship of Dr DS Rana and All India Institute of Medical Sciences in New Delhi; South India Madras Medical College Chennai, Osmania Medical College Hyderabad; West India Institute of Kidney Diseases Ahmedabad, MPUH Nadiad under stewardship of Dr. Mohan Rajapurkar; East India SCB Medical College, Government Medical College Calicut, and the institutions under the armed forces are among the other early institutions to establish a nephrology division or departments. Now, practically every major hospital, including national institutes, medical schools, and corporate/private institutions, has nephrology departments/units to serve the community, by providing service and training and engaging in research. With numerous centers performing cutting-edge interventional procedures for the benefit of patients with kidney problems, interventional nephrology is growing constantly.

In this chapter, the development of various procedures relating to clinical practice of nephrology is reviewed. Advances and in-depth focused discussions follow later in the independent chapters.

KIDNEY BIOPSY

Let us briefly trace the history of kidney biopsy, which is perhaps the first invasive interventional procedure in clinical nephrology. From the 1960s to 1970s, kidney biopsies were performed in some of the specialized centers only. Imaging the kidney was by plain radiograph of the abdomen. The lower pole of the left kidney was marked in the X-ray and the corresponding surface marking was made in the skin. The biopsy needle was Franklin modification of Vim–Silverman needle which has three parts—an outer cannula, stylet, and bifid cutting needle **(Fig. 4)**. The tip of the two arms of the bifid cutting needle has a stopper, which prevents slipping of the biopsy tissue while withdrawing the needle. The patient is positioned in prone position with sandbag under the abdomen and local anesthetic injected along the projected needle track. The position and depth of the kidney from skin surface are assessed and confirmed by using a lumbar puncture needle and noting the movement with respiration when the tip is in contact with the renal capsule. The stylet is withdrawn and the cutting needle is introduced till it reaches the tip of the cannula. The actual biopsy is a four-step procedure, which requires the patient holding his breath. The cutting needle alone is sharply pushed into the whole length, about 1.5 cm, followed by the outer cannula over the cutting needle for the same depth, followed by rotation and withdrawal of the whole unit. The biopsy tissue will be lodged within the two flanges of the cutting needle. After biopsy, care includes external pressure over the renal angle for 15–20 minutes. The sandbag offers the pressure anteriorly and the external pressure helps to reduce the chances of major bleeding. After about 12–24 hours of observation, the patient can be mobilized.

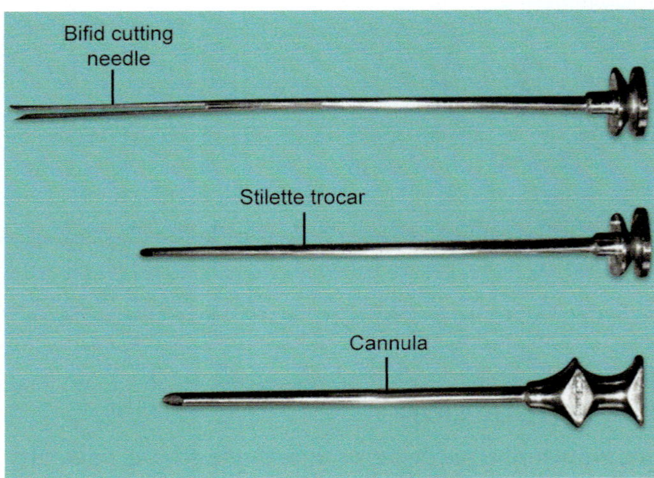

Fig. 4: Vim–Silverman biopsy needle.

Advances in kidney biopsy procedure started with crude spring-l-oaded biopsy needle. Later, more sophisticated "trucut" biopsy guns (BARD), with markings in the cannula, comfortable hand grip and trigger have been developed **(Figs. 5 and 6)**. With the advent of ultrasonography, most biopsies were done, initially after marking the skin puncture site and noting the depth of the kidney cortex from the skin. Now, it can be performed by a real-time ultrasonogram which enables the operator to visualize the needle and confirm the tip position before firing the biopsy gun. The yield of biopsy tissue and complication rates have significantly decreased, and kidney biopsies are now performed even as outpatient procedures in almost all centers.

Intermittent Peritoneal Dialysis

The next important procedure and intervention in nephrology was intermittent peritoneal dialysis (PD).

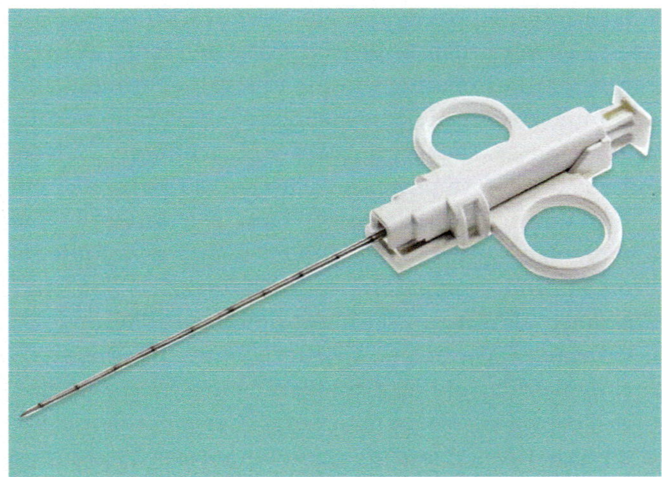

Fig. 5: Spring-loaded biopsy needle.

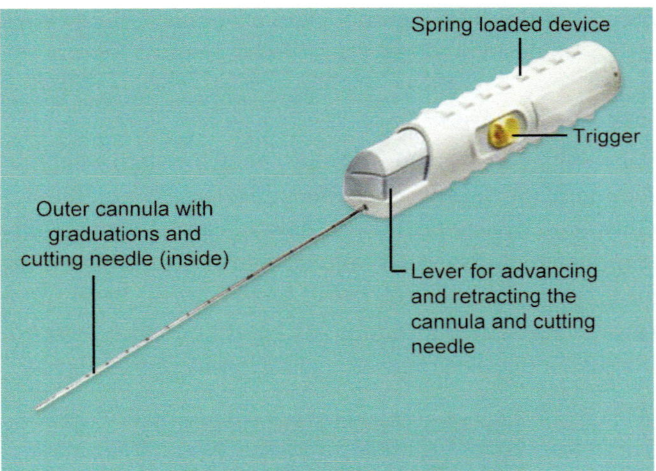

Fig. 6: Biopsy gun.

PD procedures were performed initially with improvised plastic tubes with numerous holes in one end and inserted into peritoneal cavity with the help of "trocar and canula," usually used for abdominal paracentesis in the 1960s and early 1970s. Glass bottles with PD fluid were prepared with the necessary chemicals and filtered water, in the central sterilization area. Rubber tubes with glass Y connection were improvised for the instilling and draining the fluid out of the peritoneum. In the major institutions, the procedure started initially with residents taking up "PD" as part of their thesis work. From 1970 onward, it was used as the preferred modality of treatment for acute renal failure in all major centers. By the late 1970s, presterilized thin, stiff plastic tubes with numerous holes, with introducer stylet and connecting Y tubes were made available. PD fluid was also available commercially in 500- or 1,000-mL bottles, later polythene rigid pouches, and later collapsible plastic bags. The procedure of placing the stiff catheter was performed blindly either before or after priming the peritoneal cavity with PD fluid/normal saline. A total of 40 L fluid exchanges were considered as one session of PD. Although the complications rates were higher, it was the life-saving treatment for most cases of acute renal failure. In the 1980s, silastic Tenckhoff catheters were more easily available. Uncuffed Tenckhoff catheter was used for acute PD. Being a lifesaving procedure, it is used in remote areas or smaller institutions with limited facilities for managing cases of acute kidney injury even now. The advantage is that it does not require any special equipment, and readymade catheters and sterile fluid are available.

Continuous Ambulatory Peritoneal Dialysis

Peritoneal dialysis as an option for treatment of chronic renal failure was recognized after the advent of double-cuffed silastic PD catheters which could be placed in the peritoneal cavity and retained safely for years, without causing foreign body reaction. The connecting technology for the tubing and the availability of double bags and modifications have made the procedure more acceptable. The infection rate has also significantly come down. The main advantage is that it is a gentler procedure compared to hemodialysis and can be performed by the patient himself or caregiver at home. Now, automatic cyclers are available to enable the patients to undergo the procedure during night without disturbing their sleep time. These cyclers can be programmed to administer and drain fixed volumes of fluid in the allotted time. These cyclers enable the patients to be free during daytime.

Hemodialysis Machines, Hemodialysis, and Advanced Procedures

Abel, Rowntree, and Turner in 1913 showed that it is possible to remove diffusible substances from the circulating blood of living animals by dialysis; dialysis for treating patients was developed by Willheim Kolff, using rotating drum. Subsequent developments followed, with twin coil dialyzer, flat plate dialyzers, Kiil kidney, and later, hollow-fiber artificial kidney that revolutionized the field of nephrology.

The first dialysis was started in India at the CMC, Vellore, under the leadership of Professor P Koshy in 1962. In the late 1950s/early 1960s, Dr P Koshy visited Dr Belding Scribner's dialysis unit in Seattle, USA, which was the major center doing maintenance HD in the US during that time period. He had gained confidence in using the machine and performing hemodialysis before returning to his mother institution. When the Maharajah of Hatuah, a small princely state in Bihar, approached Dr Koshy for treatment of end-stage renal disease (ESRD), a Travenol dialysis machine was procured from the US and installed in CMC, Vellore. This machine uses a twin coil dialyzer, inside a drum with warmed dialysis fluid **(Fig. 7)**. Scribner also deputed his assistant Dr Nakamoto who spent some time in Vellore to get the program going. Thus, the first patient to have received hemodialysis in India was His Highness Sri Gopeshwar Sahai, Maharaja of Hatuah **(Fig. 8)**.

In the 1970s, there were only a handful of active dialysis centers in the country. The prepared warm dialysis fluid was passed through the artificial kidney from a tank at 10–12 feet higher level by gravity **(Fig. 9)** and the blood flow was maintained through a pump for performing dialysis. Since the extracorporeal volume was high, every dialysis required priming of the system with blood. The machines have also improved from the stage of fixed volume proportionating system, to servo-controlled and later to electronically controlled system with numerous monitoring and safety features. Bicarbonate dialysis and use of reverse osmosis-treated water have become a norm throughout the country now. The developments in hydraulics system in the monitor including volumetric ultrafiltration to regulate the ultrafiltration (UF), UF modeling, safety measures in the blood pathway, and use of RO water have helped to offer smooth hemodialysis treatment. Today, although there are centers even in smaller towns, providing dialysis support to needy patients, the facility is not available in many remote areas in the country. Other more modern techniques such as hemodiafiltration (HDF), continuous renal replacement therapy (CRRT), hemofiltration (HF), and plasma exchange (PLEX) have also been developed and are available in most centers.

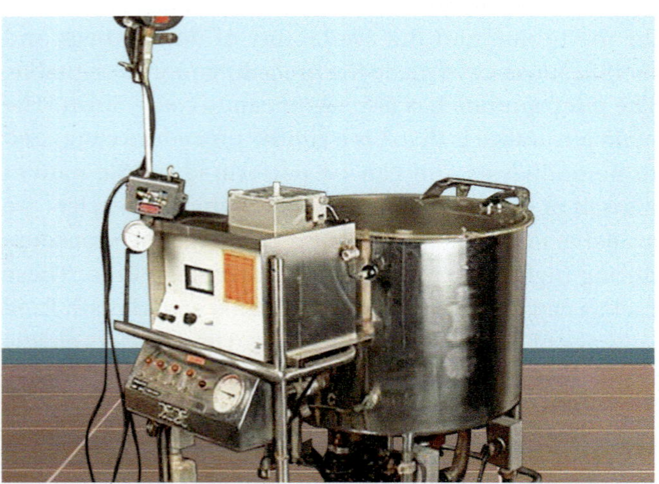

Fig. 7: Travenol dialysis machine.

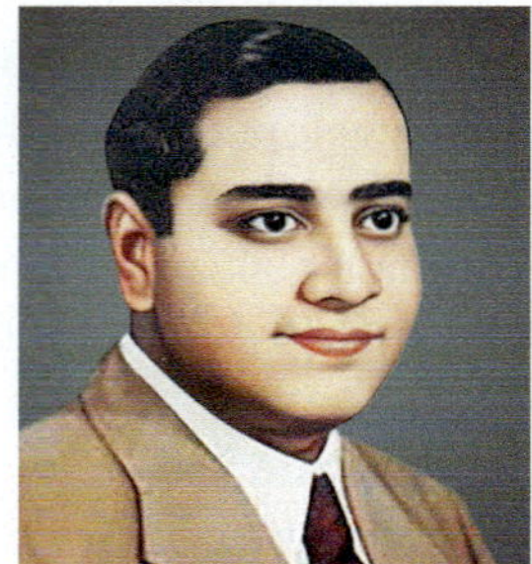

Fig. 8: First hemodialysis patient in India. H/E. (Late) Shri Gopeshwar Prasad Sahi, the erstwhile Maharaja of Hathwa (in Bihar).

Vascular Access

Vascular access is the Achilles heel for hemodialysis. An adequate vascular access is important as a lifeline for chronic dialysis. Short-term dialysis can be successfully completed using vascular catheters but for long-term access, an arteriovenous fistula (AVF) will be ideal. Permanent catheters and arteriovenous (AV) grafts can also be used, but their longevity is less than a functioning AVF.

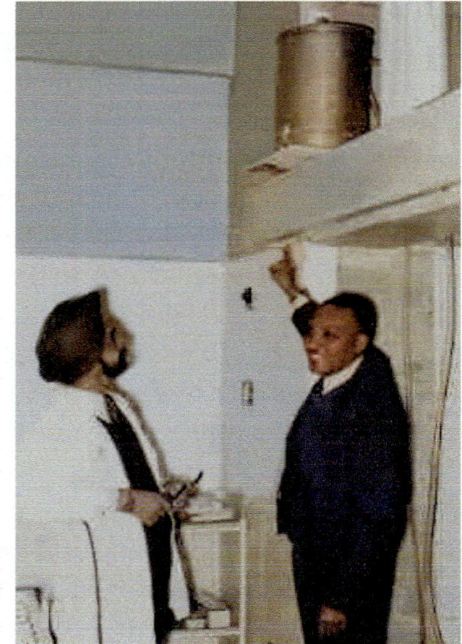

Fig. 9: Overhead tank with dialysis fluid. Tank is at a height of 11 feet connected to Kiil kidney. [Professor KS Chugh and Dr Samuel Kountz (visitor from New York), PGI, Chandigarh, 1967].

For short-term hemodialysis, only single-lumen (stiff) Teflon catheters were available in the 1970s and early 1980s. These were used as vascular access for acute renal failure. The single-lumen catheter was placed in femoral vein to take blood from the body to the artificial kidney and the blood was returned through either a good peripheral vein or another single-lumen catheter on the opposite leg. By experimenting, some of the units used both single-lumen catheters in the same femoral vein. Since these were stiff Teflon catheters, they had to be removed after each session of dialysis or by 48 hours. Residents those days had to repeatedly cannulate the femoral veins for each hemodialysis session. Later, when polyurethane double-lumen catheters were made available, subclavian and later jugular vein cannulation was possible. Initially, jugular cannulation was a blind procedure, palpating the common carotid artery and directing the guiding needle tip just lateral to the pulsation. Once the vein is identified, using a guiding needle, the larger needle is passed parallel to the guiding needle, to the same depth to reach the vein lumen. With the advent of ultrasound, the vein can be identified real time and cannulated easily. The interventions needed for double-lumen catheters include malposition, clotting, infection, hematoma, hemo/pneumothorax, etc.

Arteriovenous shunts introduced by Belding Scribner in 1960 was a modification of Alwall's bypass technique using a silicon-coated rubber tube to connect artery and vein. Scribner shunts were the earliest long-term vascular access for dialysis and were used during the 1960s to early 1980s. The AV shunt involves placing and securing a thin-walled PTFE cannula into artery and vein. Later, silastic tubing and a Teflon vessel tip were used to connect \into the radial artery and cephalic vein. The silastic tubing is taken out through a subcutaneous tunnel and the two ends of the tubes are interconnected with a Teflon connector. When clamps are released, blood flows directly from radial artery through shunt tubing to the vein **(Figs. 10 and 11)**. During dialysis, the connector is removed and the tubes connected to the blood lines. Most often, the blood flow through the extracorporeal circuit will be achieved by the patient's own blood pressure and a blood pump may not be necessary. The problems associated are infection, accidental/suicidal disconnection of the shunt connector and clotting of the shunt tubings. There are interventions to "declot" the shunt which was one of the few interventions in vascular access then. A carefully maintained shunt can function for many months to a few years. There are instances when the AV shunt has been maintained for regular dialysis for many years in the 1960s and 1970s.

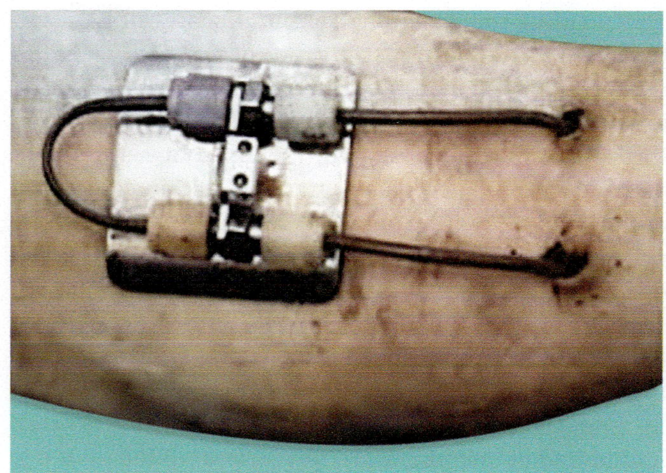

Fig. 10: Scribner shunt.

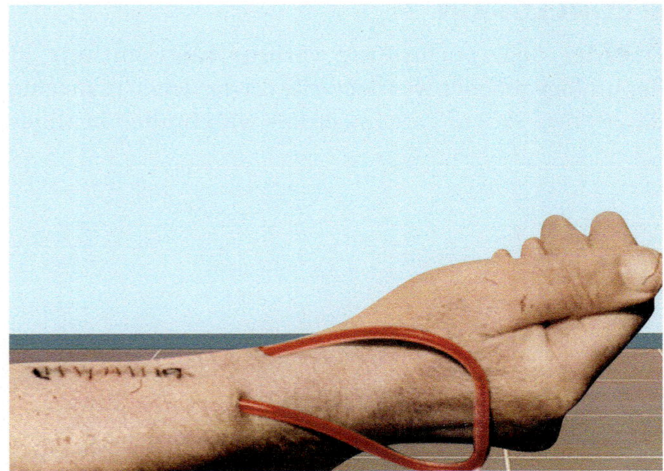

Fig. 11: Arteriovenous shunt in common use during the 1970s.

A functioning AVF is the standard vascular access these days. Both primary failure and secondary failure and vascular access dysfunction are common. Timely identification and prompt intervention can salvage the lifeline in patients on maintenance hemodialysis. This requires numerous interventions including AV fistulogram, clot lysis, thrombectomy, balloon angioplasty, stenting, and other endovascular interventions. Creation of AVF by endovascular techniques is also possible now.

RENAL TRANSPLANTATION

The first live donor kidney transplant was done in the first week of February 1971 at the CMC, Vellore.

The team of Drs KV Johny (nephrologist), Mohan Rao (urologist), and Martin Issac (anesthesiologist) were the team leaders for the successful procedure. Today, there are over 150 centers in India licensed to perform kidney transplantation. Live related, altruistic live unrelated, swap, Domino, and cadaver transplantations are being conducted. Considering the waiting list for kidney transplantation, cadaver transplantations should be encouraged. Although such transplants are taking place in a successful way in many states, some states are lagging far behind. With the advent of advanced immunosuppressive treatment, ultrasonographic evaluation, safe techniques for graft biopsy, analysis of vascular supply to the graft and interventional methods, the survival of the graft has improved.

CONCLUSION

Decades ago, performing various interventions in nephrology practice was necessity driven, when managing day-to-day patient care in centers with limited facilities and manpower. The passion of energetic nephrologists and their access to facilities in fluoroscopy and imaging methods paved the way for their greater involvement in interventional procedures. As most of the patients depend on personal finances for treatment, such innovations help to offer relatively less expensive alternatives. Interventional nephrology has now become a new subspecialty, and more nephrologists are taking up such interventions themselves rather than seeking help from already overburdened colleagues in radiology or cardiology departments.

SUGGESTED READING

1. Chugh KS. Evaluation of renal biopsy [MD (Medicine) thesis]. Chandigarh, India: Panjab University; 1958.
2. Chugh KS. World Kidney Forum—Five decades of Indian nephrology: A personal journey. Am J Kidney Dis. 2009;54(4):753-63.
3. Mohan Rao M, Pandey AP, Shastry JCM, Johny KV. Status of renal transplantation in India. Ann Acad Med Singapore. 1975;4:183-5.

CHAPTER 2

Fundamental Principles of Dialysis Vascular Access

Tushar J Vachharajani, Vaibhav Tiwari

INTRODUCTION

Planning for dialysis access is a critical step in managing patients with advanced chronic kidney disease (CKD). Early planning and timely access creation can significantly improve patient outcomes by enabling dialysis initiation with a permanent access rather than a central venous catheter (CVC).[1] The guidelines from the National Kidney Foundation-Kidney Disease Outcomes Quality Initiative (NKF-KDOQI) emphasize a patient-centered approach.[2] Patients with CKD stage 4 (estimated glomerular filtration rate <30 mL/min/1.73 m^2) should be educated about all modalities of kidney replacement therapy options, including hemodialysis, peritoneal dialysis, transplantation, and palliative care (nondialysis therapy). The goal is to achieve the "right access, at the right time, for the right patient and for the right reason," integrating patient preferences, comorbidities, and life expectancy into the access planning process.[2] Early planning allows for surgical evaluation, vessel mapping, and access maturation, thereby minimizing the need for CVC at dialysis initiation.

PATIENT EVALUATION

Comprehensive patient evaluation is the first step in planning for dialysis access. The nephrologist should begin this process when the patient is in CKD stage 4 or early stage 5, well before the need for dialysis.[2] The key components of the evaluation include the following:

- *Clinical history:* Review any history of CVCs, pacemakers, or thrombosis, as these can cause central vein stenosis and impact access site selection and choice. Determine if the patient has prior vascular surgeries or trauma to the potential access extremity. Assess comorbidities such as diabetes, peripheral vascular disease, or heart failure, which may influence access outcomes.
- *Clinical evaluation:* Examine the arms for suitable arteries and veins. Assess for the quality of pulsations in both upper extremities. Note vessel size, depth, distensibility and calcification with ultrasonography. A bedside Allen test can assess arterial blood flow to the hand if a radial artery-based fistula is planned.
- *Preserving vessels:* Avoid venipunctures and intravenous (IV) lines in veins of the preferred arm in patients with advanced CKD to preserve the veins for a future fistula. Preferably avoid transradial arterial approach interventions such as cardiac catheterization to prevent injury to the radial artery.
- *Modality decision:* Confirm the patient's dialysis modality preference. If hemodialysis is chosen, plan for a vascular access [arteriovenous fistula (AVF) or graft]; if peritoneal dialysis is chosen, coordinate peritoneal dialysis (PD) catheter placement [following the International Society for Peritoneal Dialysis (ISPD) recommendations to insert the catheter at least 2 weeks before PD start to allow for wound healing and reduce the risk of peritoneal leak].[3] A shared decision-making process will help select an appropriate access based on individual needs; e.g., an elderly patient with multiple comorbidities, poor vessels and relatively shorter life-span might be better served with a graft or even PD, whereas for a younger patient an AV fistula remains an ideal first choice.
- *Vascular mapping referral:* Arrange for preoperative vascular mapping (typically by duplex ultrasound). This imaging will measure luminal diameters of both the target artery and peripheral veins to determine an optimal site for a viable AVF. Vessels with luminal diameter of <2.5–3 mm may result into higher primary maturation failure rates.[2] For patients with a history of CVCs or pacemaker, consider a central venography or advanced imaging to rule out central vein occlusion before deciding on an ipsilateral access.

Ultrasonography of central veins can be unreliable for assessing certain aspects, but it can still provide useful information. One key feature that can be assessed is the phasic variation in blood flow, which changes with the intrathoracic pressure during the phases of inhalation and exhalation. These variations can help evaluate the central venous pressure and inform decisions regarding access or potential complications.

- *Multidisciplinary discussion:* Planning is best done collaboratively. Nephrologists, vascular surgeons, and interventional radiologists, dialysis staff and access coordinators should communicate about the patient's condition. A team approach ensures that all factors are weighed - for instance, surgical insight on whether the veins are adequate for a fistula, or whether novel approaches (like an endovascular AVF creation) could be utilized. Such multidisciplinary planning, as part of a "vascular access team," helps tailor the access plan to the individual patient.[4]

By thoroughly evaluating these aspects, the nephrologist can guide the patient to an informed choice of access that balances guideline recommendations with the patient's unique situation. The end result is a well-informed patient with a clear plan for an ideal access placement. The ultimate goal is to create the access well in advance, allowing it to mature and be available to initiate dialysis when needed.

SITE SELECTION FOR DIALYSIS ACCESS

Selecting the optimal site for dialysis access is crucial for long-term success. Site selection involves choosing which blood vessels and which limb to use for access creation, with the goals of maximizing longevity, facilitating ease of use, and preserving future access options. The key considerations include the following:

- *Upper vs. lower extremity:* In most cases, the upper extremity is preferred for hemodialysis access. The nondominant arm is often selected to preserve the dominant arm for daily activities, but vessel quality ultimately determines the choice. Within the arm, a more distal site is preferred for an initial access creation (the "distal first" approach), e.g., a wrist (radiocephalic) fistula is attempted before an elbow (brachiocephalic) fistula.[2] Using the most distal feasible site preserves proximal vessels for future accesses, if needed. If arm options are exhausted or not possible (e.g., severe bilateral central vein stenoses or arm vascular disease), thigh accesses such as a femoral fistula or graft can be considered as an alternative.
- *AVF sites:* The common fistula configurations, in order of preference, include the snuff-box fistula (near the base of the thumb), radiocephalic AVF at the wrist (connecting the radial artery to the cephalic vein), the proximal forearm fistula (using the deep communicating vein and the proximal radial or ulnar artery), the brachiocephalic AVF at the elbow (brachial artery to cephalic vein), and the brachiobasilic fistula with transposition (brachial artery to basilic vein, where the vein is tunneled superficially). A radiocephalic (wrist) fistula, often called a Brescia-Cimino fistula, is ideal due to lower risk of steal syndrome and ease of cannulation if it matures, but it requires adequately sized and quality of distal vessels. If the wrist vessels are too small or sclerosed, a mid-forearm of an upper arm fistula can be created. Fistulas require adequate arterial inflow and venous outflow; thus, vessels must meet minimal diameter criteria and be free of significant stenosis. Preoperative mapping helps confirm this.
- *AV graft (AVG) sites:* AVGs are typically placed in the arm as well, often in the upper arm if forearm veins are inadequate. A common configuration is a loop graft in the forearm, connecting the brachial artery to an antecubital or basilic vein or an upper arm AVG connecting brachial artery to proximal basilic/axillary vein via a synthetic tube. Grafts can also be placed in the upper thigh (femoral artery to vein) when arm sites are not available. When choosing a graft site, the surgeon should aim for a location that allows a straight segment for cannulation, place in the superficial layer below the skin avoiding areas with risk of kinking or compression.
- *Central venous catheter sites:* For nontunneled (temporary) or tunneled dialysis catheters, the right internal jugular vein is the preferred site for insertion.[4] This site offers a straight path to the right atrium and is associated with relatively lower complication rates. If the right internal jugular is not available, the left internal jugular is usually the second choice. Femoral vein catheters can be used, especially in acute situations or if the patient will be bedridden; they are easy to place but carry a higher infection risk when used beyond a few days. The subclavian vein should be avoided for dialysis catheters, if at all possible, due to the high risk of venous stenosis and thrombosis that

can permanently compromise veins in the ipsilateral extremity.[1]

- *Vessel preservation:* A fundamental principle of site selection is preserving veins for future access. This means no peripherally inserted central catheter (PICC) lines or unnecessary IV cannulas in upper extremity veins in patients with CKD who are more likely to progress to dialysis. Hospitalists and other providers should be made aware about the importance of protecting these veins. Additionally, if a patient already has a functioning access in one arm, blood draws, and peripheral IVs should be placed in the contralateral arm or a hand vein to avoid damage to the veins in the selected extremity for a future access placement. If a catheter is needed in a patient with a maturing fistula, usethe contralateral side or a femoral vein to avoid jeopardizing the fistula. Careful planning of site not only helps the first access succeed but also preserves a "pipeline" of sites for future accesses over the patient's lifetime.

Selecting the right site is a balancing act that considers surgical feasibility and future planning. By adhering to guidelines and by tailoring to the patient's anatomy, nephrologists and surgeons can maximize the longevity of dialysis access options for each patient.

TYPES OF DIALYSIS ACCESS

There are three main types of dialysis access for hemodialysis: AVF, AVG, and CVC. Each type has distinct characteristics, advantages, and disadvantages. In general, guidelines recommend an autogenous AVF as the first choice for chronic hemodialysis access, followed by an AVG if a fistula is not suitable, with CVCs reserved for temporary or last-resort use. The "fistula first" paradigm stems from the superior outcomes associated with fistulas.[5] However, patient factors and clinical circumstances must be considered to choose the most appropriate access. An overview of each type is given in the following text.

Arteriovenous Fistula

An AVF is a surgical connection between an artery and a vein, created to provide high blood flow for hemodialysis. Typically, a native vein (e.g., the cephalic vein) is anastomosed end-to-side to an artery (e.g., the radial artery) **(Fig. 1)**, allowing arterial pressure to dilate and thicken the vein over time. This process, called maturation, usually takes 4–12 weeks (about 6 weeks on average, but can be longer) before the fistula can be reliably used for dialysis. During maturation, the vein's diameter increases with arterialization of its walls due to a pulsatile higher-pressure flow in a low capacitance thin-walled vein.

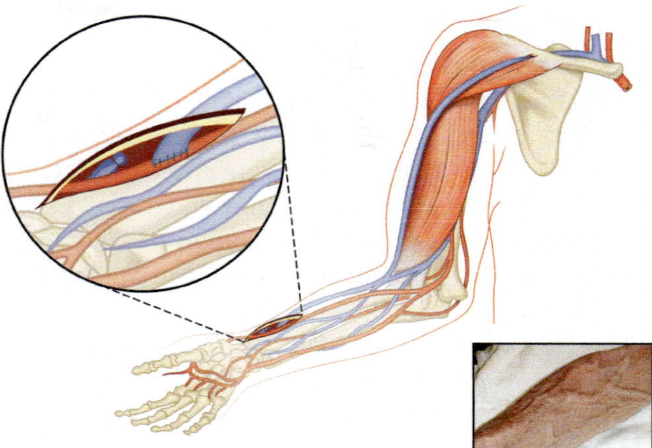

Fig. 1: Radiocephalic arteriovenous fistula (Brescia-Cimino).

- *Advantages:* AVFs have the longest survival of all access types—many can last years (average primary patency of around 3–5 years) with proper care.[6,7] They have the lowest risk of infection (since they are entirely the patient's own tissue with no foreign material) and a lower risk of thrombosis compared to grafts. They also have no implant that could degenerate. Over time, fistulas are associated with lower all-cause mortality and hospitalization rates than grafts or catheters.[7]
- *Disadvantages:* AVFs require adequate vessels and time to mature, which is often a major barrier in patients with CKD and high associated comorbidities. A high primary failure rate is common in patients with smaller luminal diameters or diseased vessels.[7] If a fistula fails to mature (no adequate flow or vein size by about 6 weeks), additional interventions (angioplasty or revision) or a new access might be needed. Since fistulas require 6–12 weeks to become usable, patients needing urgent dialysis therapy may require placement of a CVC during the interim period. In some patients (e.g., elderly individuals or those with peripheral vascular disease), an AVF may not mature or may take too long to become usable to support dialysis. Additionally, fistulas can cause hemodynamic stress: High blood flow can lead to steal syndrome (hand ischemia) or contribute to high-output cardiac failure. These issues, however, are generally manageable and less common than the complications seen with other access types.

Arteriovenous Graft

An AVG is a synthetic tube [most often made of expanded polytetrafluoroethylene (ePTFE)] that connects an artery to a vein, serving as an artificial conduit for dialysis cannulation **(Fig. 2)**. Surgically, one end of the graft is anastomosed to an artery and the other end to a vein, often creating a loop under the skin. Common configurations include a forearm loop graft or an upper arm straight graft. Unlike a fistula, the AVG does not require the patient's vein to dilate to provide immediate flow; thus, it can often be used soon after surgery—typically within 2–4 weeks, once postoperative swelling subsides, and the anastomoses heal. Newer early cannulation graft materials or designs (e.g., heparin-bonded grafts) can be used within 48–72 hours, but a standard practice is to wait for 2–3 weeks.[2]

- *Advantages:* The primary advantage of a graft is that it does not depend on the patient's veins to mature. This makes AVGs an excellent option for patients whose veins are too small or scarred and unsuitable for a fistula. Grafts can be placed and used in a shorter time frame than fistulas, so they are useful when fistula is not feasible. AVG provides adequate blood flow to support dialysis.
- *Disadvantages:* AVGs have shorter longevity than fistulas with average patency of about 1–2 years before they fail or require significant intervention.[6] They are prone to stenosis and thrombosis, especially at the venous anastomosis where neointimal hyperplasia (scar tissue) tends to develop due to the artificial material. This means grafts often require frequent interventions (angioplasty, thrombectomy, or surgical revision) to keep them open. The infection risk for grafts is higher than for fistulas, since the synthetic material can harbor bacteria. If a graft does get infected, it often needs to be removed, as simply treating with antibiotics may not eradicate an infection on the foreign material. Grafts can also develop pseudoaneurysms at needle puncture sites and carry a slightly higher risk of steal syndrome compared to fistulas. Patients must be vigilant with graft care; e.g., avoid needle sticks outside of dialysis and report any signs of infection.

Central Venous Catheter

A CVC for hemodialysis is a dual-lumen tube placed into a central vein (internal jugular, femoral, or subclavian) with its tip in the superior (or inferior) vena cava, allowing blood to be pulled and returned for dialysis **(Fig. 3)**. A nontunneled catheter is used for short-term access (days), and tunneled, cuffed catheter is used as a bridge intermediate-term access (weeks to months).[2] Tunneled catheters have a Dacron cuff that induces tissue ingrowth and anchors the catheter in the tunnel and serves as a mechanical barrier to prevent infection. Catheters can be placed at bedside or in an interventional suite, to provide an immediate access for urgent dialysis initiation or as a bridge while waiting for an AVF or graft to mature.

- *Advantages:* The main advantage of a CVC is its ease of placement and immediate availability to initiate hemodialysis therapy. Placement is less invasive than surgery (no arterial anastomosis), typically done under

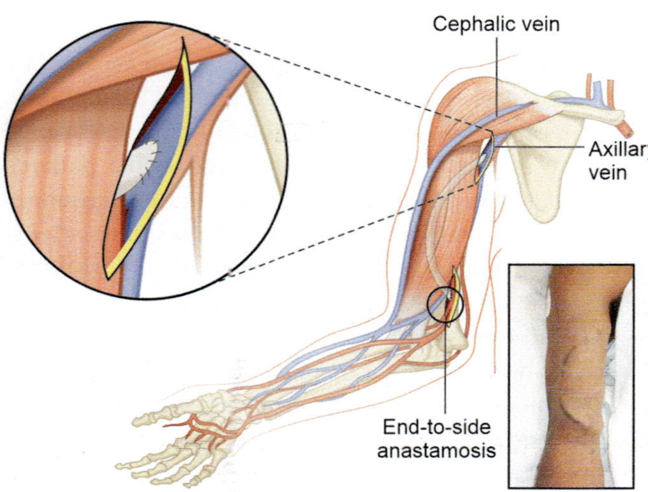

Fig. 2: Upper arm arteriovenous graft cephalic.

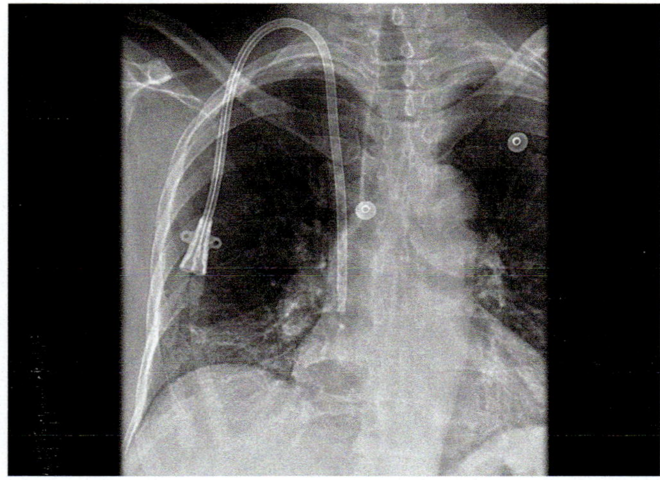

Fig. 3: Chest X-ray demonstrating right sided central venous catheter.

TABLE 1: Summary of the key features of each type of dialysis access.

Aspect	*Arteriovenous fistula (AVF)*	*Arteriovenous graft (AVG)*	*Central venous catheter (CVC)*
Composition	Native vessel (artery–vein)	Synthetic tube connecting artery–vein	Plastic catheter in a central vein
Time to use	Approximately 6–12 weeks (time to maturation)	~2–4 weeks (time to heal)	Immediate (no maturation needed)
Longevity	Longest (average 3–5+ years)	Intermediate (average 1–2 years)	Short-term (frequent replacement every 3–6 months)
Typical flow rates	350–400 mL/min (optimizes efficiency)	350–400 mL/min (slightly less than AVF)	300–350 mL/min (lower than AVF/AVG)
Infection risk	Lowest	Moderate (higher than AVF)	Highest (direct bloodstream access)
Thrombosis risk	Low–moderate	High (stenosis at graft–vein junction)	High (catheter clotting, vein thrombosis)
Maintenance	Low	Moderate–high	High (aseptic care, locks, etc.)
Ideal access	Preferred if vessels suitable	Second choice if AVF not feasible	Use only when AVF/AVG not ready/possible

local anesthesia with ultrasound guidance. Catheters can be placed in different sites [neck, chest, groin, and rarely in the lumbar region (translumbar) or through a liver (transhepatic)] and are often the first option for patients who need emergent dialysis or who have exhausted all possible sites for fistula/graft creation. A CVC is an acceptable vascular access for a patient who is likely to receive an allograft within a short time frame (generally <3 months)—a common setting with a living-related donor.

- *Disadvantages:* CVCs have the highest complication rates amongst all access types. Infection is the most serious risk—catheters provide a direct conduit for bacteria to enter the bloodstream. A CVC-related bloodstream infection, resulting in sepsis, endocarditis, osteomyelitis, and abscess formation, remains a common cause for hospitalization and increased incidence of morbidity and mortality. Intraluminal and extraluminal thrombosis is another common reason for catheter dysfunction. A CVC can develop a fibrin sheath or intraluminal clot that leads to reduced flow and inability to achieve the prescribed dialysis blood flow rate. A dysfunctional CVC can be treated with a thrombolytic agent or with an over-the-wire exchange replacement. Central vein stenosis secondary to prolonged use of CVC is another frequently encountered complication. A CVC tends to irritate the endothelium of the vessel wall leading to scarring and stenosis preventing creation of an ipsilateral fistula. As compared to an AVF or AVG, blood flow through a CVC may decline limiting dialysis efficiency. In addition, catheters can impact patient quality of life (as they protrude from the body and require daily care). For these reasons, long-term use of a catheter is discouraged and remains the least preferred vascular access in appropriate situation. The goal is usually to use a catheter as a temporary measure until a permanent access is available to support hemodialysis. Patients who dialyze with a catheter have higher mortality compared to those with a fistula or graft largely attributable to infection and complications. Hence, every effort should be made to transition patients with a catheter to a permanent access as soon as possible.

We summarized the key features of each type of dialysis access in **Table 1**.

PREOPERATIVE IMAGING AND ASSESSMENT

Before any dialysis access surgery, proper imaging and assessment of the vasculature are essential. Preoperative vessel mapping helps ensure that the chosen site has a high likelihood of success. According to guidelines, the workup for a permanent hemodialysis access should include a detailed history and physical examination, duplex ultrasound of the target arteries and veins, and evaluation of central veins in patients with risk factors (such as prior catheters or pacemakers).[8,9]

- *Duplex ultrasound mapping:* Ultrasound is the primary tool for mapping peripheral vessels. It provides measurements of vein diameter, depth from the skin, and compressibility, as well as arterial diameter. For an AVF, a minimum vessel diameter of ≥2.5–3 mm is preferred) and adequate arterial pulse. Ultrasound can also identify vein segments that might be diseased or thrombosed and unsuitable for use. Arterial evaluation checks for adequate flow and absence of significant stenosis (e.g., calcification in diabetics). Presurgery vessel mapping ensures proper selection of site and identifies underlying pathology that could potentially prevent adequate maturation and help select patient who may be ideal for AVG.

- *Central vein assessment:* If the patient has had CVC, transvenous pacemakers, or known thrombosis, imaging of the central veins (subclavian vein, brachiocephalic vein and superior vena cava) is important. Central venography (via contrast MRI, CT venogram, or conventional venogram) can identify occlusions or stenoses. As an example, subclinical central vein stenosis in a patient with past history of subclavian catheter can get unmasked as arm swelling if an ipsilateral AV access is created. Presence of significant central vein stenosis may require creating an access on the contralateral side or treating the stenosis prior to access creation.
- *Arterial assessment and Allen test:* For a wrist (radiocephalic) fistula, an Allen test or ultrasound of the palmar arch may be performed to ensure the ulnar arterial supply to the hand is adequate. Inadequate collateral flow could predispose the patient to hand ischemia after fistula creation (steal syndrome). Arterial ultrasound can also reveal if there is arterial calcification; heavily calcified arteries might not dilate or might not be compressible for hemostasis, making fistula creation difficult.
- *Cardiac evaluation:* Though not always emphasized, assessing the patient's cardiac status is relevant. Creating a large AV access increases cardiac preload and output; in patients with borderline cardiac function, a high-flow fistula (defined as >2,000 mL/min) might contribute to heart failure. In patients with significant preexisting cardiomyopathy, the close attention to the size of the anastomosis during creation is vital and preferably maintains the access blood flow between 800 and 1,200 mL/min Additionally, close monitoring of the cardiac output is recommended. Dialysis modality selection may depend on the extent of preexisting cardiac output.
- *Laboratory and other assessments:* Ensure the patient's coagulation status is managed (e.g., if on warfarin or other anticoagulants, plan perioperative management to reduce bleeding risk). Check for anemia (many patients will have anemia of CKD) as severe anemia may reduce flow turbulence and prevent fistula maturation. Addressing any active infections prior to elective access surgery is important as an active infection could seed a new graft or fistula.

POSTPROCEDURAL CARE AND FOLLOW-UP

Effective postprocedural care is crucial for ensuring access maturation and long-term function.

- *Immediate postoperative care:* Monitor the access for a palpable thrill and audible bruit. Maintain proper dressing and limb positioning to reduce swelling.
- *Patient education:* Patients should be instructed on proper care, including daily checks for the thrill and avoiding trauma or direct pressure compression to the access arm.
- *Scheduled follow-up:* Regular postoperative assessments (e.g., at 2 and 6 weeks) and duplex ultrasound evaluations are critical to document maturation and address any complications promptly.
- *Dialysis unit surveillance:* Dialysis staff should routinely check the access before, during, and after treatments to detect early signs of maturation failure.
- *Transitioning from catheters:* If a patient initiates dialysis via a CVC, a plan to switch to a permanent access should be executed as soon as the permanent access is functional.

CONCLUSION

In conclusion, planning a dialysis access is a nuanced process that requires forward thinking, patient-centered decision-making, and adherence to evidence-based guidelines. Nephrologists play a pivotal role in initiating timely access planning by educating the patient with CKD about their options, coordinating vascular evaluations, and collaborating with surgical colleagues. By following established guidelines (NKF-KDOQI for vascular access) and tailoring them to individual patient needs, we can ensure that most patients start dialysis with a well-functioning permanent access, which can lead to markedly better outcomes: Lower infection risk, fewer hospitalizations, improved dialysis efficacy, and enhanced quality of life.

Over the course of a patient's treatment, the chosen access will require ongoing care and periodic interventions. A successful dialysis access program is characterized by continuous monitoring, prompt management of complications, and planning for the next steps (be it a new access or a transition to transplant). A multidisciplinary team approach involving nephrologists, surgeons, interventional radiologists, dialysis nurses, and the patient is ideal for superior outcomes. When implemented properly, access planning and maintenance reflect individualized care: the right access in the right patient at the right time, preserved for as long as possible.

In summary, planning a dialysis access is not a one-time task but an ongoing commitment—starting in the pre-dialysis CKD phase, continuing through access creation, with lifelong surveillance. Utilizing the guidance from NKF-KDOQI, and coupling it with clinical judgment, nephrologists can influence their patient's dialysis journey, ensuring that dialysis delivery is optimized through a well-chosen and well-maintained access. The payoff is seen in better patient outcomes and a smoother path to transplantation or long-term dialysis management.

REFERENCES

1. Feldman HI, Kobrin S, Wasserstein A. Hemodialysis vascular access morbidity. J Am Soc Nephrol. 1996;7(4):523-35.
2. Lok CE, Huber TS, Lee T, Shenoy S, Yevzlin AS, Abreo K, et al. National Kidney Foundation. KDOQI Clinical Practice Guideline for Vascular Access: 2019 Update. Am J Kidney Dis. 2020;75(4 Suppl 2):S1-S164.
3. Chow KM, Li PK, Cho Y, Abu-Alfa A, Bavanandan S, Brown EA, et al. ISPD Catheter-related Infection Recommendations: 2023 Update. Perit Dial Int. 2023;43(3): 201-19.
4. Santoro D, Benedetto F, Mondello P, Pipitò N, Barillà D, Spinelli F, et al. Vascular access for hemodialysis: current perspectives. Int J Nephrol Renovasc Dis. 2014;7:281-94.
5. Lok CE. Fistula First Initiative: advantages and pitfalls. Clin J Am Soc Nephrol. 2007;2(5):1043-53.
6. Arhuidese IJ, Orandi BJ, Nejim B, Malas M. Utilization, patency, and complications associated with vascular access for hemodialysis in the United States. J Vasc Surg. 2018;68(4):1166-1174.
7. Ghimire A, Lloyd AM, Szigety S, Merino JL, Alibhai K, Winkelaar G, et al. Prospective analysis of arteriovenous fistula performance in the context of competing risks. Kidney 360. 2025;6(2):272-83.
8. Chlorogiannis DD, Bousi SE, Zachiotis M, Chlorogiannis A, Kyriakoulis I, Bellos I. Pre-operative ultrasound mapping before arteriovenous fistula formation: an updated systematic review and meta-analysis. J Nephrol. 2024;37(2):281-92.
9. Teodorescu V, Gustavson S, Schanzer H. Duplex ultrasound evaluation of hemodialysis access: a detailed protocol. Int J Nephrol. 2012;2012:508956.

CHAPTER 3

Setting Up Training in Interventional Nephrology in Resource-Limited Settings

Vineet Behera, Umesh B Khanna, Sandeep Mahajan

INTRODUCTION

Interventional nephrology (IN) has rapidly emerged as a critical subspecialty within nephrology, focusing on the procedural and diagnostic aspects essential to the management of patients with kidney diseases, particularly those on dialysis. Traditionally, nephrologists have relied on radiologists, surgeons, or vascular specialists for procedures such as vascular access creation and maintenance, peritoneal dialysis (PD) catheter insertions, and biopsies. However, with the increasing burden of chronic kidney disease (CKD), particularly in resource-limited settings like India, the need for nephrologists to be equipped with interventional skills has become more apparent than ever before.[1]

INTERVENTIONAL NEPHROLOGY AS A NECESSARY SPECIALTY

The last two decades have witnessed the maturation of IN from a concept to a structured clinical discipline. The driving force behind this evolution has been the rising number of patients with end-stage kidney disease (ESKD), the increasing complexity of renal replacement therapies, and the logistical and financial inefficiencies of outsourcing essential procedures.[2] Studies have shown that nephrologist-performed procedures lead to faster access salvage, lower central venous catheter infection rates, and greater patient satisfaction. IN is uniquely positioned to enhance patient outcomes by providing:[3]

- *Timely interventions:* Nephrologists are often the first point of contact and can intervene early when access dysfunction arises.
- *Cost-effectiveness:* IN procedures, when done in-house, reduce dependence on radiology or surgery, cut down delays, and lower costs.
- *Continuity of care:* Nephrologists are intimately familiar with the patient's access history, offering personalized procedural care.
- *Improved outcomes:* Early access salvage, reduced catheter dependence, and timely catheter placements translate to better morbidity and mortality outcomes.

INTERVENTIONAL NEPHROLOGY IN INDIA

India is home to over 800 million people at risk of CKD due to diabetes, hypertension, and lifestyle changes. Approximately 2.2 lakh new patients are estimated to require dialysis annually, yet less than 40% of these receive long-term care. The challenges faced by nephrologists in India include delayed referrals, limited surgical access creation services, high catheter-related bloodstream infections, and dialysis dependency. Timely interventions, such as early fistula creation, catheter salvage, and real-time PD catheter insertions, can significantly reduce morbidity and mortality.[4] These procedures, if performed promptly by nephrologists, avoid the delays of scheduling with overburdened radiology and surgical departments. Furthermore, with the National Dialysis Program under the Pradhan Mantri National Dialysis Programme expanding access to dialysis, the volume of patients requiring interventions will rise exponentially.[5]

CHALLENGES FOR INTERVENTIONAL NEPHROLOGY

Despite the clear benefits, IN has not gained equal traction in developing countries, where health systems are often underfunded, and access to specialized care is uneven.[3]

- *Human resource deficiency:* There is a scarcity of trained nephrologists, and an even smaller number are trained in interventional procedures. Most nephrology training programs in India do not include comprehensive hands-on training in these techniques.

- *Inadequate infrastructure:* Many dialysis centers operate without dedicated procedural rooms or imaging guidance (e.g., fluoroscopy), which are essential for safe and effective interventions.
- *Regulatory barriers:* There is ambiguity in the regulatory framework about whether nephrologists can perform certain procedures, especially those traditionally done by surgeons or radiologists.
- *Financial constraints:* Government funding is often insufficient to develop full-scale interventional laboratories. Patients, too, may be unable to afford the costs of procedures if not covered under national insurance schemes.
- *Regional disparities:* Rural areas are particularly affected, with most interventional services concentrated in tier-1 and tier-2 cities.

MANPOWER AND SKILL REQUIREMENTS

Setting up an IN service requires trained personnel across multiple domains. In a resource-limited setting, a tiered manpower approach can be considered to maximize efficiency.[6]

- *Interventional nephrologist:*
  - Should have undergone focused training in IN techniques such as arteriovenous fistula (AVF) cannulation, tunneled dialysis catheter insertion/removal, PD catheter insertion, angiography, and access salvage procedures.
  - Currently, formal fellowship programs are limited in India. Thus, partnerships with established IN centers or international observership can be a feasible alternative.
- *Trained dialysis technicians/nurses:*
  - Should be skilled in assisting procedures, maintaining sterile fields, handling imaging equipment, and postprocedure monitoring
  - May be upskilled through short courses or hands-on workshops
- *Radiology/ultrasound technician:* In settings without interventional radiology, a trained nephrologist may perform ultrasound-guided procedures; however, dedicated imaging support enhances efficiency.
- *Biomedical technician:* For maintaining and troubleshooting equipment, including fluoroscopy and C-arm units, if available.
- *Support staff:* For patient movement, logistics, documentation, and inventory management.

INFRASTRUCTURE REQUIREMENTS[6,7]

Establishing an IN laboratory does not necessarily require high-end radiology suites or catheterization laboratories. In a resource-limited setting, a *modular, scalable design* can be used, as shown in **Figure 1**.

- *Physical space:*
- A procedure room of around 200–300 sq ft
- Adjacent recovery area for patient observation
- *Essential equipment:*
  - Ultrasound machine with vascular probe (7–10 MHz)
  - Minor OT table or fluoroscopy-compatible table
  - Sterile instrument trays for catheter placements and arteriovenous fistula (AVF) interventions
  - Central oxygen and suction lines
- *Advanced equipment:*
  - Mobile C-arm with digital subtraction angiography (DSA) for angioplasty or thrombectomy
  - ECG monitor, defibrillator, crash cart
- *Consumables:*
  - Tunneled and nontunneled dialysis catheters (various lengths and calibers)
  - Guidewires, peel-away sheaths, dilators
  - Sterile gowns, drapes, chlorhexidine, local anesthesia
- *Radiation safety:* Lead aprons, thyroid shields, and radiation badges (if using fluoroscopy)
- *Infection-control protocols:*
  - Autoclaving unit or access to central sterile services
  - Proper disposal of sharps and biomedical waste

The IN suite may be planned keeping in mind the above requirements, as shown in **Figure 2**. The infrastructure should be developed with modularity in mind, enabling gradual expansion from basic catheter insertion services to more complex interventions.

REQUISITES FOR A GOOD INTERVENTIONAL LABORATORY SETUP[6,7]

A well-functioning IN laboratory requires more than just equipment—it must have systems in place to ensure safety, efficiency, and quality.

- *Patient safety systems:*
  - Preprocedure evaluation checklist
  - Antibiotic prophylaxis protocols
  - Postprocedure observation charts

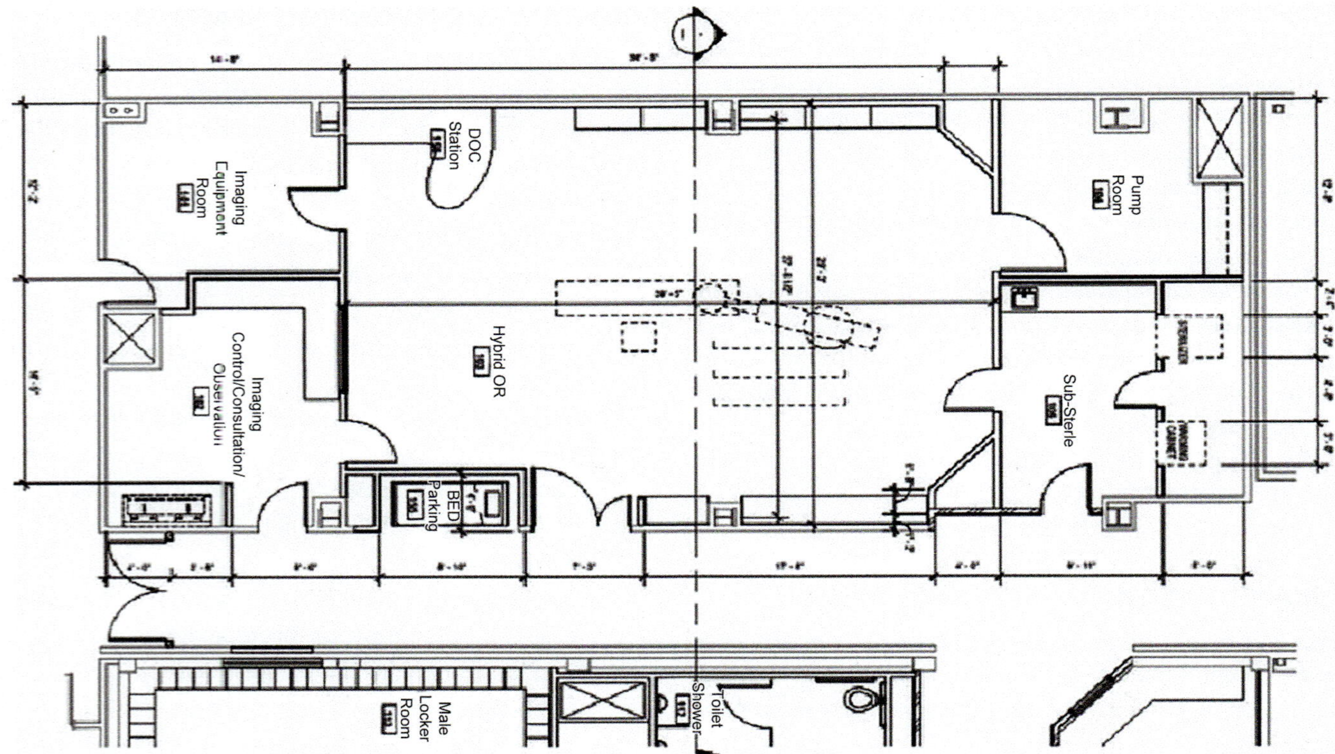

Fig. 1: Sample plan for a IN center with various facilities. (IN: interventional nephrology)

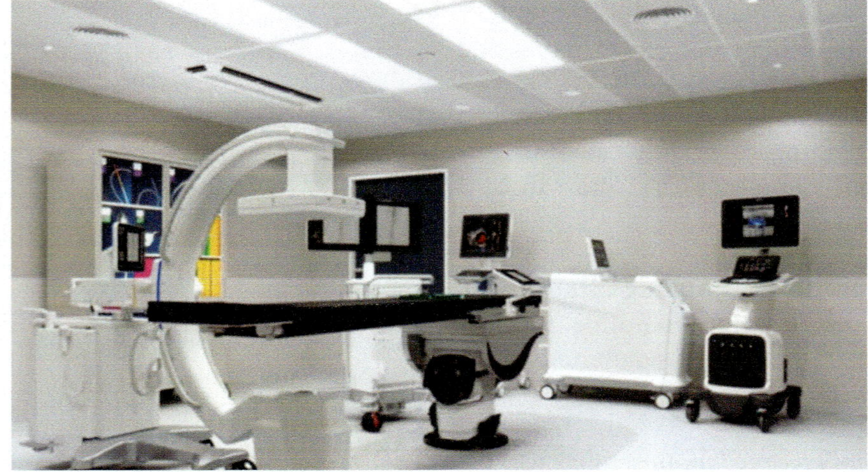

Fig. 2: A modern interventional suite with various equipment.

- *Procedural protocols:*
  - Standard operating procedures (SOPs) for each intervention
  - Emergency handling guidelines (e.g., bleeding, pneumothorax)
- *Audit and quality control:*
  - Monthly review of complications, infections, and outcomes
  - Root cause analysis of adverse events
  - Benchmarking with national/international standards

- *Documentation and data management:*
  - Procedure logs
  - Complication records
  - Inventory tracking for consumables
- *Training and accreditation:*
  - Periodic workshops
  - Credentialing of nephrologists for specific procedures

LEVELS OF INTERVENTIONAL NEPHROLOGY SETUP IN LIMITED SETTINGS[8]

In resource-poor contexts, all interventional centers cannot be fully equipped and all procedures cannot be started at once. A tier-wise approach is prudent:

- *Level I (basic interventions):*
  - Temporary and tunneled catheter insertions
  - Acute PD catheter insertions (percutaneous/surgical)
  - Ultrasound-guided vein mapping
  - Kidney biopsy
- *Level II (intermediate interventions):*
  - All basic interventions of level I
  - Fluoroscopy-guided tunneled catheter placements
  - AVF creation
  - Basic AVF venoplasty (USG guided)
  - PD catheter insertion
- *Level III (advanced/complex interventions):*
  - All basic and interventions of levels I and II
  - Angioplasty of stenosed AVFs/AVF thrombectomy
  - Other complex endovascular interventions
  - Central vein angioplasty
  - AVF superficialization/repair procedures
  - PD catheter repositioning/removal

Level III centers may be a full-fledged advanced center with most facilities and equipment acting as training centers or referral centers from lesser echelons, as shown in **Figure 3**. Each center may look after a region/state and may be located in a major medical college of national repute/or state-of-art tertiary hospital. Level II centers may perform intermediate interventions and may look after a city or small state, being located in big medical colleges or leading hospitals. Level I centers may be peripherally located centers in each hospital or dialysis center doing basic interventions, done by all nephrologists.

TRAINING IN INTERVENTIONAL NEPHROLOGY[2,5]

Training in IN has evolved significantly, with structured programs, fellowships, and dedicated societies playing a key role in advancing skills and standardizing practices. There are various levels of training available in IN, ranging from introductory workshops to formal fellowship programs. Basic training often includes observational learning

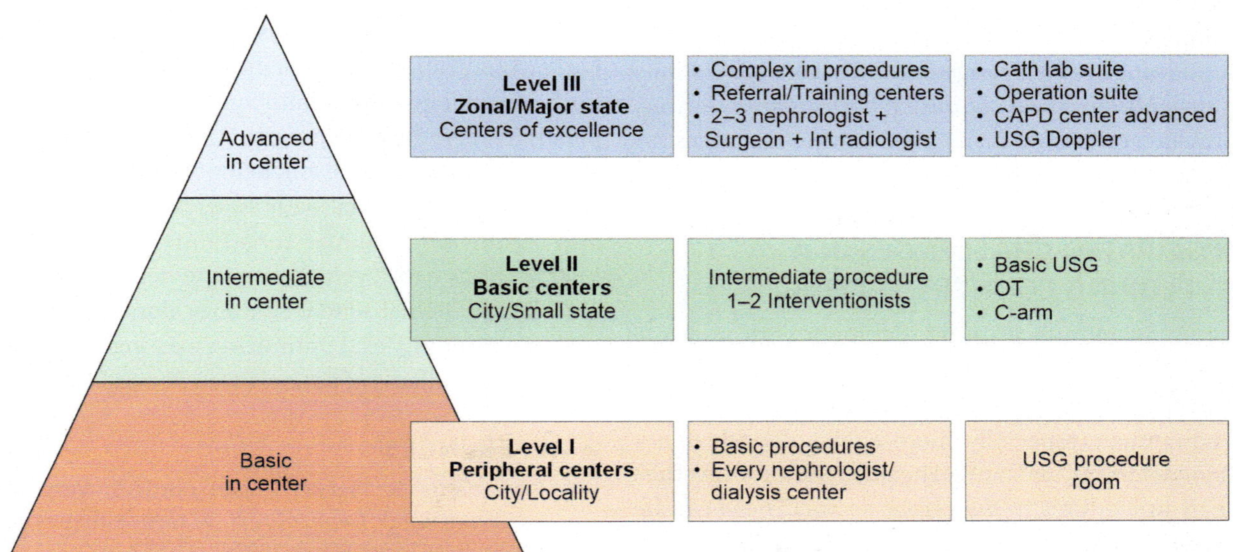

Fig. 3: Three-tier system of IN facility, ideally suited for low resource setting.
(CAPD: continuous ambulatory peritoneal dialysis; IN: interventional nephrology; USG: ultrasonography)

and simulation-based workshops aimed at familiarizing nephrologists with essential procedures such as vascular access ultrasound, tunneled dialysis catheter placement, and PD catheter insertion. Intermediate and advanced training levels involve supervised hands-on experience with procedures such as angioplasty, thrombectomy, and stent placement for dysfunctional dialysis accesses.

Fellowships in IN provide comprehensive exposure and are typically 3–12 months long. These are offered by select academic centers, especially in the United States, India, and parts of Europe. Fellows receive rigorous training in vascular access management, endovascular procedures, and imaging techniques under the guidance of experienced mentors. Hands-on training remains a cornerstone of IN education. Workshops at major nephrology conferences often incorporate simulation models, cadaver laboratories, and live demonstrations. These sessions allow participants to practice needle techniques, catheter placements, and use of fluoroscopy, fostering skill development in a controlled environment.

The "Train the Trainer" model is also gaining prominence, especially in regions with limited access to structured programs. This model empowers experienced interventional nephrologists to become educators themselves, ensuring the sustainability of skill transfer and the growth of the specialty globally. IN societies such as ASDIN (American Society of Diagnostic and Interventional Nephrology) and AVATAR (Association of Vascular Access and InTerventionAl Renal) play pivotal roles in promoting education, establishing procedural standards, and supporting credentialing efforts. These organizations facilitate collaboration, conduct certification exams, and provide continuing medical education resources for nephrologists at all career stages.

ANTICIPATED CHALLENGES IN A DEVELOPING COUNTRY SETTING[4,5]

Setting up an IN unit in India is fraught with multiple logistical and systemic challenges:

- *Cost and funding:* This includes high initial investment in equipment (especially fluoroscopy units) which is a major deterrent, and limited health insurance coverage for IN procedures in the public sector. These can be handled by seeking funds/CSR (Corporate Social Responsibility) partnerships, utilizing government schemes like PMJAY for dialysis patients, or sharing infrastructure with existing departments (radiology/surgery).
- *Training and skill development:* Few centers offer formal IN fellowships in India. There is also lack of mentorship and hands-on training. Possible solutions include encouraging national nephrology societies (e.g., AVATAR-IN, ASDIN) to initiate structured workshops, use simulation-based training modules, and form an IN consortia for collaborative skill-sharing.
- *Resistance from specialties and institutional hurdles:* Resistance from surgical or radiology departments fearing encroachment is a common phenomenon. Moreover, delay in approvals for purchasing capital equipment is a frequent problem. These can be tackled by fostering interdisciplinary collaboration with joint protocols, highlighting cost and time savings to hospital administration, and by showing the benefit of collaboration.
- *Infection control and sterility:* There is a risk of procedure-related infections due to substandard sterility in some centers. Possible solutions include adopting strict aseptic protocols, regular staff training and audits, and other infection-control measures
- *Patient perception:* Patients may have greater trust in procedures performed by surgeons or radiologists. Community education and success stories can help shift this perception.

CONCLUSION

Setting up an IN setup in a resource-limited environment is not without challenges, but the rewards are substantial—for both patients and healthcare systems. IN enhances patient care, reduces dependency on other departments, and improves the overall efficiency of nephrology practice. In countries like India, with an escalating CKD burden and significant resource constraints, nephrologist-led interventions can revolutionize care delivery. The future of IN lies not in high-end technology alone but in capacity building, training, and optimizing existing infrastructure to serve the millions of patients who depend on it.

REFERENCES

1. Efstratiadis G, Platsas I, Koukoudis P, Vergoulas G. Interventional nephrology: a new subspecialty of nephrology. Hippokratia. 2007;11(1):22-4.
2. Asif A, Byers P, Vieira CF, Roth D. Developing a comprehensive diagnostic and interventional nephrology

program at an academic center. Am J Kidney Dis. 2003; 42:229-33.
3. Niyyar VD, Beathard G. Interventional nephrology: opportunities and challenges. Adv Chronic Kidn Dis. 2020; 27(4):344-9.
4. Ramachandran R, Bhargava V, Jasuja S, Gallieni M, Jha V, Sahay M, et al. Interventional nephrology and vascular access practice: A perspective from South and Southeast Asia. J Vasc Access. 2022;23(6):849-60.
5. Jasuja S, Jha V, Rana DS, Sagar G, Gallieni M, Bahl A, et al. Building Interventional Nephrology Skills in India: A Decade-Long Journey by the AVATAR Foundation. Kidney Int Rep. 2025;10(4):983-7.
6. Vachharajani TJ, Moossavi S, Salman L, Wu S, Maya ID, Yevzlin AS, et al. Successful models of interventional nephrology at academic medical centers. Clin J Am Soc Nephrol. 2010;5(11):2130-6.
7. Rasmussen RL. Establishing an interventional nephrology suite. Semin Nephrol. 2002;22(3)237-41.
8. Vachharajani TJ, Kim YS, Riella M, Harris D, Jha V; International Society of Nephrology Interventional Nephrology Working Group. International Society of Nephrology's initiative on interventional nephrology minimum training and program-building standards in resource-limited countries. Kidney Int. 2020;98(5):1067-70.

SECTION

2 Vascular Anatomy and Radiology

CHAPTER 4

Vascular Anatomy for Dialysis Access

Edwin Mervin Fernando, Shamnad P

INTRODUCTION

Access for dialysis is the lifeline of a patient on hemodialysis. A basic understanding of vascular anatomy is essential for an interventional nephrologist, who is going to create and manage dialysis vascular access. Interpretation of an ultrasound (USG) Doppler or a fluoroscopic image is far superior when the interventionist has an adequate understanding of the vascular anatomy, especially of the upper limb, thorax, and femoral vessels. In this chapter, we shall look into the essential anatomy with focus on its clinical implications.

VASCULAR ANATOMY OF UPPER LIMB AND THORAX

Thoracic Aorta

After arising from the left ventricle, the thoracic aorta runs posterior to the pulmonary artery and ascends upward to form the arch of the aorta. The arch gives rise to three branches: (1) Right brachiocephalic artery, (2) left common carotid artery, and (3) left subclavian artery. Beyond the arch, the aorta then continues as the descending aorta, which descends laterally to the vertebral column at the onset. As it descends, it moves to the midline and becomes anterior to the spine at the level of the bifurcation of the aorta into the common iliacs.

Brachiocephalic Artery

The brachiocephalic artery is the first branch of the aortic arch, which arises at the level of the second right intercostal cartilage. It then ascends obliquely upward and backward to reach the right sternoclavicular junction, where it divides into the right common carotid and the right subclavian artery. There is no brachiocephalic artery on the left side of the body. But when it comes to veins, there are brachiocephalic veins on both sides.

Common Carotid Artery

The right common carotid artery, as mentioned earlier, originates from the right brachiocephalic trunk. On the other hand, the left common carotid artery originates as a direct branch of the arch of aorta. Both the right and left common carotid arteries have similar courses in the cervical region. They run upward obliquely and divide into the internal and external carotid arteries at the level of the upper border of the thyroid cartilage, which also corresponds to the 4th cervical vertebrae.

Subclavian Artery

As mentioned earlier, the right subclavian artery originates from the brachiocephalic trunk and the left subclavian arises as a direct branch, from the arch of aorta. The subclavian artery then travels laterally from its origin between the head of anterior and middle scalenus muscle. When it crosses the first rib, it continues as the axillary artery. The subclavian vein lies anterior to the scalenus anterior muscle.

Clinical implication 1: *This anatomical arrangement makes the cannulation of the subclavian vein[1] easier, as the vein lies very close to the posterior aspect of the medial one third of the clavicle, anterior to the subclavian artery.*

Arteries of the Upper Limb

Axillary Artery

The axillary artery is the main artery of the upper limb and is a continuation of the subclavian artery. It extends from the lateral border of the first rib to the lower border of the teres major. It then continues as the brachial artery in the arm. The axillary artery is divided into three parts based on its relationship with the teres minor muscle—the part which lies superior, posterior, and inferior to teres minor muscle.

Brachial Artery

The brachial artery is the continuation of the axillary artery beyond the lower margin of the teres major muscle. This artery runs in the medial compartment of the arm in the initial segment, later while it descends it becomes midline. At a point slightly below the elbow, it divides into the radial and ulnar arteries. The brachial artery is closely related to the median nerve. The median nerve lies lateral to the brachial artery in the initial third of the brachial artery, and lies medial to it in the distal third.

Accessory brachial artery: This artery can be mistaken for the brachial artery when a brachial arteriovenous fistula (AVF) is planned. It originates from the initial part of the brachial artery and then rejoins the brachial artery distally, just above the elbow. We can differentiate the accessory brachial artery from the brachial artery by the difference in caliber between the two and by tracing the relationship of the brachial artery with the median nerve.

Ulnar Artery

The ulnar artery is the main artery of the forearm and is the larger of the two terminal branches of the brachial artery. From its origin just below the elbow, it runs downward and medially to reach the ulnar side and then travels along the ulnar border to the wrist, where it divides into two terminal branches—one superficial and the other deep. These superficial and deep branches help in the formation of superficial and deep palmar arch.

Radial Artery

The radial artery arises from the brachial artery at the level of the neck of the radius in the cubital fossa. Being the smaller of the two branches of the brachial artery, the radial artery is considered the principal artery of the hand rather than the forearm. In the forearm, the artery lies in the anterior compartment and runs along radius bone just deep to the deep fascia. It can be felt readily against the bone making it easily identifiable during AVF creation.

The Palmar Arches

There are two palmar arches—a superficial palmar arch and deep palmar arch.[2] The superficial palmar arch is predominantly formed by the ulnar artery, with a small contribution from the radial artery. In some individuals, this superficial palmar arch is incomplete. Superficial palmar arch is more distal than deep palmar arch.

The deep palmar arch is an arterial network predominantly formed from the terminal branch of the radial artery. Unlike the superficial palmar arch, the deep palmar arch is a complete arch with contribution from the deep terminal branch of the ulnar artery via deep palmar branch. The deep palmar arch is more proximal than distal and lies on the metacarpal bones.

Clinical implication 2: *Before creating a radiocephalic AVF, it is imperative to confirm the patency of the palmar arch using the modified Allen's test.[3] The modified Allen's test tests the patency of the ulnar artery. The palm is blanched by tightly occluding the radial and ulnar arteries at wrist in a tight grasp. A patent ulnar artery is indicated by the return of normal color to the blanched palm within 5–15 seconds of releasing the pressure on ulnar side alone, keeping the radial side occluded. The patency of the ulnar artery is a must for preventing limb ischemia post-AVF creation.*

Veins of the Upper Limb

Discussion of the venous system of the upper limb should start from the distal end and proceed caudally. The peripheral veins of the upper limb are of two types: (1) Superficial and (2) deep veins. The superficial veins begin from two irregular venous plexuses: One in the palm, known as the volar venous plexus, and the other in the dorsum, known as the dorsal venous plexus. For dialysis access creation, the superficial veins are used, as they are contained within the subcutaneous tissue and deep fascia. In addition, they do not accompany any arteries, thus making the cannulation safer and easier. On the other hand, the course of the deep veins are closely concordant to major arteries. For example, radial veins lie on either side of the radial artery and accompany it along the entire course of the artery. This is why the deep veins are also called vena comitans (accompanying vein).

Basilic Vein

The basilic vein is a superficial vein that arises from the dorsal venous plexus on the back of the hand. It then ascends to the medial side of the forearm, assuming a posteromedial position in the entire forearm. In the arm, it ascends through the medial compartment, retaining a posteromedial position. After ascending through the medial bicipital sulcus, the basilic vein pierces the brachial fascia and in joins the brachial vein in the proximal third of the arm to form the axillary vein. Because of its posteromedial location and the course in the arm, brachiobasilic AVFs prove to be difficult for cannulation and may need transposition of the basilic vein.

Cephalic Vein

The cephalic vein begins initially on the dorsum of the hand on the radial side, and then it ascends curving around the radial border to come to the ventral side of the forearm. It then ascends upward to reach the ventral surface of the elbow where the medial cubital vein connects the basilic and cephalic veins. The cephalic vein then ascends caudally in the anterior compartment along the lateral side (lateral bicipital sulcus) and in the upper arm, it runs in deltopectoral groove. It then passes under the clavicle, taking a sharp curve to pierce the clavipectoral fascia, to join the axillary vein and form the subclavian vein. The cephalic arch refers to the final arch of the cephalic vein before terminating as the axillary vein.

Clinical implication 3: *The cephalic arch* ***(Fig. 1)*** *is a common site for vascular access dysfunction because of its unique morphology and anatomic characteristics.*[4] *Stenosis of the cephalic arch segment is very common, especially in long-standing high-flow brachiocephalic AVFs. The overall prevalence of cephalic arch stenosis is 15%.*

Axillary Vein

The axillary vein is formed by the union of the basilic vein and the brachial veins. Anatomically, it begins at the inferior border of the teres major muscle, then it accompanies the axillary artery in the axillary fossa. At the outer border of the first rib, it joins with the cephalic vein to form the subclavian vein.

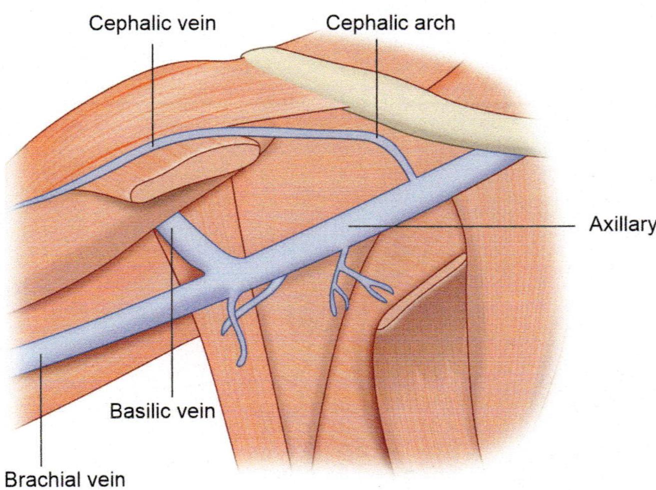

Fig. 1: Cephalic arch.

Subclavian Vein

The subclavian vein is a direct continuation of the axillary vein. It runs from the outer border of the first rib to the medial border of the anterior scalene muscle. The internal jugular vein (IJV) joins with the subclavian vein at the medial border of the anterior scalene muscle to form the brachiocephalic vein. The subclavian vein lies anterior to scalenus anterior muscle and follows the course of the subclavian artery, which lies posterior to the scalenus anterior muscle. At the medial border of the scalenus anterior, the external jugular vein joins the subclavian vein. The thoracic duct joins the subclavian vein at a point very near to the point where the IJV joins the subclavian vein. The subclavian vein passes behind the clavicle as it courses centrally.

External Jugular Vein

The external jugular vein receives the greater part of its blood from the exterior of the cranium and the deep parts of the face. One can trace the external jugular vein originating from the substance of the parotid gland at the level of angle of the mandible running perpendicularly down the neck in the direction of a line drawn from the angle of mouth to the middle third of the clavicle at the posterior border of sternocleidomastoid. At the lower end, it pierces the posterior border of the sternocleidomastoid, perforates the deep fascia and ends in the subclavian vein just lateral or anterior to the scalenus anterior muscle. The vein is covered by the platysma, the superficial fascia, and the integument.

This vein usually has two valves—the upper one is 4 cm above the clavicle and the lower is just at the entry into the subclavian vein. The portion of the vein between these two valves is often dilated and hence called the sinus.

Internal Jugular Vein

The IJV **(Fig. 2)** originates in the posterior compartment of the jugular foramen at the base of the skull, where it forms a slight dilation known as the superior bulb. From there, it descends vertically along the side of the neck, maintaining a position lateral to the internal carotid artery at its origin and lateral to the common carotid artery as it continues downward, gradually becoming more superficial. This predictable course makes the IJV cannulation relatively straightforward.

At the root of the neck, the IJV joins the subclavian vein just lateral to the sternoclavicular joint, to form the brachiocephalic vein. Before this union, it expands again, creating the inferior bulb. The vagus nerve, enclosed within the carotid sheath, runs posterior to both the IJV and the common carotid artery.

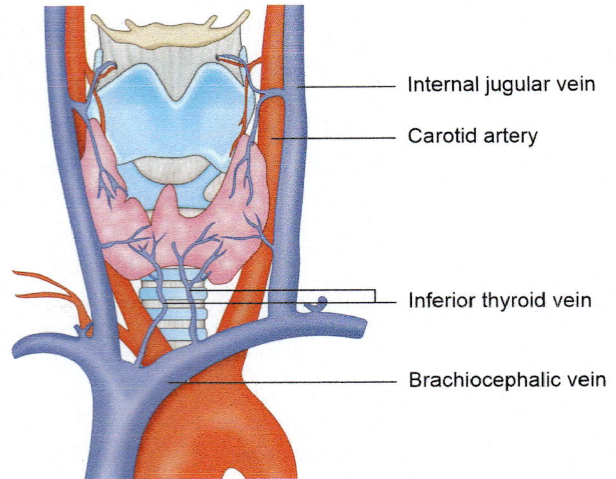

Fig. 2: Vascular anatomy of the neck.

Clinical implication 4 (Fig. 3): *The anatomical positioning of the IJV can vary.*[5] *While it is most commonly lateral to the artery, it may also be positioned anteriorly, medially, or extremely lateral, affecting the access during medical procedures. Due to these variations, ultrasound guidance (USG) has become the gold standard for IJV cannulation, particularly for procedures such as hemodialysis catheter insertion. By providing real-time visualization, USG minimizes the risk of arterial puncture and other complications, significantly improving the procedural safety and accuracy.*

A thorough knowledge of both the normal and variant anatomy of the IJV, along with the use of ultrasound, is essential for ensuring successful and safe venous access insertion.

Brachiocephalic Vein

The brachiocephalic veins are paired large vessels located at the root of the neck, formed by the convergence of the internal jugular and subclavian veins on each side. While they share a similar origin, their anatomical relationships differ considerably.

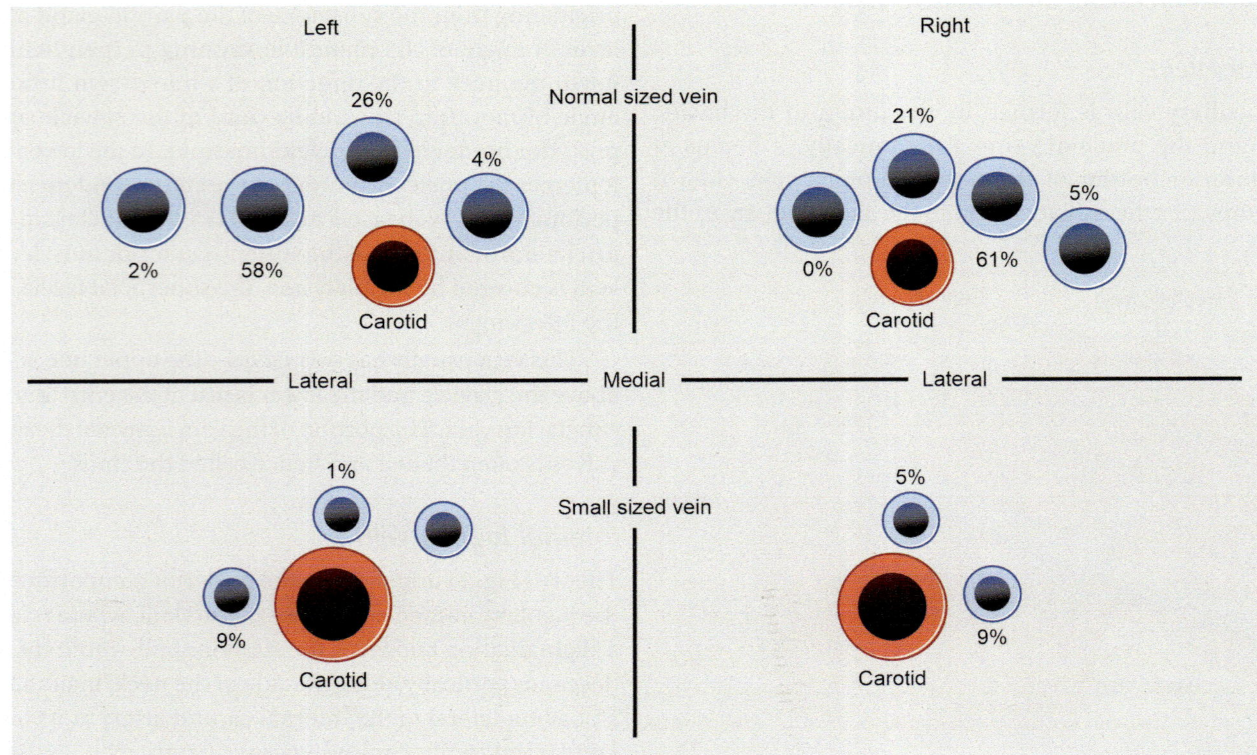

Fig. 3: Variations in internal jugular vein.

The *right brachiocephalic vein* **(Fig. 1)** is a short, approximately 2.5 cm long vessel that begins behind the sternal end of the clavicle. It descends almost vertically and unites with the left brachiocephalic vein just below the first rib's cartilage, near the right border of the sternum, forming the superior vena cava. It is situated anterior and to the right of the brachiocephalic artery. On its right side, the pleura separate it from the apex of the lung. Any injury or perforation to this vein can result in bleeding into the pleural cavity, potentially leading to serious complications.

The *left brachiocephalic vein* **(Fig. 1)** measures approximately *6 cm* in length. It originates behind the sternal end of the clavicle and travels in an oblique downward and rightward direction behind the upper half of the manubrium, eventually reaching the sternal end of the first right costal cartilage. Here it joins the right brachiocephalic vein to become the superior vena cava.

The left brachiocephalic vein receives the *left superior intercostal vein,* which drains the upper intercostal veins on the left side. When a central venous obstruction/stenosis occurs near the junction of these veins, the left superior intercostal vein may serve as an important collateral pathway. In response to the increased blood flow, this vein often enlarges considerably.

Clinical implication 5: *Visualizing the anatomical course of the left brachiocephalic vein* ***(Fig. 4)*** *is crucial when placing a left-sided tunneled hemodialysis catheter, especially during the insertion of the peel-away sheath. An inadvertent downward force at this stage could pierce the brachiocephalic vein,[6] potentially causing fatal bleeding. Therefore, it is always advisable to monitor the tip of the dilator under C-arm guidance to ensure proper positioning and direction, thereby preventing this serious complication.*

Azygos Venous System

The azygos venous system is composed of the *azygos vein,* the *hemiazygos vein,* and the *accessory hemiazygos vein.*

- *Azygos vein:* The azygos vein **(Fig. 5)** originates opposite the second lumbar vertebra. It ascends through the aortic hiatus and continues upward until it reaches the level of the fourth thoracic vertebra where it arches forward over the root of the right lung and empties into the superior vena cava. It receives blood from both the subcostal and intercostal veins. Notably, the upper three or four intercostal veins coalesce to form the superior intercostal vein, which subsequently drains into the azygos vein.
- *Hemiazygos vein:* The hemiazygos vein **(Fig. 5)** ascends on the left side of the vertebral column, beginning at the diaphragm's left crus (at the level of L2 vertebra). As it enters the thorax and reaches approximately the ninth thoracic vertebra, it crosses the midline posterior to the aorta, esophagus, and thoracic duct to join the azygos vein. It primarily drains the lower intercostal and subcostal veins.

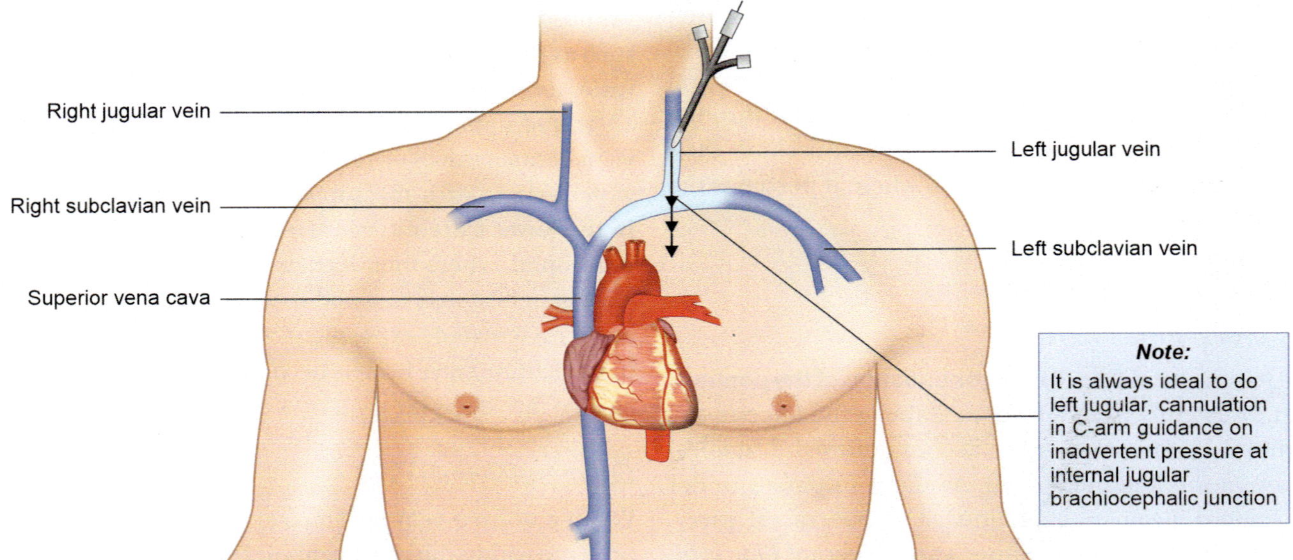

Fig. 4: Anatomical course of the left and right brachiocephalic veins and their relevance in tunneled hemodialysis catheter placement.

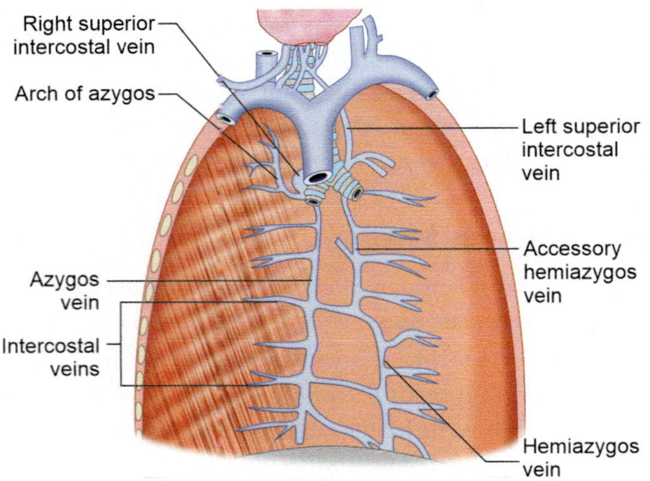

Fig. 5: Anatomy of azygos system.

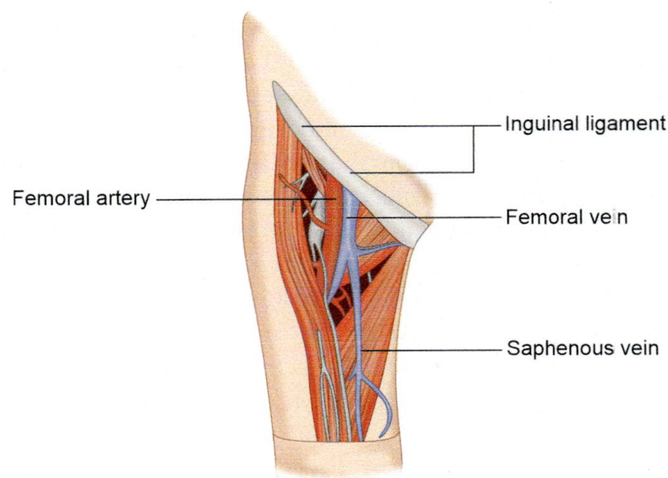

Fig. 6: Femoral triangle.

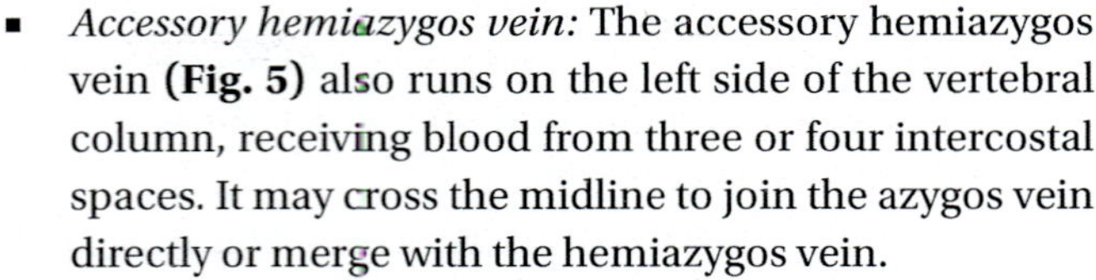

- *Accessory hemiazygos vein:* The accessory hemiazygos vein **(Fig. 5)** also runs on the left side of the vertebral column, receiving blood from three or four intercostal spaces. It may cross the midline to join the azygos vein directly or merge with the hemiazygos vein.

Note: This venous system serves as an important collateral pathway for venous return from the thoracic wall, particularly in cases of central vein stenosis.

Arteries of the Lower Limb

Femoral Artery

The femoral artery **(Fig. 6)** is a continuation of the external iliac artery. It begins at the mid-inguinal point, just behind the inguinal ligament. Thus, the inguinal ligament marks the boundary between the external iliac and femoral arteries. The artery exits the femoral triangle through its apex, passing beneath the sartorius muscle. It then continues into the popliteal fossa, where it becomes the popliteal artery.

Veins of the Lower Limb

Femoral Vein

The femoral vein **(Fig. 6)** is a continuation of the popliteal vein. It extends from a level just above the knee to the inguinal ligament where it accompanies the femoral artery in the femoral sheath. As the vein passes under the inguinal ligament, it lies medial to the femoral artery. Beyond this point, it continues as the *external iliac vein.* This anatomical relationship is crucial for vascular access, surgical procedures, and understanding venous circulation in the lower limb.

Venous Valves

Unlike the arterial system, which operates under high pressure, the venous circulation is a low-pressure system without a strong driving force to propel blood flow. Many small peripheral veins collapse when they are not filled with blood. Blood movement through these veins largely depends on muscle contractions and a network of one-way valves. These valves, composed of delicate leaflet pairs, prevent the backward flow of blood. The regions where valves are located often appear slightly widened. While venous valves are commonly found in certain locations, such as the proximal cephalic vein, their exact distribution varies among individuals.

In the upper extremities, all peripheral and central veins contain valves up to the level of the innominate veins, which, along with the superior vena cava, lack valves.[7] In the lower extremities, valves are frequently visible on ultrasound, where their leaflets can be seen opening and closing in response to blood flow. When an arteriovenous access is created, exposing a vein to arterial pressure, these delicate valve leaflets become permanently flattened against the vein wall.

Collateral Veins

When a normal vein develops an obstructive lesion, the pressure within the vein begins to rise. An elevated venous pressure predisposes to the development of new or collateral veins. These veins bypass an area of obstruction; in doing so, they tend to deviate from the usual course of the normal vein. This is one of the primary reasons that it is important to be able to recognize normal venous pathways and locations. These anomalous veins tend to be more tortuous than normal. Their course is more random and they tend to come off of the main channel at odd angles. Collateral veins serve as a hallmark sign that an obstructive lesion is present. Collateral veins tend to be more fragile than the other veins. They are prone to rupture and are often multiple in number.

CONCLUSION

Now that we have a good understanding of the relevant anatomy, we will be able to delve into the fascinating world of interventional nephrology with greater ease and understanding. Our understanding will further be strengthened as we practically see these vessels during ultrasound screening, fistulogram interpretations, and while doing procedures.

REFERENCES

1. Capobianco SM, Fahmy MW, Sicari V. Anatomy, Thorax, Subclavian Veins. In: StatPearls [Internet]. Treasure Island (FL): StatPearls Publishing; 2025.
2. Gellman H, Botte MJ, Shankwiler J, Gelberman RH. Arterial patterns of the deep and superficial palmar arches. Clin Orthop. 2001;(383):41-6.
3. Agarwal T, Agarwal V, Agarwal P, Thakur S, Bobba R, Sharma D. Assessment of collateral hand circulation by modified Allen's test in normal Indian subjects. J Clin Orthop Trauma. 2020;11(4):626-9.
4. Echefu G, Shivangi S, Dukkipati R, Schellack J, Kumbala D. Contemporary review of management techniques for cephalic arch stenosis in hemodialysis. Ren Fail [Internet]. 2023;45(1):2176166.
5. Lim CL, Keshava SN, Lea M. Anatomical variations of the internal jugular veins and their relationship to the carotid arteries: a CT evaluation. Australas Radiol. 2006;50(4):314–8.
6. Kang SH, Kim AY, Do JY. Hemodialysis catheter malpositioned into the mediastinum: Lessons from two cases. Semin Dial. 2021;34(3):252-6.
7. Asif A, Agarwal AK, Yevzlin A, Wu S, Beathard GA. Interventional Nephrology, 1st edition. New York: McGraw Hill/Medical; 2012. p. 752.

CHAPTER 5

Ultrasound/Doppler for Vein Mapping

Nikhil Chaudhari

CASE VIGNETTE

A 56-year-old male patient who is a case of chronic kidney disease (CKD) stage 5 on maintenance hemodialysis is not able to undergo hemodialysis through his left radio-cephalic arteriovenous fistula (AVF). He had undergone AVF creation surgery 4 months back. He had to rely upon his central venous catheter for his hemodialysis. Can we modify his clinical outcome by a simple test of ultrasound vein mapping? What could be the reason for nonmaturation of his autogenous arteriovenous (AV) access?

Answer: Vein mapping test is a simple ultrasound test, which is noninvasive and quick. On vein mapping ultrasound for the patient, it was found that a small tributary of cephalic vein was anastomosed with the radial artery instead of main cephalic vein the forearm. Main cephalic vein was anatomically situated posterior to this branch and it was missed by the operating surgeon. This must have caused technical difficulty for the surgeon and morbidity to the patient. His fistula did not mature as there was a segment of reduced caliber vein anastomosed to the artery. He had to undergo second corrective surgery for his AV access which involved creation of the fresh anastomosis with the main cephalic vein proximally. Routine preoperative vein mapping can help to decide target vessels for the anastomosis and avoid such complication and morbidity caused to the patient.

INTRODUCTION

This chapter will take you through the basics to the challenges faced during ultrasound vein mapping for assessment of patients and achieving desirable outcome of AV access procedure.

NEED FOR VEIN MAPPING

Ultrasound is being increasingly utilized in many centers, as it is readily available and cheap but its major advantage is that skilled operator can detect a need for further imaging to assess central vein patency in the form of contrast venography, which can help in detecting central venous stenosis or occlusion. Literature that evaluates the role of preoperative noninvasive ultrasound in AV access procedures provides convincing evidence to support the use of duplex ultrasound to identify potential blood vessels prior to a hemodialysis access operation.[1] Vein mapping also helps in planning of the procedure and patient counseling. Currently, there is increasing evidence that preoperative duplex ultrasound can not only increase the utilization of native AVF for dialysis access, but also allow proper selection of a target vessel with adequate luminal diameter to improve dialysis access outcome.[2] Mihmanli et al. randomized 124 patients undergoing assessment for fistula construction into preoperative physical examination alone or evaluation with ultrasound alone. The rate of primary nonfunction was 5.6% in the ultrasound group compared with 25% in patients undergoing physical examination.[3] The routine use of intraoperative DUS mapping after regional anesthesia is recommended to determine the optimal access site for chronic hemodialysis access. Identifying additional access options not seen with physical examination and preoperative DUS mapping will provide end-stage renal disease patients with more fistula options and hence, a longer access life span for a lifelong disease.[4] Intraoperative evaluation is mandatory as brachial plexus block can alter the results of preoperative vein mapping.[4]

TABLE 1: Guidelines for vessel mapping.

Criteria	*Statement*	*Recommendation*	*Quality of evidence*
Vessel mapping	KDOQI suggests selective preoperative ultrasound in patients at high risk of AV access failure **(Table 2)** rather than routine vascular mapping in all patients	Conditional	Low
Which imaging study?	KDOQI considers it reasonable to use various imaging studies as needed to evaluate the suitability of vessels for AV access creation such as ultrasonography for peripheral vessels (including intraoperative ultrasound) and venography for suspected central vein occlusion, while considering the patient's clinical circumstances and residual kidney function	No recommendation	Expert opinion
Vessel diameter	KDOQI considers it reasonable that while there is no minimum diameter threshold to create an AVF, arteries and veins of <2 mm in diameter should undergo careful evaluation for feasibility and quality to create a functioning AVF	No recommendation	Expert opinion
Vessel characteristics	KDOQI considers it reasonable to evaluate multiple characteristics of vessel quality for AVF creation (size, distensibility, flow, etc.)	No recommendation	Expert opinion

(AVF: arteriovenous fistula; KDOQI: Kidney Disease Outcomes Quality Initiative)

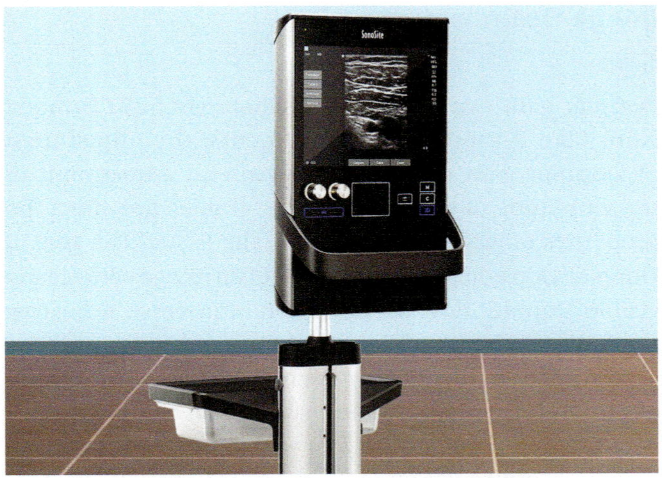

Fig. 1: Miniature portable ultrasound machine.

WHAT THE GUIDELINES SAY (TABLE 1)[5]?

There are various guidelines for standardizing assessment of the upper limb veins and most commonly used are KDOQI guidelines. Simplified in a tabular form above.

TABLE 2: Examples of risk factors for which vessel mapping may be beneficial.[5]

Clinical problem	*Risk factors*
Fistula failure	Elderly age, female, comorbidities (e.g., peripheral vascular disease, coronary artery disease), small pediatric patients
Peripheral vessel damage	*Ipsilateral:* PICC insertion, other iatrogenic (e.g., venipuncture), self-inflicted (e.g., IVDU), disease states (e.g., vasculitis), radial artery harvesting for CABG
Central venous stenosis	Multiple CVCs; prolonged CVC duration; cardiac implantable electronic device; PICC; surgery or trauma to neck, chest, upper extremity
Limitations to physical examination	Morbid obesity, suboptimal conditions (e.g., patient dehydrated or vasoconstricted), poor skin integrity, patient refusal

(CABG: coronary artery bypass grafting; CVC: central venous catheter; IVDU: intravenous drug users; PICC: peripherally inserted central catheter)

KNOW YOUR MACHINE

With advancement in the technology, ultrasound machine has become a miniature tool in the form of portable unit, which is far more convenient for the surgeon, to perform vein mapping in preoperative area or in the OPD **(Fig. 1)**. Linear array probe of 8–12 MHz is used for the scans. There is a mark on the probe to know the orientation of the image. Scan is performed with the mark being kept on the left side of the operator for uniformity.

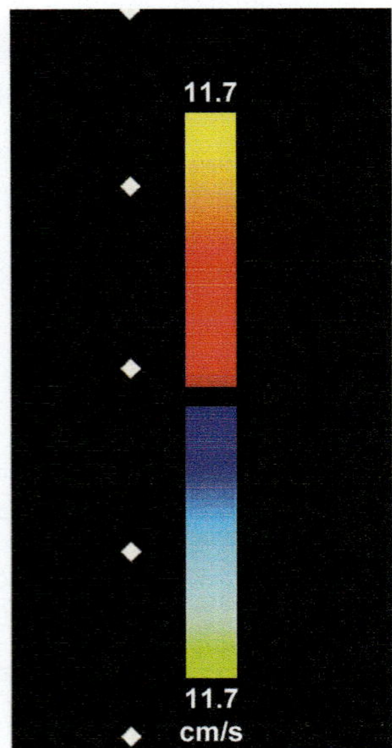

Fig. 2: *Example of color scale key:* Numbers represent velocity range displayed. Upper color (red) represents flow toward transducer. Lower color (blue) represents flow away from transducer.

Doppler Modalities

Color

Color Doppler covers information about the velocity of moving objects over a typical B-mode image. A sample volume is placed over an area of interest. The machine then uses the frequency and amplitude of the returning echoes from pulsed interrogation of that region to display information regarding flow in the given area. The machine assigns different colors depending on the direction of flow, also known as phase shift. This is traditionally assigned as red for flow toward the transducer or blue for flow away from the transducer **(Fig. 2)**.

Pulsed Wave

Pulsed-wave (PW) Doppler is used for determining frequency shifts within a specific area of interest. To do this, the user uses B-mode imaging to set the location of a sample volume or "gate" for interrogation with pulsed wave Doppler. The device then transmits short sound pulses and waits for the returning echo. Since the speed of sound in soft tissues is known, the device can vary the period during which it is "listening" for returned echoes based on the expected time, the sound will need to travel to return to the transducer. PW Doppler can then isolate frequency shifts from the sample volume, which is displayed in graphical form with frequency on the y-axis and time on the x-axis **(Fig. 3)**.

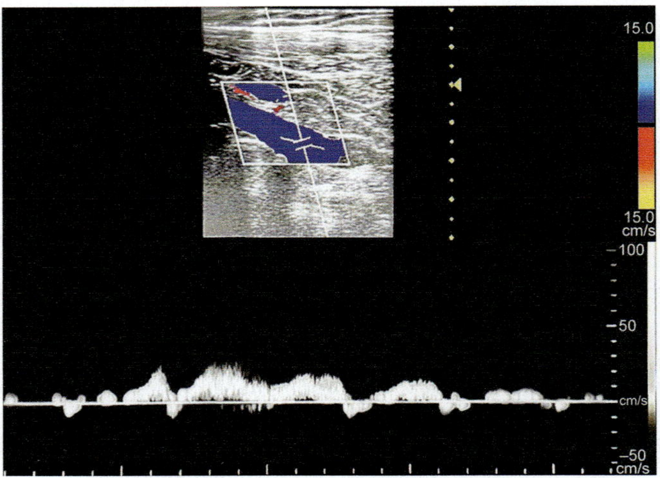

Fig. 3: Pulsed-wave imaging of a subclavian vein.

Image Optimization

Gain

Doppler gain can be adjusted separately from B-mode gain. Like B-mode gain adjustments, the adjustment of Doppler gain causes a receiver end adjustment of the amplitude of returning signals. It does not affect the properties of waves transmitted to the tissue. The goal of Doppler gain adjustment is to obtain an image with clearly visible Doppler flow in the region of interest. Adjusting the gain too high will lead to increased noise and the appearance of flow in nonvascular regions. Adjustment of gain too low will preclude visualization of flow where it is present. In practice, the best way to optimize gain is to increase it until color artifacts appear in nonvascular areas ("blooming") and then decrease it slightly.

Pulse Repetition Frequency/Scale

Changing the pulse repetition frequency (PRF) brings changes the number of pulses transmitted from the probe over a 1-second period. The higher the PRF, the higher the scale of velocities that can be detected. If the area of interest contains velocities higher than the upper limit of the Doppler scale, aliasing will occur, causing loss of directional and velocity information. For low velocities, lowering the scale will increase the sensitivity to low-velocity blood flow and improve the relative detection of differences in flow.

In some cases, setting the scale at a predetermined level on color Doppler can help identify the point at which the flow characteristics change such as at a stenotic area of a vessel. The machine will display velocities up to the limit of the set scale, at which point an area of aliasing will be apparent as velocities increase rapidly through the stenotic portion of the vessel. This can help the sonographer quickly identify the point at which velocities exceed a preset value.

PREREQUISITES FOR ULTRASOUND VEIN MAPPING

- Warm ambient temperature of the room
- Vein mapping preferably should be done before dialysis of the patient and not immediately after dialysis so that patient should not be in dehydrated state.
- Examine upper limbs in sitting position as depicted in the figure and central veins in supine position **(Fig. 4)**.

TECHNIQUE

Venous Study

The entire upper extremity is evaluated, starting from the cephalic vein in the forearm to the cephalic and basilic veins in the upper arm. A tourniquet is sequentially placed at the midforearm, antecubital area, and at the upper arm, and the cephalic, basilica, and brachial vein diameters are measured throughout their course up to their insertion into the subclavian or axillary veins. The arm is scanned proximal to distal, with and without a tourniquet. Veins should be thin walled, vary in size with respiration, collapse completely on compression with the transducer, and augment with distal compression. Essential parameters which are measured include vessel depth, internal diameter with and without the tourniquet, continuity with the deep system and the presence of any stenosis or thrombosis. Veins should dilate by approximately 50% by the use of a tourniquet. The draining and central veins are assessed for stenosis or thrombosis by analysis of the waveform for changes in respiratory phasicity and transmitted cardiac pulsatility. However, it is important to note that ultrasonography offers only indirect evaluation of central venous vasculature; therefore, additional techniques may be needed, particularly among patients with a history of central venous catheter use **(Figs. 5A and B)**.

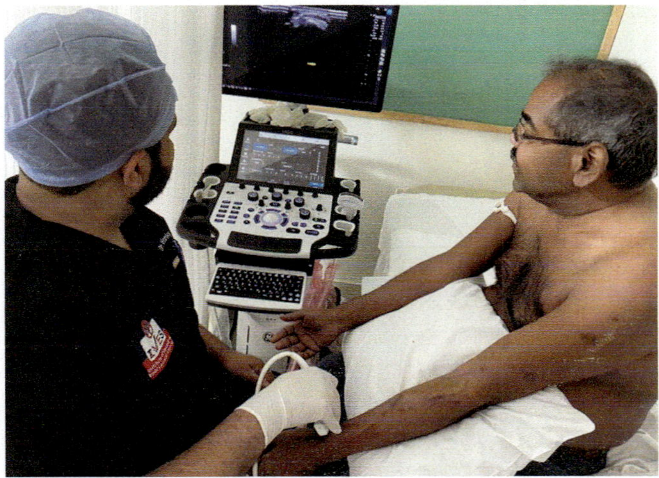

Fig. 4: Position of the patient for vein mapping.

Arterial Study

The arm is again scanned proximal to distal. Diameters of radial, ulnar, and brachial artery should be measured. Calcification and abnormal arterial wall thickening should be recorded. Recordings are made on another suitable chart **(Fig. 6)**. The arterial waveform should also be evaluated both proximally and distally and, in particular, at the site of the proposed AVF. Peak systolic velocities should be recorded. The normal waveform should be triphasic high-resistance flow with no evidence of dampening, which could indicate a proximal stenosis.

CRITERIA FOR SUCCESSFUL AVF CONSTRUCTION

Arterial Diameter

The normal diameter of the radial artery ranges from 2 to 3.5 mm. Unfortunately, there is limited literature on the influence of arterial diameter and vessel quality on fistula success rates. Wong et al.[6] showed that a luminal diameter of <1.6 mm was associated with early fistula failure and Malovrh[7] reported that a diameter of <1.5 mm was associated with a success rate of only 45%. Similarly, Lemson et al.[8] observed significantly smaller mean preoperative radial artery diameters among patients with failed forearm fistulae compared with successful fistulae (1.9 vs. 2.8 mm). A minimum diameter of 2 mm has been proposed by Silva et al.[9] and adopted by other investigators.[10] Above this minimal diameter there seems to be no correlation between arterial diameter and fistula success.[10] Peak systolic velocity (PSV) of the proposed inflow artery is easier to measure and has also been evaluated as a predictor of a successful AVF.

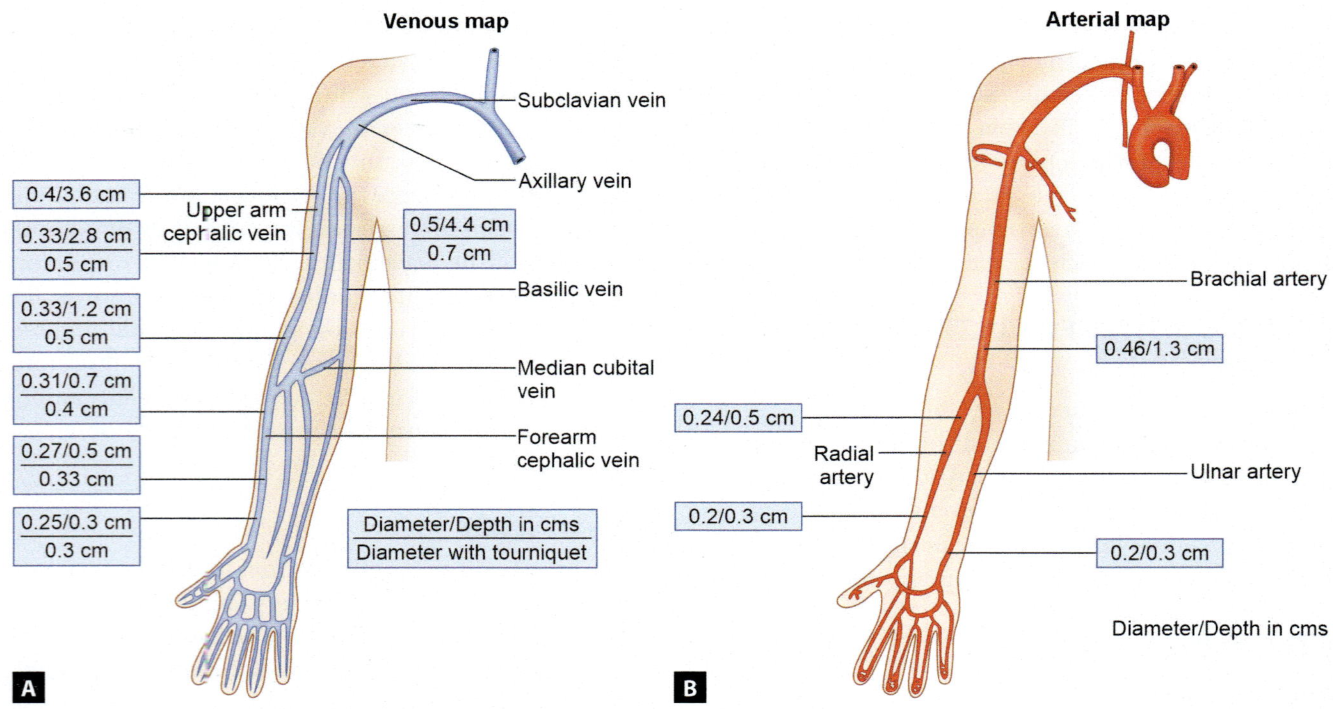

Figs. 5A and B: (A) Venous and (B) arterial charts for vein mapping report depicting diameter and the depth.

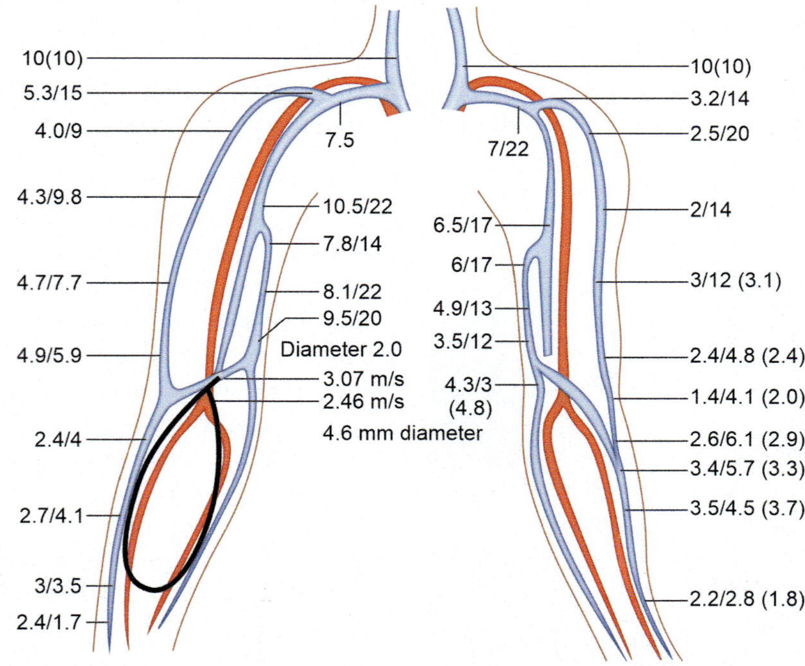

Fig. 6: Depiction of the chart and measurements of diameter with and without augmentation. Depth is written in brackets.

Venous Diameter

Mendez[11] analyzed 44 consecutive patients who underwent preoperative vein mapping prior to wrist AVF construction. Successful maturation of the fistula was achieved in 22 patients (50%) and was significantly higher if the preoperative cephalic vein diameter was >2.0 mm. In these studies, venous measurements were undertaken without a tourniquet, demanding the application of a very precise pressure by the transducer during scanning to achieve accurate results. Although a precise threshold for minimal vein diameter in successful fistulae has not been established, most clinical studies use a cut off value of 2.5 mm for AVF, and 4.0 mm for synthetic grafts as suggested by Silva et al.[9] The ability of a vein to dilate is also an important predictor of a successful fistula. Measurements of venous diameter should be taken with and without augmentation with a tourniquet. Malovrh[12] found that venous diameter increased by an average of 48% in patients with successful fistulae compared with only 11.8% in fistulae that failed. Similarly, Hou et al. found that the outcome of wrist radiocephalic AVF survival would be significantly improved through the use of cephalic vein with venous distensibility >0.52 mm.[13]

The study of the entire vascular territory performed with color Doppler ultrasound, within a multidisciplinary team of nephrologists and vascular surgeons, is associated with high rates of autologous access and very low rates of primary failure and maturation failure (almost unprecedented in the literature).[14] Other criteria such as hyperemia response of artery, flow volume in artery/vein and PSV have doubtful value in predicting AV access maturation.

CONCLUSION

- There is increasing evidence that routine preoperative duplex ultrasound reduces the rate of primary fistula failure and unnecessary surgical exploration.
- Ultrasound increases the utilization of native AVF and allows proper selection of suitable target vessels of adequate diameter.
- A minimum arterial diameter of 2 mm is associated with successful radiocephalic fistula formation. Below this diameter, the ability of an artery to increase flow and dilate will determine fistula success.
- Most clinical studies use a threshold value for minimal venous diameter of 2.5 mm for AVF and 4 mm for prosthetic grafts. There is no clear data for various levels of autologous AV access in terms of minimum diameter of vein/artery.
- Contrast venography is an essential investigation if there is suspicion of central vein stenosis.

PRACTICE POINTS

- Vein mapping ultrasound is a must before planning AV access for the patients performed with and without augmentation.
- Vein mapping has to be repeated in the OR before starting the procedure.
- Diameter of artery and vein has a definite impact on the success of the AVF creation and maturation; however, cut-off points are different for different type of AV access.
- There are no definite criteria in the guidelines.

Recommendations:

- *Radiocephalic AVF:* Cephalic vein 2 mm without augmentation (male/female) and radial artery >2 mm (inner diameter)
- *Brachiocephalic AVF:* Cephalic vein 2.5 mm with augmentation and brachial artery 2.5 mm
- *AV graft:* Axillary vein 4 mm after augmentation and brachial artery >2.5 mm

REFERENCES

1. Robbin ML, Gallichio MH, Deierhoi MH, Young CJ, Weber TM, Allon M. US vascular mapping before hemodialysis access placement. Radiology. 2000;217(1):83-8.
2. Lin PH, Bush RL, Chen C, Lumsden AB. What is new in the preoperative evaluation of arteriovenous access operation? Semin Vasc Surg. 2004;17(1):57-63.
3. Mihmanli I, Besirli K, Kurugoglu S, Atakir K, Haider S, Ogut G, et al. Cephalic vein and hemodialysis fistula: surgeon's observation versus color Doppler ultrasonographic findings. J Ultrasound Med. 2001;20(3):217-22.
4. Hui S, Folsom R, Killewich L, Vu M, Li C, Michalek J, et al. A comparison of preoperative and intraoperative vein mapping sizes for arteriovenous fistula creation. J Vasc Surg. 2017;65(1):e11-2.
5. Lok CE, Huber TS, Lee T, Shenoy S, Yevzlin AS, Abreo K, et al. KDOQI clinical practice guideline for vascular access: 2019 update. Am J Kidney Dis. 2020;75(4):S1-164.
6. Wong V, Ward R, Taylor J, Selvakumar S, How TV, Bakran A. Factors associated with early failure of arteriovenous fistulae for haemodialysis access. Eur J Vasc Endovasc Surg. 1996;12(2):207-13.
7. Malovrh M. Non-invasive evaluation of vessels by duplex sonography prior to construction of arteriovenous fistulas

for haemodialysis. Nephrol Dial Transplant [Internet]. 1998;13(1):125-9.
8. Lemson MS, Leunissen KML, Tordoir JHM. Does preoperative duplex examination improve patency rates of Brescia-Cimino fistulas? Nephrol Dial Transplant. 1998;13(6):1360-1.
9. Silva J, Hobson RW, Pappas PJ, Jamil Z, Araki CT, Goldberg MC, et al. A strategy for increasing use of autogenous hemodialysis access procedures: impact of preoperative noninvasive evaluation. J Vasc Surg. 1998;27(2):302-8.
10. Lockhart ME, Robbin ML, Allon M. Preoperative sonographic radial artery evaluation and correlation with subsequent radiocephalic fistula outcome. J Ultrasound Med. 2004;23(2):161-8.
11. Mendes RR, Farber MA, Marston WA, Dinwiddie LC, Keagy BA, Burnham SJ. Prediction of wrist arteriovenous fistula maturation with preoperative vein mapping with ultrasonography. J Vasc Surg. 2002;36(3):460-3.
12. Pajek J, Malovrh M. Preoperative ultrasound still valuable for radio-cephalic arteriovenous fistula creation? J Vasc Access. 2017;18:S5-9.
13. Hou G, Hou Y, Sun X, Yin N, Feng G, Yan Y, et al. Venous distensibility is more important than venous diameter in primary survival of autogenous radiocephalic arteriovenous fistulas. J Vasc Access. 2020;21(6):963-8.
14. Ibeas J, Roca-Tey R, Vallespín J, Moreno T, Moñux G, Martí-Monrós A, et al. Spanish clinical guidelines on vascular access for haemodialysis. Nefrologia. 2017;37:1-191.

CHAPTER 6

Renal Ultrasound

Yimeng Zhang, Shalabh Srivastava, Sarah McCloskey, James Andrews

INTRODUCTION

Ultrasonography is an expanding field with increasing clinical practice globally. It does not use any ionizing radiation and is noninvasive, therefore it is a safe modality to evaluate the kidneys and urinary tract. Point-of-care ultrasound allows nephrologists to evaluate patients at the bedside, forming an extension of physical examination. This allows for real-time examination for a wide range of indications including abdominal or flank pain, renal dysfunction, detection and follow-up of masses in the urinary tract, renal stones as well as other pathologies described in this chapter.

EQUIPMENT

A low-frequency 3–6 MHz curvilinear transducer.

PREPARATION FOR KIDNEY ULTRASOUND SCANNING

- Kidney ultrasound is typically performed with the patient in the lateral decubitus position. In emergency settings, the supine position is often preferred. For those undergoing ultrasound as part of a native renal biopsy, the prone position is commonly used.
- Enhancing the visibility of the kidneys can often be achieved by having the patient raise their arms above their head and take a deep breath in.
- To obtain optimal views of the collecting system and bladder, it is recommended that the patient consumes approximately 500 mL of fluid 1 hour before the scan, ensuring that they avoid micturition. If a urinary catheter is present, it should be clamped for 1–2 hours prior to scanning.

LOCATING THE KIDNEYS

The kidneys are located deep to the posterolateral lower rib cage within the paravertebral gutters. They sit between the levels of T12 and L4 vertebrae. The superior poles of the kidneys are tilted slightly posterior and medial with respect to the inferior poles.

The right kidney lies inferior and posterior to the right lobe of the liver. It is covered anteriorly by the liver and inferiorly by the right colic flexure and duodenum. The most effective approach for scanning the right kidney is through the intercostal spaces from the posterolateral side or mid-axillary line, utilizing the liver as an acoustic window.

The left kidney lies posterior and inferior to the spleen, with the stomach overlapping the front of the upper pole. Its lower half is covered by the descending colon and left colonic flexure, which passes around its anterior surface. Like the right, the left kidney is best scanned through a posterolateral approach using the intercostal spaces and spleen as an acoustic window. The left kidney is generally located higher and posterior compared to the right, making it more challenging to scan due to the intervening gas.

Start scanning both kidneys in longitudinal views. Once a clear image is acquired, fan the probe to cover the entire organ. Rotate the probe 90° to examine the kidney in the transverse plane, scanning from pole to pole. Both kidneys should be scanned routinely for comparison and to identify any anatomical variations.

Abnormalities in Kidney Location

- *Renal agenesis:* One kidney is absent, while the contralateral kidney may be enlarged.
- *Ectopic kidneys:* One or both kidneys may be located outside the normal renal fossa, often in the pelvis, but they may be obscured by bowel gas.

Renal Size

Kidneys can be measured in three dimensions: Length, width, and thickness **(Fig. 1)**. The longitudinal scan is

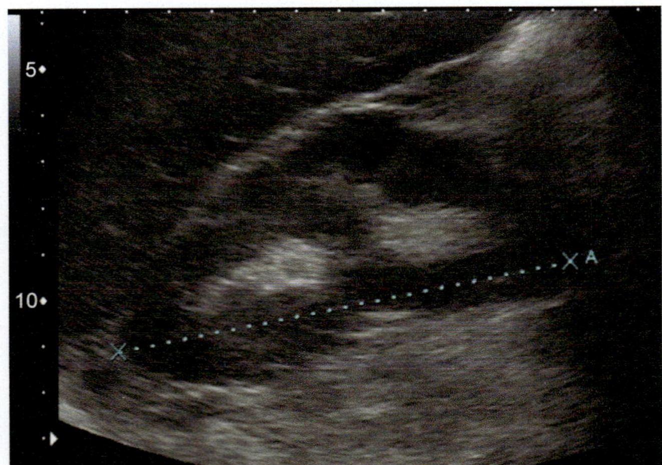

Fig. 1: Normal right kidney measuring 10.7 cm.

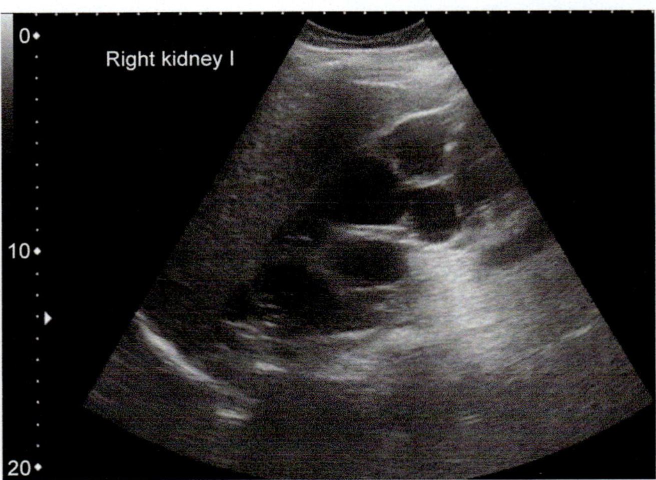

Fig. 2: Polycystic kidneys containing multiple hypoechoic cysts with no internal shadows.

ideal for measuring renal length. Freeze the image and measure the maximum length from pole to pole. For width and thickness, the transverse view is most effective.[1]

Normal renal dimensions:

- *Length:* 9–12 cm
- *Width:* 4–7 cm
- *Thickness:* 3–5 cm

Small Kidneys

Causes of bilateral small kidneys include:

- Chronic renal diseases such as glomerulonephritis, renal artery stenosis, reflux nephropathy, and chronic pyelonephritis
- Aging
- Low body weight or height

Enlarged Kidneys

Renal enlargement can be seen in conditions like acute glomerulonephritis, hydronephrosis, and amyloidosis. Renal masses or cysts, such as in polycystic kidney disease,[2] can also cause the kidneys to appear enlarged **(Fig. 2)**.

APPEARANCE OF THE KIDNEYS ON ULTRASOUND

The kidneys are bean-shaped with a smooth surface. It is not uncommon for older patients to exhibit surface indentations. Pyelonephritis can also cause such indentations. The parenchyma of the left kidney often forms a bulge beneath the spleen's border, creating a "dromedary hump".

Anatomical variants:

- *Horseshoe kidney:* The two kidneys are connected at their lower poles by a parenchymal isthmus, forming a U-shape.
- *Duplication of the collecting system:* This developmental abnormality results in two ureters.
- *Extrarenal pelvis:* In about 10% of individuals, the renal pelvis lies outside the renal hilum. The renal pelvis is formed by the major calyces and the extrarenal pelvis can appear dilated, leading to a false impression of urinary obstruction.

Renal Parenchyma and Sinus

The kidneys consist of three main layers: The cortex, the medulla (collectively referred to as the renal parenchyma), and the renal sinus. The kidneys and adrenal glands are encased in a dense fibrous capsule called Gerota's fascia. Just beneath this capsule is the cortex, which typically measures 5–7 mm in thickness and decreases with age. The columns of Bertini are projections of cortical tissue that extend into the medulla. These columns separate the 8–10 renal pyramids, which have a characteristic hypoechoic appearance on ultrasound. This is especially prominent in younger patients and can be mistaken for renal cysts.[3]

The apex of each renal pyramid forms a papilla, which excretes urine into a corresponding minor calyx. Several minor calyces converge to form the major calyces, which then merge to form the renal pelvis. The latter tapers through the renal hilum into the proximal ureter. The transition between the renal pelvis and ureter is the ureteropelvic junction (UPJ), which is a common site of obstruction from ureterolithiasis. This is typically at the level of the hilum, where blood vessels, lymphatics, and ureters pass through. Collectively, the minor and major calyces, intrarenal blood vessels, and surrounding fat tissue constitute the renal sinus, which is the hyperechoic central region of the kidney.

The collecting system and ureters are usually not visible on ultrasound unless hydronephrosis is present. The ureters descend across the psoas muscle, crossing the common iliac vessels at the pelvis brim and then anteriorly and medially to empty into the bladder via the ureterovesical junctions (UVJs) at the two superior corners of the trigone. In severe urinary retention, the distended bladder can extend to the level of the umbilicus.

Circumscribed Lesions

- *Hyperechoic:*
    - *Angiomyolipomas:* These are benign tumors, round, homogeneous, well-circumscribed masses. They are typically within the renal parenchyma containing blood vessels, muscle tissue, and fat. They are usually solitary and asymptomatic, if multiple and bilateral can be associated with tuberous sclerosis.
    - Renal scars
    - Calcifications **(Fig. 3)**
- *Isoechoic:* Renal cell carcinoma (RCC)
- *Hypoechoic:*
    - Intracystic hemorrhage
    - Abscess: Appears with irregular margins and possible bright internal echoes
- *Echo-free: Simple cysts* **(Fig. 4)**: Smooth, thin-walled, round or oval-shaped cysts with posterior acoustic enhancement. These may be solitary or multiple. Cysts are classified by their location: Pararenal, cortical, or parapelvic. Cysts that have irregular borders, septations, calcifications, or heterogenous echo density should be referred for further evaluation.

Polycystic Kidney Disease

Polycystic kidney disease is a hereditary condition with multiple cysts of various sizes, with compression and thinning of the renal parenchyma, leading to the eventual replacement of renal parenchyma by cysts.

Renal Cancer

Renal cancer has a varied appearance on ultrasound. Any unexplained mass or disruption of the renal architecture should be considered for referral for further imaging. Smaller RCCs can be hyperechoic and may be mistaken with angiomyolipomas; however, they tend to be less well defined. Larger RCCs may show cystic degeneration, calcification, and disorganized blood flow on color Doppler.

Intrarenal Hematomas

Intrarenal hematomas can appear as hyperechoic, isoechoic, or hypoechoic, depending on their stage. Acute hematomas may appear heterogenous and hyperechoic, becoming more hypoechoic or cystic over time. Subcapsular hematoma appears as a crescent-shaped fluid collection between the renal parenchyma and capsule.

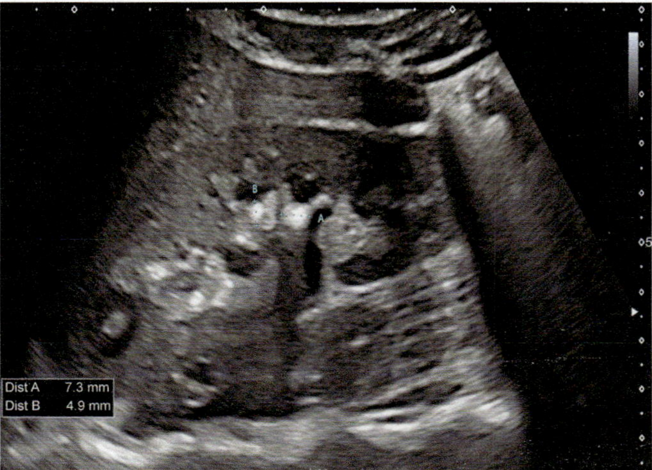

Fig. 3: Renal calcification/urolithiasis.

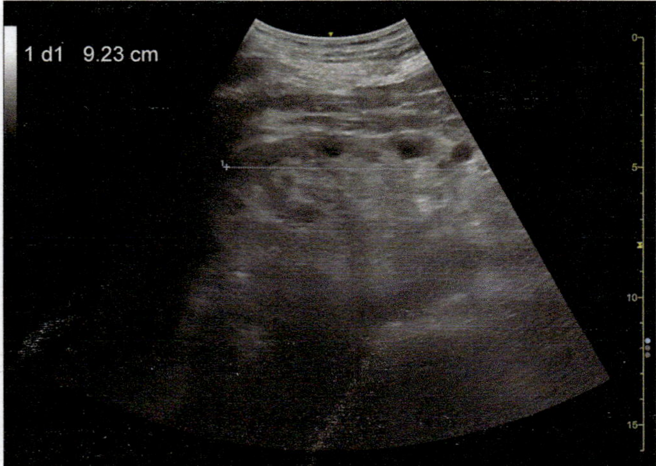

Fig. 4: Simple cyst at the lower pole in an atrophic kidney.

Diffuse Changes

In health, the renal parenchyma is relatively hypoechoic and appears less echogenic than the adjacent liver or spleen.[4]

- *Cortical atrophy* (**Fig. 5**):
  - Length usually <9 cm depending on body size
  - Length and echogenicity can be normal
  - Cortical thinning with accentuation of lobulation
  - Sign of chronic kidney disease due to the loss of functional tissue
- *Medullary disease:* Increased echogenicity leading to greater corticomedullary differentiation, which may suggest sloughing of the papillae **(Fig. 6)**

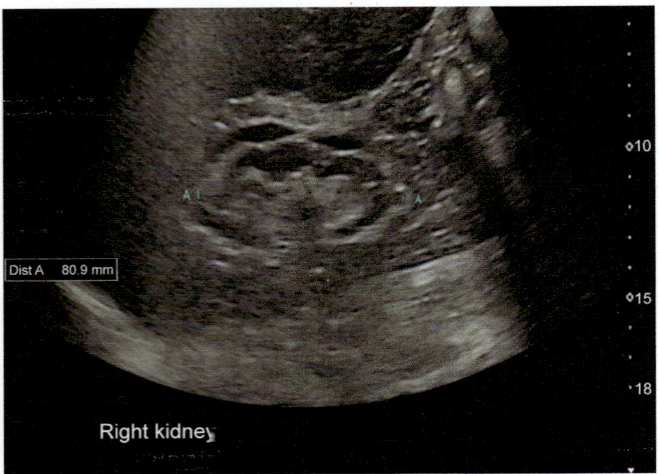

Fig. 5: Reduced corticomedullary differentiation demonstrating cortical atrophy in a small kidney.

- *Diffusely increased cortical echogenicity:*
  - Increased renal echogenicity is a nonspecific finding but can represent several underlying conditions.
  - Causes include various renal conditions associated with inflammation or swelling or the renal cortex or chronic kidney disease such as:
    - Acute glomerulonephritis
    - Diabetic nephropathy
    - HIV nephropathy
    - Renal amyloidosis
    - Sickle cell disease
  - Chronic glomerulonephritis leads to a decrease in renal size. The echogenicity of the parenchyma is uniformly increased. There may be loss of definition of the medullary pyramids with an indistinct corticomedullary junction.

Hydroureteronephrosis (Figs. 7 and 8)

Ultrasound imaging of hydronephrosis will demonstrate a dilated pelvicalyceal system. The severity can be classified into mild, moderate, or severe or graded from 1 to 4 based on sonographic criteria:

- *Grade 1:* Dilated renal pelvis with no calyceal dilatation with thinning of the parenchyma
- *Grade 2:* Dilatation of the renal pelvis and calyces with thinning of the parenchyma
- *Grade 3:* Cystic dilatation of the renal pelvis with a thin rim of parenchyma
- *Grade 4:* Parenchyma no longer demonstrated

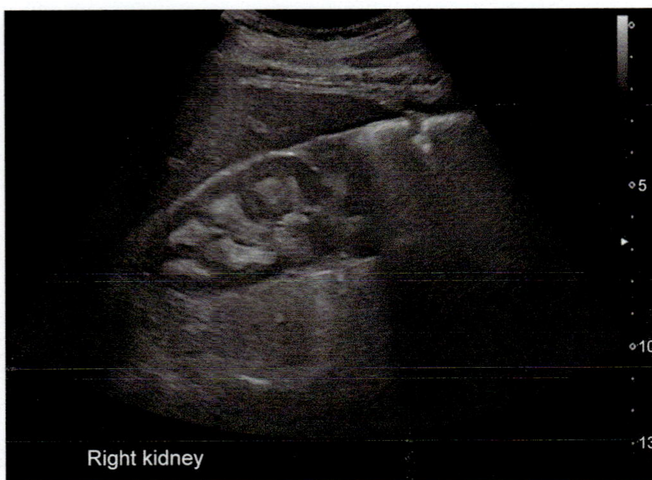

Fig. 6: Medullary nephrocalcinosis.

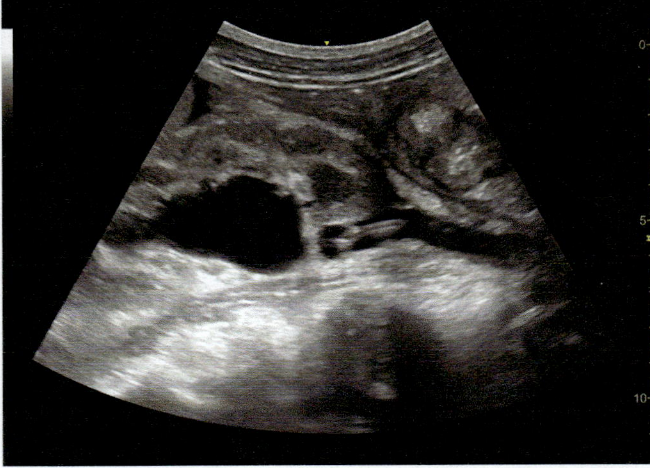

Fig. 7: Native left proximal ureter around blocked urinary stent and hydronephrotic kidney.

Thinning of the renal cortex in the context of hydronephrosis usually implies chronicity.

Once hydronephrosis is identified, further scanning or imaging is often required to further assess to determine the underlying cause. Always scan the lower urinary system. Dilation of the renal pelvis does not always indicate obstruction. A dilated renal pelvis can be a normal variant in some people; other causes include pregnancy, large diuresis, reflux disease, and papillary necrosis. A very full bladder may result in a bilaterally prominent pelvicalyceal system; this should be reassessed post-void for change in the degree of pelvicalyceal dilatation. Conversely, dehydration may prevent the development of hydronephrosis. Scanning may be repeated after hydration.

Ureterolithiasis

The cause of nephrosis, including ureterolithiasis, may not always be identifiable on ultrasound, with CT imaging of the abdomen and pelvis being the gold standard for stone evaluation. Small stones can often be undetectable on ultrasound, and ureteral stones are generally difficult to visualize.

On ultrasound, calculi typically appear as bright, echogenic foci accompanied by posterior shadowing. In the renal sinus, the echo may be indistinguishable from the surrounding fat, and stones can sometimes be identified purely by the shadow. Ureteral stones are most commonly located at the UVJ. To visualize this area effectively, the ultrasound gain settings should be adjusted to make the bladder appear entirely black, while the structures behind the bladder should display varying shades of gray. Additionally, color Doppler can reveal a "twinkling artifact", characterized by alternating colors behind the stone, simulating turbulent blood flow.

Ureteric jets, which represent the normal periodic reflux of urine into the bladder, are commonly observed in well-hydrated individuals. These jets appear as brief bursts of low-level echoes from the vesicoureteral junction (VUJ) and can be seen on color Doppler as a sudden burst of color within the bladder lasting a few seconds. In cases of obstruction, no jet will be detected. With partial obstruction, the jet may show a variety of patterns, including increased or decreased flow, or even a continuous, dribbling jet.

ULTRASONOGRAPHY OF THE BLADDER

To begin the scan, position the probe transversely above the symphysis pubis and angle it caudally. Rotate the transducer 90 to examine the bladder longitudinally along the midline, just above the symphysis pubis. Tilt the probe to visualize the entire bladder **(Figs. 9 and 10)**.

Normal Anatomy

The bladder appears as an echogenic cavity within the pelvis. Under normal conditions, the bladder empties completely during voiding. However, in older individuals with detrusor dysfunction, there may be a residual volume ranging from 5 to 100 mL. Bladder volume can be estimated using the following formula, which includes a correction factor for the bladder's ellipsoid shape:

$$\text{Bladder volume} = 0.75 \times \text{width} \times \text{length} \times \text{height}$$

(all in millimeters)

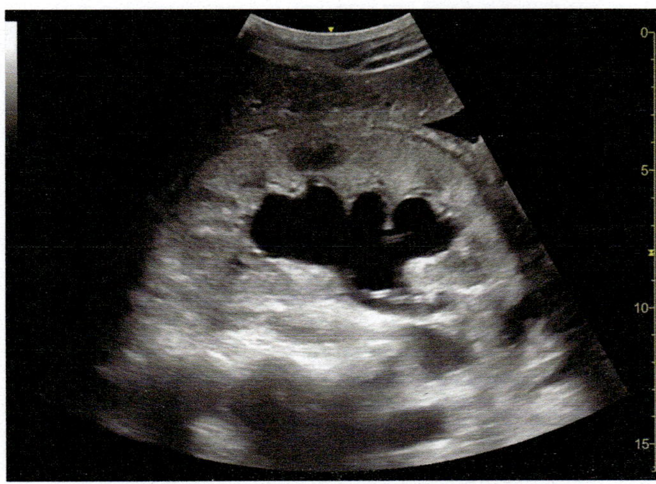

Fig. 8: Hydroureteronephrosis without stent.

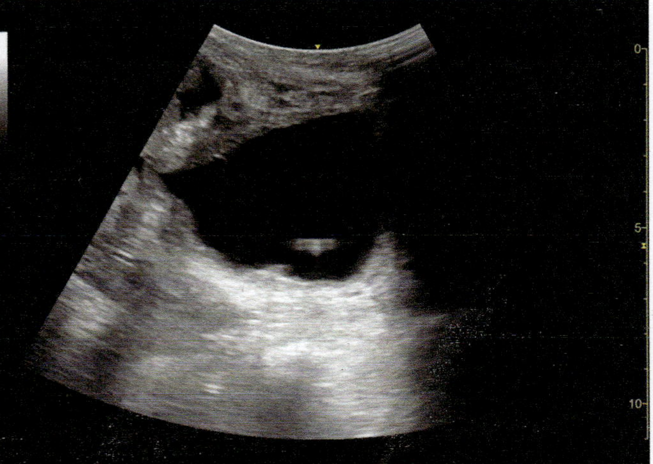

Fig. 9: Urinary bladder with a stent in situ.

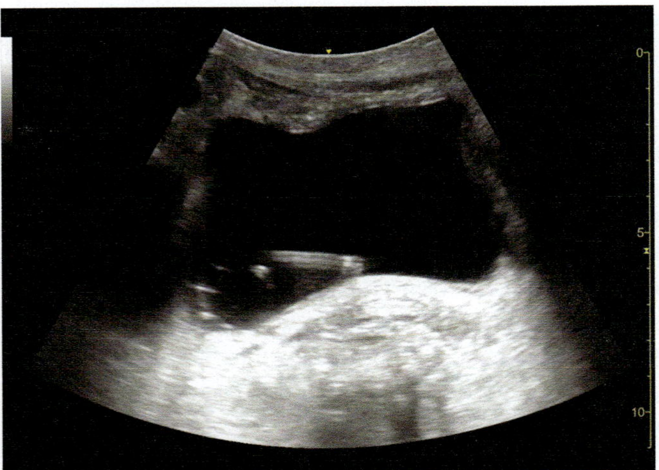

Fig. 10: Transverse bladder with a urinary stent.

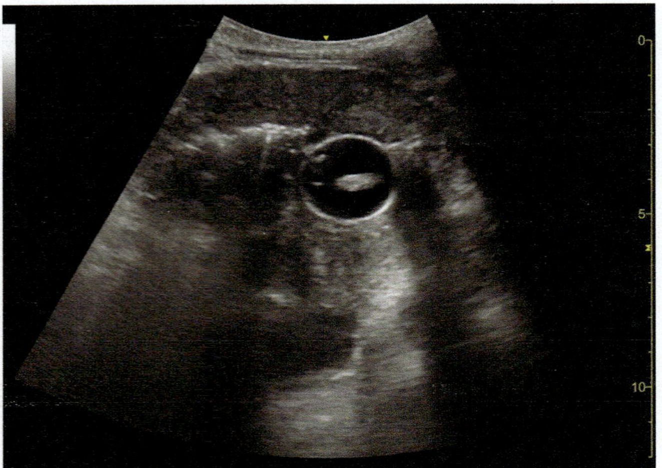

Fig. 11: Longitudinal bladder post-catheter insertion for macroscopic hematuria. Grossly thickened bladder wall superiorly, inflated bladder catheter balloon next to air within the remainder of bladder. Transitional cell carcinoma (TCC) confirmed on cystoscopy.

Pathology

Bladder outlet obstruction is characterized by a bladder containing more than 100–150 mL of urine after an attempt to void. In addition to volume measurement, ultrasound can often identify conditions such as prostatic hypertrophy or neoplasm, diffuse thickening of the bladder wall from detrusor hypertrophy, and/or the presence of bladder diverticula. Additionally, bladder stones and neoplasms can be detected during the scan **(Fig. 11)**.

CONCLUSION

The increased accessibility and widespread use of portable ultrasound has allowed it to be successfully used as an adjunct in clinical decision making. An appreciation of normal renal anatomy and ultrasound appearance is crucial in detection of variants and pathological features. There remains a significant intra and interoperator variability with subjective interpretations of imaging, highlighting the importance of formal education and additional training. Cross-sectional imaging such as CT or MRI scans may be required to assist in obtaining a definitive diagnosis.

REFERENCES

1. Rad PM, Abbasi B, Valizadeh N, Hatami F, Tohidinezhad F, Gharehbaghi Z. Evaluation of normal renal size and its influencing factors: A cross-sectional study on the adult population of Mashhad. Caspian J Intern Med. 2022;13(3):623-33.
2. Connolly JA, Dean AJ, Hoffmann B, Jarman RD (Eds). Emergency Point-of-Care Ultrasound, 2nd edition. New York: Wiley; 2017.
3. Kang TL, Bailitz J (Eds). Clinical Ultrasound: A How-to Guide. Boca Raton, FL: CRC Press; 2015.
4. Block B. Abdominal Ultrasound: Step by Step, 3rd edition. Thieme; 2015.

CHAPTER 7

Interventional Radiology

Oladunni O Akin-Akintayo, Daniel Rubin, Ram Kishore Gurajala

INTRODUCTION

Interventional radiology (IR) is one of the most dynamic fields of medicine, with constantly evolving procedures and new technologies aimed at growing and advancing established techniques and treatments. This field of IR aims to provide safe and effective treatment to patients using minimally invasive techniques. The first documented procedure in the field was in January 1964 when Charles Dotter performed dilatation of the left superficial femoral artery in an 82-year-old woman with limb ischemia and gangrene of the lateral three toes with documented clinical and imaging improvement.[1] Since then, the field has expanded beyond vascular procedures to include vascular and nonvascular interventions spanning all systems of the body.

Expertise in all imaging modalities is a foundational skill for an interventional radiologist with the IR professional leveraging this skill in performing image-guided procedures. This is a crucial distinguishing factor from other professionals and when appropriately harnessed, results in better outcomes for an interventional radiologist. Like most image-guided interventions, most procedures in IR are based on the fundamental principle of the Seldinger technique which was originally described by Sven Ivar Seldinger for replacing direct puncture angiography with catheter-based angiography.[2] Using a modification of the Seldinger technique and expertise of image guidance, an interventional radiologist can access and place catheters or stents within the renal collecting system, the renal vessels, and other areas safely and effectively.

ROLE OF INTERVENTIONAL RADIOLOGY IN INTERVENTIONAL NEPHROLOGY

The field of interventional nephrology arose from the need for vascular access in patients on hemodialysis and was initially performed by nephrologists.[3] With involvement of other specialties such as radiology and surgery, the scope of interventional nephrology has expanded beyond dialysis access to include other interventions for various renal pathologies. Using minimally invasive techniques, interventional radiologists now perform procedures such as percutaneous nephrostomy tube placement, renal tumor ablations, embolization, and arteriovenous fistula (AVF) creation, amongst others. All interventions are done under image guidance and with minimal access which is the hallmark of IR.

PREPROCEDURE

Appropriate workup and patient selection are crucial in IR. Prior to the procedure, laboratory investigations including complete blood count, comprehensive metabolic profile, clotting profile, and other indicated investigations are reviewed and optimized accordingly. Cross sectional imaging such as CT scans, MRI, or ultrasound scans are ordered when indicated, to determine appropriateness of intervention, accessibility of lesions, and preprocedural planning.

Informed consent is obtained after discussion of the procedure including risks, benefits, and short- and long-term complications of the procedure. As with all interventions, the benefits of a procedure should always outweigh the risks or at least be comparable.

PROCEDURES

- *Dialysis access and dialysis access interventions:*
    - Tunneled dialysis catheter placement:
        - *Indications:*
            - Temporary access for hemodialysis
            - Short-term hemodialysis access in patients with a newly created AVF pending fistula maturation, healing, or management of

existing dialysis access malfunction or complications, e.g., clotted AVFs
  - Permanent hemodialysis access in patients with no feasibility of creation of other means of permanent hemodialysis
- *Procedure:* Tunneled dialysis catheters provide immediate central venous access for patients needing long-term dialysis. Typically, the right internal jugular vein is preferred; however, other veins including subclavian, external jugular, and even common femoral veins can also be used. Less common approaches such as translumbar or transhepatic access can also be utilized when the aforementioned access sites have been exhausted.

  The technical aspects would be discussed under Chapter 12.

  The final catheter position is confirmed by fluoroscopy **(Figs. 1A and B)**. The catheter is immediately ready for use which is a major advantage of the tunneled hemodialysis catheters.
- *Complications:*
  - Bleeding
  - Infection
  - Pneumothorax, air embolism
  - Central vein stenosis, thrombosis, or occlusion

- *Venoplasty:*
  - *Indication:* Venoplasty is sometimes indicated in patients with central vein stenosis **(Figs. 2A and B)** related to multiple prior central venous catheters. In addition to limiting options for central venous catheter placement, AVF function may be compromised if the stenosis is on the same side as the AVF, due to elevated venous pressures and decreased blood flow. In extreme cases of severe stenosis or near-occlusion,

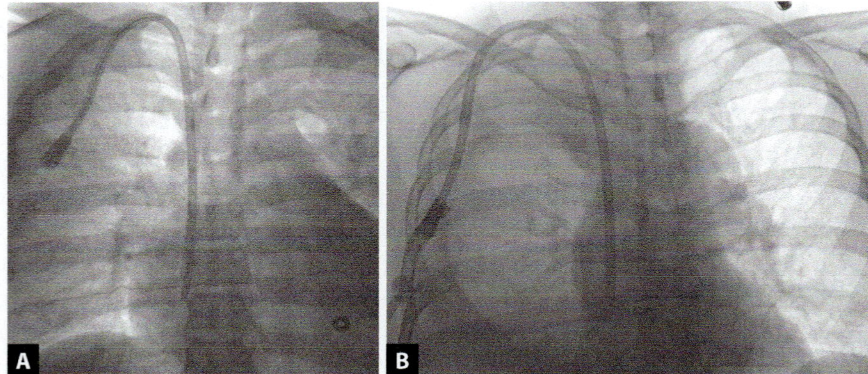

Figs. 1A and B: Frontal spot views of the chest with right internal jugular vein approach tunneled dialysis catheters, each with tip terminating in the right atrium.

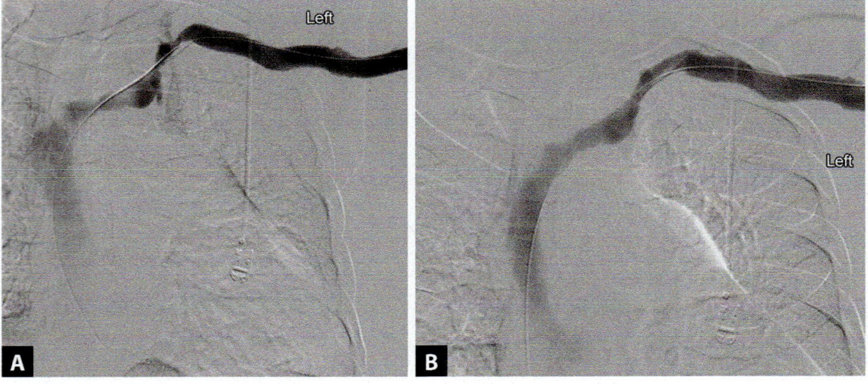

Figs. 2A and B: Central venogram of the proximal left arm and chest showing a segment of severe stenosis at the left innominate vein with improvement following balloon venoplasty (B).

patients may present with facial and/or upper extremity swelling with development of collateral veins often in the cervical region and chest wall.
    - *Procedure:* Percutaneous transluminal angioplasty is often the first line of treatment for hemodynamically significant central vein or peripheral venous stenosis. The technical aspects would be discussed under Chapters 20 and 26.2.
    - *Complications:*
        - Hematoma or bleeding
        - Infection
        - Central vein dissection
        - Restenosis
- Arteriovenous fistulogram and arteriovenous fistulogram interventions, i.e., angioplasty, thrombolysis
    - *Indications:*
        - *Dialysis access issues:* Difficulty with cannulation, excessive bleeding after hemodialysis, decreased flow rate during hemodialysis, etc.
        - Concern for stenosis
        - Clotted AVF
        - Nonmaturing AVF
    - *Procedure:* Arteriovenous fistulogram interventions are discussed in Chapter 26.2. **Figures 3A and B** show an example of upper extremity fistula stenosis before and after balloon angioplasty.
    - *Complications:*
        - Hematoma
        - Bleeding
        - Vessel dissection
- *Endovascular AVF creation:*
    - *Indication:* Permanent access for hemodialysis patients with end-stage renal disease
    - *Procedure:* Initially attempted by Scribner in the early 1960s, AVF creation involves establishing a communication between an artery and a vein for permanent dialysis access.[3] This remains the preferred hemodialysis access for end-stage renal disease patients. For a long time, the procedure was performed surgically by vascular surgeons; however, more recently percutaneous AVF (pAVF) creation by interventional radiologists is gradually gaining eminence.
    Both surgically and percutaneously created AVF have similar results with the additional benefit of lack of a surgical scar with percutaneous creation.[4]
    - *Complications:* As with other transarterial interventions, complications of pAVF are rare and include:
        - Hematoma
        - Bleeding
        - Vessel dissection
- *Peritoneal dialysis catheter placement:*
    - *Indications:* Peritoneal dialysis allows for in-home dialysis; however, proper patient selection and adequate planning are necessary to ensure an optimal outcome. The most common indications include:
        - Inability to obtain vascular access for hemodialysis
        - Children especially <2 years as a bridge to renal transplant or due to difficulty obtaining vascular access
        - Patients with cardiac disease, e.g., heart failure, shown decrease in hospitalizations

    Despite these, peritoneal dialysis may not be feasible in patients with extensive abdominal surgeries due to possibility of adhesions,

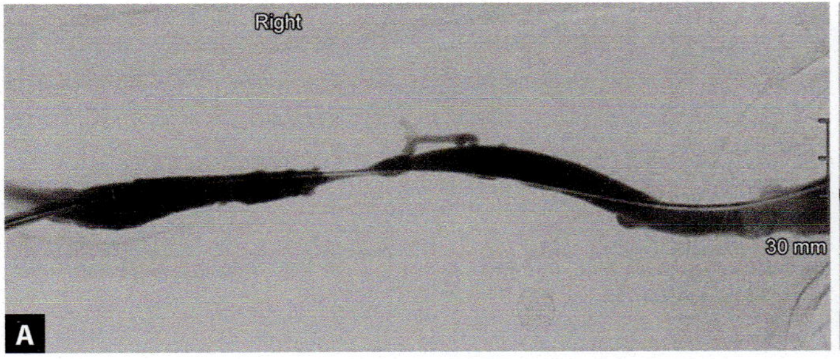

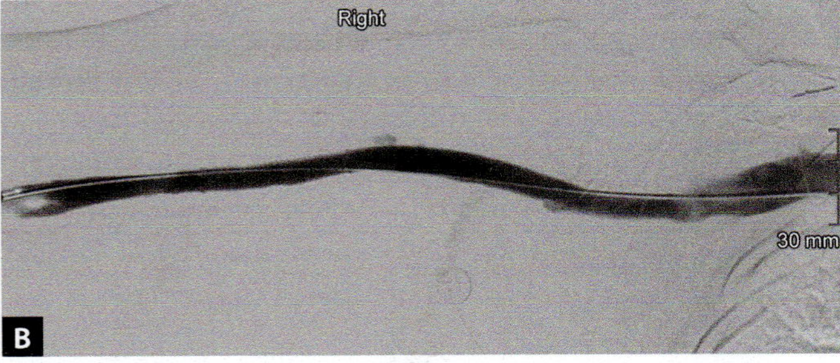

Figs. 3A and B: Right upper extremity arteriovenous fistulogram showing a short segment severe stenosis in the outflow tract with resolution following ballon venoplasty (B).

patients with enterocutaneous fistulas, or obese patients.[5]

- *Procedure:* The procedure is a sterile procedure which is often performed under ultrasound and fluoroscopic guidance by an interventional radiologist or by a laparoscopic surgeon.
- *Complications:*
  - Bleeding
  - Bowel injury
  - Pericatheter infection or leakage
  - Peritonitis

- *Renal drainage procedures:* Percutaneous nephrostomy, nephroureteral catheter, internal ureteral catheter.
  - *Indications:* While there are numerous indications for image-guided percutaneous nephrostomy access, the two most common indications are urinary obstruction and urinary diversion. Other indications include collecting system access for percutaneous intervention (i.e., nephrolithotomy or stricture dilation) and pre- or postureteral surgical interventions in order to assist with healing.
  - *Procedure:* Access is obtained into the renal collecting system, usually under ultrasound or sometimes fluoroscopic guidance. Ideally, a posterior approach is employed, and a lower pole calyx is punctured with an introducer needle. A catheter is thereafter placed using a modified Seldinger technique. Typically, an 8 or 10 French catheter is large enough for adequate drainage and the locking mechanism decreases the risk of accidental dislodgement. **Figure 4A** illustrates the different types of renal drainage catheters with the corresponding fluoroscopic views also shown in **Figure 4B**. Depending on the indication for catheter placement, additional or alternative catheters or stents can be placed either at the time of initial collecting system access or during future exchanges. For example, a nephroureteral catheter (which is placed in the same fashion as a percutaneous nephrostomy, with the additional step of placing a wire into the bladder and deploying the specialized stent over the wire, with the stent's distal loop within the bladder and proximal loop within the renal pelvis) may be placed if long-term internal drainage is needed with the potential to convert an internal–external percutaneous nephroureteral catheter to a fully internal ureteral catheter or stent.
  - *Complications:*
    - Massive hemorrhage (<4%)
    - Perirenal bleeding
    - Urinary infection, sepsis
    - Pneumothorax
    - Hematuria
    - Urinary extravasation
    - Catheter-related problems (including dislodgement, encrustation/obstruction)

- *Oncologic procedures*: Tumor ablation (percutaneous thermal ablation) and tumor embolization
  - Tumor ablation
    - *Indications:* Ablation for renal tumors may be performed effectively and safely even in patients with multiple comorbidities. Clinical guidelines include thermal ablation as an alternative for high surgical risk patients with localized tumors that are 4.0 cm or smaller. According to the 2021 American Urology Association guidelines, clinicians should consider renal tumor ablation as an alternate approach for the management of cT1a (defined as 4 cm or smaller) solid renal masses. For patients who elect thermal ablation, a percutaneous technique is preferred over a surgical approach whenever feasible to minimize morbidity.[6] Tumor size and location are the two most critical aspects in determining targets for percutaneous ablation. Ideally, the tumor should be <4 cm in size and studies have decreased technical success as tumor size increases.[7] The location of the tumor is also important as tumor proximity to the collecting system, bowel, or other adjacent organs may create technical challenges which may require additional measures (such as hydro dissection) to avoid nontarget thermal injuries. Exophytic renal tumors typically provide the safest and least complicated ablations. In addition to appropriate tumor candidacy, a critical part of preprocedure planning is to determine approach, patient position, and modality of image guidance.
    - *Procedure:* Ultrasound and CT guidance are the two most common methods of image guidance with ultrasound providing the advantage of

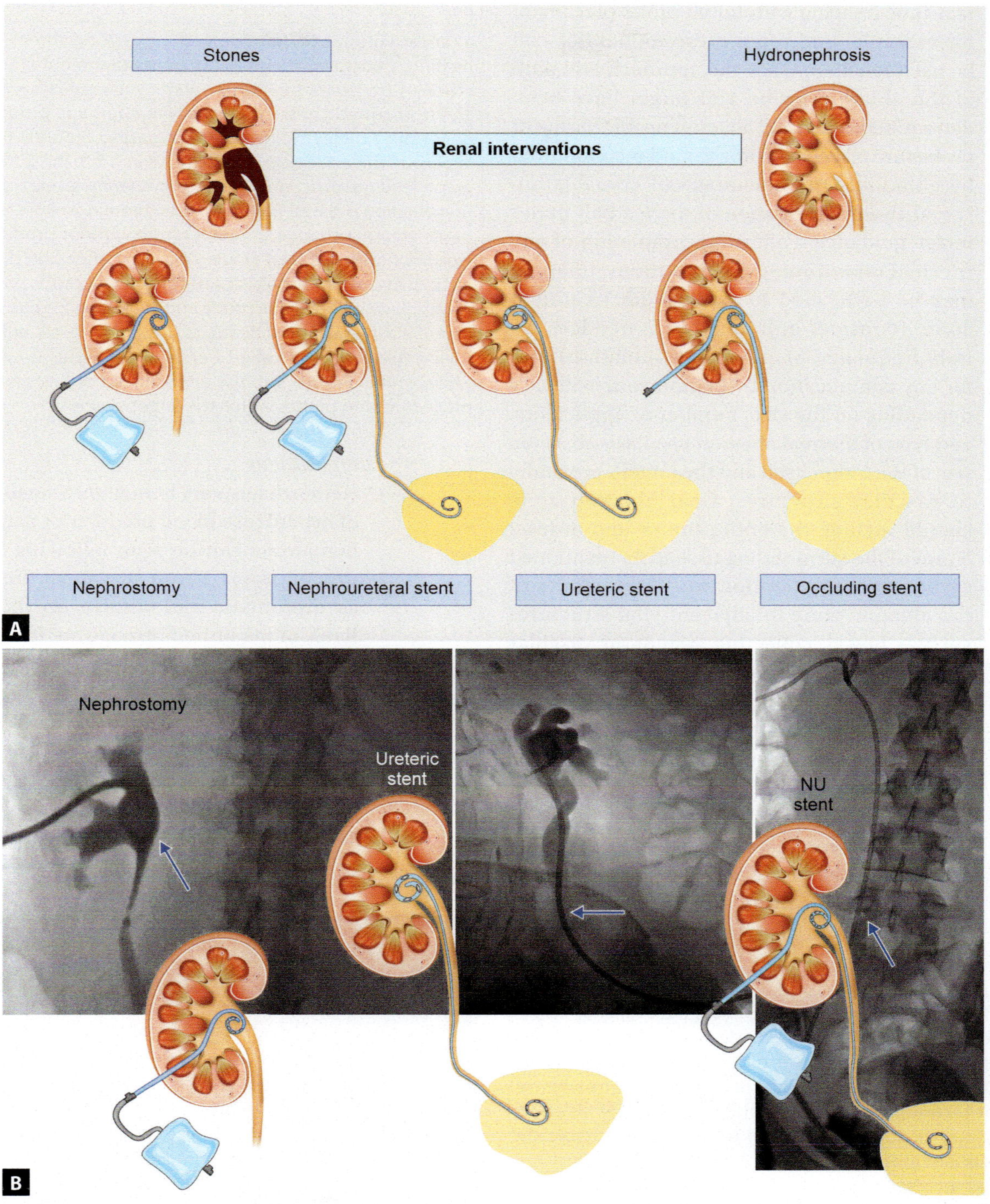

Figs. 4A and B: (A) Most common types of renal drainage catheters/stents. An occluding stent is often utilized to maximize drainage of a segment of the urinary system, typically in order to promote healing by diverting urine from a damaged or injured portion of the urinary system/bladder. (B) Fluoroscopic images from left to right: A nephrostomy catheter with tip coiled within the renal pelvis (blue arrow), a ureteric stent with one end coiled within the renal pelvis and body of the stent within the ureter (blue arrow), a nephroureteral (NU) catheter with a percutaneous catheter portion, one proximal coil within the renal pelvis, body of the stent within the ureter (blue arrow) and the distal portion of the stent within the urinary bladder.
Source: With permission from Dr Ram Gurajala, MD and IR4U.

real-time imaging with initial probe placement for example, and often these modalities can be used together. Once the approach and path of the ablation probe and target have been determined, a thermal ablation needle/probe or probes are placed with image guidance, followed by ablation. One advantage of cryoablation is real-time visualization of the ice ball under image guidance. Following completion of any thermal ablation, post-treatment imaging may be performed to assess both treatment zone (contrast-enhanced CT needed for radiofrequency or microwave ablation) and for any complications. Ablation zone will vary depending on the size, number of applicators, and type of thermal ablation used as well as the size of the lesion itself and the target's proximity to vascular structures. Goal ablation zone should include the entire tumor and at least 5 mm of the surrounding tissue.[8] As mentioned earlier, careful attention to the proximity of the ablation zone to adjacent vital structures such as bowel, collecting system, or vascular structures is imperative. If a tumor is <1 cm from bowel for example, interventions should be performed to increase the distance such as altering patient's position or percutaneous instillation of fluid or air (hydrodissection or pneumodissection). Tumors <1 cm from the ureter may require ureteral displacement or retrograde pyeloperfusion—temporary ureteral stent placement through which either room temperature or cooled fluid is gradually instilled during ablation.[9,10]

Across different types of thermal ablation, the overall principle of tissue destruction via image-guided percutaneous probe placement is the same; however, differences in the underlying mechanism of thermal ablation modalities lead to slightly different techniques and considerations. Thermal ablation refers to destruction of tissue with the use of heat (typically radiofrequency or microwave) or cold (cryoablation) by inducing irreversible thermal cellular injury.[11] Radiofrequency ablation is performed by using a generator to create impedance controlled alternating electrical current, which induces tissue heating around multilined needle electrodes placed within the target, resulting in active frictional heating and immediate coagulative necrosis of heated tissue. Nonelectric thermal diffusion (conductive heating) also occurs and results in

Contd...

Contd...

a larger volume of cell death than beyond direct electric heating.[12] Microwave also heats target tissue but is based on efficient frictional heating of water molecules by wavelike electromagnetic energy. Microwave energy is produced by generating dielectric hysteresis (rotating dipoles) from the exposed tip of a needlelike probe (antenna) into the surrounding tissue, leading to frictional heating of water molecules in tissue.[12] Cryoablation is based on the physics through which expanding gases create a change in temperature without production of work or transfer of heat (Joule–Thomson effect). In particular, gas expansion (argon) within a needlelike cryoprobe produces a heat sink which cools the probe and creates an ice ball which in and of itself induces cell death, as does the process of thawing, giving rise to the so-called freeze–thaw cycles used during cryoablation. **Figure 5** shows a renal mass during an ablation procedure with probes within the target tumor.

- *Complications:*
  - Hemorrhage (very frequently a small amount of hyperdense blood products or perinephric hematoma can be seen following ablation procedures). These are most frequently asymptomatic and resolve on their own. Rates of major hemorrhage are low, ranging from 0 to 2%.[13,14]
  - Hematuria
  - Pneumothorax (upper pole tumors)
  - Abscess
  - Thermal injury to bowel (including delayed perforation, fistula formation to kidney)
  - Thermal injury to collecting system (including ureteral stricture, urinoma, or obstruction)

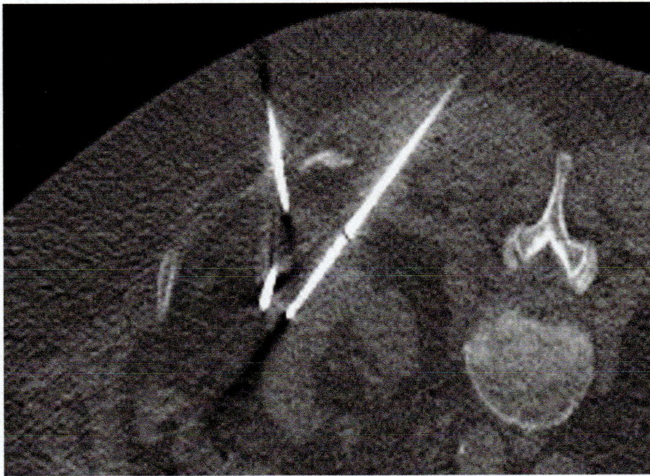

Fig. 5: An intraprocedural CT scan during an ablation procedure with probes within the target renal tumor.

- Tumor embolization
  - *Indications:* Transcatheter renal artery tumor embolization may be utilized as an adjunct or primary treatment. As an adjunct, tumor embolization can be performed prior to ablation to reduce bleeding complications and improve ablation efficacy (by reducing vascularity and heat sink and increasing tumor ischemia). Combined embolization and thermal ablation have been proven safe and effective in smaller studies, although current data regarding demonstrating superiority is lacking.[15,16] As an adjunct to presurgical resection, tumor or main renal artery embolization may be performed in those with extensive vascular involvement or in patients who refuse blood transfusions. As a primary treatment, tumor embolization is most frequently performed in the cases of palliation and symptom relief such as hematuria or flank pain of renal masses including advanced stage renal cell carcinoma (RCC).[17] The most frequent tumor embolization involves angiomas, particularly angiomyolipomas (AMLs). Embolization can be used as primary treatment of symptom relief (flank pain, hematuria, mass effect) or most commonly those with ongoing or prior rupture or bleeding. Due to a high rate of spontaneous hemorrhage, prophylactic embolization is recommended for AML >4 cm or in patients who are pregnant or planning to become pregnant. AMLs >4 cm have been shown to be associated with spontaneous hemorrhage (50–60%).[17]
  - *Procedure details:* Catheterization and angiography of the target renal artery are performed followed by embolization. The choice of embolic material may depend on the underlying disease process. For example, preferred embolic materials for AML treatment include ethanol-lipiodol, polyvinyl alcohol (PVA) particles or Onyx liquid embolic. Some authors discourage use of coil embolization as this may induce collateral feeding vessels in the setting of AML as well as preclude future access should recurrence occur. In terms of palliative tumor treatment, the embolic choice should penetrate into tumor vascular bed which includes categories such as particle embolization but also may include liquid embolics such as NBCA (N-butyl cyanoacrylate) glue and ethanol which are known to cause permanent small vessel/capillary bed occlusion/sclerosis. With nonselective renal artery embolization, operator comfort and procedure length are often a consideration with embolic agent choice. Following embolization, postembolization angiography is typically performed to confirm treatment adequacy.
  - *Complications:*
    - Hemorrhage or arterial injury
    - Postembolization syndrome can be seen in nonselective renal artery embolization
    - Abscess formation
    - Nontarget embolization, transvenous embolism including pulmonary thromboembolism. Also, certain embolic materials carry their own risk; ethanol, e.g., has severe risk of spinal cord ischemia and skin and bowel injury should there be nontarget embolization into the systemic arterial side (reflux into aorta).

CONCLUSION

Much like the field of IR, the field of interventional nephrology is one built off a foundation of innovation, image guidance, and minimally invasive effective treatments. As a result, the scope of interventional nephrology (and IR as a whole) is continuously expanding with constant introduction of newer techniques and procedures. The fundamental principles of image guidance and minimal access however remain unchanged, thus making expertise in image interpretation an essential skill for an interventional radiologist. More important, however, is understanding the appropriate indications for a procedure, when to intervene or not to intervene, and the potential complications. With these critical pieces of knowledge, we can safely and effectively perform the well-established procedures highlighted in this chapter as well as be equipped to safely and effectively carry out any future procedures or innovations that may be developed.

REFERENCES

1. Dotter CT, Judkins MP. Transluminal Treatment of Arteriosclerotic Obstruction. Circulation. 1964;30(5):654-70.

2. Varon J, Nyman U. Sven-Ivar Seldinger: The revolution of radiology and acute intravascular access. Resuscitation. 2007;75(1):7-11.
3. Sachdeva B, Abreo K. The History of Interventional Nephrology. Acv Chronic Kidney Dis. 2009;16(5):302-8.
4. Tyagi R, Ahmed SS, Navuluri R, Ahmed O. Endovascular Arteriovenous Fistula Creation: A Review. Semin Interv Radiol. 2021;38(05):518-22.
5. Lambie M, Davies S. An update on absolute and relative indications for dialysis treatment modalities. 2023;16(Suppl 1):i39-i47.
6. Campbell SC, Clark PE, Chang SS, Karam JA, Souter L, Uzzo RG. Renal Mass and Localized Renal Cancer: Evaluation, Management, and Follow-Up: AUA Guideline: Part I. J Urol. 2021;206(2):199-208.
7. Zagoria RJ, Traver M, Werle DM, Perini M, Hayasaka S, Clark PU. Oncologic Efficacy of CT-Guided Percutaneous Radiofrequency Ablation of Renal Cell Carcinomas. AJR Am J Roentgenol. 2007;189(2):429-36.
8. Joe WB, Zarzour JG, Gunn AJ. Renal Cell Carcinoma Ablation: Preprocedural, Intraprocedural, and Postprocedural Imaging. Radiol Imaging Cancer. 2019;1(2):e190002.
9. Schmit GD, Kurup AN, Weisbrod AJ, Houston Thompson R, Boorjian SA, Thomas Wass C, et al. ABLATE: a renal ablation planning algorithm. AJR Am J Roentgenol. 2014;202(4):894-903.
10. Abdelsalam ME, Matin SF, Ahrar K. Ablation of renal cell carcinoma. In: Image-Guided Interventions. Philadelphia: Elsevier; 2020. pp. 823-35.e4 (Chapter 101).
11. Goldberg SN, Grassi CJ, Cardella JF, Charboneau JW, Dodd GD, Dupuy DE, et al. Image-guided Tumor Ablation: Standardization of Terminology and Reporting Criteria. Journal of Vascular and Interventional Radiology. 2005; 20(7):S377-90.
12. Higgins LJ, Hong K. Renal Ablation Techniques: State of the Art. Am J Roentgenol. 2015;205(4):735-41.
13. Gervais DA, McGovern FJ, Arellano RS, McDougal WS, Mueller PR. Radiofrequency ablation of renal cell carcinoma: part 1, Indications, results, and role in patient management over a 6-year period and ablation of 100 tumors. AJR Am J Roentgenol. 2005;185(1):64-71.
14. Wah TM, Irving HC, Gregory W, Cartledge J, Joyce AD, Selby PJ. Radiofrequency ablation (RFA) of renal cell carcinoma (RCC): experience in 200 tumours. BJU Int. 2014;113(3):416-28.
15. Terauchi M, Yamashiro T, Sawamura S, Koyama S, Nakaigawa N, Kondo K, et al. Combining Transarterial Embolization and Percutaneous Cryoablation for Early-Stage Renal Cell Carcinoma: Embolization Materials and Impacts of Tumor Size. Tomography. 2024;10(11):1767-79.
16. Gunn AJ, Mullenbach BJ, Poundstone MM, Gordetsky JB, Underwood ES, Rais-Bahrami S. Trans-Arterial Embolization of Renal Cell Carcinoma prior to Percutaneous Ablation: Technical Aspects, Institutional Experience, and Brief Review of the Literature. Curr Urol. 2018;12(1):43-9.
17. Li D, Pua BB, Madoff DC. Role of embolization in the treatment of renal masses. Semin Interven Radiol. 2014; 31(1):70-81.

CHAPTER 8

Preoperative Evaluation of Arteriovenous Fistula

Shalini Priya, Vidhi Singla, Vinant Bhargava

CASE SCENARIO

A 45-year-old male, known hypertensive, chronic kidney disease (CKD) stage V, presented with complaints of pedal edema and shortness of breath. After relevant investigations (hemoglobin 8.2 g/dL, serum urea 189 mg/dL, creatinine 12.2 mg/dL), he was initiated on hemodialysis through the right internal jugular nontunneled dialysis catheter.

After stabilization, arteriovenous fistula (AVF) creation was planned for future access. Arteriovenous mapping of bilateral upper limbs and USG Doppler of bilateral neck veins were done. Due to unfavorable anatomy of cephalic vein in left wrist (presence of accessory veins and small diameter of main cephalic vein) and cephalic vein thrombosis in right wrist, he was taken up for left brachiocephalic fistula with a good postoperative thrill and bruit. After 6 weeks, he underwent successful cannulation and dialysis through the same and the fistula is still functional without any intervening complications at 1 year follow-up.

This signifies the importance of preoperative assessment as in our case, this exempted unnecessary attempt at radiocephalic fistula creation which would have resulted in primary fistula failure and inconvenience to the patient.

INTRODUCTION

As the life expectancy of a chronic kidney disease (CKD) patient on maintenance hemodialysis is increasing, the creation and maintenance of hemodialysis vascular access is becoming more challenging.[1] Vascular and access are medical words that mean "a way to get to your blood". Vascular means blood and access means a way to get there.[2] The intricacies of selecting an appropriate vascular access route are pivotal, not only for the immediate success of the therapeutic intervention but also for safeguarding the patient's long-term health and well-being. The ultimate determinant of success in vascular access for hemodialysis is a circuit that allows consistent and uninterrupted delivery of the prescribed hemodialysis. Attainment of right access in the right patient at the right time for the right reason is a more patient-centered approach. For each successful vascular access, we need to have four plans: (1) Vessel preservation, (2) insertion/creation, (3) contingency, and (4) succession plans.[3]

The preoperative evaluation is not a cursory glance at the patient's medical history but a comprehensive and multifaceted assessment including a complete history, physical examination, and ultrasonographic vessel assessment.[4] Such an evaluation requires a keen understanding of the vascular system and an appreciation of the unique circumstances of each patient, including their medical history, the condition of their vasculature, and the expected outcome.[5,6]

ACCESS TYPES

In the realm of vascular access, a nuanced understanding of the four primary types as discussed in **Table 1**—AVFs, arteriovenous grafts (AVGs), arteriovascular shunts, and central venous catheters (CVCs)—is crucial. The selection among these options is not merely a matter of preference but a critical decision that hinges on a delicate balance between the advantages and disadvantages of each type to meet patient-specific needs and treatment goals.[7-10]

PREOPERATIVE EVALUATION FOR ARTERIOVENOUS FISTULA

The history **(Table 2)** is a key factor in determining the site of creation of AVF and expected maturation time and in foreseeing the complications that may develop over time **(Video 1)**.

History for Hemodialysis Catheter Procedures

- Recent history of fever, chills, positive blood cultures, antibiotic treatment

TABLE 1: Different types of vascular access.

Vascular access	*Types*	*Advantages*	*Disadvantages*
Arteriovenous fistula	• Direct arteriovenous fistula • Transposition fistula	Less infections and thrombosis and their longevity compared to other forms of access	• Requires skilled personnel • Requires more maturation time
Arteriovenous graft	Bovine polytetrafluoroethylene (PTFE) graft	Less maturation time	More chances of infection and thrombosis
Arteriovenous shunt		Less time for maturation	• Costly procedure • Outdated
Central venous catheter	Tunneled cuffed and noncuffed	Immediate use	Increased risk of bloodstream infections and venous stenosis

TABLE 2: History.

Chronic illness	• Diabetes, coronary artery disease, peripheral vascular disease, neuropathies, obesity • Presence of pacemakers, cardiac prosthetic valves, inferior vena cava filters
Conditions that can increase the risk of bleeding postoperatively	Coagulopathies, thrombocytopenia, anticoagulant, or antiplatelet medications
History of allergy	Allergies to narcotics, benzodiazepines, local anesthetic agent, radiocontrast dye, latex, heparin

- *Previous history of hemodialysis (central veins) catheters:* Number, location, timing, possible problems encountered on catheter placement[11]
- Presence of any signs of central vein stenosis, swelling of the face, arm, breast, collateral veins

Physical Examination

The objective of doing a physical examination is to select the most ideal blood vessels that maximize the chances of placement of an AV access and eventually maturation and reducing the primary failure rate. Frequent phlebotomies, peripherally inserted central catheter (PICC) lines, and a high prevalence of comorbid conditions including diabetes, obesity, and vascular disease in advanced CKD and end-stage renal disease (ESRD) patients are some of the challenges that serve as barriers toward getting a mature AV access.[12,13]

Latest Kidney Disease Outcomes Quality Initiative (KDOQI) 2019 guidelines on vascular access recommend greater emphasis and training in preoperative clinical examination to assess patients and their vessels prior to placement of vascular access.[11]

For preoperative purposes, the physical examination can be broken down into three parts as shown in **Box 1**.

MODALITIES OF EVALUATION

Ultrasonography is an excellent noninvasive tool offering a real-time visualization of the venous system. It should be done via the linear probe, minimum frequencies of 7 MHz for the B-mode examination and 5 MHz for the Doppler study.[16] Although historically a minimal venous diameter of 2.5 mm and a minimal arterial diameter of 2.0 mm in the upper extremities had been proposed as the preferred vessel sizes for creation of an AVF, this has not been validated in actual studies. KDOQI has revised the vascular access guideline recently and recommend to have no minimum threshold for vein and arterial diameter to create an AVF; however, vessels <2 mm should be carefully evaluated for creation and maturation **(Video 2)**.[11,14]

Arterial Doppler Examination (Table 3)[13,17,18]

Arterial Doppler examination is shown in **Table 3**.

Venous Examination

Ideally, veins should be thin walled, vary in size with respiration especially subclavian vein, collapse completely on compression with transducer, and augment with proximal compression by ~50% by use of tourniquet.[17] Vein diameter (minimum 2.5 mm) before and after proximal vein compression has been proposed to be suitable for access creation.[17,19]

If the veins are deeper than 6 mm, the distance from the skin surface should be recorded to assist in planning for superficialization. All abnormalities should be noted including venous stenosis, branches of veins near the future AVF site, or sclerotic, thick-walled veins. A vein with a proximal diameter (at the site of the venous

BOX 1: Preoperative evaluation.

1. *General examination:*
   - Peripheral pulse; all pulses in upper extremity (axillary, brachial, radial, and ulnar) should be evaluated and recorded; whether normal (2+), diminished (1+), or absent (0)
   - *Blood pressure in both arms should be measured:* Difference of 20 mm Hg or greater in systolic blood pressure is suggestive of subclavian artery stenosis in the low pressure arm
2. *Arterial evaluation*:
   - *Modified Allen test*: It helps to confirm the patency of the palmar arch and thereby the collateral circulation to the hand. Normally, the ulnar artery is able to support the arterial circulation to hand through palmar arch even in the presence of decreased radial artery flow.[12,14]
   - *Method:* The patient is asked to make a fist, and pressure is applied over both the ulnar and the radial arteries to occlude them. Once the fist is opened, the hand should appear blanched or pale **(Figs. 1A and B)**. Then, pressure is alternately released from both the arteries and the hand monitored for return of color; this is called modified Allen test.[13]
   - *Barbeau test:* By using a pulse oximeter probe on tip of a hand digit. Adequate manual occlusion of arteries is signaled by loss of pulse waveform. Return of pulse waveform as each artery is released signals patency of that artery. If either ulnar or radial artery has decreased patency, a wrist AVF should not be created.[15]
3. *Evaluation of veins*: Examination for evidence of previous central venous catheterization, signs of trauma or surgery of the arm, chest, or neck, previous AV access surgery. The presence of arm edema, collateral veins, or differential extremity size should prompt an evaluation of the central vein.

   A tourniquet is placed sequentially at the upper extremity, and the veins are visually inspected to determine the diameter, the distance of the vein from the skin surface, and the length of a straight venous segment suitable for cannulation.[12,13,15]

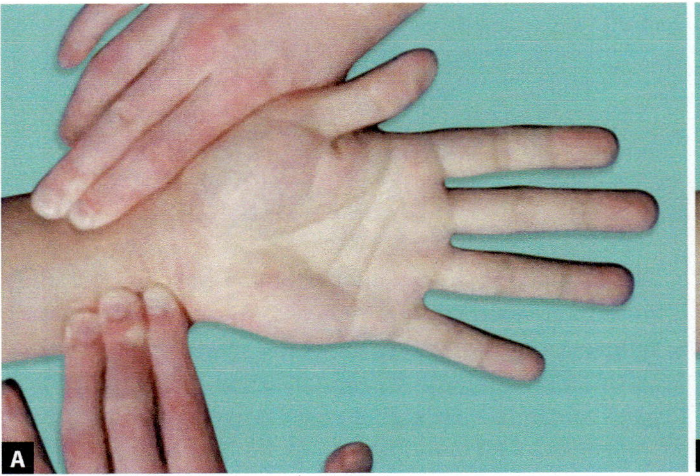

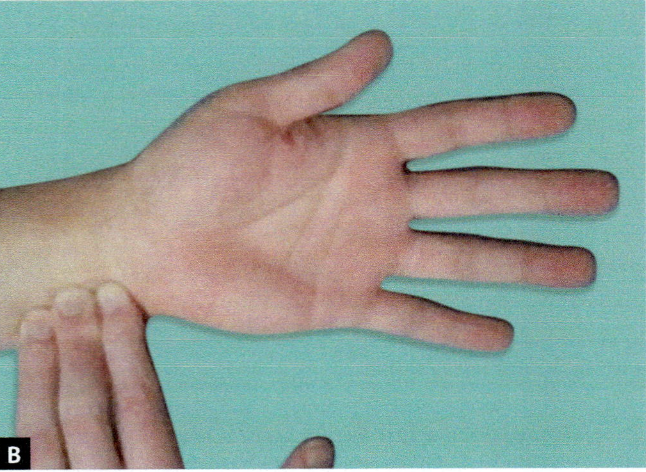

Figs. 1A and B: Modified Allen test. (A) Blanching of hand on compression of ulnar and radial arteries; (B) Hyperemic response on release of ulnar compression demonstrating patency.

TABLE 3: Arterial evaluation by ultrasonography and Doppler.[17]

Internal diameter	Minimum 2 mm and borderline 1.5 mm for arterial blood flow before and after reactive hyperemia test
	Normal flow is triphasic high-resistance flow with no dampening. **Figure 2** shows reactive hyperemic response to clenched fist (A) and on releasing (B) simulating response after AVF creation
Condition of vessel wall	To look for calcification

anastomosis) of at least 4 cm is ideally recommended for graft placement.[11,19,20]

Preoperative mapping decreases unsuccessful surgical explorations from 11 to 0%, and the AVF placement rate increased from 32 to 58%.[13] The proportion of fistulas placed increased to 64% with preoperative vascular mapping as compared to 34% in the historical controls.[18] The major limitations to use of ultrasound are operator skill and subjective interpretation of vessel lumen size.

A major limitation of ultrasonography is indirect evaluation of central venous vasculature. They are assessed

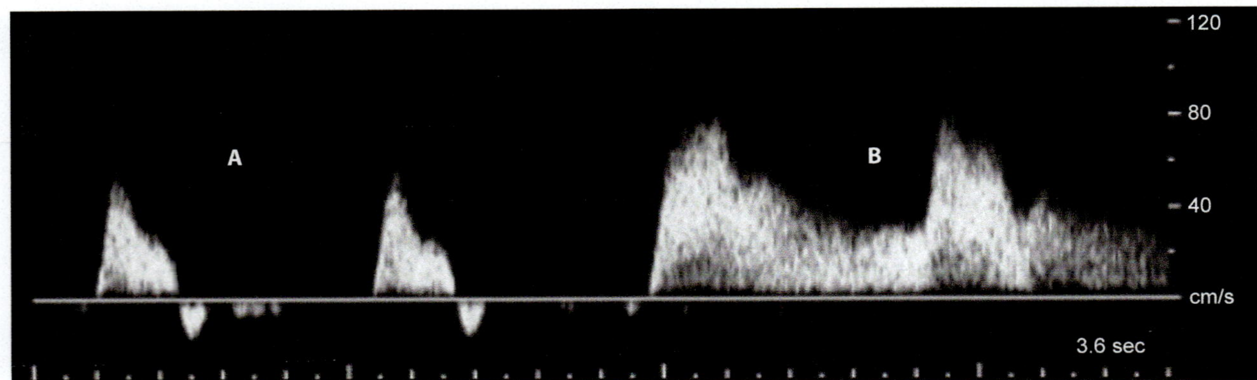

Fig. 2: Radial artery waveform during clenched fist (A) and on release showing a hyperemic response (B).

TABLE 4: Other modalities for preoperative evaluation.

Modality	*Advantage*	*Disadvantage*
CT venography/ angiography[18]	Offers comprehensive three-dimensional mapping of both the venous and arterial systems	Use of contrast agent and risk of radiation exposure
Ferumoxytol MR angiography (FeMRA)[24]	• Newer gadolinium contrast for use in chronic kidney disease (CKD) patients • FeMRA can better detect peripheral and central vessel stenosis than Doppler US	• High cost • Trained personnel • Not readily available
CO_2 angiography[25-28]	Non-nephrotoxic, nonallergenic, easily eliminated by the lungs, and is relatively inexpensive	Risks of neurotoxicity and cardiac arrhythmias
Artificial intelligence (AI)[29]	Offering the potential to automate and refine the interpretation of diagnostic images	Trained personnel required

for stenosis or thrombosis by analysis of the waveform for changes in respiratory phasicity and transmitted cardiac pulsatility. Thus, additional techniques may be required to fully delineate the central venous system among patients with a history of CVC use.[20,21]

HARDWARE FOR EVALUATION

The landscape of preoperative vascular evaluation has been profoundly transformed by technological advancements in diagnostic imaging, heralding a new era of precision and reliability in vascular access planning. At the forefront of this revolution are high-resolution ultrasound machines, which have become indispensable tools in the clinician's arsenal.

Various modalities **(Table 4)** offer comprehensive three-dimensional mapping of both the venous and arterial systems, providing a detailed blueprint that aids in surgical planning and decision-making. The choice of evaluation technique is a judicious one, balancing the need for detailed vascular information against those associated with contrast use in imaging.[21-23]

CONCLUSION

The primary objective of preoperative vascular mapping prior to creation of an AV access is to reduce the primary failure rate and to increase the cumulative patency rates of created AV access with few or no additional interventions.[4] Though preoperative vessel mapping increases AVF creation, there is limited and conflicting evidence regarding the effect of vessel mapping on AVF maturation.[18] It is essential to differentiate an increase in the number of AVFs created from an increase in mature fistulas that are successfully used for dialysis. Though it could be reasonably concluded that a preoperative strategy to identify suitable vessels for AVF creation would translate into decreased early failure rates and an increased proportion of prevalent patients dialyzing with an AVF, it may not always be the case.[18,24]

Future research should focus on prospective, randomized controlled trials to evaluate the benefits of preoperative mapping on the creation, maturation, and patency of AVF. With a lack of strong evidence supporting one-vessel mapping technique over another, an individualized approach should be taken, in consideration with the patient's risk factors and advantages and disadvantages of each mapping technique. A combination of one or more technique(s) individualized to each patient may be the best suitable approach.

REFERENCES

1. Lawson JH, Niklason LE, Roy-Chaudhury P. Challenges and novel therapies for vascular access in haemodialysis. Nat Rev Nephrol. 2020;16(10):586-6.
2. UpToDate. Vascular Access: A comprehensive resource that discusses the evaluation of patients with chronic kidney disease for dialysis access, highlighting the importance of a detailed and complete assessment. [online] Available from Vascular.org [Last accessed June, 2025].
3. Trerotola SO. KDOQI Clinical Practice Guideline for Vascular Access 2019 Update: Kinder, Gentler, and More Important Than Ever. J Vasc Interv Radiol. 2020;31(7):1156-7.
4. Van Klei WA, Grobbee DE, Rutten CL, Hennis PJ, Knape JT, Kalkman CJ, et al. Role of history and physical examination in preoperative evaluation. Eur J Anaesthesiol. 2003;20(8):612-8.
5. Vascular Access 2006 Work Group. Clinical practice guidelines for vascular access. Am J Kidney Dis. 2006; 48(Suppl 1):S248-73.
6. Ethier J, Mendelssohn DC, Elder SJ, Hasegawa T, Akizawa T, Akiba T, et al. Vascular access use and outcomes: an international perspective from the Dialysis Outcomes and Practice Patterns Study. Nephrol Dial Transplant. 2008;23(10):3219-26.
7. Lok CE, Huber TS, Lee T, Shenoy S, Yevzlin AS, Abreo K, et al. KDOQI clinical practice guideline for vascular access: 2019 update. Am J Kidney Dis. 2020;75(4 Suppl 2):S1-164.
8. Vascular Access 2006 Work Group. Clinical practice guidelines for vascular access. Am J Kidney Dis. 2006; 48(Suppl 1):S176-247.
9. Asif A, Ravani P, Roy-Chaudhury P, Spergel LM, Besarab A. Vascular mapping techniques: advantages and disadvantages. J Nephrol. 2007;20(3):299-303.
10. Malovrh M. Native arteriovenous fistula: preoperative evaluation. Am J Kidney Dis. 2002;39(6):1218-25.
11. Patel ST, Hughes J, Mills JL Sr. Failure of arteriovenous fistula maturation: an unintended consequence of exceeding dialysis outcome quality initiative guidelines for hemodialysis access. J Vasc Surg. 2003;38(3):439-45.
12. Abreo K, Amin BM, Abreo AP. Physical examination of the hemodialysis arteriovenous fistula to detect early dysfunction. J Vasc Access. 2019;20(1):7-11.
13. Salman L, Beathard G. Interventional nephrology: physical examination as a tool for surveillance for the hemodialysis arteriovenous access. Clin J Am Soc Nephrol. 2013;8(7):1220-7.
14. Allon M, Robbin ML. Increasing arteriovenous fistulas in hemodialysis patients: problems and solutions. Kidney Int. 2002;62(4):1109-24.
15. Beathard GA. An algorithm for the physical examination of early fistula failure. Semin Dial. 2005;18(4):331-5.
16. Robbin ML, Gallichio MH, Deierhoi MH, Young CJ, Weber TM, Allon M. US vascular mapping before hemodialysis access placement. Radiology. 2000;217(1):83-4.
17. Malovrh M. The role of sonography in the planning of arteriovenous fistulas for hemodialysis. Semin Dial. 2003;16(4):229-303.
18. Asif A, Cherla G, Merrill D, Cipleu CD, Tawakol JB, Epstein DL, et al. Venous mapping using venography and the risk of radiocontrast-induced nephropathy. Semin Dial. 2005;18(3):239-42.
19. Won YD, Lee JY, Shin YS, Kim YS, Yoon SA, Hahn ST, et al. Small dose contrast venography as venous mapping in predialysis patients. J Vasc Access. 2010;11(2):122-7.
20. Ascher E, Gade P, Hingorani A, Mazzariol F, Gunduz Y, Fodera M, et al. Changes in the practice of angioaccess surgery: impact of dialysis outcome and quality initiative recommendations. J Vasc Surg. 2000;31(1 Pt 1):84-92.
21. Silva MB Jr, Hobson RW 2nd, Pappas PJ, Jamil Z, Araki CT, Goldberg MC, et al. A strategy for increasing use of autogenous hemodialysis access procedures: impact of preoperative noninvasive evaluation. J Vasc Surg. 1998;27(2):302-7.
22. Allon M, Lockhart ME, Lilly RZ, Gallichio MH, Young CJ, Barker J, et al. Effect of preoperative sonographic mapping on vascular access outcomes in hemodialysis patients. Kidney Int. 2001;60(5):2013-20.
23. Kian K, Wyatt C, Schon D, Packer J, Vassalotti J, Mishler R. Safety of low-dose radiocontrast for interventional AV fistula salvage in stage 4 chronic kidney disease patients. Kidney Int. 2006;69(8):1444-9.
24. Stoumpos S, Tan A, Hall Barrientos P, Stevenson K, Thomson PC, Kasthuri R, et al. Ferumoxytol MR Angiography versus Duplex US for Vascular Mapping before Arteriovenous Fistula Surgery for Hemodialysis. Radiology. 2020;297(1):214-22.
25. Cho KJ. Carbon dioxide angiography: scientific principles and practice. Vasc Specialist Int. 2015;31(3):67-80.
26. Sharafuddin MJ, Marjan AE. Current status of carbon dioxide angiography. J Vasc Surg. 2017;66:618-37.
27. Heye S, Maleux G, Marchal GJ. Upper-extremity venography: CO_2 versus iodinated contrast material. Radiology. 2006;241(1):291-7.
28. Ehrman KO, Taber TE, Gaylord GM, Brown PB, Hage JP. Comparison of diagnostic accuracy with carbon dioxide versus iodinated contrast material in the imaging of hemodialysis access fistulas. J Vasc Interv Radiol. 1994; 5(5):771-5.
29. Kordzadeh A, Esfahlani SS. The role of artificial intelligence in the prediction of functional maturation of arteriovenous fistula. Annals Vasc Dis. 2019;12(1):44-9.

CHAPTER 9

Imaging for Peritoneal Dialysis Catheter Placement

Anantharam Jairam, (Gp Cpt) Vijoy Kumar Jha

INTRODUCTION

Continuous ambulatory peritoneal dialysis (CAPD) is one of the modes of renal replacement therapy (RRT) for end-stage kidney disease (ESKD) patients in which vessel-rich peritoneum is utilized as a semipermeable membrane for blood filtration. A tunneled catheter is placed through the abdominal wall into the peritoneal cavity with an ideal tip position in the most dependent part of the pelvis, ideally the rectouterine space in females and rectovesical space in males. Multiple approaches including blind percutaneous, open surgical, laparoscopic, and fluoroscopy techniques have been utilized for placing CAPD catheters. Imaging techniques have become standard of care in placing a CAPD catheter and during follow-up for diagnosis of complications.

Various imaging techniques in the setting of CAPD catheter insertion are discussed in the following text.

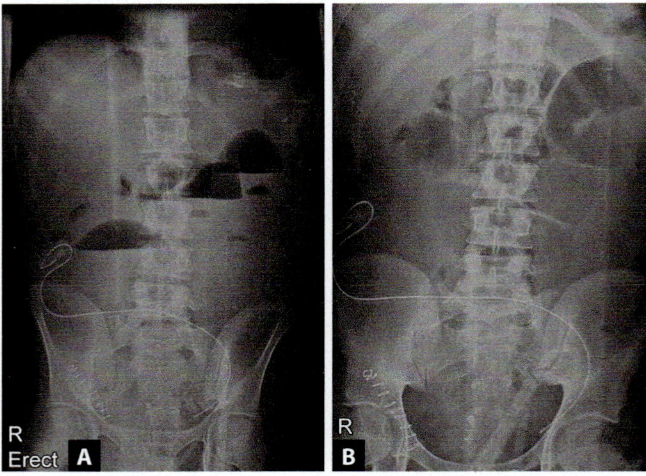

Figs. 1A and B: Plain radiography after CAPD catheter insertion. X-ray abdomen erect view including KUB showing catheter tip in the left pelvis with exit site and the extraperitoneal part on the right side. (CAPD: continuous ambulatory peritoneal dialysis)

PLAIN RADIOGRAPHY

Plain radiography can be used to see the catheter position after blind percutaneous catheter insertion. In a normal case, it will show the catheter path inside the abdominal cavity tracking into the pelvis **(Figs. 1A and B)**.

Plain radiography is the most easily available and cheapest investigation but has limited value. It may be useful in identifying complications such as bowel obstruction, constipation, and migration of catheters. Fecal loading can lead to catheter displacement or dysfunction. It may also identify some other complications such as advanced encapsulating sclerosing peritonitis (ESP), perforation, pneumoperitoneum, extraperitoneal collections, peritoneal calcifications, and hydrothorax (in case of communication between pleural and peritoneal cavity). It may not be as sensitive and specific for diagnosing leaks and other complications as compared to computed tomography. In a retrospective study, radiological parameters predicted functional catheter problems and the need for surgical intervention. These parameters were evaluated from plain abdominal X-ray taken 2 days after catheter placement where 110 swan neck double-cuff Missouri curled peritoneal dialysis (PD) catheters were used.[1] Pneumoperitoneum has been detected in 11–34% of patients undergoing CAPD but in a majority of the cases, patients remain asymptomatic. The specificity of finding subdiaphragmatic air on an erect chest X-ray in gastrointestinal perforation is much lower in PD patients.[2]

ULTRASONOGRAPHY

Ultrasonography is a very useful and noninvasive procedure used for assessing the patient before and during the CAPD insertion, evaluating catheter malfunction and any pleuroperitoneal communication, leakage, and herniation, and also for detecting and monitoring infections. Contrast-enhanced ultrasound (CEUS) can detect leakage, herniation, and catheter malfunction.[3] It is more cost-effective than other imaging modalities and is also radiation-free. The following points are to be adhered to while doing USG in these patients:

- We should use a high-frequency linear probe (7–13 MHz) and a medium-low-frequency convex transducer (2.5–6 MHz).
- The site to be probed should be disinfected and the exit site needs to be covered with a sterile film dressing.
- There should not be any air bubbles between the film and the skin to avoid distorting the signal.
- The catheter is to be visualized in a short axis at the exit site, which will appear as a circular structure with an anechoic lumen.

While doing CAPD catheter insertion, a medium-frequency (10–12 MHz) vascular probe is to be used to know the thinning of the rectus sheath to localize the medial and lateral border of the rectus muscle and also to locate the inferior epigastric artery. 1-cm thickness of the rectus muscle is considered adequate for the reception of the entire deep cuff. The inferior epigastric artery is well known for its considerable anatomical variation but usually located near the middle of the rectus muscle and against the posterior rectus sheath.[4] Normally on USG, visceral peritoneum moves freely against the parietal peritoneum. A clear double-line image of the parietal peritoneum is seen formed by the posterior rectus sheath and the parietal peritoneum separated by a thin layer of fat **(Figs. 2A and B)**. In the area having adhesions, a single line or no line will be seen. It can also detect which side of the abdomen adhesions exist.

The sonographic sign suggestive of tunnel infection is the presence of a hypo/anechoic collection >2-mm diameter existing between the catheter wall/cuff and the surrounding tissues. Few radiologists have also proposed a 1-mm cutoff. While differentiating infectious episodes from leakage, the color Doppler module (300–800 Hz) would identify an increase in color signal in case of infections.[3] Depending on the availability, USG could be used for early recognition of tunnel infection with or without the deep cuff involvement. The severity of the involvement prognosticates short-term recurrence and the need for aggressive medical therapy or removal of the PD catheter.[5] The presence of USG findings suggestive of tunnel infection at the segment of the catheter between the superficial and deep cuffs predicts secondary peritonitis episodes in 62.5% of cases.[6] Tunnel infections with cuff involvement are very less responsive to antibiotic therapy and may require catheter removal. Clinical experience suggests that the color Doppler signal without any hypoechoic collection predicts the diagnosis of early infection. Although no concrete data are available yet, patients on antibiotic therapy show a reduction in the size of both hypoechoic collection and local hypervascularization. Currently, there is no evidence to support the role of USG as a screening modality for diagnosing asymptomatic tunnel infections. However, the clinical utility of USG in the diagnosis and management of CAPD catheter-related infections remains indisputable.

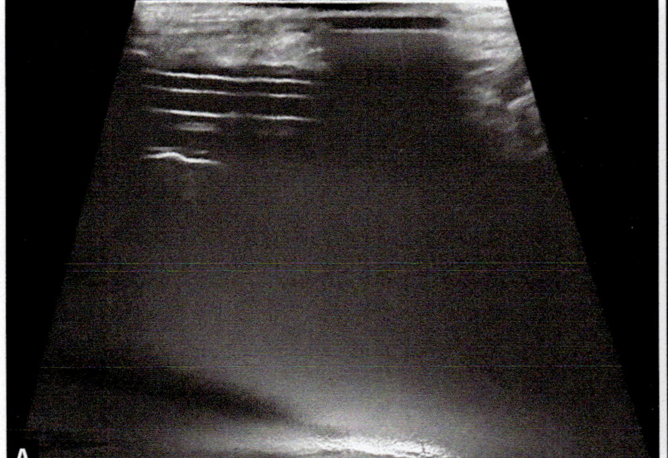

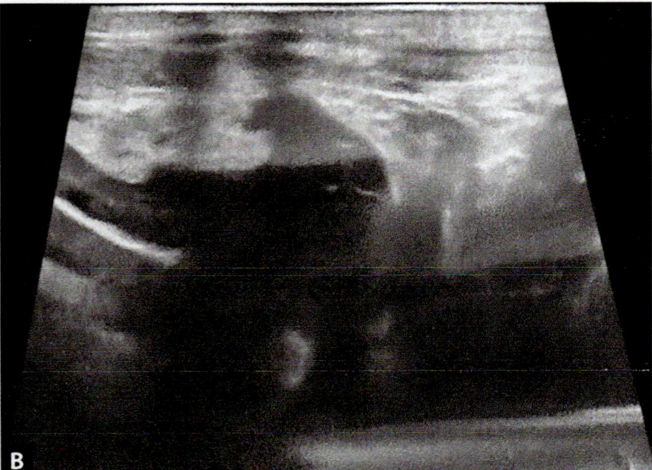

Figs. 2A and B: (A) Ultrasonography (USG) of the abdomen showing the extraperitoneal part with double-line image; (B) USG of the abdomen showing the intra-abdominal portion of the catheter.

For the diagnosis of ESP, USG performed with the presence of dialysate fluid is considered sensitive, which shows peritoneal thickenings, fibrinous strands, and dilated peristaltic small bowel loops. Peritoneal thickness is a nonspecific feature for prolonged CAPD treatment and can be present in ESP, increased age, larger body height, and obese individuals. There is uncertainty regarding when to discontinue CAPD based on peritoneal thickness and a biopsy may be considered which has potential complications.[7]

FLUOROSCOPY

During Catheter Insertion

Under fluoroscopy guidance, the needle position is easily confirmed by the instillation of a contrast agent. Due to the expansion of dye into small spaces between the visceral and parietal peritoneum, a spider-like image develops. Insertion of the long guidewire and its formation as a large curve crossing the midline confirms that the wire is against the parietal peritoneum. It also suggests that it is neither in the bowel lumen nor a recess formed under bowel loops or any adhesions. In the case of bowel loop perforation, as the sheath is retracted, the outline of the visceral lumen will occur. It is very important to detect the needle penetration into other organs or any spaces outside the peritoneum. Smaller needle penetration usually does not damage the bowel wall and will not require any surgical repair.[8]

When the location of the needle and guidewire is confirmed, a dilator and then a dilator with a split sheath are advanced over the guidewire. The catheter is advanced through the split sheath till the deep cuff reaches the anterior surface of the rectus muscle. The deep cuff is placed below the external rectus sheath and a suture may be applied to secure the position. Thereafter catheter is tunneled laterally to an exit site **(Figs. 3A and B)**.

Contrast administration will confirm free flow into the peritoneum and will become more dilute and move quickly into surrounding spaces. Sometimes, the contrast will fill limited space if lying in position near a large flat surface, but fluoroscopy images after 15 seconds of contrast injection will reveal the progression of contrast to large peritoneal space and confirm the appropriate position of the catheter.

Outflow Failure and Catheter Migration

Omental attachment is the most common cause of outflow failure and catheter migration, when there is no restriction in the inflow of fluid into the peritoneum. This attachment happens principally to the side holes of the catheter. With the use of fluoroscopy, repositioning of the PD catheter is being done using a long guidewire so that the catheter can be brought into the anterior peritoneal space. The long flexible guidewire forms a loop that can fit into anterior peritoneal space only when advanced into this straight or coiled Tenckhoff catheter. In the case of coiled catheters, the guidewire follows the spiral of the coil and should not exit through the side hole. Formation of a large coil, when the guidewire is advanced very far enough, will free the

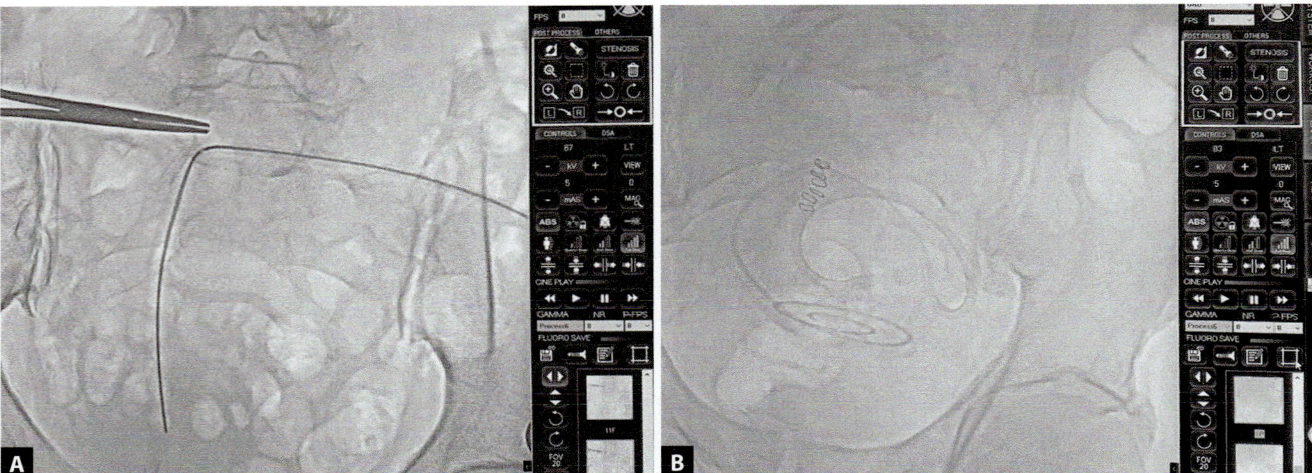

Figs. 3A and B: (A) Fluoroscopy-guided catheter insertion with imaging done after putting a straight Tenckhoff catheter with the catheter tip in the right pelvis and an extraperitoneal portion including exit site on the left side; (B) Fluoroscopy-guided catheter insertion with imaging done after putting a coiled Tenckhoff catheter with a coiled catheter in the pelvis.

omental attachments from the catheter tip and bring it into anterior peritoneal space. The contrast administration after the CAPD catheter placement will show a free outflow of contrast with extension from the catheter quickly. In case of migration and outflow failure, the contrast sometimes is viewed in a completely isolated space even after inspecting the image after 15 seconds of contrast administration. Laparoscopic removal of adhesions, omentectomy, and placement of a new catheter may be the other options in case it is not getting corrected with guidewire manipulation. The old catheter can be replaced with a new catheter using the same site for the deep cuff and peritoneal entry by placing a guidewire into the old catheter, removing the old catheter, placing a dilator/split sheath over the guidewire and placing a new catheter through the split sheath. The split sheath is directed in different directions once the guidewire is removed so the same track of the old catheter is avoided.[4]

COMPUTED TOMOGRAPHY

Computed tomography (CT) is usually performed with both intravenous (IV) and oral contrast for evaluating the complications of CAPD. In CT peritoneography, the iodinated contrast medium is administered via the indwelling CAPD catheter into the peritoneal cavity. 1 mL/kg of nonionic contrast material is mixed with 30 mL/kg of dialysate fluid and then injected into the peritoneal cavity through the PD catheter. The individual is then asked to move around for about 30 minutes and then a scan is performed. This time allows the mixture to get distributed around the peritoneal cavity in a supine position though any position may be used while undergoing the investigation. Approximately 30–55% of the dialysate is distributed within the pelvis around the bowel and mesentery with only 1–3% in the lesser sac in the supine position.[9] A few indications of CT peritoneography are dialysate leak into the abdominal wall or any soft tissue, adhesions or loculated collections/abscesses, hernias, ultrafiltration failure, and issues with fluid exchanges. Intra-abdominal abscesses appear as unopacified fluid collections and the path and site of dialysate leaks are better viewed in CT peritoneography and are considered superior to CT scans. IV and oral contrast CT are used preferably for intestinal obstruction, pancreatitis, or bowel ischemia. In all these cases, altered enhancement of these structures may be obscured by the opacified dialysate on CT peritoneography **(Figs. 4A and B)**. Even residual dialysate obscures inflammatory changes in the mesentery if any and thereby it is difficult to interpret as the dialysate fluid may cause thickening of the intestinal and gallbladder wall. CT is advantageous to rule out other intra-abdominal causes and collections amenable to drainage. It is more sensitive to detect early stages of peritoneal calcification, which may be present in ESP, and tuberculosis (TB) infections of mesothelioma. IV contrast has the potential risk of nephrotoxicity in patients with residual renal function.

MAGNETIC RESONANCE IMAGING

Magnetic resonance imaging (MRI) is not recommended in routine practice due to the uncertain risk of nephrogenic systemic fibrosis from gadolinium exposure within the peritoneal cavity. Other disadvantages are its cost, lack of availability, and inferior spatial resolution compared to CT. It can be of value as it has multiplanar capability and a lack of ionizing radiation exposure. Gadolinium-based contrast mixed with the dialysate into the peritoneal cavity can be utilized for T1-weighted imaging with no IV or oral contrast. T2-weighted imaging can be used for fluid collections without the gadolinium exposure.[10] MR peritoneography may provide detailed information about the dialysate leakage and is considered safer with no risks associated with nephrotoxic contrast agents and radiation exposure. The extraperitoneal tungsten tip of the Tenckhoff catheter is MRI-compatible and may cause some susceptibility artifacts if the tip is lying over the imaging area.

SCINTIGRAPHY

Scintigraphy is not used in routine clinical practice. Before the use of CT peritoneography, it was used with an intraperitoneal injection of a radioisotope for the imaging of any hernial complication or to detect any pleuroperitoneal fistula secondary to CAPD procedure. It is considered a cheap and less invasive procedure for determining the site of dialysate leakage and diagnosing any predisposing factors for hernia. Also, it may help in detecting a few complications without any clinical features at an earlier stage. The patients can be monitored for several hours following the instillation of labeled dialysate because initially, negative scintigrams may become positive after a few hours of ambulation. To confirm extraperitoneal leakage, postdrainage images are also very useful. Besides, it is relatively safer with low radiation exposure.[11]

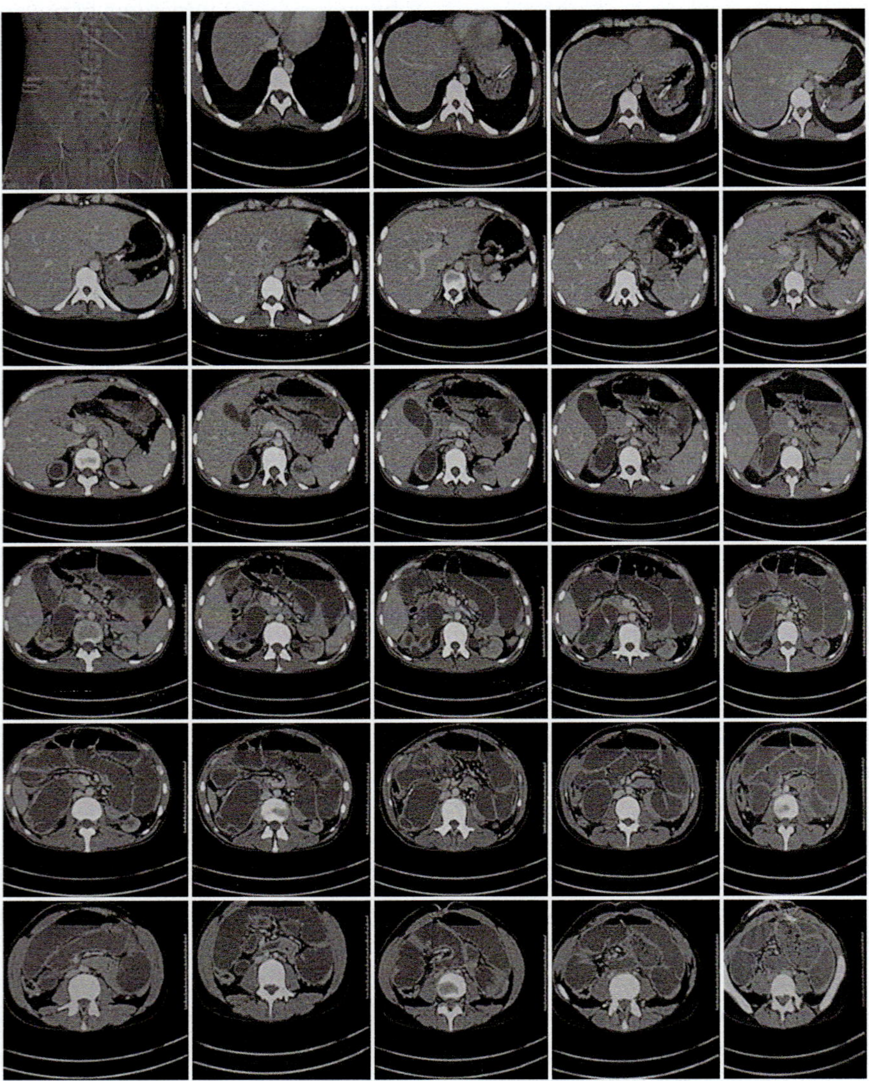

Fig. 4A

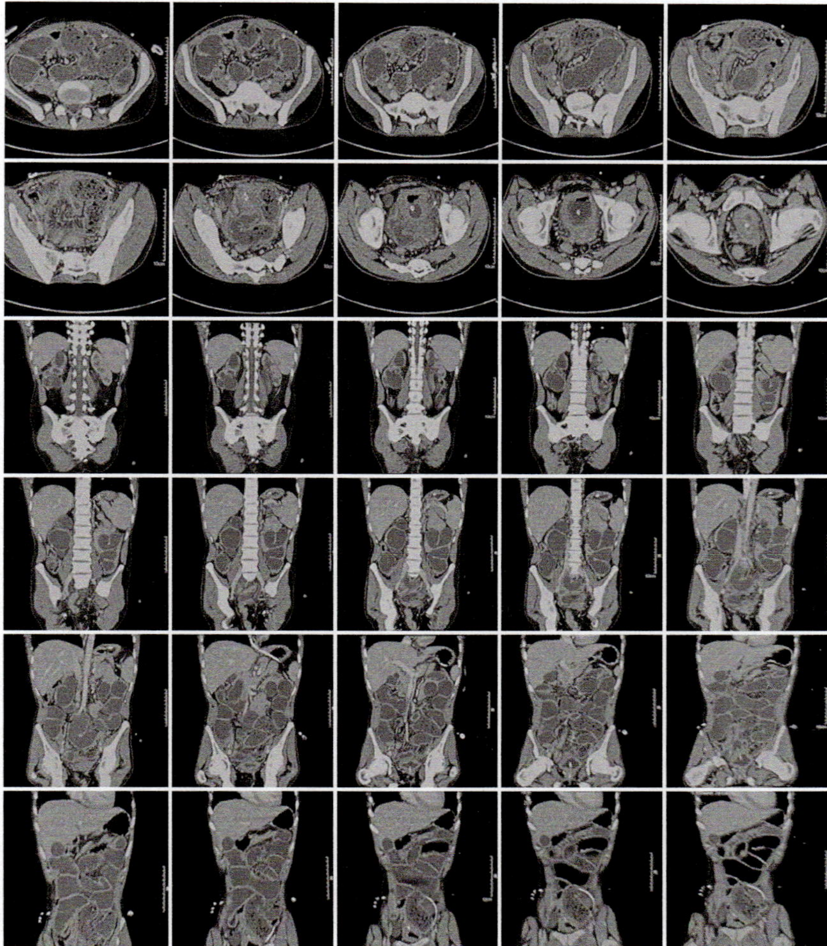

Fig. 4B

Figs. 4A and B: CECT abdomen in axial and coronal sections, showing catheter tip in the left iliac fossa with multiple bowel loops with air–fluid levels with transition zone at the distal ileum (in a patient with intestinal obstruction). The image also shows right pelvic ureteric junction obstruction causing gross hydronephrosis and cortical thinning. (CECT: contrast-enhanced computed tomography)

CONCLUSION

Imaging has a definitive role in the initial placement of CAPD catheter and follow up management of patients on CAPD. Various imaging modalities like plain radiography, ultrasound, CT peritoneography, fluoroscopy, and MRI have its own merits and weaknesses. While CT scans can reveal thickening and calcification of the peritoneum, CT peritoneography can be useful for assessing fluid leaks and adhesions. Fluoroscopy, a type of real time X ray imaging is used to guide the placement and manipulation of peritoneal dialysis catheters. It enables a percutaneous approach which is less invasive than open surgery. Adequate knowledge of CAPD and its complications are essential for early recognition of complications through accurate interpretation of imaging studies.

REFERENCES

1. Bammens B, Peeters D, Jaekers J, Claes KJ, Evenepoel P, Kuypers D, et al. Postimplantation X-ray parameters predict functional catheter problems in peritoneal dialysis. Kidney Int. 2014;86(5):1001-6.
2. Saunders RN, Veitch PS, Nicholson ML. Pneumoperitoneum in CAPD Peritonitis. JR Soc Med. 2004;97(1):28-9.
3. Nardelli L, Scalamogna A, Castellano G. Utility of ultrasonographic examination in catheter related infections in peritoneal dialysis: A clinical approach. J Nephrol. 2023; 36(7):1751-61.

4. Ash S, Sequeira A, Narayan R. Imaging and peritoneal dialysis catheters. Semin Dial. 2017;30(4):338-46.
5. Szeto C, Li PK, Johnson DW, Bernardini J, Dong J, Figueiredo AE, et al. ISPD catheter-related infection recommendations: 2017 update. Perit Dial Int. 2017;37(2):141-54.
6. Plum J, Sudkamp S, Grabensee B. Results of ultrasound-assisted diagnosis of tunnel infections in continuous ambulatory peritoneal dialysis. Am J Kidney Dis. 1994;23: 99-104.
7. Goldstein M, Carrillo M, Ghai S. Continuous ambulatory peritoneal dialysis: A guide to imaging appearances and complications. Insights Imaging. 2013;4(1):85-92.
8. Abreo K, Sequeira A. Bowel perforation during peritoneal dialysis catheter placement. Am J Kidney Dis. 2016;68:312-5.
9. Twardowski ZJ, Tully RJ, Ersoy FF, Dedhia NM. Computerized tomography with and without intraperitoneal contrast for determination of intraabdominal fluid distribution and diagnosis of complications in peritoneal dialysis patients. ASAIO Trans. 1990;36(2):95-103.
10. Prokesch RW, Schima W, Schober E, Vychytil A, Fabrizii V, Bader TR. Complications of continuous ambulatory peritoneal dialysis: findings on MR peritoneography. Am J Roentgenol. 2000;174(4):987-91.
11. Tokmak H, Mudun A, Turkmen C, Sanli Y, Cantez S, Bozfakioglu S. The role of peritoneal scintigraphy in the detection of continuous ambulatory peritoneal dialysis complications. Ren Fail. 2006;28(8):709-13.

SECTION 3

Vascular Access Creation for Hemodialysis

CHAPTER 10

Arteriovenous Fistula Creation

10.1 SURGICAL ARTERIOVENOUS FISTULA

Yogita Sharma, AK Bhalla, Ashwani Gupta, Sanjiv Jasuja

"A surgeon is not defined by the cut of the scalpel, but by the precision of thought behind it."

CASE SCENARIO

A 62-year-old female with a 10-year history of poorly controlled hypertension and a background of ischemic heart disease presents to the nephrology clinic for evaluation. She has recently progressed to *end-stage renal disease (ESRD)*, with an estimated glomerular filtration rate (eGFR) of 6 mL/min/1.73 m^2. She reports increasing fatigue, reduced urine output, and episodes of volume overload requiring frequent hospitalizations.

Given the need for initiating hemodialysis in the near future, the plan is to establish a *permanent vascular access*. A physical examination reveals that the veins in her left arm are small and poorly palpable, likely due to a prior history of multiple intravenous cannulations during hospital stays.

To assess vascular suitability, a *Doppler ultrasound mapping* of the upper limbs is performed. The right cephalic vein is found to be of good caliber (≥2.5 mm) with a corresponding radial artery of adequate diameter and flow.

How would you proceed further?

INTRODUCTION

In hemodialysis, two primary forms of permanent vascular access are available: Arteriovenous fistula (AVF) and arteriovenous graft (AVG). Whenever possible, the AVF is preferred for long-term dialysis access, as long as it is compatible with the patient's end-stage kidney disease (ESKD) life-plan and broader treatment goals, and when patient-specific factors are favorable for its creation.

Compared to AVGs, a mature and functional AVF is typically associated with fewer complications such as thrombosis, reduced primary patency, and a lower need for subsequent interventions, making it the access of choice for patients starting hemodialysis.[1] However, successful creation of an AVF requires appropriate arterial and venous anatomy, along with sufficient time to allow for proper maturation before it becomes usable.

SELECTION OF ARTERIOVENOUS FISTULA SITE

The type of AVF should be referred to by the specific artery and vein that are involved.[2] Although various anatomical configurations of AVFs can be created, most fall into a few standard categories:

- *Radial-cephalic fistula (RCF):* Connecting the radial artery to the cephalic vein at the wrist
- *Forearm basilic fistula:* Involving the basilic vein and either the radial or the ulnar artery at the wrist
- *Brachial-cephalic fistula (BCF):* Joining the brachial artery and cephalic vein in the proximal forearm
- *Brachial-basilic fistula (BBF):* Connecting the brachial artery with the basilic vein in the upper arm
- *Lower extremity fistulas:* Typically involving the superficial femoral artery and the saphenous or femoral/popliteal veins in the thigh

Among these, the RCF tends to have a lower blood flow compared to more proximal fistulas. Nevertheless, it is often selected as the initial access point, as it preserves the proximal vascular structures for future use if needed.

The surgical creation of AV access types is guided by the fundamental principles of vascular surgery. Ideally, the nondominant arm is chosen first if both arms present equally suitable vessels. Access creation should start distally and progress proximally if necessary, and whenever possible, autogenous AVFs are preferred over prosthetic AVGs due to better outcomes.[3]

When using native vessels, the following sequence is generally recommended:

1. Direct AV anastomosis (native fistula)
2. Venous transposition procedures
3. Venous translocation if needed

Following these principles, the order of preferred access creation typically includes:

1. RCF
2. BCF or a proximal radial artery-based fistula
3. BBF
4. Forearm AVG
5. Upper arm AVG

Less commonly, transpositions involving the basilic or brachial veins in the forearm may also be considered if primary options are not feasible.

ANESTHESIA OPTIONS FOR ARTERIOVENOUS FISTULA SURGERY

Options for anesthesia at the time of AVF creation include:

- Local anesthesia
- Regional block
- General anesthesia (rare, special cases)

It is preferable to avoid the use of general anesthesia in this patient population. In most cases, AVF creation can be successfully performed under regional or local anesthesia, with or without the addition of intravenous sedation.

Some studies suggest that brachial plexus blocks may be advantageous by inducing regional sympathetic blockade, leading to arterial and venous vasodilation. This venodilation effect appears to enhance the success rates of AVF creation and subsequent use.[4-8]

Antimicrobial prophylaxis: This is indicated at the time of the surgical creation. Single-dose cephalosporin (Cephazolin 2 g) is administered prior to incision. Only if the patient is on a temporary/tunneled cuffed catheter is it preferable to place them on a short course of oral antibiotic (Cephalexin 500 mg BD for 5 days).

SURGICAL TECHNIQUES FOR ARTERIOVENOUS FISTULA CREATION

Arteriovenous fistula can be created using any of the following techniques of anastomosis:

- End-to-side anastomosis
- Side-to-side anastomosis
- End-to-end anastomosis (rare use)

RADIAL-CEPHALIC ARTERIOVENOUS FISTULA PROCEDURE

The preferred site on the forearm is identified where there is minimal displacement of the cephalic vein across any plane (mediolateral or anteroposterior). A safe distance from the wrist is maintained to preserve options for future endovascular procedures.

- Typically, a lazy-S shaped incision is made **(Fig. 1)**, with the curves directed toward the artery and vein that have been previously mapped with ultrasound.
- The arms of the S-shaped incision can be extended as needed to achieve adequate exposure of the venous segment while carefully protecting the radial cutaneous nerve of the forearm and the superficial branch of the radial nerve.
- The distal segment of the vein is carefully dissected, with minimal handling and manipulation confined to the adventitia to avoid vein injury **(Fig. 2)**.

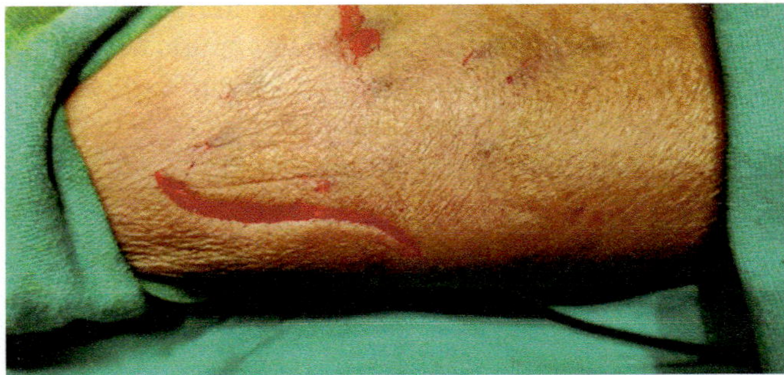

Fig. 1: Lazy-S shaped incision is made.

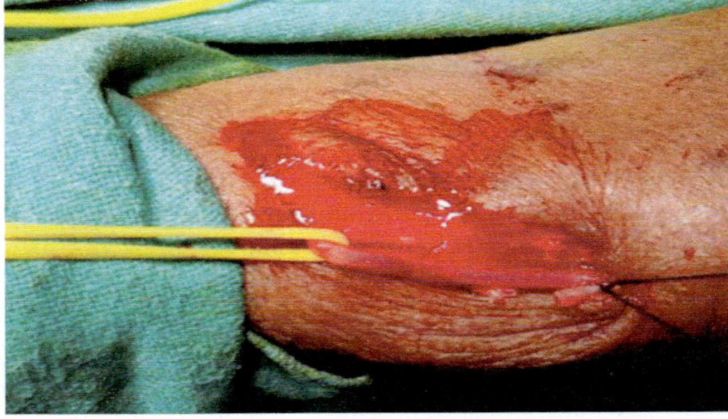

Fig. 2: The cephalic vein is dissected and mobilized. Side branches are ligated and divided.

- A longitudinal incision is made through the antebrachial fascia to expose the radial artery, located medial to the flexor carpi radialis muscle or tendon **(Fig. 3)**. It is preferable to leave the artery largely undisturbed, freeing only the portion necessary for anastomosis after the vein dissection and site assessment **(Video 1)**.
- Marking the vein before division helps maintain its orientation during anastomosis **(Fig. 4)**. An arteriotomy is made (4–6 mm) using blade scalpel no. 11 **(Fig. 5)** in manner to create roughly 30–45° intersectioning conduit **(Fig. 6)**.
- Polypropylene sutures (sizes 6-0, 7-0, or 8-0) are typically used to perform the anastomosis **(Video 2) (Figs. 7 to 9)**.
- Various anastomotic techniques can be utilized, including end-to-side (vein end to artery side), back-straight (p-SLOT), side-to-side, line onlay, or piggyback configurations.
- Ensuring that the vein lies without any undue tension or twisting is critical, as this minimizes turbulence-induced shear stress and promotes optimal fistula function **(Fig. 10)**.

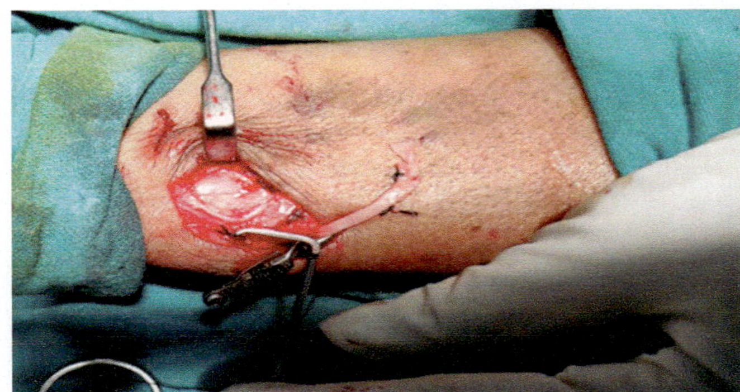

Fig. 3: A longitudinal incision is made through the antebrachial fascia to expose the radial artery.

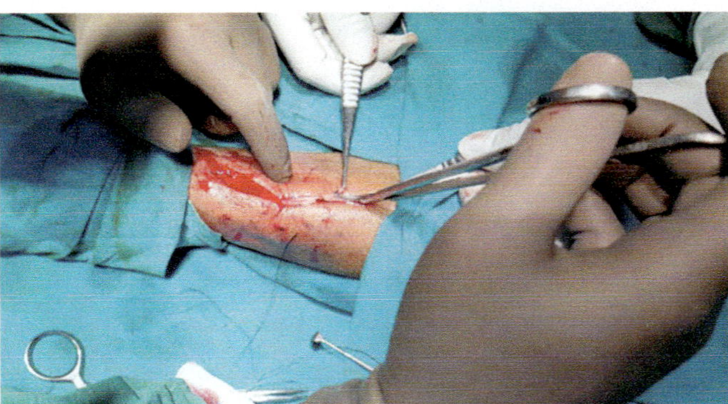

Fig. 4: The vein is transected and spatulated **(Fig. 5)**.

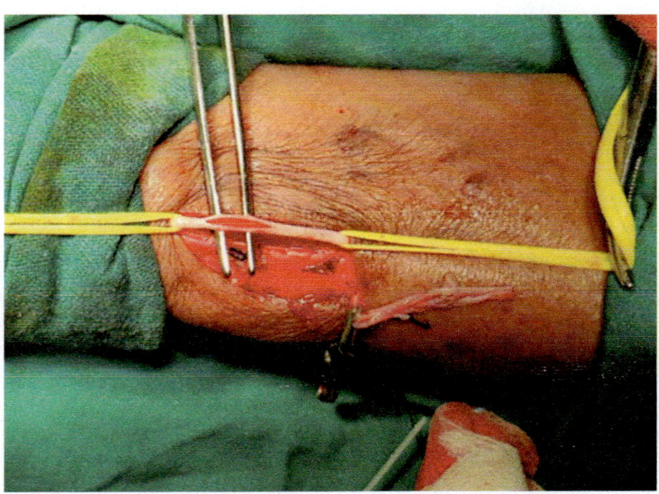

Fig. 5: An arteriotomy is made (4–6 mm) using blade scalpel no. 11 **(Fig. 6)**.

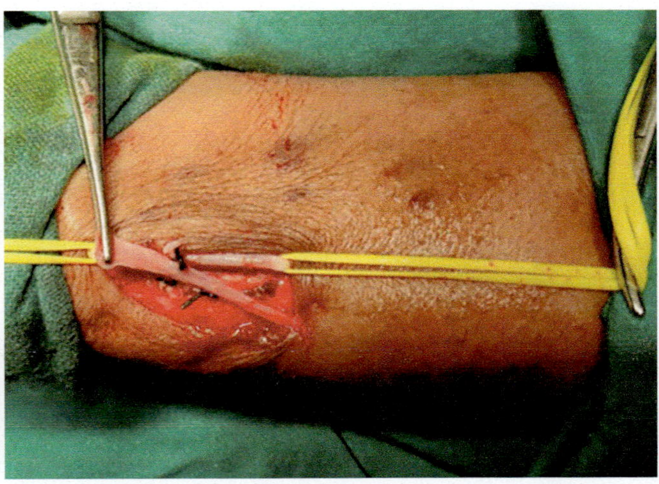

Fig. 6: The arteriotomy is made in a manner to create roughly a 30–45° for intersectioning conduit.

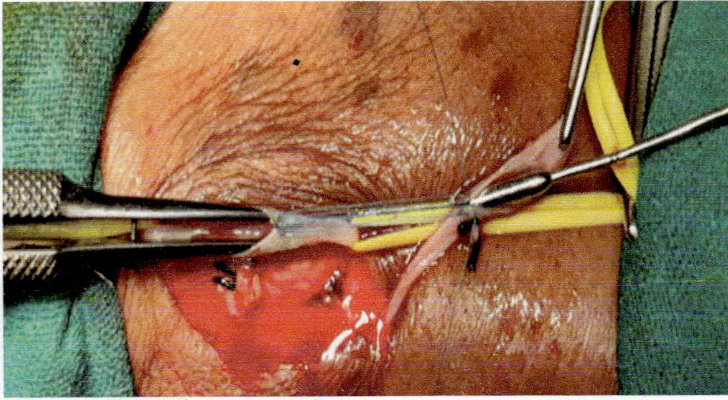

Fig. 7: An end-to-side anastomosis is made between the vein and the artery using 6-0 or 7-0 polypropylene sutures.

- After completing the anastomosis, check for immediate thrill or bruit to confirm the patency and functionality of the fistula.

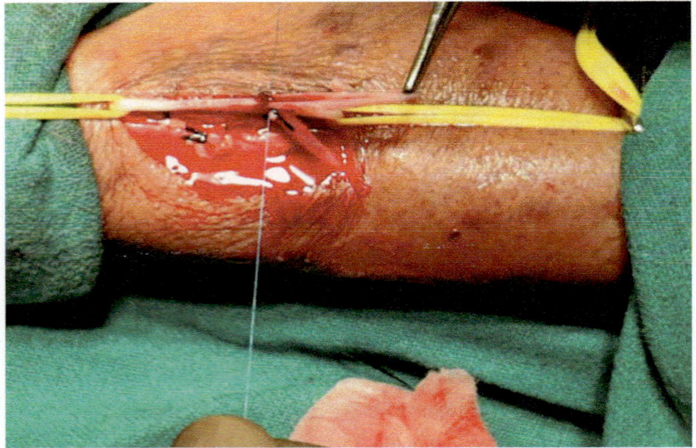

Fig. 8: The apex is anastomosed with the parachute technique of suturing.

- Achieve hemostasis carefully and close the wound in layers, avoiding compression over the fistula.

Brachial-Cephalic Arteriovenous Fistula

The autogenous BCF is the connection of the end of the cephalic vein to the brachial artery at the level of the antecubital fossa.

Steps:

1. Confirm that the cephalic vein and brachial artery are suitable for fistula creation at the level of the antecubital fossa using preoperative ultrasound mapping.
2. Make a single transverse incision at the antecubital fossa if the brachial artery and cephalic vein are close together **(Fig. 11)**.
3. If the vessels are not adjacent, tunnel the cephalic vein toward the brachial artery to allow a tension-free anastomosis.

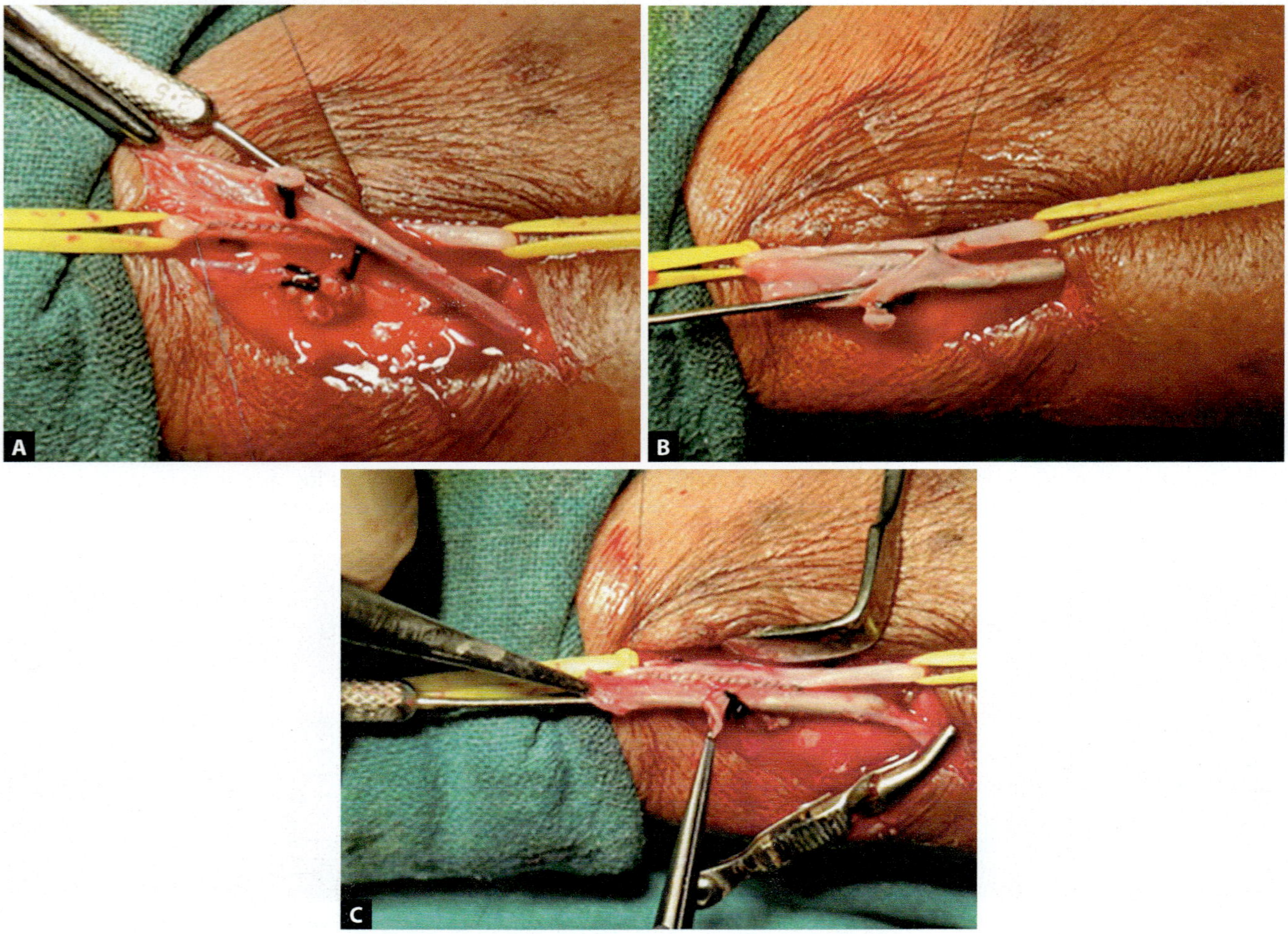

Figs. 9A to C: Either side of arteriovenous anastomosis is secured using running sutures.

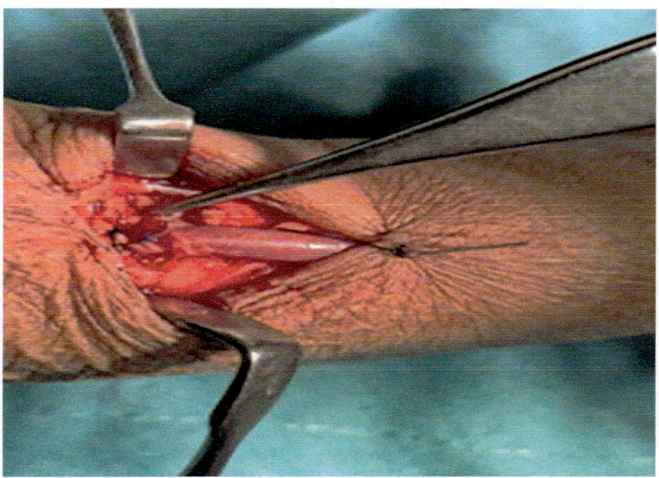

Fig. 10: The vascular loops are removed after completing the anastomosis.

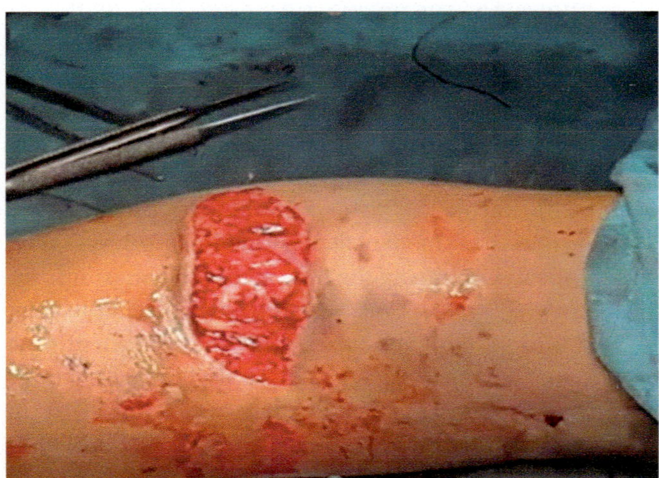

Fig. 11: A single transverse incision is made at the antecubital fossa.

4. Carefully dissect and mobilize the cephalic vein with minimal handling to avoid injury **(Video 3)**.
5. Isolate and control the brachial artery, taking care to preserve surrounding structures.
6. Create a limited arteriotomy in the brachial artery to help regulate flow volume and reduce the risk of developing high-flow complications such as aneurysm formation or steal syndrome.
7. Perform an *end-to-side anastomosis* between the end of the cephalic vein and the side of the brachial artery.
8. Use fine vascular sutures (e.g., polypropylene 6-0 or 7-0), ensuring a tension-free and rotation-free connection.
9. After completing the anastomosis, check for immediate thrill or bruit to confirm the patency and functionality of the fistula.
10. Achieve hemostasis carefully and close the wound in layers, avoiding compression over the fistula.

When the proximal radial artery is appropriate for use, creating a proximal radial artery–cephalic vein fistula becomes a good alternative, offering a lower risk of developing steal syndrome. A major concern with BCFs is their tendency to produce high-flow rates, leading to complications such as aneurysm formation and steal phenomenon. To minimize these risks, it is important to limit the size of the arteriotomy during BCF creation and, whenever feasible, to prefer the proximal radial artery for inflow.[9]

Brachial-Basilic Arteriovenous Fistula

The *BBF* serves as an excellent upper arm access option when the cephalic vein is unsuitable. Due to the basilic vein's deep, medial positioning and its proximity to branches of the medial antebrachial cutaneous nerve, *transposition or superficialization* is typically required to make the vein accessible for dialysis use.[10] Both *single-stage and two-stage transposition techniques* are practiced, and current literature does not consistently favor one method over the other.[11]

One-stage procedure:

- In this procedure, both the creation of the AVF and the transposition of the basilic vein are performed in a single operation.
- This approach is preferred when the basilic vein is sufficiently large and the surgeon is confident in achieving a tension-free anastomosis.
- The basilic vein is mobilized and transposed to a more superficial position in the arm, where it is then directly anastomosed to the brachial artery.
- The advantage of this method is that it provides immediate access to the fistula, allowing for quicker maturation and use once the fistula becomes functional.
- This approach is generally quicker, with fewer surgical interventions, and is associated with a shorter recovery time for the patient.

Two-stage procedure:

- It is typically employed when the basilic vein is initially too deep, small, or unsuitable for immediate transposition.

- In the first stage, the AVF is created, and the basilic vein is left in its deep position, often with some portion of the vein placed in a more accessible location for future transposition.
- The fistula is allowed to mature over a period of weeks to months.
- Once the vein has matured sufficiently, the second stage involves transposing the basilic vein to a more superficial position in the arm, where it is then connected to the brachial artery for use.
- This approach offers the advantage of allowing the vein to enlarge and strengthen before transposition, which can improve the overall outcomes of the fistula, but it requires two separate procedures and a longer waiting time for full functionality.

INTRAOPERATIVE COMPLICATIONS

- *Rotation of the vein:*
  - It is crucial to avoid rotation before performing anastomosis.
  - Mark the ventral side of the vein with methylene blue to maintain orientation.
  - If rotation is detected after anastomosis:
    - *Option 1:* Redo the anastomosis.
    - *Option 2:* Divide the vein and create a veno-venous anastomosis (less preferred in small veins during second-stage procedures).
  - Prefer redoing the anastomosis when the vein is small.
- *Kinking of the vein:*
  - It is caused by excessive mobilization of the vein or sharp bends from subcutaneous tissue compression
  - It can be prevented by adjusting vein length appropriately before anastomosis.
  - If kinking occurs:
    - Release the surrounding subcutaneous tissue to relieve tension.
    - If unresolved, redo the anastomosis.
- *Thrombosis:*
  - It is a rare intraoperative complication.
  - Its causes include:
    - Poor vessel handling.
    - Atherosclerotic plaques at the anastomosis site
    - Prolonged anastomosis time
    - Underlying prothrombotic conditions
  - Preventive measures:
    - Select an anastomosis site away from plaques.
    - Handle vessels delicately by the adventitia.
  - If thrombosis persists despite proper technique:
    - Abandon the procedure and evaluate for a hypercoagulable state.

Intraoperative Assessment of Arteriovenous Fistula

- *Clinical signs of flow:* Once the arteriovenous anastomosis is completed and clamps are released, immediate clinical assessment is crucial. A palpable *thrill*—a buzzing or vibrating sensation over the fistula—should be felt on light touch. This thrill indicates good blood flow through the anastomosis and into the outflow vein. Additionally, an audible *bruit* can often be heard over the fistula using a stethoscope, suggesting turbulent flow, which is expected immediately post-surgery. The absence of a thrill or bruit raises suspicion for technical issues like anastomotic narrowing, kinking of the vein, or thrombosis, and may warrant immediate correction.
- *Role of intraoperative Doppler or flow measurement:* Intraoperative Doppler ultrasound provides an objective assessment of fistula function during surgery. It helps in visualizing the flow across the anastomosis, identifying stenosis, or detecting any kinks in the vein. In addition, *flow measurements* (such as transit time flowmetry) can be used to quantify blood flow rates through the fistula. A flow rate >300–500 mL/min intraoperatively is generally considered favorable for maturation. Use of Doppler and flow measurement techniques can enhance surgical decision-making and may improve early AVF success rates by identifying problems before completing the operation.

POSTOPERATIVE CARE AND MONITORING

The patients should be counseled regarding the following:

- Maintain proper hygiene and keep the surgical dressing dry and clean. Elevate the limb to help reduce swelling.
- Maintain stable blood pressure to ensure adequate blood flow through the newly created access.
- Perform self-checks on the AVF by palpating for a "thrill" (a buzzing sensation) at least twice a day. Immediately report if the thrill is absent.
- Monitor the access arm for changes in color, size, temperature, or sensation, as these may indicate infection, ischemia, or bleeding.

- Avoid using the arm with the vascular access for drawing blood, inserting intravenous lines, or measuring blood pressure.
- Protect the access arm by avoiding tight clothing, straps, compression, contact sports, trauma, or lifting heavy objects.
- Once the dressing is removed and the surgical wound has healed, start prescribed arm exercises. These exercises promote vein dilation and improve blood flow, helping fistula maturation, particularly for distal AVFs (though they are less helpful for AVGs).[12,13]
- Discuss and adhere to a regular postoperative follow-up plan, which should be explained thoroughly to both dialysis and nondialysis patients.

Monitoring by the healthcare professionals: The maturation of an AVF is a critical determinant of its long-term functionality for hemodialysis. Clinical research has demonstrated that a skilled practitioner can predict the maturation of a newly formed AVF with over 80% accuracy using physical examination alone.[13-15]

- A physical examination of a newly formed AVF should be conducted within 4–6 weeks after creation.
- This early assessment is crucial for evaluating fistula maturation and promptly identifying any complications.
- Extended waiting does not improve the likelihood of successful AVF function or recovery.[16]

Duplex ultrasound (DUS) plays a pivotal role in assessing AVF development, particularly around the 6-week post creation.[17] A mature AVF is generally defined by the fulfillment of the widely recognized "rule of six" criteria:

- *Vein diameter:* The body of the AVF should have a minimum internal diameter of 6 mm.
- *Blood flow rate:* Flow through the AVF should be at least 600 mL/min.
- *Depth from skin surface:* The AVF should lie no deeper than 0.5–0.6 cm to facilitate easy cannulation.
- *Length of the access segment:* A cannulation segment of 5–6 cm is necessary to allow for safe and effective two-needle dialysis.

In addition to evaluating these core parameters, a detailed DUS examination is strongly recommended to identify anatomical or hemodynamic abnormalities that may contribute to early AVF failure. Such thorough assessments are instrumental in guiding personalized management strategies and planning timely interventions, thereby improving the chances of salvaging or optimizing the vascular access.

CONCLUSION

Arteriovenous fistula creation is the preferred method for long-term hemodialysis access due to its superior patency and lower complication rates. Successful outcomes depend on careful patient selection, preoperative vessel mapping, appropriate surgical technique, and structured postoperative care.

Distal AVFs, particularly the radial-cephalic type, are prioritized to preserve proximal sites. The use of regional anesthesia and intraoperative flow assessment enhances surgical success. Early monitoring using clinical examination and duplex ultrasound is vital for detecting maturation issues and guiding timely intervention.

A patient-centered, stepwise approach ensures durable vascular access and supports optimal dialysis delivery.

REFERENCES

1. Lok CE, Huber TS, Lee T, Vachharajani TJ, Valentini RP, National Kidney Foundation. KDOQI Clinical Practice Guideline for Vascular Access: 2019 Update. Am J Kidney Dis. 2020;75:S1.
2. Sidawy AN, Gray R, Besarab A, Henry M, Ascher E, Silva Jr M, et al. Recommended standards for reports dealing with arteriovenous hemodialysis accesses. J Vasc Surg. 2002;35:603.
3. Macsata RA, Sidawy AN. Hemodialysis access general considerations and strategies to optimize access placement. In: Sidawy AN, Perler BA (Eds). Rutherford's Vascular Surgery and Endovascular Therapy, 9th edition. Philadelphia, PA: Elsevier; 2019. pp. 2291-8.
4. Aitken E, Jackson A, Kearns R, Steven M, Kinsella J, Clancy M, et al. Effect of regional versus local anaesthesia on outcome after arteriovenous fistula creation: a randomised controlled trial. Lancet. 2016;388:1067.
5. Ismail A, Abushouk AI, Bekhet AH, Abunar O, Hassan O, Khamis AA, et al. Regional versus local anesthesia for arteriovenous fistula creation in end-stage renal disease: a systematic review and meta-analysis. J Vasc Access. 2017;18:177.
6. Cerneviciute R, Sahebally SM, Ahmed K, Murphy M, Mahmood W, Walsh SR. Regional Versus Local Anaesthesia for Haemodialysis Arteriovenous Fistula Formation: A Systematic Review and Meta-Analysis. Eur J Vasc Endovasc Surg. 2017;53:734.
7. Lo Monte AI, Damiano G, Mularo A, Palumbo VD, Alessi R, Gioviale MC, et al. Comparison between local and regional

anesthesia in arteriovenous fistula creation. J Vasc Access. 2011;12:331.

8. Reynolds TS, Kim KM, Dukkipati R, Nguyen TH, Julka I, Kakazu C, et al. Pre-operative regional block anesthesia enhances operative strategy for arteriovenous fistula creation. J Vasc Access. 2011;12:336.
9. Leake AE, Winger DG, Leers SA, Gupta N, Dillavou ED. Management and outcomes of dialysis access-associated steal syndrome. J Vasc Surg. 2015;61:754.
10. Sidawy AN, Spergel LM, Besarab A, Allon M, Jennings WC, Padberg Jr FT, et al. The Society for Vascular Surgery: clinical practice guidelines for the surgical placement and maintenance of arteriovenous hemodialysis access. J Vasc Surg. 2008;48:2S-25S.
11. Cooper J, Power AH, DeRose G, Forbes TL, Dubois L. Similar failure and patency rates when comparing one- and two-stage basilic vein transposition. J Vasc Surg. 2015;61:809-16.
12. Dember LM, Beck GJ, Allon M, Delmez JA, Dixon BS, Greenberg A, et al. Effect of clopidogrel on early failure of arteriovenous fistulas for hemodialysis: a randomized controlled trial. JAMA. 2008;299:2164-71.
13. Robbin ML, Chamberlain NE, Lockhart ME, Gallichio MH, Young CJ, Deierhoi MH, et al. Hemodialysis arteriovenous fistula maturity: US evaluation. Radiology. 2002;225:59-64.
14. Leon C, Asif A. Physical examination of arteriovenous fistulae by a renal fellow: does it compare favorably to an experienced interventionalist? Semin Dial. 2008;21(6): 557-60.
15. Leon C, Orozco-Vargas LC, Krishnamurthy G, Choi KL, Mercado C, Merrill D, et al. Accuracy of physical examination in the detection of arteriovenous graft stenosis. Semin Dial. 2008;21(1):85-8.
16. Robbin ML, Greene T, Cheung AK, Allon M, Berceli SA, Kaufman JS, et al. Arteriovenous fistula development in the first 6 weeks after creation. Radiology. 2016;279(2):620-9.
17. Clinical practice recommendations for needling of arteriovenous fistulae and grafts for haemodialysis. 2021.

10.2A ENDOVASCULAR ARTERIOVENOUS FISTULA: MAPPING AND CREATION

Adrian P Sequeira, Rashid Sharaf, Vinant Bhargava

"Don't just climb the ladder, chart a new path"

INTRODUCTION

The radiocephalic (RC) arteriovenous fistula (AVF) is the first and distal-most vascular access considered in the access algorithm. Though preoperative vessel mapping is frequently obtained prior to AVF creation, primary failure and poor maturation are vexing problems. Juxta-anastomotic stenosis is a common cause of nonmaturation.[1] This is caused by neointimal hyperplasia (NIH) and inadequate outward remodeling. Factors responsible for these include surgical trauma, abnormal shear stress, and torsional stress.[2] Sheer stress is influenced by the anastomotic angle which should ideally be 30–50° for RC AVFs.[3,4] Surgical trauma occurs from clamping and suturing which damage the endothelial lining. Torsional stress occurs as the cephalic vein must be moved in three different directions to meet the radial artery.[2] Dissection of the vein from its surrounding tissue damages the vasa vasorum.[5] In fact, newer surgical techniques such as radial artery deviation and reimplantation (RADAR) and modified no-touch technique have shown better patency results as they do not involve mobilization or skeletonization of the vein.[6]

The viability of percutaneous AVF (pAVF) came from the observation that penetrating injuries to the body causing AVFs do so without extravasation. This implied that in such situations if vessels were in proximity and properly aligned, blood would flow from the high-pressure artery into the low-pressure vein without bleeding even though the vessels are not sutured. In addition, they rarely close spontaneously.[7,8]

The development of percutaneous catheter-based devices now enables the creation of fistulas without exposing the patient to the complications and morbidity of a surgical fistula. pAVF is a novel percutaneous technique of AVF creation, with two devices approved for use in the United States—*WavelinQ* (Becton, Dickinson and Company; Franklin Lakes, NJ) and *Ellipsys* (Medtronic, Minneapolis, MN). WavelinQ utilizes the radial artery and radial vein, ulnar artery and ulnar vein, and the interosseous vessels, while Ellipsys uses the proximal radial artery (PRA) and a venous perforator [deep communicating vein (DCV)]. These are *proximal forearm fistulas with a side-to-side anastomosis*. Their high physiologic maturation rates are due to the avoidance of aspects of the surgical procedure that promote NIH.[7,9] In addition, the long preprocedural wait times as well as medical clearance that was previously needed for a surgical AVF are nonexistent. The *pAVF does not compete with a surgical AVF creation but provides a new anatomic location for AVF creation*[10] **(Fig. 1)**.

ANATOMY

The upper extremity venous drainage consists of two systems: Superficial and deep venous systems **(Fig. 2)**. The superficial venous system is primarily composed of the basilic and cephalic veins in the forearm and upper arm. The deep venous system comprises paired radial and ulnar veins (*vena comitans*) which drain into the brachial vein in the upper arm. In addition, there are anterior and posterior interosseous deep veins that drain into the ulnar vein. These two systems communicate via a perforator vein in the forearm, located just distal to the antecubital fossa with *flow normally from the superficial to the deep system.* The presence of a perforator vein is essential for successful pAVF creation as it serves as the conduit for arterialized venous blood from the deep venous system to reach the superficial venous system, *i.e., direction of flow is reversed.* The maturation of superficial veins allows for cannulation of the cephalic, basilic, median cubital, median cephalic or basilic, or a combination of two veins, thereby broadening the cannulation zone. This limits the complications from repetitive single-site cannulation.[11]

Patient Selection

Percutaneous AVF is an ideal option for patients who would prefer to avoid surgery or with contraindications to surgery. In the current algorithm, a surgical RC AVF is given first preference. If this is not feasible, then an pAVF is the next option before more proximal fistulas are considered. It should not be attempted in patients with nonpatent

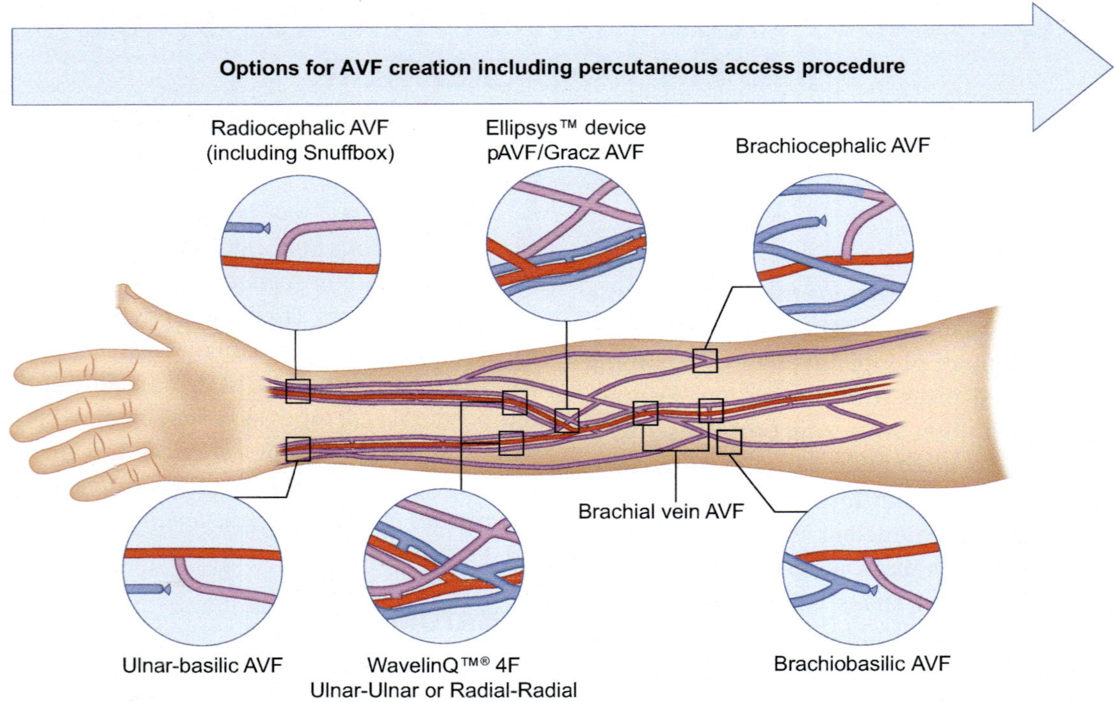

Fig. 1: Preference and order of (from distal to proximal) access placement in the upper limb. (AVF: arteriovenous fistula)

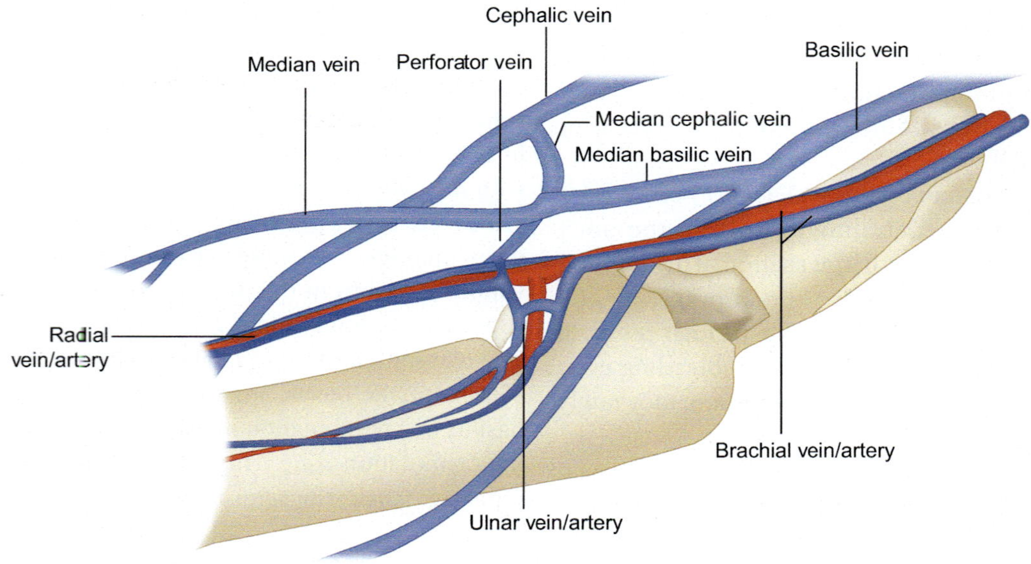

Fig. 2: Anatomy of the superficial and deep venous system of the upper extremity.

outflow veins or in patients with flow-limiting transmural arterial calcification. Further patients with a pacemaker/ defibrillator or a prior tunneled dialysis catheter may need a venogram to rule out central stenosis. Congestive heart failure with ejection fraction (EF) <20%, and coagulopathy are contraindications.

Vessel Mapping

Assessment of vascular anatomy and patency should be performed to determine if the patient is a candidate for pAVF creation. Criteria for pAVF eligibility depend upon the device used but are similar for both WavelinQ and Ellipsys systems. Vein mapping is done with a tourniquet.

Eligible candidates using the WavelinQ system must have cephalic and basilic vein with diameters ≥2.5 mm, a patent perforator with diameter ≥2 mm, brachial artery and vein with diameter ≥2 mm, an ulnar artery/vein pair with diameter ≥2 mm, or a radial artery/vein pair with diameter ≥2 mm. Additionally, there must be <2 mm of separation between the target vessels. These vessels must not be tortuous. Multiple sites including the brachial artery/vein, ulnar artery/vein, or radial artery/vein can be used to introduce the WavelinQ catheters if they are sufficiently wide (≥2 mm).

With the Ellipsys system, eligible patients must have a PRA and a straight perforator vein with diameter ≥2 mm and with <1.5 mm of separation between the target artery and vein. Proximity of vessels is paramount to a successful AVF creation due to the mechanism of the Ellipsys system (i.e., a single and direct puncture of the adjacent target vessels).

Other things to be aware of during mapping are:[12]

- Depth of the superficial veins—in anticipation of superficialization
- Antecubital vein anatomy and its variants
- Perforator veins and its variants
- Is there a high brachial bifurcation? The radial artery is more mobile and difficult to cannulate with the Ellipsys system in this case.
- Note aberrant branches or anatomic variations of brachial artery.
- Identify the recurrent radial artery (to avoid targeting it).

Transmural calcification of the artery at the site of the anastomosis: This will result in technical failure.[13] At the present time, it is unclear what degree of calcification presets a problem.[13] Compressible arteries with mild or moderate intimal or medial calcification may be considered.[14]

Evidence of competitive flow: Are deep brachial veins larger in diameter than superficial veins?

Besides this, one must also perform:

- A Barbeau test to confirm a patent palmar arch
- Blood pressure measurements in both arms to rule out proximal artery stenosis

Generally, 25–30% of patients have unsuitable anatomy for either of the two devices.[15] The primary limiting factors are perforator vein size and patency of superficial veins.[16]

Procedure

Percutaneous AVF creation is performed with local anesthesia and moderate sedation (midazolam and fentanyl). A brachial plexus block is preferred but not essential. It induces arterial and venous dilation and reduces spasm. Additionally, brachial plexus block may also minimize patient discomfort and prevent elbow flexion (from neuromuscular excitation) during the radiofrequency (RF) pulse application with the WavelinQ system. Elbow flexion results in catheter movement and misalignment leading to pseudoaneurysm formation and inability to create the anastomosis.[7] The arm may also be immobilized with a dedicated arm board and Velcro straps to prevent elbow flexion. The nerve block also minimizes IV analgesia requirements.[13]

WavelinQ

Using the WavelinQ system, the brachial artery and vein in the mid-upper arm are accessed using a micro puncture kit. One should exhibit caution to avoid stimulation or cause injury to the median nerve in this area. Thereafter, 6 Fr vascular sheaths are inserted into the brachial artery and vein. An arteriogram is performed to study the anatomy **(Fig. 3)**. A guidewire is passed through both vessels and directed toward the ulnar artery and vein (or radial artery and vein) with the aid of an angled catheter. The short segment of the ulnar artery between the brachial artery bifurcation and the origin of the interosseus artery (i.e., common ulnar artery) is the location for an ulnar–ulnar

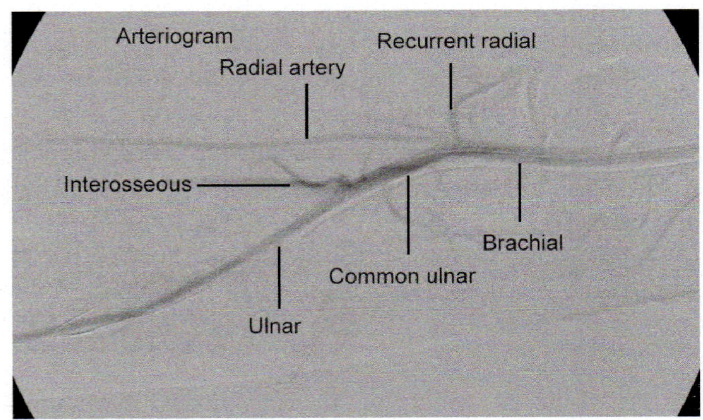

Fig. 3: Arteriogram showing arterial branches of the upper extremity.

pAVF.[7] This fistula is preferred by some operators, as the proximity of the ulnar vein to the perforator vein may improve flow to the superficial venous system. Advancing the wire using a brachial approach may also prove challenging due to the presence of venous valves. As such, using a stiffer guidewire may aid in navigation.

Alternatively, when using a *4 Fr* system (this was developed to enhance safety and allow for access of smaller vessels), catheters can be inserted from the wrist through either the ulnar artery/vein or the radial artery/vein. An antiparallel approach via brachial artery and radial or ulnar veins can also be done.

Once the arterial and venous catheters are positioned at the creation site, magnets in both the catheters help align them. Precise alignment is achieved with microadjustments of the catheter and confirmed with an orthogonal view. Once aligned, a spring-loaded RF electrode in the venous catheter is activated which momentarily contacts the ceramic backstop on the arterial catheter to form the fistula. The RF pulse takes only 0.7 seconds and causes a momentary spasm of the arm. This results in 5 mm × 1 mm side-to-side anastomosis.[9] An arteriography is repeated once the anastomosis is formed confirming technical success and ruling out extravasation. The lateral brachial vein, just central to the perforator vein, is often coil (6–8 mm diameter, 7–15 cm length) embolized at this point to aid in flow diversion to the superficial veins.[13] The decision is subjective and based on observed flow patterns on the postcreation angiogram.[13] Flow in the brachial artery should be >400–500 cc/min (per original studies) but now operators are aiming for >800 cc/min.[14] The other important consideration besides flow is that the spectral doppler should show low-resistance waveforms **(Figs. 4A and B)**. Once the sheaths are removed, vessels are manually compressed with brachial artery needing 15 minutes while veins needing 5 minutes.[13]

A benefit of the WavelinQ AVF is that it spares the proximal vessels enabling an Ellipsys device pAVF. Another benefit is the option of choosing between three creation sites, especially for those with vascular calcification, tortuous perforator, or need for vessel preservation.[17] The challenging task of this device is getting into the wrist veins and traversing venous valves retogradely.[13,17]

Ellipsys

With the Ellipsys system, the median basilic or cephalic vein is accessed in the distal upper extremity with a micropuncture kit. A guidewire is inserted through a *6 Fr* vascular sheath and navigated into the perforator vein. The guidewire and sheath are positioned adjacent to the PRA to facilitate direct puncture. A micropuncture needle is advanced from the perforator into the PRA followed by the guidewire. The Ellipsys catheter is then advanced over the guidewire into the PRA. Upon activation, thermal energy is delivered by the catheter which results in the formation of a 4 mm × 2 mm elliptical anastomosis between the perforator vein and PRA.[18] Angioplasty of the anastomosis and perforator is then performed using a 4 or 5 mm × 2 cm balloon. This was found to resolve spasm and reduce early thrombosis rate, the number of maturation procedures, and the time to maturation.[19] The entire procedure is done under ultrasound (US). Brachial artery flow has been alluded to above.

There is no need to provide antiplatelet agents post-procedure.

LEARNING CURVE AND PROCEDURE TIME

It takes 5–10 cases to become comfortable with both devices.[20] The average procedure time is less with the Ellipsys device (15–20 minutes vs. 60–80 minutes with WavelinQ).[21]

COMPLICATIONS

Complication rates are small ranging from 3 to 8% with WavelinQ.[7,9] They were largely related to brachial artery access using the 6 Fr system.[18] These include pseudoaneurysm formation of brachial artery (1–3%; **Fig. 5**), brachial artery periarterial hematoma (6%), brachial artery dissection (1–2%), brachial artery thrombus (3%), and one case of fistula formation between brachial artery and vein. Other complications include device breakage (3%), closure device embolization (3%), and steal syndrome (1–2%).

2.5% device-related complications and 5.8% procedure-related complications have been noted with the 4 Fr WavelinQ system.[17] No arterial or venous access complications were noted and the frequency of brachial artery complications was lower compared to the 6 Fr system.[17]

A complication rate of 0–2.5% has been reported with the Ellipsys device.[22] They have mainly occurred with a single group of authors.[18]

FOLLOW-UP AND CLINICAL MATURITY

Follow-up after creation is important to ensure maturity. Initial follow-up varies but is usually at 2 weeks when flow

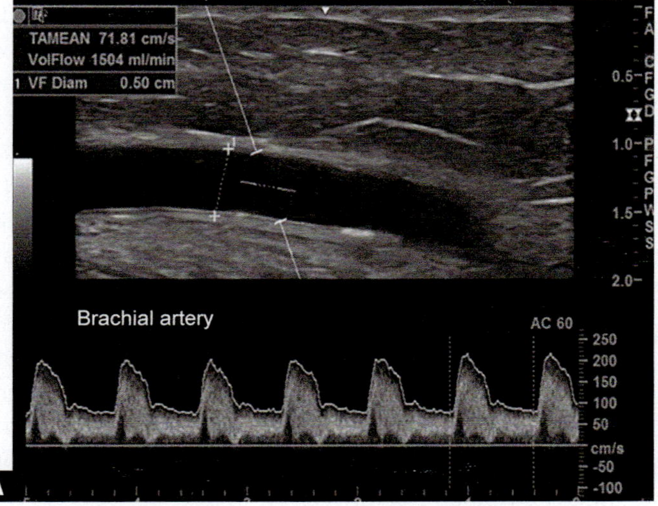

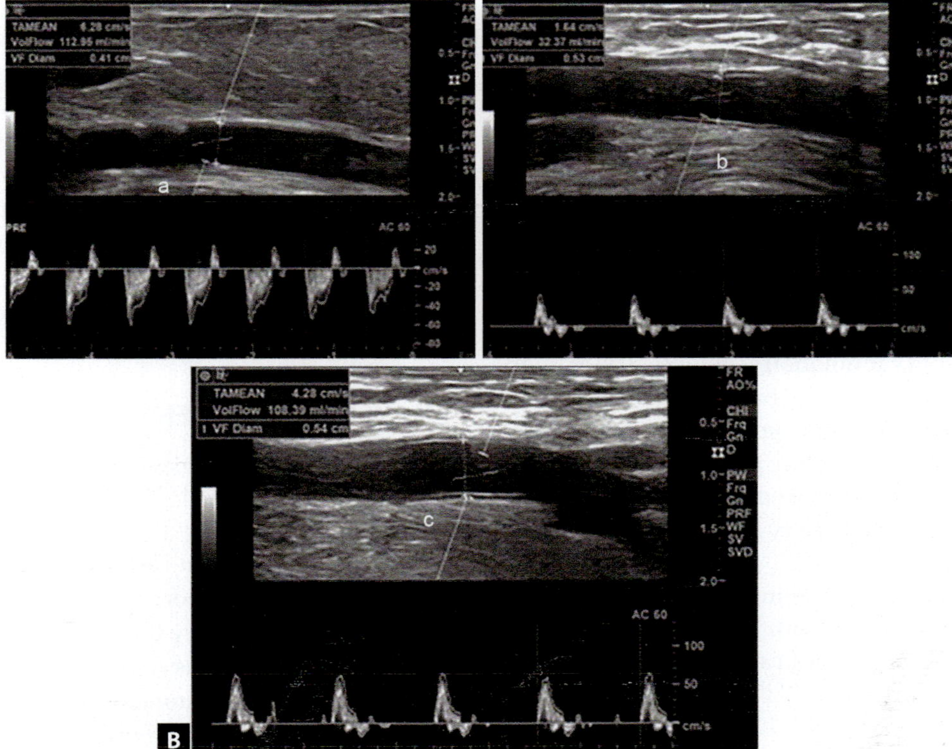

Figs. 4A and B: (A) Example of low-resistance waveform after fistula creation (monophasic with prolonged downstroke in late systole and diastole with pan-diastolic forward flow); (B) a, b, c: Examples of high-resistance waveforms: Sharp upstroke and brisk downstroke biphasic waveform with diastolic reversal of flow.

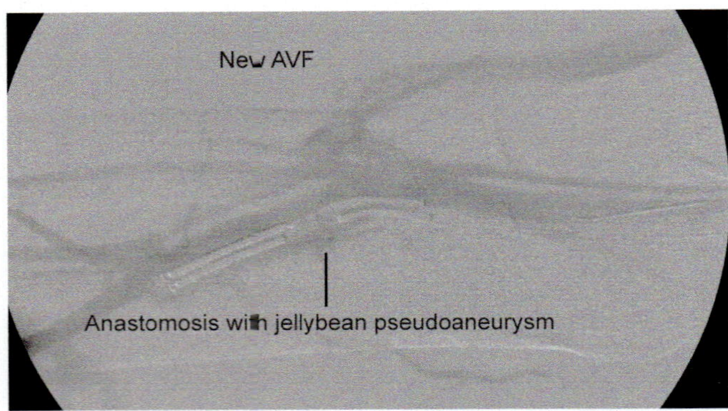

Fig. 5: WavelinQ pAVF creation with a pseudoaneurysm. (AVF: arteriovenous fistula)

in the brachial artery, deep brachial veins, and outflow superficial veins as well as depth and diameter are noted. If brachial blood flow is <400–500 mL/min immediately after creation, then follow-up is in 1 week with angioplasty of the inflow. This is a juxta-anastomotic stenosis of the perforator which directs flow into the deep venous system or a preanastomotic stenosis of the artery.[22]

If brachial artery flow >1 L/min but target vein cephalic vein has <500 mL/min flow, then coil a brachial vein (brachial veins may have flow >200–300 mL/min, diameter >4 mm) or band the median basilic vein.[13] If the target vein is the basilic vein, then band the median cephalic vein or band one of the brachial veins. If the target vein is <5 mm, then consider balloon-assisted maturation (BAM) with a 6 mm balloon. If depth >6 mm, then consider transposition or lipectomy. Follow-up is in 1–2 weeks after each maturation procedure.

pAVF is suitable for cannulation when the cannulation segment is 5 mm in diameter, depth <6 mm, with brachial artery flow of >500 mL/min for a single outflow vein and >700 mL/min for split cannulation segments. The primary end points in the pivotal studies (brachial artery >500 mL/min, target vein diameter 4 mm) were found unsuitable for two needle cannulations in many practices and needed a combination of maturation procedures and transposition to further increase brachial artery flow and vein diameter while decreasing depth.[19]

Generally, dual outflow systems take longer to mature (up to 10 weeks) versus that with a single outflow (up to 6 weeks). The number of maturation interventions per patient-year range from 0.2 to 2.7.[18]

PATENCY RATES AND DURABILITY

For the Ellipsys system, primary patency (time to first secondary procedure) rates at 1 year are low (54%) simply because of additional procedures to mature the fistula.[22] Maturation procedures are performed in 67% of patients.[23] The mean time to maturation is 40 days.[23]

5-year follow-up data of the pivotal Ellipsys population (n = 107) reveal that the fistulas have good functional patency and are durable with low procedure rates to maintain functional patency.[19] The assisted primary patency rates (time to first thrombosis) at 1, 2, and 5 years are 81%, 79%, and 74%, respectively. Secondary/cumulative patency rates (time to abandonment) at 1, 2, and 5 years are 89.5%, 88.4%, and 82%, respectively. Functional patency rate (ability to cannulate with two needles and perform hemodialysis) was 92% throughout the 5 years. Maintenance procedures were needed to treat complications from sustained use. Fistula dysfunction and cannulation injury were predominant in the inflow and cannulation zones. Thrombosis (6%) occurred more often in patients with single outflow vein. Arm swelling (5%) occurred in those with central vein stenosis. The number of procedures per patient year was 0.32 (excluding maturation procedures). Primary failure rate is 3%.[23]

A primary patency rate of 69% at 1 year was noted in the pivotal NEAT trial.[9] 2-year data is now available for the 4 Fr WavelinQ system (n = 112).[13] Maturation procedures are performed in 45% of patients. Cumulative patency rates at 1 and 2 years are 94% and 91.7%, respectively. Functional patency rates at 1 and 2 years are 95.7% and 92.7%, respectively. Maintenance procedures were predominantly angioplasty followed by thrombectomies. The number of procedures per patient-year was 0.51 (excluding maturation procedures). The median time to maturation is 95 days (51–231 days). The primary failure rate is 10%.

NEW DEVELOPMENTS

There are two other catheter-based pAVF techniques that are being developed. The one that is further along at this point is the Velocity (Venova Medical) which relies on delivering an implant through a single venous access at the junction of the perforator vein and the PRA that allows distal radial artery flow but also at the same time excludes the deep venous circulation allowing more rapid maturation with fewer interventions.

The second device is the ePATH (Pathfinder Medical) system. This system is still in its early phase of development. It requires an arterial and venous access leading to the deep venous system of the forearm followed by sharp needle canalization of the artery from the vein with the help of a curved needle and a homing device. Balloon angioplasty is used to create a track between the artery and the vein.

Another technique that has been described involves accessing the median cubital vein and tracking the needle down through the perforator vein to the PRA where it is cannulated. Once the PRA has been cannulated, angioplasty with a balloon is used to create a track fistula. Another similar technique, called *VAST HD* (Venous Arterialization Simplified Technique for percutaneous HemoDialysis access), requires the use of snares in the artery and vein and then percutaneously passing a 21G needle through the open snares. A guidewire is then passed through the needle. The needle is removed, and each snare grabs each end of the wire to bring it out through sheaths. A 3.5 mm × 40 mm balloon is then passed over the guidewire to angioplasty the anastomosis.[24]

CONCLUSION

Percutaneous AVF is an exciting innovation that has expanded anatomic options for fistula creation. Preprocedural wait times are short and these can be performed by trained interventional nephrologists. These fistulas overcome many of the issues noted with surgical fistulas while offering additional cannulation sites. They do not interfere with the creation of future surgical fistulas. Success depends on proper patient selection and follow up. These fistulas tend to have lower primary patency rates but high secondary patency rates. Primary failure rate is much lower compared to surgical fistulas. Next generation devices have made their entrance. They hope to overcome some of the technical issues noted with first generation devices.

REFERENCES

1. Beathard GA, Litchfield T, Jennings WC. Two-year cumulative patency of endovascular arteriovenous fistula. J Vasc Access. 2020;21(3):350-6.
2. Quencer KB, Arici M. Arteriovenous Fistulas and Their Characteristic Sites of Stenosis. Am J Roentgenol. 2015;205(4):726-34.
3. Xu W, Lu G, Tang W, Gong L, Lu J. Comparison of different anastomosis angles in radiocephalic fistula with modified functional end-to-side anastomosis. Int Urol Nephrol. 2023;55(12):3237-43.
4. Yang CY, Li MC, Lan CW, Lee WJ, Lee CJ, Wu CH, et al. The Anastomotic Angle of Hemodialysis Arteriovenous Fistula Is Associated With Flow Disturbance at the Venous Stenosis Location on Angiography. Front Bioeng Biotechnol. 2020;8:846.
5. Loesch A, Dashwood MR. Vasa vasorum inside out/ outside in communication: a potential role in the patency of saphenous vein coronary artery bypass grafts. J Cell Commun Signal. 2018;12(4):631-43.
6. Xiaohe W, Yuanyuan Z, Zhen L, Guocun H. A modified no-touch technique for anastomosis to create a radiocephalic arteriovenous fistula. J Vasc Surg Cases Innov Tech. 2021;7(4):686-90.
7. Rajan DK, Ebner A, Desai SB, Rios JM, Cohn WE. Percutaneous creation of an arteriovenous fistula for hemodialysis access. J Vasc Interv Radiol. 2015;26(4):484-90.
8. Radosa CG, Radosa JC, Weiss N, Schmidt C, Werth S, Hofmockel T, et al. Endovascular Creation of an Arteriovenous Fistula (endoAVF) for Hemodialysis Access: First Results. Cardiovasc Interv Radiol. 2017;40(10):1545-51.
9. Lok CE, Rajan DK, Clement J, Kiaii M, Sidhu R, Thomson K, et al. Endovascular Proximal Forearm Arteriovenous Fistula for Hemodialysis Access: Results of the Prospective, Multicenter Novel Endovascular Access Trial (NEAT). Am J Kidney Dis. 2017;70(4):486-97.
10. Berland TL, Clement J, Griffin J, Westin GG, Ebner A. Endovascular Creation of Arteriovenous Fistulae for Hemodialysis Access with a 4 Fr Device: Clinical Experience from the EASE Study. Ann Vasc Surg. 2019;60:182-92.
11. Abdel Aal AK, Jefferson X, Klusman C, Garcia L, Hassanein H, Abdel Aal T, et al. Devices and Techniques for Percutaneous Creation of Dialysis Arteriovenous Fistulas. Semin Interv Radiol. 2022;39(1):66-74.
12. Khawaja AZ, Tullett KAJ, Jones RG, Inston NG. Preoperative assessment for percutaneous and open surgical arteriovenous fistula creation in patients for haemodialysis. Clin Kidney J. 2021;14(1):408-17.
13. Klein E, Repko B, Alvarez A, Inston N, Jones R, Rajan DK. Multi-Center Two-Year Patency Outcomes of Endovascular Arteriovenous Fistulas (endoAVF) Created with a 4 French System. Cardiovasc Interv Radiol. 2024;47(8):1045-54.
14. Wasse H, Alvarez AC, Brouwer-Maier D, Hull JE, Balamuthusamy S, Litchfield TF, et al. Patient selection, education, and cannulation of percutaneous arteriovenous fistulae: An ASDIN White Paper. J Vasc Access. 2020;21(6): 810-7.
15. Wasse H. Place of Percutaneous Fistula Devices in Contemporary Management of Vascular Access. Clin J Am Soc Nephrol. 2019;14(6):938-40.
16. Popli K, Dittman JM, Amendola MF, Plum J, Newton DH. Anatomic suitability for commercially available percutaneous arteriovenous fistula creation systems. J Vasc Surg. 2021;73(3):999-1004.
17. Berland T, Clement J, Inston N, Kreienberg P, Ouriel K, Wavelin QFI. Percutaneous arteriovenous fistula creation

with the 4F WavelinQ EndoAVF System. J Vasc Surg. 2022;75(3):1038-46.e3.
18. Choinski KN, Sundick SA, Rao AG, Ting W, Faries PL, Tadros RO. The Current Role of the Percutaneous Arteriovenous Fistula for Hemodialysis Access. Surg Technol Int. 2020; 37:217-24.
19. Hull JE, Jennings WC, Cooper RI, Narayan R, Mawla N, Decker MD. Long-Term Results from the Pivotal Multicenter Trial of Ultrasound-Guided Percutaneous Arteriovenous Fistula Creation for Hemodialysis Access. J Vasc Interv Radiol. 2022;33(10):1143-50.
20. Shahverdyan R, Beathard G, Mushtaq N, Litchfield TF, Nelson PR, Jennings WC. Comparison of Outcomes of Percutaneous Arteriovenous Fistulae Creation by Ellipsys and WavelinQ Devices. J Vasc Interv Radiol. 2020;31(9):1365-72.
21. Lie G, Ahmed N, Shah N, Eleti S, Lam S, Elsaadany A, et al. Adapting a Dialysis Service for Delivery of Percutaneous Arteriovenous Fistulas. Radiographics. 2022;42(6):1795-811.
22. Mallios A, Bourquelot P, Franco G, Hebibi H, Fonkoua H, Allouache M, et al. Midterm results of percutaneous arteriovenous fistula creation with the Ellipsys Vascular Access System, technical recommendations, and an algorithm for maintenance. J Vasc Surg. 2020;72(6):2097-106.
23. Hull J, Deitrick J, Groome K. Maturation for Hemodialysis in the Ellipsys Post-Market Registry. J Vasc Interv Radiol. 2020;31(9):1373-81.
24. Lobato M, Hernandez Vaquero JA, Fonseca JL. Percutaneous endovascular arteriovenous fistula creation for hemodialysis access using "off-the-shelf" conventional devices. J Vasc Surg Cases Innov Tech. 2020;6(4):664-5.

10.2B ENDOVASCULAR ARTERIOVENOUS FISTULAS: OPTIONS, MAINTENANCE, AND SALVAGE

Sarvanan Balamuthuswamy, Vijayaprakash Sreenarasimhaiah

INTRODUCTION

Surgically created arteriovenous fistulas (AVFs) were the preferred arteriovenous access for initiating and maintaining hemodialysis in end-stage kidney disease patients. AVF creation has traditionally been tasked with vascular surgeons, though a few nephrologists perform surgically created fistulas. Hence, there was a need to create AVFs with a percutaneous modality that could increase the number of operators who create fistulas.

The concept of pAVF creations was based on the unique anatomy of the perforator veins in the upper extremity. A comprehensive review of the forearm venous anatomy is important to understand the logic behind the flow dynamics in an pAVF. Perforating veins are communications between the extremities' superficial and deep venous systems. There are 9–16 perforating veins in each upper extremity, and several perforator veins disappear in the muscles. The perforators that are in consideration for an pAVF are those that communicate between the radial and ulnar veins and the cephalic and basilic veins. The deep veins (radial and ulnar veins) communicate through these perforators to the cephalic and basilic veins; the radial veins usually communicate with the cephalic venous system, and the ulnar venae communicate with the basilic system. The concept of pAVFs was to create a side-to-side anastomosis between the radial or ulnar artery and one of its venue commitments with flow directed from the deep veins through the proximal forearm perforators to the upper arm superficial veins. The flow into the upper arm veins is limited by the same factors that determine flow in a maturing AVF, including the flow in the radial artery, the diameter of the perforator vein, and the length of the deep vein and the perforator vein before it feeds into the more prominent cephalic or basilic vein.

IMPORTANCE OF VESSEL MAPPING

A detailed vessel mapping using ultrasound is critical before planning for the procedure. The general recommendations on venous diameters are 2 mm for the radial or ulnar vein at the point of anastomosis creation, 2 mm for the perforator vein, and 2.5 mm for the outflow cephalic and basilic veins. The radial and ulnar arteries are recommended to be >2 mm and the brachial artery to be 4 mm or more. The perforator vein should communicate directly from the radial or ulnar veins to the superficial venous system. In addition to a comprehensive ultrasound vein mapping, there could be additional information if a venogram is done from the radial or ulnar vein to assess the preferential flow into the superficial veins instead of the deep venous system in the upper extremities **(Figs. 1A and B)**. If the flow is not seen preferentially in the superficial system without occluding the brachial veins, there would be a high likelihood that brachial venous embolization might be needed eventually for maturation **(Figs. 2A and B)**.[1]

LIMITATIONS OF CURRENT TECHNOLOGY IN CREATING pAVF

Heat energy is a common denominator in both Food and Drug Administration (FDA)-approved techniques for creating pavers. Heat-induced vessel spasms have been reported in the arteries and the perianastomotic deep vein, limiting forward flow into the upper arm cephalic veins. The other reported complications include arterial rupture, hematomas, and hand swelling from increased

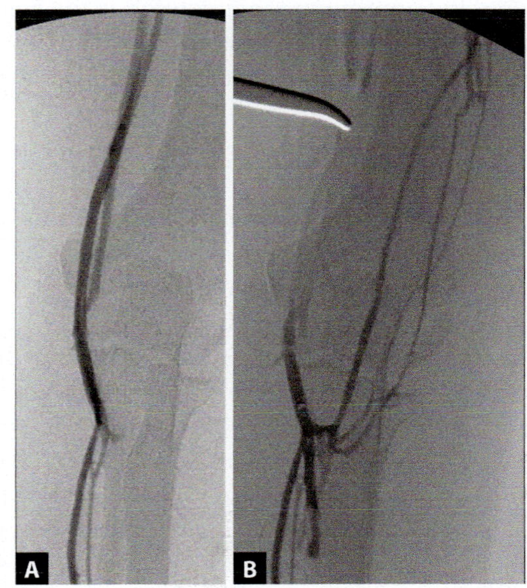

Figs. 1A and B: (A) Venogram performed from the radial vein with preferential flow into the upper arm deep venous system; (B) Venogram with brachial venous occlusion.

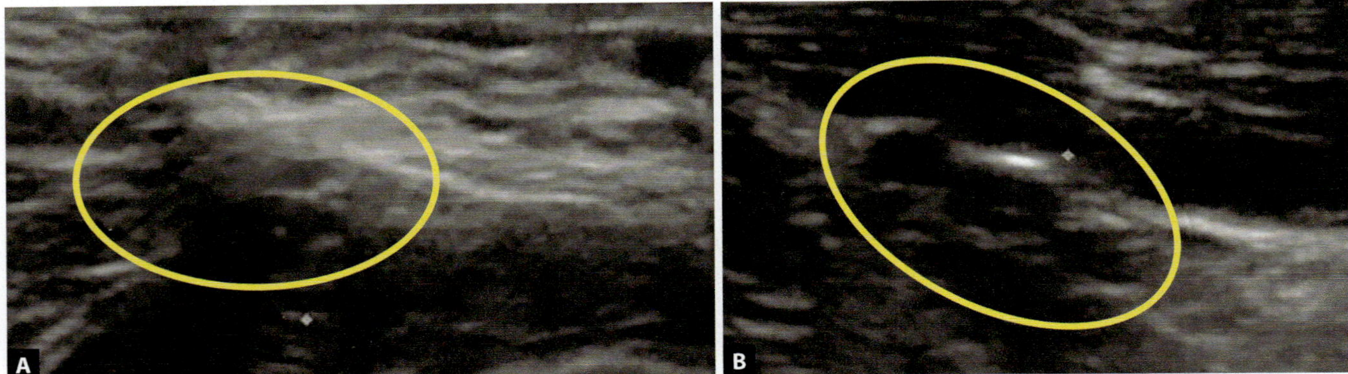

Figs. 2A and B: Paired radial and ulnar veins, and venae comitantes.

retrograde venous flow. The most common side effect was hematoma at the brachial artery cannulation site for the WavelinQ device prior to the approval of the 4 Fr system. An average of two to three interventions are required during the first year after access creation for maturation efforts, which include embolization of the brachial veins, ligation of the proximal basilic vein, superficialization of the cephalic or basilic veins, venous angioplasty of the anastomosis, and deep venous stenosis. Hence, there has been a need to explore newer pAVF techniques that do not utilize heat to create AV anastomosis.

Maturation Assistance of pAVF

After creating the pAVF, regular follow-up with ultrasound evaluation and appropriate intervention is the lynchpin for facilitating the timely maturation of AVF. The minimal maturation criteria required to attempt cannulation of the pAVF for hemodialysis include:

- Brachial artery flow volume >800 mL/min for multiple target venous outflow
- Brachial artery flow volume >500 mL/min for single target venous outflow
- Target cannulating vein diameter ≥5 mm
- Target cannulating vein depth <5 mm

After the creation of pAVF, an ultrasound duplex evaluation is performed before discharging the patient to obtain the baseline values. The patient needs to be seen about 1–2 weeks after the initial creation of AVF and assessed with ultrasound to obtain volume flow in the brachial artery as well as the superficial target veins in the arm and if indicated in the brachial veins, especially for the WavelinQ AVF. The flow volumes obtained in the artery and veins are based on the assumption that artery inflow = venous outflow; hence, the arterial flow value should approximately match the sum of the venous outflow values. The depth of the target vein also needs to be measured to assess the feasibility of cannulation with dialysis needles. Thereafter, the follow-up depends on the maturation process and the need for intervention, on an average every 2–4 weeks until the AVF can be used for hemodialysis by cannulating using two 16- or 15-gauge needles **(Flowchart 1)**.

pAVF interventions are performed preferably via the arterial approach with the insertion of slender 5–6 Fr sheaths into the retrograde direction via the distal radial or ulnar arteries depending on the site of anastomosis or in the antegrade direction via the brachial artery segment in the distal arm region. Angioplasty balloons of size 5–6 mm diameter ranging from compliant balloons to high-pressure noncompliant balloons as well as cutting balloons can be used depending on the severity and extent of the stenosis. Interventions like coil embolization for obliterating the competing veins are usually approached via the superficial outflow veins or the deep veins like the brachial, ulnar, or radial veins. If the target veins are located at a deeper plain >5 mm, superficialization with either surgical technique or using percutaneous liposuction technique will facilitate easy cannulation of the target veins without causing any infiltration hematoma.

Cannulation of pAVF

The ultimate success for an pAVF creation is the end-point ability to use the fistula for hemodialysis with the insertion of two needles **(Figs. 3 and 4)**. The ability to effectively cannulate and use the pAVF for hemodialysis is as important as executing the endovascular techniques successfully to create the access itself. The cannulation technique varies to a considerable extent and can be quite

Flowchart 1: Basic algorithm for follow-up evaluation of pAVF.

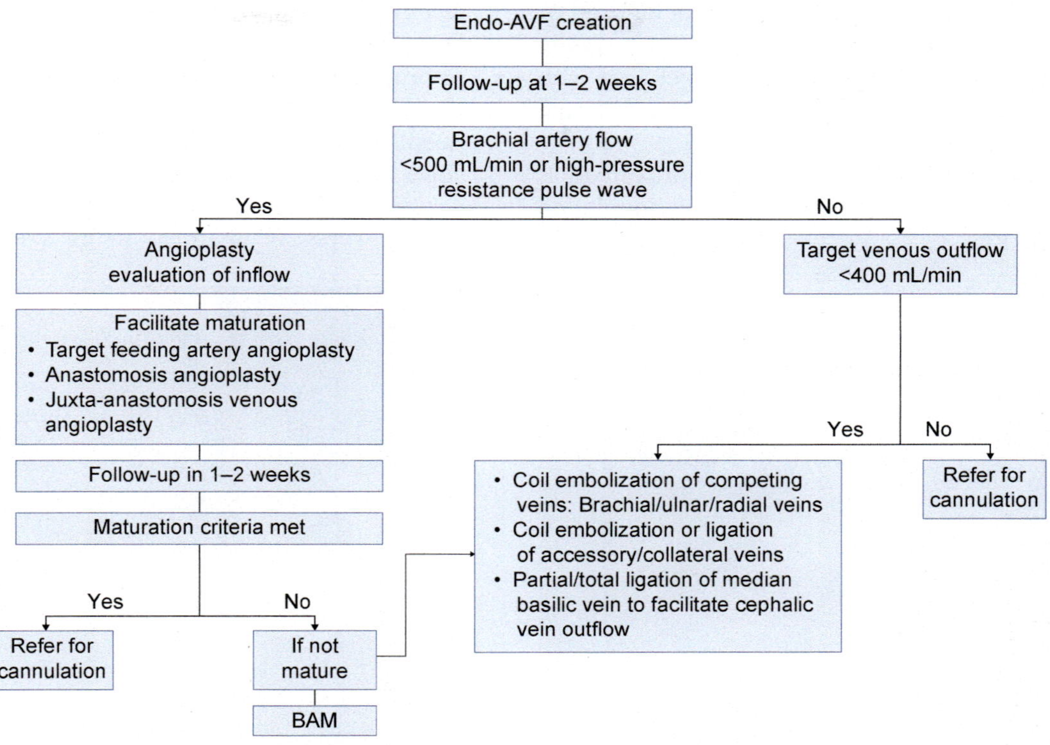

(AVF: arteriovenous fistula; BAM: balloon-assisted maturation)

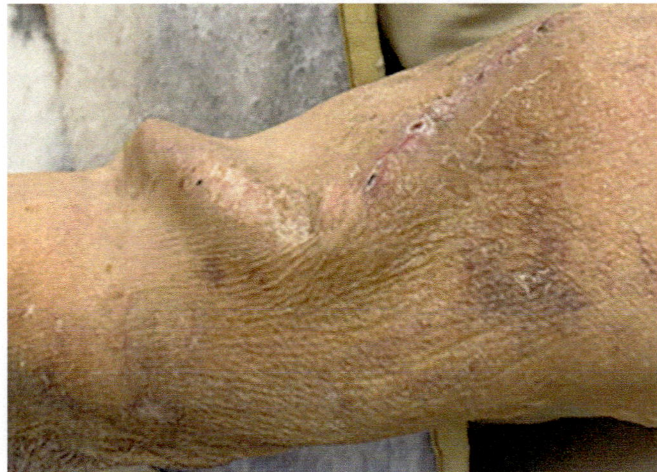

Fig. 3: Surgically created B-C AVF.
(AVF: arteriovenous fistula; B-C: brachiocephalic)

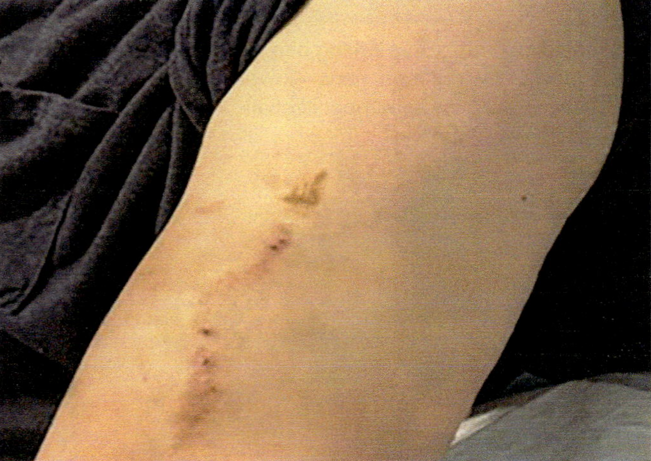

Fig. 4: WavelinQ ulnar pAVF with cephalic vein outflow.

challenging compared to the traditional surgically created AVF (sAVF).

The novel pAVF differs considerably from the traditional sAVF in the following aspects:

- pAVF is usually a low-flow access.
- It lacks surgical marks or scars as landmarks.
- Target veins of pAVF are not readily visible.
- Physical examination features are usually more subtle.

CANNULATION TECHNIQUES

The following guidelines are helpful in achieving successful two-needle cannulation for hemodialysis:

- Assessing maturation and marking the cannulation zones or targets. A skin-marking pen can be used or *henna* can be applied over the target vein to guide cannulation **(Fig. 5)**. Photos of the target area with marking can be stored in the smart phone and shared with the cannulation dialysis staff **(Fig. 6)**.
- *Use of tourniquet:* Applying tourniquet proximally is imperative to augment the target vein for cannulation **(Figs. 7 and 8)**.
- *Cannulating at a shallow angle of 25–35°:* Following this technique is crucial in preventing backwall infiltration **(Figs. 9A and B)**.
- Appropriate length and type of cannulation needles. Many of these fistulas require the use of short-length needles like 3/5" long needle, especially while using superficial veins in the arm and target veins present across the elbow region or in the proximal forearm region. Types of needles—using a flexible plastic

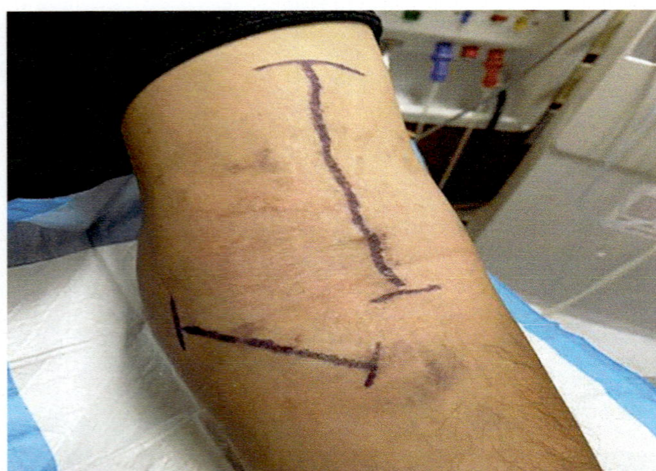

Fig. 5: Marking with skin-marking pen. WavelinQ ulnar pAVF with marked target cannulation veins—lower median basilic venous segment across elbow and upper cephalic venous segment.

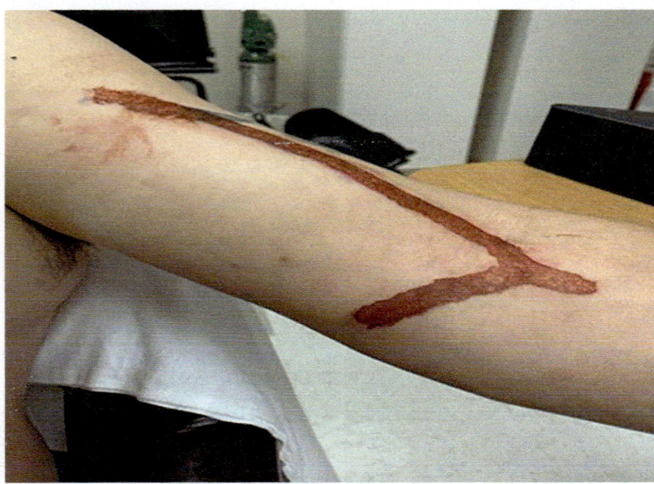

Fig. 6: Marking by applying henna. Ellipsys pAVF with marked target cannulation veins—lower median basilic venous segment across elbow and upper cephalic venous segment.

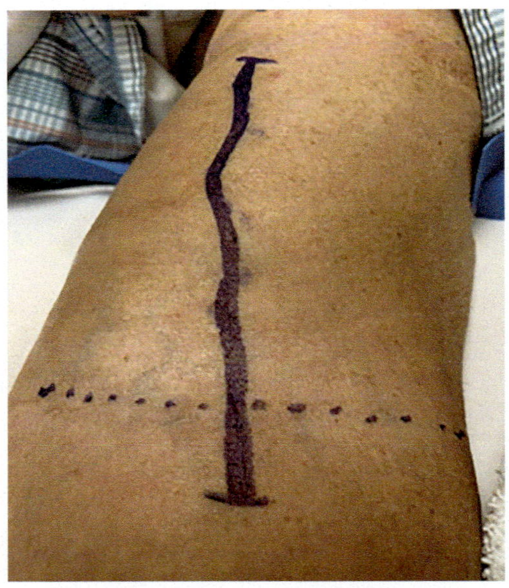

Fig. 7: WavelinQ ulnar pAVF with cephalic vein outflow (Without torniquet).

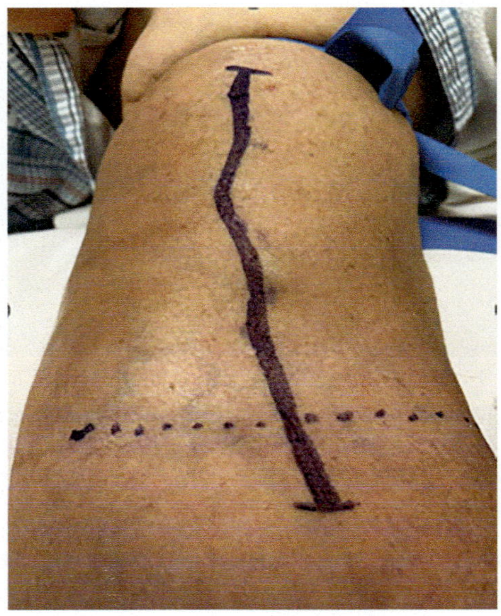

Fig. 8: WavelinQ ulnar pAVF with cephalic vein outflow. With torniquet.

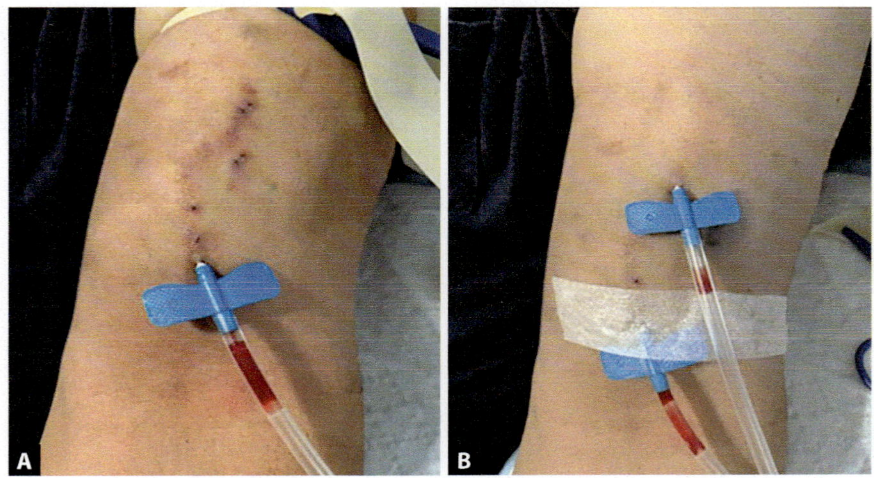

Figs. 9A and B: (A) Shallow angle cannulation using short-length needles; (B) WavelinQ ulnar pAVF with cephalic vein outflow—shallow angle cannulation.

cannulation needle has advantage over metal needles, it being safe with far less complications.

- Applying only gentle pressure while cannulating; otherwise, the use of high pressure will result in backwall infiltration and hematoma formation.
- Graduated approach to cannulation by using larger gauge to lower gauge needles.
- Rope ladder and buttonhole techniques are the usual methods for cannulation, with the buttonhole technique having a better advantage while cannulating at unconventional locations.
- Ultrasound guidance during cannulation provides a much-added advantage, which can lower the complications to a great extent with the pocket point-of-care ultrasound (POCUS) device being an important tool for the successful cannulation of pAVF.
- *Using lower pump speed:* Dialing down the hemodialysis pump speed can be done to avoid endovascular trauma and hematoma.

CANNULATION CHALLENGES

Since pAVFs do not have a scar that is seen in sAVFs and are non-high-flow fistulas, dialysis technicians could find it challenging to cannulate them. Cannulation injuries and infiltrations are not uncommon during the initial cannulations on some patients. Cannulation experts have been employed by the two companies that offer these devices to train technicians in dialysis clinics. These cannulation experts have hand-held ultrasounds to find the vein and cannulate them with reasonable success.

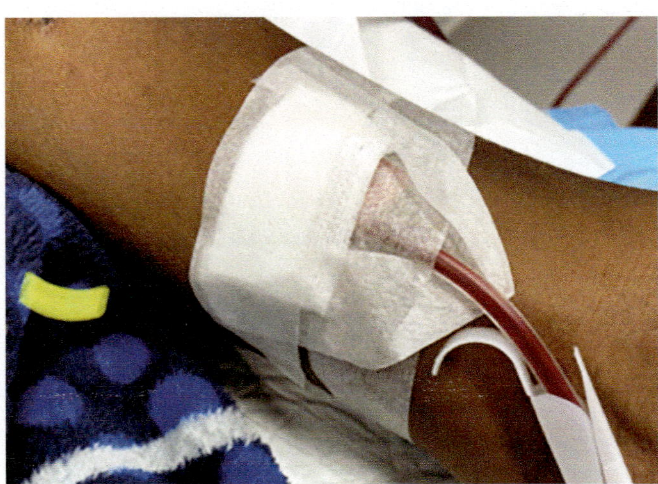

Fig. 10: Successful cannulation of the pAVF.

Hence, while there are new technologies to create AVFs, the industry would have to commit to resources to sustain the true potential of this new approach **(Figs. 10 to 12)**.

pAVF MONITORING AND TROUBLESHOOTING

Getting an access flow at the brachial artery after creation is recommended. A flow of at least 500 mL/min suggests a successful maturation after creation. Follow-up access ultrasound with flow measurement should be done at 4 weeks if the initial flow is >500 mL/min. If the initial flow is <500 mL/min, a repeat scan would be needed in 2 weeks post creation, and the expectation would be 500 mL/min.

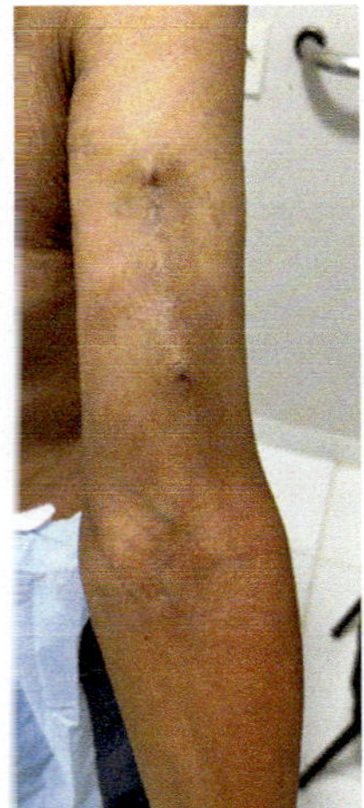

Fig. 11: pAVF 2 years after creation being cannulated with buttonholes on the cephalic vein.

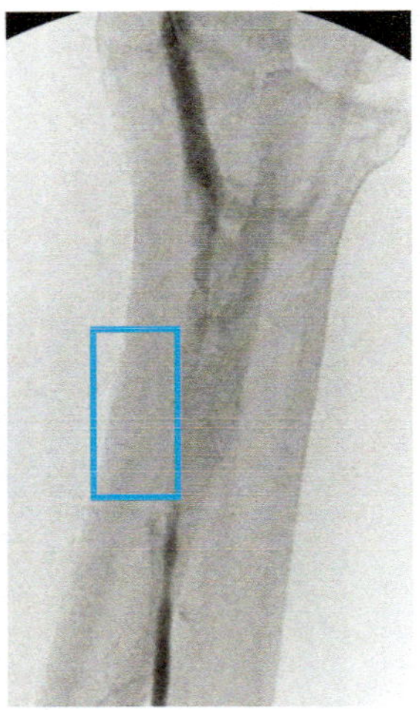

Fig. 13: Deep vein stenosis.

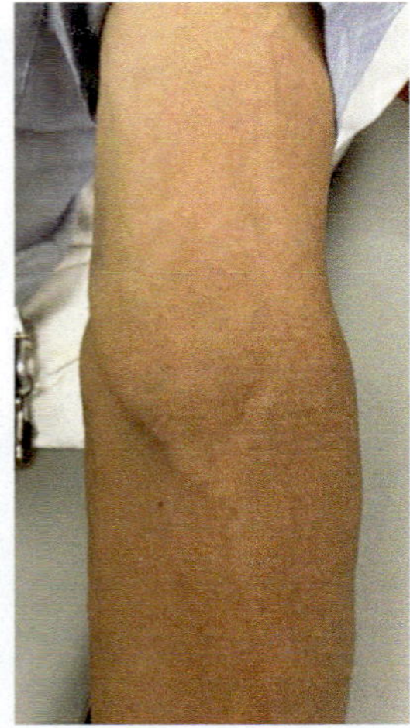

Fig. 12: pAVF with Y cannulation option at the proximal basilic vein and cephalic vein.

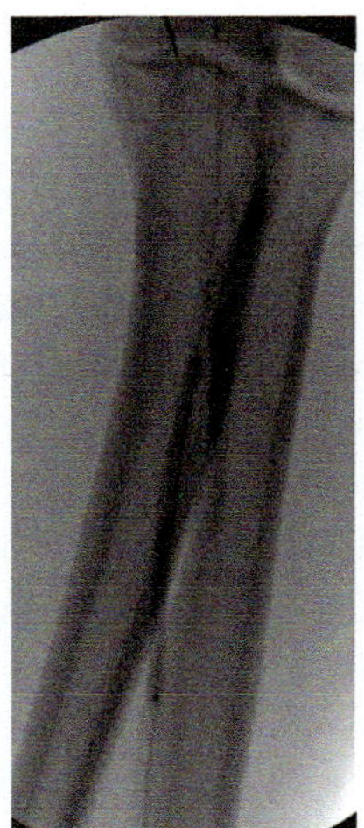

Fig. 14: Balloon angioplasty of deep venous stenosis.

Cannulation readiness ultrasound would be done again in 6 weeks. Most fistulas would achieve cannulation readiness at the end of 6 weeks. If the net brachial arterial flow is >500 mL/min and cephalic or basilic venous system is less than 75% of that flow, there might be more flow diverted into the brachial or retrograde veins. This could be due to deep/perforator vein stenosis or a more direct contiguous flow into the deep veins. This could be addressed with angioplasty of the deep/perforator stenosis with a high-pressure balloon and, at times, a cutting balloon. If there is more dominant flow into the brachial veins, flow could be diverted by embolizing the brachial vein with dominant flow volume. Flow improvement should be appreciated with a 2-week postprocedure ultrasound. If there are cannulation difficulties despite adequate flow, there might be a need to superficialize the cephalic or basilic vein, for which surgical support would be required. Since the anastomosis is at the proximal forearm, a longer venous segment would be available for superficializing and cannulation **(Figs. 13 to 16)**.[2]

MAINTENANCE OF ARTERIOVENOUS FISTULA

Maintenance of a functionally patent AVF for hemodialysis assisted with clinical monitoring and surveillance program is equally important as executing various techniques to successfully create the AVF itself. Most of the AVFs

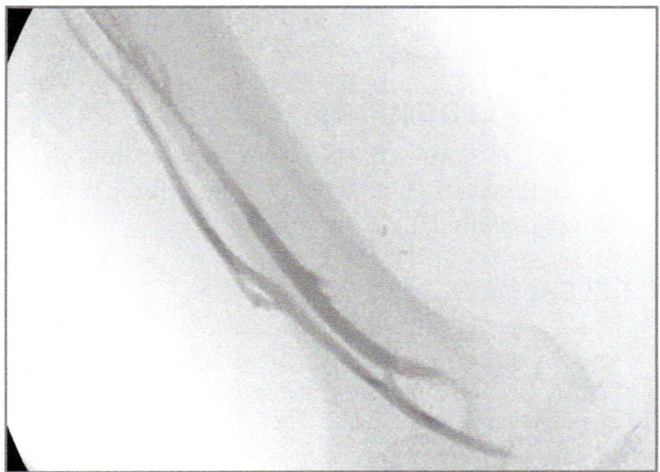

Fig. 15: Angiogram revealing dominant deep venous flow in the paired brachial veins.

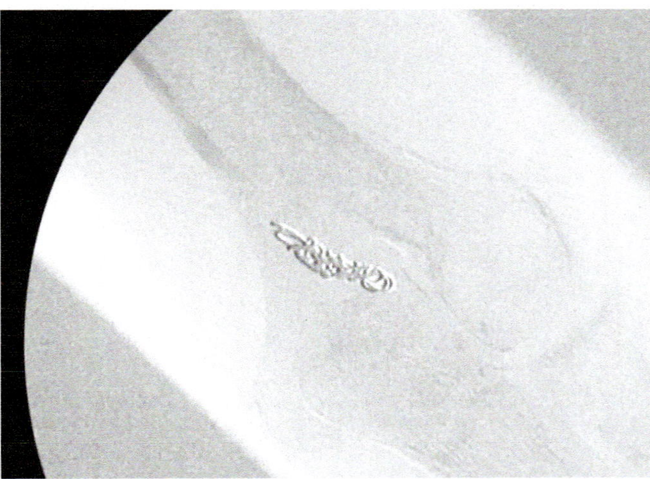

Fig. 16: Embolization done at brachial veins.

with dysfunction have an anatomic problem due to the development of neointimal hyperplasia causing stenosis in the access circuit, which can present as a single lesion or multiple lesions affecting the same access. These stenotic lesions commonly involve the access circuit at the inflow segment (arterial anastomosis and juxta-arterial anastomosis venous segment), venous outflow segment of the AVF due to the disruption in the laminal flow resulting from anatomical variations (cephalic venous arch segment and swing segment angulation involving the transposed basilic venous segment), and at the access cannulation sites due to abnormal remodeling with fibrotic transformation. Being a well-known fact that vascular access dysfunction leads to increased patient morbidity as well as mortality, early detection of AVF dysfunction due to stenosis and timely intervention will help to maintain the functional patency of the access and also prevent the occurrence of access failure with thrombosis.

The AVF function can be evaluated by using clinical monitoring on a regular basis to detect access dysfunction, which can be combined with surveillance methods when indicated to provide additional information. The clinical monitoring used for AVF evaluation includes the use of physical examination of the access, monitoring for clinical problems during dialysis sessions, and monitoring Kt/V values. The surveillance methods available for monitoring include intra-access dynamic blood flow study, measuring static dialysis venous pressure, duplex ultrasound access flow assessment, and using Vasc-Alert (VA) system. The AVF surveillance methods unlike clinical monitoring require specialized equipment, especially trained staff, and repeated measurement to obtain prospective trend analysis rather than using a single isolated abnormal value. Prospective observational studies have consistently demonstrated that physical examination performed by trained personnel is an accurate method for the diagnosis of fistula stenosis. The Kidney Disease Outcomes Quality Initiative (KDOQI) clinical practice guideline for vascular access recommends that physical examination be performed on all mature AVFs routinely on a weekly basis, with such monitoring also being recommended by the Society for Vascular Surgery and, therefore, should be part of all surveillance protocols of the vascular access. Due to the paucity of unequivocal benefits and conflicting data available from observational as well as nonrandomized studies, routine primary surveillance monitoring of AVF followed by pre-emptive angioplasty is currently not recommended without the presence of clinical indicators suggestive of AVF dysfunction. Using a systematic multipronged approach facilitates the evaluation and timely intervention to ensure a prolonged functional survival of the AVF.

WORKFORCE OPTIMIZATION

Since vascular surgeons were the only resource to create AVFs, there is an unrealistic burden and expectation to achieve an optimal start (patients starting hemodialysis with an AVF) rate of over 50%. Less than 20% of patients starting hemodialysis do so with an AVF, and 50% of patients remain on renal replacement therapy (RRT) with a catheter at 6 months since initiation. With this new technique, interventional nephrologists and radiologists could join the workforce that creates AVFs, and that could potentially decrease the burden on vascular surgeons and improve access to high-quality care for our patients.

CONCLUSION

pAVFs are a novel technique for creating AVFs facilitated by two FDA-approved devices. There is an increased need to create more fistulas before initiating RRT as the status quo, even in developed nations. pAVFs are not an alternative to surgically created fistulas. However, optimizing the increased need for better patient care would be an additional technique since the data supports good long-term outcomes. The cost of the catheter can be prohibitive in many parts of the world. However, novel endeavor creation techniques and devices could lower the cost of these procedures for adoption across developing nations.

ACKNOWLEDGMENTS

I would like to thank Dr Mawla for sharing images on vessel mapping and Manu S Bala for performing detailed edits and formatting the script.

REFERENCES

1. Wasse H, Alvarez AC, Brouwer-Maier D, Hull JE, Balamuthusamy S, Litchfield TF, et al. Patient selection, education, and cannulation of percutaneous arteriovenous fistulae: An ASDIN White Paper. J Vasc Access. 2020; 21(6):810-7.
2. Franco G, Mallios A, Bourquelot P, Jennings W, Boura B. Ultrasound evaluation of percutaneously created arteriovenous fistulae between radial artery and perforating vein at the elbow. J Vasc Access. 2020;21(5):694-700.

CHAPTER

11 Arteriovenous Graft Placement

Ambarish Satwik, Pranay Pawar

CASE SCENARIO

A 64-year-old gentleman, a known case of chronic kidney disease for 12 years and a renal transplant failure, presented to the vascular surgery outpatient department (OPD) for an access creation. His access history was a left radiocephalic fistula, a left brachiocephalic fistula, and a right basilic vein transposition. All these accesses functioned well for 2 years each, and ultimately he proceeded for a renal transplant. Unfortunately, his transplant failed 4 months ago. On examination, his axillary veins on both arms were normal and he only had a history of right internal jugular vein (IJV) cannulation for a Permacath 10 years ago. He was undertaken for a left arteriovenous graft surgery with a tapered 4–6 mm × 30 cm expanded polytetrafluoroethylene (ePTFE) graft from the left brachial to left axillary vein. The procedure was uneventful and the graft was deemed usable after 2 weeks.

INTRODUCTION

The aim of permanent hemodialysis access should be to provide repeated access to the circulation with minimal complications. Historically, arteriovenous fistulas (AVFs) were strongly promoted by societal guidelines because of their association with lower mortality, lower complications, and lower costs. The 2019 Kidney Disease Outcomes Quality Initiative (KDOQI) guidelines stated that care decisions surrounding hemodialysis access are often complex and should be individualized to promote patient-centric care using a multidisciplinary team comprised of the treating nephrologist, vascular surgeon, radiologist, and access nurses.[1] This statement challenged the "fistula first" initiative that autogenous AVFs were the best access type due to their high primary failure rate and their usefulness in the high-risk and geriatric population. The use of arteriovenous prosthetic graft (AVG) is usually offered when autogenous vascular accesses are exhausted or when the expected duration of hemodialysis is less than 2 years. This chapter aims to review the AVG, the planning of its placement, the different anatomic locations and types, and the common complications associated with this access.

EVALUATION AND PLANNING

Arteriovenous grafts are made by interposing a graft (prosthetic or biologic) between an artery and a vein. The graft is usually made of a synthetic material, e.g., polytetrafluoroethylene/polyester or decellularized bovine or cadaveric artery. The main benefits of AVGs are a relatively safe and quick surgery with a shorter cannulation time (24 hours to 2 weeks depending on the type of graft material). The disadvantages include and are not limited to lower patency rates as compared to autogenous fistulas, higher infection rates, and higher steal rates leading to distal ischemia.[2]

The patient evaluation for creation of an AV graft mirrors that of an AVF. A detailed history with emphasis on prior central venous catheter placement, arterial line placement, cardiac rhythm devices, and prior dialysis vascular access should be elicited. A medical history to identify cardiac and vascular diseases, heart failure, malignancy, and pulmonary hypertension should be taken as the presence of these can affect the choice of access placement.

A focused and detailed physical examination is paramount in ensuring good clinical outcomes in patients who are to undergo an AVG placement. Evaluation of arterial pulses, differential blood pressures, Allen's test to establish the integrity of the palmar arch, documentation of prior access-related surgical sites and signs of central vein stenosis/occlusion like arm or face edema, dilated or collateral veins on the chest should be done. Usually, if the procedure is being performed by a vascular surgeon, a detailed arterial and venous duplex is performed to note vessel diameter, flow rates, stenosis, occlusions, calcifications, and aberrant anatomy. A differential blood pressure of >20 mm Hg would indicate a proximal subclavian or axillary artery stenosis and it would warrant further imaging or the access surgery can be performed on the contralateral limb. Since AV grafts have a higher incidence of steal syndrome, it would be prudent to place them to the contralateral side of the internal mammary artery harvest in cases of patients who are post-coronary artery bypass graft (CABG), as it could lead to coronary steal syndrome and eventual severe angina.[1,3-6]

LOCATION

During the creation of AVFs, the nondominant arm should be used first; however, previous surgical procedures should be kept in mind while choosing a site for placing an AV graft. The sites that can be used for AV graft placement are given in the following text.

Forearm

Forearm is usually the most common access site with a loop configuration. The arterial inflow is taken from the brachial artery and outflow to the median cubital vein, cephalic vein, basilic vein, or brachial vein. Occasionally, a straight tapered graft can be used taking the radial or ulnar artery as inflow, with outflow into any of the above-mentioned veins.

Arm

In the arm, the inflow is taken from the brachial artery and outflow is given to the axillary vein by a straight graft configuration. The proximal brachial artery can also be used in a loop configuration as well.

Chest

Arteriovenous grafts in the chest are usually placed when all upper and lower limb access sites are exhausted. The options in these cases are usually a "necklace" graft from the ipsilateral axillary artery to the contralateral axillary vein or a loop graft from the ipsilateral axillary artery to the ipsilateral axillary vein, with the loop formed on the anterior chest wall.

Lower Limb

The grafts in the lower limb are fashioned in a loop configuration with the inflow being from the common or superficial femoral artery and the outflow to the superficial femoral or the saphenous vein.

Novel Sites

Once all the above sites have been exhausted, some novel procedures that have been described are axillary artery to right atrium graft, brachial artery to jugular vein graft, and axillary artery to common iliac vein graft. These configurations are usually reported as anecdotal case reports.[7,8]

GRAFT TYPES

Arteriovenous grafts can be made of prosthetic and the recently available biologic materials. Initially, Dacron grafts were used, but due to their poor patencies and complication, their use has been abandoned for ePTFE grafts. A few of the graft types are listed below.

Standard Wall Polytetrafluoroethylene Graft

The wall thickness of a standard wall PTFE graft is 0.64 mm and is the most commonly used graft.

Thin Wall Polytetrafluoroethylene Graft

The wall thickness of a thin wall PTFE is 0.37 mm, and the advantages of these grafts are that they are more flexible.

Heparin-bonded Polytetrafluoroethylene Grafts

One of the concerns of the standard grafts was graft thrombosis, and heparin-bonded grafts were introduced to address this issue. There are many studies that were done, but the data is equivocal with regard to their improved patency as compared to the standard grafts.

Tapered Grafts

The standard AV grafts are straight 6 mm grafts. One of the concerns with this graft size is the high incidence of steal syndrome and high output cardiac failure as compared to autogenous fistulas. The configuration is commonly 4 mm for the arterial end and 6–7 mm for the venous end. This reduces the size of the arterial anastomosis and theoretically reduces the incidence of the above-mentioned complications.

Early Cannulation Grafts

Early cannulation grafts have a multilayer structure that allows cannulation after 24 hours as the graft has a self-sealing property. This is in stark difference to the standard PTFE grafts that need a 2–3 week "implantation" period to allow ingrowth. These grafts are especially useful for patients to avoid dialysis cannulas and lines that could lead to infection.

HeRO Graft

The Hemodialysis Reliable Outflow (HeRO) graft is a new graft that has been introduced to address the issue of outflow in patients with central vein stenosis. The graft essentially is comprised of two parts: (1) 6 mm PTFE grafts and (2) nitinol-reinforced silicone single- lumen venous outflow component. The PTFE graft is anastomosed to the brachial artery and the venous outflow component is placed in the superior vena cava (SVC) or the right atrium. An adaptor then attaches both of these components to each other.

Biologic Grafts

Cryopreserved femoral vein, bovine carotid artery, mesenteric vein, and tissue-engineered grafts have been studied and used in few centers. These grafts, if available freely, could take the place of prosthetic grafts in the near future.[9,10]

COMPLICATIONS

The complications related to the formation of AV grafts can be local complications and can be flow-related ones. It is pertinent to recognize these problems and identify them early and treat them.

Bleeding

Bleeding is most commonly seen via the needle holes while using the standard ePTFE graft and less with the early cannulation graft. Local pressure and hemostatic agents usually help resolve these issues. Sometimes, hematomas can form around the anastomosis in the early postoperative period around the anastomotic sites and must be explored. Graft tunnel hematomas can also occur and are usually managed conservatively. In standard wall PTFE grafts, it is important not to stretch the graft too much while tunneling it as it can lead to anastomotic site bleeding.

Seroma

"Weeping", i.e., ultrafiltration of plasma across the graft, can occur in the early postoperative period and is usually managed conservatively.

Pseudoaneurysm

Arteriovenous grafts are notorious for this complication, and this usually occurs by needling the graft in the same place repeatedly. Avoiding this technique and using the "rope ladder" technique of graft access and providing adequate compression can help in avoiding pseudoaneurysms. Small pseudoaneurysms can be managed with guided compression and thrombin injections, but larger ones would require graft ligation, removal, repair, or endovascular stent graft placement across the defect.[11]

Infection

Approximately 20% of AV graft access loss is due to infection with *Staphylococcus aureus* and less commonly with *Staphylococcus epidermidis*, these being the most common causative organisms. Risk factors remain hematomas, pseudoaneurysms, skin infections, and bloodstream infections. Removal of the graft (total or partial) remains the mainstay of treatment, although very rarely graft conservation can be looked at where infection is very localized.[12]

Dialysis Access-associated Steal Syndrome

Physiologic vascular steal occurs in all the patients with AV grafts, but approximately 4–5% will have it in severity that would necessitate further intervention. The symptoms usually manifest within 2–7 days after creation and can vary from cool extremities to severe pain and minor tissue loss. In these scenarios, it is important to image the arterial tree and document evidence of steal. If revascularization is not possible, then ligation of the graft is done to establish flow before any permanent damage is done to the extremity. Sometimes, a proximal subclavian artery stenosis can be unmasked and stenting it may improve the distal circulation. Other options for revascularization include distal revascularization-interval ligation (DRIL) procedure, revision using distal inflow (RUDI), proximalization of arterial inflow (PAI), and proximal stenting. It is very important to screen patients well prior to any surgery, so that this complication is avoided.[13,14]

Ischemic Monomelic Neuropathy

Ischemic monomelic neuropathy (IMN) is a very rare condition affecting less than 1% of vascular access creations. It occurs immediately after the access creation and is characterized by profound motor and sensory deficits in the absence of any vascular compromise. It is usually due to underperfusion of the vascular nervosum leading to permanent axonal damage. The treatment of this condition is urgent ligation of the graft. Any delay in treatment can lead to permanent nerve damage.[15]

Limb Swelling

Limb swelling secondary to graft placement can be due to stenosis/occlusion of the central veins, and this gets unmasked due to the placement of a high-flow graft. The treatment is usually endoluminal angioplasty of the central veins.

GRAFT DYSFUCNTION AND FAILURE

Arteriovenous grafts need to be monitored like AVFs for flow rates and evidence of recirculation. Grafts are more prone to thrombosis and failure as compared to AVFs. The thrombosis rate is between 55 and 77% annually, and almost 90% are due to neointimal hyperplasia causing stenosis, almost always in the venous outflow. An important point to note while creation is to always construct a longer venous anastomosis.

Immediate graft failures are usually always due to technical issues, be it poor anastomosis technique, graft kink, or poor tunneling. These need to be surgically corrected. Delayed graft thrombosis is usually due to venous outflow stenosis or ingraft stenosis and needs regular monitoring and treatment.[16]

Clinical Presentation and Evaluation

Clinical monitoring tools such as poor thrill, abnormal auscultation, difficulty in needling, thrombus aspiration, prolonged bleeding from needle sites, poor dialysis flow rate, and sustained fall (>2 units) in delivered Kt/V in spite of adequate dialysis prescription can point toward graft flow abnormalities and should be investigated with imaging, which could be ultrasound Doppler or diagnostic angiograms. These sites of stenosis are:

- Venous anastomosis stenosis (most common)
- Ingraft stenosis
- Peripheral draining vein stenosis
- Central vein stenosis
- Arterial anastomosis stenosis

Stenosis once identified must be treated. Percutaneous transluminal angioplasty is the first line of treatment and can be done preemptively in lesions that are identified. Covered stent graft placement can also be performed at the venous end to cover the intimal hyperplasia stenosis. Surgical revision of the venous end by performing a patch angioplasty is also a well-described durable option. The introduction of the drug-eluting balloons has shown promising results in these patients.[17-19]

GRAFT THROMBOSIS

The management of graft thrombosis is not standardized and is more in line with local practices. Some of the options are given in the following text.

Percutaneous Thrombectomy

Percutaneous thrombectomy can be done by using lytic drugs in conjunction with mechanical clot disruptors/suction devices. Once the thrombus is aspirated and cleared, the underlying lesion is identified and addressed by angioplasty or stenting. Some of the devices used are the Penumbra suction device, AngioJet device, and EKOS device.

Surgical Thrombectomy

Surgical thrombectomy is a relatively simple procedure that involves a small incision on the graft and then by using a Fogarty catheter to remove the thrombus. An on-table angiogram can be done which would help in identifying the venous stenosis, which is followed by a patch angioplasty or a jump graft to a healthier segment of vein.[20]

CONCLUSION

An AV graft is a good option for a patient on chronic hemodialysis, either as an initial choice or as a secondary one when all other accesses have failed. Adequate preoperative evaluation and planning go a long way in ensuring a graft with good hemodynamics. Monitoring of the graft is important and will help in elongating its life. Recognition of complications and their prompt treatment will ensure good graft patencies.

REFERENCES

1. Lok CE, Huber TS, Lee T, Shenoy S, Yevzlin AS, Abreo K, et al. KDOQI clinical practice guideline for vascular access: 2019 update. American Journal of Kidney Diseases. 2020;75(4):S1-64.
2. Al Shakarchi J, Houston G, Inston N. Early cannulation grafts for haemodialysis: a systematic review. J Vasc Access. 2015;16(6):493-7.

3. Lok CE, Allon M, Moist L, Oliver MJ, Shah H, Zimmerman D. Risk equation determining unsuccessful cannulation events and failure to maturation in arteriovenous fistulas (REDUCE FTM I). J Am Soc Nephrol. 2006;17(11):3204-12.
4. Misskey J, Hamidizadeh R, Faulds J, Chen J, Gagnon J, Hsiang Y. Influence of artery and vein diameters on autogenous arteriovenous access patency. J Vasc Surg. 2020;71(1):158-72.
5. Malovrh M. Native arteriovenous fistula: preoperative evaluation. Am J Kidney Dis. 2002;39(6):1218-25.
6. Malovrh M. Non-invasive evaluation of vessels by duplex sonography prior to construction of arteriovenous fistulas for haemodialysis. Nephrol Dial Transplant. 1998;13(1):125-9.
7. Miller CD, Robbin ML, Barker J, Allon M. Comparison of arteriovenous grafts in the thigh and upper extremities in hemodialysis patients. J Am Soc Nephrol. 2003;14(11):2942-7.
8. Liechty JM, Fisher T, Davis W, Oglesby WC, Bennett M, Grimsley B, et al. Experience with chest wall arteriovenous grafts in hemodialysis patients. Annals Vasc Surg. 2015;29(4):690-7.
9. Glickman MH. HeRO vascular access device. Semin Vasc Surg. 2011;24(2):108-12.
10. Lawson JH, Glickman MH, Ilzecki M, Jakimowicz T, Jaroszynski A, Peden EK, et al. Bioengineered human acellular vessels for dialysis access in patients with end-stage renal disease: two phase 2 single-arm trials. The Lancet. 2016;387(10032):2026-34.
11. Pandolfe LR, Malamis AP, Pierce K, Borge MA. Treatment of hemodialysis graft pseudoaneurysms with stent grafts: institutional experience and review of the literature. Semin Intervent Radiol. 2009;26(2):89-95.
12. Fysaraki M, Samonis G, Valachis A, Daphnis E, Karageorgopoulos DE, Falagas ME, et al. Incidence, clinical, microbiological features and outcome of bloodstream infections in patients undergoing hemodialysis. Int J Med Sci. 2013;10(12):1632.
13. Lazarides MK, Staramos DN, Kopadis G, Maltezos C, Tzilalis VD, Georgiadis GS. Onset of arterial 'steal' following proximal angioaccess: immediate and delayed types. Nephrol Dial Transplant. 2003;18(11):2387-90.
14. Leake AE, Winger DG, Leers SA, Gupta N, Dillavou ED. Management and outcomes of dialysis access-associated steal syndrome. J Vasc Surg. 2015;61(3):754-61.
15. Thermann F, Kornhuber M. Ischemic monomelic neuropathy: a rare but important complication after hemodialysis access placement-a review. J Vasc Access. 2011;12(2):113-9.
16. Harms JC, Rangarajan S, Young CJ, Barker-Finkel J, Allon M. Outcomes of arteriovenous fistulas and grafts with or without intervention before successful use. J Vasc Surg. 2016;64(1):155-62.
17. Beathard GA. Angioplasty for arteriovenous grafts and fistulae. Semin Nephrol. 2002;122(3):202-10.
18. Kouvelos GN, Spanos K, Antoniou GA, Vassilopoulos I, Karathanos C, Matsagkas MI, et al. Balloon angioplasty versus stenting for the treatment of failing arteriovenous grafts: a meta-analysis. Eur J Vasc Endovasc Surg. 2018;55(2):249-56.
19. Lookstein RA, Haruguchi H, Ouriel K, Weinberg I, Lei L, Cihlar S, et al. Drug-coated balloons for dysfunctional dialysis arteriovenous fistulas. New Engl J Med. 2020;383(8):733-42.
20. Tordoir JH, Bode AS, Peppelenbosch N, van der Sande FM, de Haan MW. Surgical or endovascular repair of thrombosed dialysis vascular access: is there any evidence?. J Vasc Surg. 2009;50(4):953-6.

CHAPTER 12

Tunneled Cuffed Catheter Insertion

Prashant C Dheerendra, Karthikeyan Balasubramanian, Denis Dawle Tirkey

CASE SCENARIO

Mr XYZ, a 64-year-old male, diabetic and hypertensive, was initiated on maintenance hemodialysis via right internal jugular vein (IJV) tunneled cuffed catheter (TCC). The TCC was removed after 6 months following left radiocephalic arteriovenous fistula (AVF) maturation. Two years later, he developed fistula thrombosis. He continued hemodialysis via a temporary hemodialysis catheter in the right IJV. He developed catheter-related bloodstream infection (CRBSI) a few weeks later. The temporary hemodialysis catheter was removed and adequate antibiotics were administered as per culture sensitivity. He is planned for a TCC insertion, but the right IJV is stenotic. Which is the preferred vein for TCC insertion?

INTRODUCTION

Renal replacement therapy for end-stage renal disease (ESRD) includes options like renal transplantation, hemodialysis, and peritoneal dialysis. The best access methods for hemodialysis are arteriovenous fistulas (AVF), followed by arteriovenous grafts (AVG). When these options are not feasible, cuffed or uncuffed central venous catheters (CVC) are used.[1]

Tunneled CVCs are designed to travel through a subcutaneous tunnel and terminate away from the venotomy site. These catheters have a cuff that secures them within the subcutaneous tissue, enhancing stability and reducing the risk of infection.[2]

TUNNELED CUFFED CATHETER—A NECESSARY EVIL

Most patients begin hemodialysis in an emergent situation, often relying on temporary hemodialysis catheters or tunneled cuffed catheters (TCC). An arteriovenous (AV) access has not been created or it is not usable at the time of dialysis initiation. Additionally, the lack of trained physicians in remote areas further limits the feasibility of establishing AVFs, making catheters a more common initial choice for dialysis access.[3]

WHEN IS A TEMPORARY CATHETER PREFERRED OVER TUNNELED CUFFED CATHETER?

Temporary dialysis catheters, while considered a last resort, can be lifesaving for ESRD patients facing urgent situations like fluid overload or refractory hyperkalemia without a functioning AV access. The Kidney Disease Outcomes Quality Initiative (KDOQI) guidelines from 2019 recommend their use for patients needing dialysis for less than 2 weeks.[4]

The right IJV is the preferred insertion site, but the femoral vein may be more practical for orthopneic patients who cannot lie down or in cases of coagulopathy.[5]

Financial constraints and limited availability of expertise can further necessitate the use of these catheters.[6]

WHEN SHOULD TUNNELED CUFFED CATHETER BE USED?

- *AVF or AVG not ready:* AVF or AVG are created but not yet usable when dialysis is needed
- *AVF or AVG complications:* Major infiltration injury or cellulitis affecting AV access, requiring temporary nonuse
- *Multiple failed AV accesses:* Patients with several prior failed AV accesses and no viable options left
- *Poor vessels preventing AVF creation due to inflow and outflow problems:* Lack of options due to severe arterial occlusive disease or central venous obstruction
- *Temporary modality switch:* A temporary switch from another modality due to complications, expecting a return once resolved

- *Impending living donor transplant:* Patients confirmed for a living donor transplant within 90 days who require dialysis
- *Acute complications:* Acute transplant rejection or other urgent complications requiring immediate dialysis
- *Clinical deterioration:* Conditions that may worsen with AV access, like severe heart failure or nontreatable skin lesions
- *Limited life expectancy:* Patients with a limited life expectancy who may not benefit from permanent access
- *Informed patient choice:* Competent patients, such as elderly individuals at high risk for AV access failure, who opt not to pursue permanent access after informed consent.[4]

Is USG Guidance Necessary for Tunneled Cuffed Catheter Insertion?

Numerous studies highlight the safety and effectiveness of ultrasound-guided TCC insertion compared to traditional landmark techniques. Benefits include lesser number of attempts for successful vein cannulation, avoidance of arterial punctures, and higher success rates.[7]

This method ensures better guidewire positioning and lowers the risk of complications like excessive bleeding, hematoma, and pneumothorax. For ESRD patients who struggle to lie supine, have altered anatomy, or are obese, ultrasound guidance is especially advantageous.

Is Fluoroscopy Essential?

Fluoroscopic guidance for TCC insertion is beneficial, ensuring accurate positioning of the guidewire, dilators, and catheter.[8] A catheter tip in the mid right atrium (RA) is the optimal position for adequate flows and decreased complication. Fluoroscopy makes the achievement of this position more predictable. It confirms that the angle between the venotomy site and tunnel allows for unobstructed blood flow.[9,10] Additionally, this technique enables simultaneous venogram, venoplasty, removal of fibrin sheaths, etc.

However, disadvantages include radiation exposure for patients and healthcare workers, as well as reliance on cardiac catheterization laboratories, which may be overloaded with urgent cases. In nephrology departments lacking dedicated catheterization laboratories, TCC insertion can still be performed with precautions, followed by a chest X-ray for verification. In complex cases such as left IJV TCC insertion,[11] multiple access failures, central vein stenosis, etc., fluoroscopy is advisable. Thus, prioritizing laboratory resources for these cases enhances patient safety and procedural success.

TECHNIQUE OF TUNNELED CUFFED CATHETER INSERTION INTO RIGHT INTERNAL JUGULAR VEIN (VIDEO 1)

The steps involved in TCC insertion into the right IJV will be described in detail. Except for a few changes, similar considerations apply to insertion into other veins.

A few points need to be kept in mind to improve success rates and decrease complications:

- Entering the vein with a smaller gauge needle (21G) is preferable. In case of an inadvertent arterial puncture, the resulting hematoma is smaller and allows for further attempts at vein cannulation. Using an 18G needle may result in a hematoma that might compress the vein and preclude further attempts at cannulation. Also, the sheath that is used after venipuncture to maintain venous access allows measurements to be made on table.
- Select the length of the catheter to be used after taking measurements on table. This will maximize the possibility that the tip is close to its ideal location in mid-RA.
- Positioning the guidewire in the IVC confirms a correct venipuncture and adds safety to the procedure. It also provides purchase for the dilators and peel away sheath during the procedure.

Preprocedure Workup

Explain the procedure and its risks and obtain an informed consent. Assess bleeding risk. Withhold anticoagulant and antiplatelets for the desired period prior to procedure. Scan the neck veins prior to the procedure to get a proper idea about the anatomy and size. Check for compressibility of the vein.

Preparation

Use continuous ECG, BP, and saturation monitoring during the procedure. Paint and drape the patient. Prepare the US probe in a sterile manner. Administer local anesthesia.

Venipuncture

Puncture the vein under USG guidance using 21G needle. A micropuncture kit consisting of 21G needle, 0.18" guidewire, and 5 Fr sheath with dilator can be used for vein puncture.

There are two methods to enter the vein: (1) A short-axis, out-of-plane method and (2) an oblique axis, in-plane method.

Short-axis, Out-of-plane Method

Place the probe along the short axis of the vein so that it is seen as a circular structure. Enter the skin a few millimeters away from the probe ("out of plane"). Advance the needle while fanning the ultrasound probe such that the needle tip is constantly visualized.[12] The vein becomes tented by the needle before becoming circular/oval again on USG. Aspiration of dark venous blood at this point means that the vein has been entered. The needle tip is visualized inside the vein. A "haptic" feedback is appreciated on entering the vein and one develops a feel for it over time. Insert the 0.018" guidewire into the needle and vein. Confirm the guidewire in superior vena cava (SVC)/RA using fluoroscopic guidance. Secure the 5 Fr sheath and remove the guidewire and dilator. Confirm blood flow from the sheath and flush with saline. Conscious sedation can be administered through the sheath at this point in time.

Oblique-axis, In-plane Method

Hold the probe midway between the short axis and long axis of the vein. The vein will be seen as an oblong structure. Insert the needle into the skin at the lateral end of the probe ("in plane") and advance the needle under constant vision into the vein. Once the vein is entered, the remaining steps are identical. As opposed to the needle tip that is visualized in the previous method, the whole of the needle is visualized by using this method.[13]

Measurements

Place mosquito forceps at an approximate surface location of mid RA on the patient's chest and confirm on fluoroscopy image. Mark the location and measure the distance to skin entry site. Decide the catheter length and mark the appropriate cuff and exit site locations. Mark the tunnel and anesthetize the skin over the tunnel. Choose the correct length of the catheter and open the kit.

Guidewire Insertion

Under fluoroscopic guidance, maneuver the 0.038" guidewire (from the catheter kit) into the inferior vena cava (IVC). Note the guidewire markings when the tip is in mid-RA. Subtle adjustments to the measurements taken above can be made if needed. Making the J tip of the guidewire point outward and asking the patient to inspire deeply help to get the wire into the IVC. Remove the 5 Fr sheath and make a 1-cm incision from the guidewire extending laterally. Perform blunt dissection to create a subcutaneous "pocket" around the guidewire. Insert the first dilator into the vein and secure the guidewire.

Tunnel Creation

Incise the skin carefully at the exit site mark. Use untoothed forceps to extend the tunnel. Get the tunneler out through the lateral end of the neck incision. In some cases, if the patient has tough subcutaneous tissue, a few subtle nicks can be given. One should be mindful while using sharp instruments while doing the procedure. Disconnect the tunneler and position the cuff as marked previously.

Tunneled Cuffed Catheter Insertion

Remove the first dilator (from the venotomy site) and maintain compression to prevent bleeding while keeping the guidewire in place. Insert the second dilator and dilate the subcutaneous tissue and venotomy. Smooth movement of guidewire within the dilator reassures that they are correctly positioned. Advance the peel-away sheath under fluoro guidance (after removal of the second dilator). Remove the dilator (the one present in the peel-away sheath) and guidewire together. Advance the catheter into the sheath and peel away the sheath. Check proper position and for any catheter kinks on fluoroscopy. Check for proper flow and flush the lumens with saline. Lock both lumens with the recommended volume of heparin. Secure the catheter with sutures. Use compressive dressing if needed and change within 24 hours to a noncompressive dressing.

An "over-the-wire" insertion of TCC without using the peel-away sheath is possible with catheters that are available with a stiffening stylet being included with the kit.

Variations of the Procedure for Other Veins

The left IJV vein has a curved path to the RA and left-sided insertions are more prone to complications. The authors prefer an "over-the-wire" insertion of TCC for left IJV catheters.

The left-sided and right external jugular vein (EJV) insertions generally need a longer length (23 or 27 cm tip to cuff length) of the catheter compared to the right IJV (19 or 23 cm).

Femoral TCCs are the longest (36–55 cm) among the usually used veins.

Taking the measurements on table is especially important as one size does not fit all.

Order of Preference of Veins for Tunneled Cuffed Catheter Insertion

The NKF-KDOQI guidelines recommend the right IJV as the first choice for hemodialysis catheters due to its easy identification, straighter course to RA, larger size, and lower complication rates.[14,15] If the right IJV is unavailable, alternatives include the left IJV and subclavian veins, which have higher complication risks, central stenosis, and thrombosis.[16,17] Because of high risk of central vein stenosis with subclavian vein catheters, they should generally be avoided.

The right EJV is a viable option as well, as it is easy to access, located close to the surface, and has similar blood flow to the IJV. Studies have found right EJV performing better than the left IJV for tunneled dialysis catheters, especially in terms of catheter patency and ease of removal.[18]

Femoral catheters can be used when neck veins are exhausted, with similar infection rates to neck catheters while subclavian veins are a last resort due to complications.[16,17,19] Other options, like the left EJV and lumbar veins, should only be considered by experienced doctors as a last resort.

Postcatheter Insertion Care

Taking good care of TCCs once inserted is crucial for preventing problems like infections and dysfunction. Some important steps to follow are as follows:

- Keep the catheter dressing clean and dry.
- Stitches at the neck incision are removed after 7–10 days and those at the exit site are kept for 3–4 weeks.
- Ensure that the insertion site is clean, and the dialysis team needs to change the dressing every dialysis session for the first 2 weeks and then weekly afterward.
- Waterproof dressings can help keep the site clean.
- Keep the caps and clamps tightly closed when not in use, and only allow the dialysis care team to use the catheter for blood draws or medications.
- Inspect the area around the catheter for soreness or redness whenever the dressing is changed.
- Monitor Kt/V and urea reduction ratio (URR) values for dialysis adequacy.

COMPLICATIONS OF TUNNELED CUFFED CATHETER INSERTION

Pneumothorax

Pneumothorax occurs due to accidental puncture of the lung during insertion. It can be prevented by constant monitoring of vitals and using ultrasound and fluoroscopic guidance for accurate placement. Treatment includes continuous monitoring for respiratory distress and administration of supplemental oxygen and in severe cases may require chest tube placement.

Hemorrhage

Excessive bleeding from insertion site leads to hemorrhage. Adequate hemostasis during insertion and avoiding unnecessary trauma to surrounding tissues can prevent it. It can be managed by applying direct pressure to control bleeding. Surgical intervention may be needed if bleeding persists.

Catheter Malposition

The catheter tip is in an incorrect position. Confirm placement via imaging (e.g., X-ray) or perform procedure under fluoroscopic guidance which also helps to reposition.[20]

Infection (Local/Systemic)

Localized or systemic infection can occur postinsertion. For prevention, maintain a strict aseptic technique during dressing changes. Educate patients on hygiene practices. Blood culture sensitivity and administration of appropriate antibiotics are required. Catheter removal may be necessary in case of tunnel infection, fungal catheter-related bloodstream infections (CRBSIs), metastatic infection, or recurrent or persistent infections.

Thrombosis

Thrombosis is the formation of a clot within the catheter, either intraluminal or at the tip. It can be avoided by use of adequate volume of anticoagulant lock solutions (heparin or sodium citrate) for the catheter. Thrombolytic therapy can be used if appropriate. Catheter replacement may be necessary in refractory cases.

Catheter Fracture

Catheter fracture can lead to leaks or embolism. Regular inspection of the catheter for wear is needed. Avoid excessive pulling on the catheter. Monitor for signs of breakage. Replace the catheter if a fracture is confirmed.

Fibrin Sheath

After catheter insertion, a fibrin sheath can form within 24 hours, made of fibrinogen, lipoproteins, albumin, and coagulation factors.[21] Over time, white blood cells and microorganisms attach, leading to infection risk. Collagen and smooth muscle cells further encase the catheter, potentially disrupting blood flow and causing thrombosis.[22] To manage this, fibrin sheath stripping[23] or catheter exchange with balloon disruption can restore function.[4]

Stenosis of Central Vein

Narrowing of the vein where the catheter is placed leads to stenosis.[24] It will need intervention if symptomatic.

Embedded Catheter

Many case reports describe tunneled catheters that remain embedded or tethered to the vein despite cuff dissection. Approaches to manage this include open surgery for direct removal, cutting and burying the catheter when removal is not feasible, and endoluminal dilatation to loosen the catheter for easier extraction.[25]

REMOVAL OF TUNNELED CENTRAL CATHETER (VIDEO 2)

Preparation

Gather necessary equipment: Sterile gloves, antiseptic solution (e.g., chlorhexidine), sterile gauze, mosquito forceps or a blunt dissection tool, and a sterile dressing. Explain the procedure to the patient and obtain informed consent.

Positioning

Position the patient comfortably, usually in a supine position with the catheter site easily accessible.

Aseptic Technique

Perform hand hygiene and wear sterile gloves and gown. Clean the catheter insertion site with an antiseptic solution.

Suture Removal

If applicable, remove any sutures holding the catheter in place using sterile scissors or mosquito forceps.

Dissection of the Fibrosed Cuff

Provide local anesthesia around the cuff subcutaneously.

Use a blunt dissection tool or mosquito forceps to carefully dissect around the cuff. Apply gentle pressure to separate the cuff from the surrounding tissue without damaging either.

Manual Removal

Once the cuff is freed, gently pull the catheter out in a straight motion while asking the patient to breathe out and hold in expiration. If resistance persists, do not apply pull and reassess for additional adhesions or fibrotic tissue.

Site Management

After removal, apply gentle pressure with sterile gauze to control any bleeding.

CONCLUSION

Tunneled cuffed catheter insertion is a fundamental procedure for nephrologists and they need to be proficient in routine performance of the same. Attention to detail and safety are important. Developing competence with the procedure translates into better outcomes for the patients over the long term.

REFERENCES

1. Bagul A, Brook NR, Kaushik M, Nicholson ML. Tunnelled catheters for the haemodialysis patient. Eur J Vasc Endovascular Surg. 2007;33(1):105-12.
2. El Khudari H, Ozen M, Kowalczyk B, Bassuner J, Almehmi A. Hemodialysis catheters: Update on types, outcomes, designs and complications. Semin Intervent Radiol. 2022; 39(1):90-102.
3. Kher V. Tunneled central venous catheters for dialysis - A necessary evil? Indian J Nephrol. 2011;21(4):221-2.
4. Lok CE, Huber TS, Lee T, Shenoy S, Yevzlin AS, Abreo K, et al. KDOQI Clinical Practice Guideline for Vascular Access: 2019 Update. Am J Kidney Dis. 2020;75(4):S1-164.
5. Parienti JJ, Thirion M, Mégarbane B, Souweine B, Ouchikhe A, Polito A, et al. Femoral vs jugular venous catheterization and risk of nosocomial events in adults requiring acute renal replacement therapy: A randomized controlled trial. JAMA. 2008;299(20):2413.

6. Khanna U. The economics of dialysis in India. Indian J Nephrol. 2009;19(1):1.
7. Rabindranath KS, Kumar E, Shail R, Vaux EC. Ultrasound use for the placement of haemodialysis catheters. Cochrane Database Syst Rev. 2011;(11):CD005279
8. McGee DC, Gould MK. Preventing complications of central venous catheterization. N Engl J Med. 2003;348(12):1123.
9. Taal MW, Chesterton LJ, McIntyre CW. Venography at insertion of tunnelled internal jugular vein dialysis catheters reveals significant occult stenosis. Nephrol Dial Transplant. 2004;19(6):1542-5.
10. Koroglu M, Demir M, Koroglu B, Sezer MT, Akhan O, Yildiz H, et al. Percutaneous placement of central venous catheters: comparing the anatomical landmark method with the radiologically guided technique for central venous catheterization through the internal jugular vein in emergent hemodialysis patients. Acta Radiologica. 2006;47:43-7.
11. Yevzlin AS, Song GU, Sanchez RJ, Becker YT. Fluoroscopically guided vs modified traditional placement of tunneled hemodialysis catheters: Clinical outcomes and cost analysis. J Vasc Access. 2007;8(4):245-51.
12. Kamata T, Tomita M, Iehara N. Ultrasound-guided cannulation of hemodialysis access. Ren Replace Ther. 2016;2:7.
13. Rossi UG, Rigamonti P, Tichà V, Zoffoli E, Giordano A, Gallieni M, et al. Percutaneous ultrasound-guided central venous catheters: the lateral in-plane technique for internal jugular vein access. J Vasc Access. 2014;15(1):56-60.
14. Vascular Access Work Group. Clinical practice guidelines for vascular access. Am J Kidney Dis. 2006;48(Suppl 1): S248-73.
15. Bannon MP, Heller SF, Rivera M. Anatomic considerations for central venous cannulation. Risk Manag Healthc Policy. 2011;4:27-39.
16. Agarwal AK. Central vein stenosis. Am J Kidney Dis. 2013;61(6):1001-15.
17. Trerotola SO, Kuhn-Fulton J, Johnson MS, Shah H, Ambrosius WT, Kneebone PH. Tunneled infusion catheters: increased incidence of symptomatic venous thrombosis after subclavian versus internal jugular venous access. Radiology. 2000;217(1):89-93.
18. Wang P, Wang Y, Qiao Y, Zhou S, Liang X, Liu Z. A retrospective study of preferable alternative route to right internal jugular vein for placing tunneled dialysis catheters: Right external jugular vein versus left internal jugular vein. PLoS One. 2016;11(1):e0146411.
19. Marik PE, Flemmer M, Harrison W. The risk of catheter-related bloodstream infection with femoral venous catheters as compared to subclavian and internal jugular venous catheters: a systematic review of the literature and meta-analysis. Crit Care Med. 2012;40(8):2479-85.
20. Schwab SJ, Beathard G. The hemodialysis catheter conundrum: hate living with them, but can't live without them. Kidney Int. 1999;56(1):1-17.
21. Faintuch S, Salazar GM. Malfunction of dialysis catheters: management of fibrin sheath and related problems. Tech Vasc Interv Radiol. 2008;11(3):195-200.
22. Miller LM, MacRae JM, Kiaii M, Clark E, Dipchand C, Kappel J, et al. Hemodialysis Tunneled Catheter Noninfectious Complications. Can J Kidney Health Dis. 2016;3:2054358116669130.
23. Angle JF, Shilling AT, Schenk WG, Bissonette EA, Stadtlander KS, Hagspiel KD, et al. Utility of percutaneous intervention in the management of tunneled hemodialysis catheters. Cardiovasc Intervent Radiol. 2003;26(1):9-18.
24. MacRae JM, Ahmed A, Johnson N, Levin A, Kiaii M. Central vein stenosis: a common problem in patients on hemodialysis. ASAIO J. 2005;51(1):77-81.
25. Field M, Pugh J, Asquith J, Davies S, Pherwani AD. A stuck hemodialysis central venous catheter. J Vasc Access. 2008;9(4):301-3.

Vascular Access Creation for Hemodialysis by Nontunneled Catheters

Shahbaj Ahmad, Smriti Sinha

INTRODUCTION

Nontunneled dialysis catheters (NTDC) are noncuffed, short-term catheters meant to be used for few days to weeks as access for hemodialysis (HD). The procedure is quick and can be carried out bedside; hence, NTDC are often used as the first vascular access for kidney failure patients needing urgent HD. In patients with acute kidney failure (AKI) requiring HD, they are the most common vascular access. In chronic kidney disease (CKD) patients, an arteriovenous fistula (AVF) is recommended as the best option due to its lower infection and complication rates. Despite this, in incident dialysis patient population, nontunneled catheters remain the most common vascular access. In a study from the United States, 80% of incident dialysis patients had a central venous catheter.[1] The scenario is very similar in Southeast Asia wherein 50–80% of incident dialysis patients, especially from middle- and low-income groups, had a NTDC.[2] The current recommendations suggest that in patients who are unlikely to recover in near future or need HD for more than 14 days, it is better to change to a tunneled cuffed catheter (TCC) at the earliest.

Indications for Nontunneled Catheter Insertion

- Urgent start of HD in a patient with no other vascular access like AVF or arteriovenous graft (AVG)
- Complications of AVF such as thrombosis, extravasation, hematoma, or infection
- Patient planned for peritoneal dialysis
- Patient planned for renal transplant within the next 2 weeks
- Nondialysis procedures such as plasmapheresis
- In acute diseases, where renal recovery is anticipated, e.g., acute kidney injury, acute rejection
- Contraindication to TCC insertion like sepsis or coagulopathy
- Financial constraints, lack of facility, or expertise for TCC insertion.

Preferred Location

Veins accessible for cannulation include bilateral internal jugular vein (IJV), external jugular vein (EJV), subclavian vein, and femoral veins. The right IJV is the most preferred site as it has a short straight course to heart. Left-sided IJV/EJV has a long tortuous course, making it difficult to cannulate with higher rates of catheter thrombosis and central venous stenosis/thrombosis. Subclavian vein is the least preferred vein as the rate of stenosis following NTDC insertion may be as high as 50%. Since the upper limb veins drain into the subclavian vein, so chances of symptomatic central venous stenosis manifesting as ipsilateral limb edema following AVF construction increase significantly. While selecting the vein for NTDC insertion, future prospect for AVF/AVG must be taken into consideration. Femoral veins are easy to cannulate with least complication rates but were discouraged as they were thought to have a high infection rate. The Cathesdia study[3] has partially challenged it. It showed that in critically ill patients, femoral catheters had similar catheter-related bloodstream infection (CRBSI) rates to IJV catheters. In the subgroup of patients with body mass index (BMI) >28.4 kg/m^2, there was significantly increased risk of catheter colonization with femoral versus internal jugular catheters. Patients in the lowest BMI tertile (<24.2 kg/m^2) had a significantly reduced risk of catheter colonization with femoral versus internal jugular nontunneled catheters. Femoral vein may be chosen as the preferred site for NTDC in few special circumstances like patients with severe pulmonary edema who cannot lie down supine or in Trendelenburg position, patients with severe hyperkalemia, when USG guidance is unavailable in patients with deranged bleeding or coagulation profile, or an inexperienced operator. Femoral site does not have serious complications of hemothorax or pneumothorax.

Catheter Size and Length

Nontunneled catheters are mostly 15–20 cm long. The choice of the catheter depends on the insertion vein and intended catheter tip position. The ideal tip position of a nontunneled catheter inserted via the jugular vein is superior vena cava–right atrium (RA) junction. As these catheters are made of stiffer materials, there is a higher risk of cardiac tamponade if placed more deeply into the RA.[4] Femoral catheters should ideally reach the inferior vena cava (IVC); hence, a longer catheter of at least 20 cm length should be preferred. In adult patients, a catheter size of 11.5–13 Fr is recommended depending upon the vein diameter size. In pediatric population, formulas have been made for calculation of the size of the catheter, by taking into account the height and weight of child.[5] The National Kidney Foundation Kidney Disease Outcomes Quality Initiative (NKF-KDOQI)[6] guidelines have given weight-based suggestion of catheter size. The size of a nontunneled catheter in children >10 kg is 7–8 Fr. In children >40 kg, it is recommended to insert adult size catheters of 11.5–12.5 Fr.

One study published by Andropoulos et al.[7] suggested the insertion length of the catheter as (height in cm/10): 1 for patients <100 cm in height, and (height in cm/10): 2 for patients >100 cm in height. The catheters available from various manufacturers in India have a fixed wing, so the intravascular length cannot be changed. The author, Shahbaj Ahmad, had used special non-tunneled catheters (UNIQATH),[8] which had movable fixation wings, allowing the intravascular length to be adjusted to the required one. However, this is not currently available in India.

GUIDEWIRES

The modified Seldinger technique involves passing the catheter over the guidewire, so an appropriate guidewire is necessary. The ones that come with the catheter kit are usually J-tipped and mostly made of steel. However, a few manufacturers provide guidewires made of Nitinol. The latter is an alloy that has shape memory and is kink-resistant. This provides added safety from inadvertent vascular injury.

TECHNIQUE OF CATHETER INSERTION

Nontunneled catheters can be inserted using anatomical surface markings or ultrasound guided. Traditionally, central line insertion was carried out blindly using surface anatomy landmarks. The artery was palpated, and vein position was guessed as per its relation to the artery. However, there can be variations. Up to 40% patients can have a deviation from the most common superior-lateral positioning of the IJV to carotid artery with variation being more on the left side.[9] In patients with a history of previous cannulation, surgery or radiation to neck and upper thorax, there can be vein thrombosis or stenosis. Using the "blind" technique for cannulation has a success rate of 60–93% and a mechanical complication rate of 5–19%.[10] Complication rates are more with inexperienced operators and obese or cachexic patients and congenitally abnormal vasculature. Use of ultrasound for central vein insertion has drastically decreased complication rates and improved outcomes. The current practices strongly recommend insertion of a central venous catheter under ultrasound guidance to minimize complications and improve success rates. In emergent conditions where ultrasound is unavailable, the femoral vein and the right IJV without a history of cannulation can be punctured without USG guidance. USG guidance should especially be used in patients with history of multiple prior cannulations, neck surgery, if left IJV or EJV is being cannulated, or with thrombocytopenia or coagulopathy. Ultrasound helps detection of any immediate postprocedure complications such as catheter malposition, hematoma because of mistaken arterial puncture, pneumothorax (sliding pleura sign), and hemothorax.

STEPS OF CENTRAL LINE INSERTION USING POCUS

The standard sterile procedure of central line insertion is carried out with the additional step of screening for best vein for access. However, a technique that must be mastered with practice is the technique of holding the USG probe with the nondominant hand while the dominant hand is used for needle insertion, all the while keeping our eyes on the screen for monitoring real-time movement of the needle. In the beginning, an assistant can help with holding the transducer. For ease of explanation, the steps of point-of-care ultrasound (POCUS) guided right IJV insertion have been enumerated.

1. Ultrasound of the right neck to look for position, distensibility, and compressibility of the right IJV, tracing it down to below clavicle to ensure that there is no thrombosis/narrowing of the vein. By tilting the lower end of the transducer in the upward direction, it is possible to trace the deeper end of IJV and

visualize the joining of the subclavian vein to form the brachiocephalic vein. Color Doppler and spectral Doppler may also be used to confirm the patency of the veins **(Figs. 1 and 2)**.

2. The patient should be positioned in Trendelenburg position and the head should be rotated to the contralateral side at an angle of approximately 45°. The operator must familiarize with the anatomical boundary of the lesser supraclavicular triangle.
3. Preparation of the table with all the required equipment and materials in the sequence in which they are used during the procedure **(Fig. 3)**. This becomes especially important when insertion is done using anatomical landmarks.
4. Draping and cleaning of the area of insertion.
5. Cleaning of the transducer with 2% chlorhexidine and then in a sterile manner applying jelly on top of the transducer. Covering the probe with either a sterile transducer cover or sterile gloves. Use of routine systemic antimicrobial prophylaxis before catheter insertion is not recommended.[11]
6. Visualizing the vein by placing the transducer perpendicular to the vessels (co-axial view). It is ideal to adjust the probe to place the image of the vein at the center of the screen **(Fig. 2)**.
7. After giving local anesthetic, the introducer needle is punctured through the skin by entering 2–3 mm above the transducer and entering at a more acute angle of 60°. This can be adjusted in real time by visualizing the needle on screen and guiding it to enter the vein superiorly at the 12 o'clock position (preferably). The advancing needle tip will create an indentation on the superior venous wall when it reaches it, which can be visualized on the ultrasound **(Fig. 4)**.
8. Once the needle position is confirmed inside the lumen by aspirating blood **(Fig. 5)**, the guidewire is inserted **(Fig. 6)**, and the position of the same inside the vein can be confirmed by visualizing the vein in transverse **(Fig. 7)** and longitudinal **(Fig. 8)** sections. The guidewire should enter resistance-free

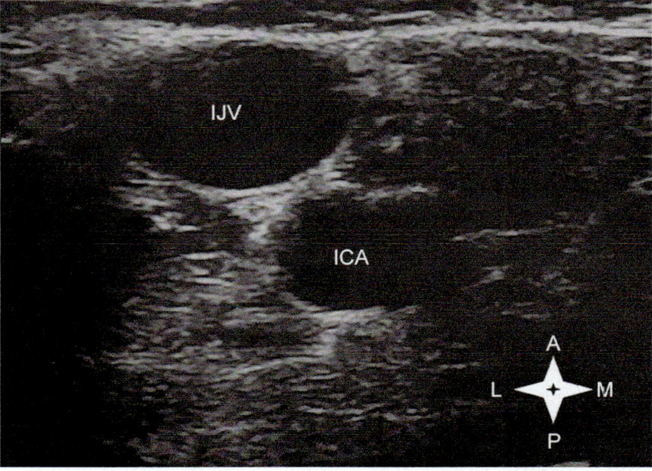

Fig. 2: Radiological anatomy of the neck for nontunneled catheter insertion. (ICA: internal carotid artery; IJV: internal jugular vein)

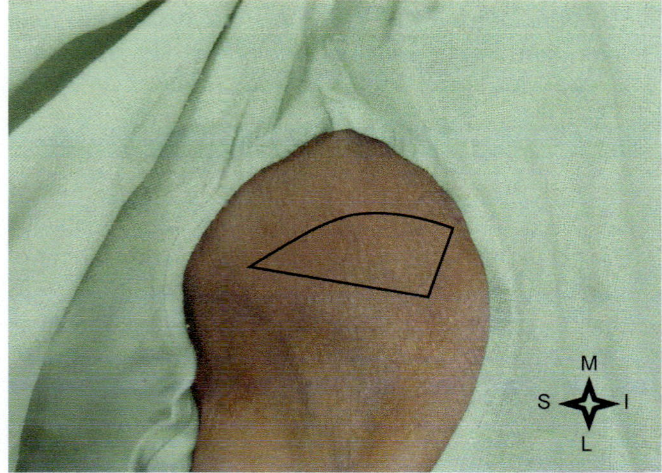

Fig. 1: Anatomical landmarks of the lesser supraclavicular triangle. Medial border: Lateral border of the sternal head of the sternocleidomastoid muscle. Lateral border: Medial border of the clavicular head of the sternocleidomastoid muscle. Inferior border: Superior surface of the medial side of the clavicle.

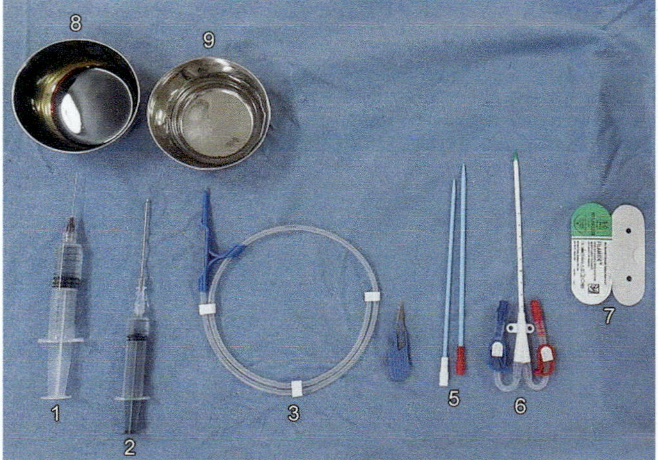

Fig. 3: Necessary equipment for nontunneled catheter insertion. Keys: 1. Syringe loaded with 2% xylocaine, 2. Introducer needle loaded over the syringe, 3. 0.035" guidewire, 4. Scalpel, 5. Fascial dilators, 6. Precurved double-lumen catheter, 7. Nylon suture 3.0, 8. Bowl with Betadine solution, 9. Bowl with normal saline.

and should be advanced to a length greater than the catheter. At this stage, it is a good idea to visualize the passage of the guidewire into the brachiocephalic vein to exclude the possibility of the guidewire passing into the subclavian vein or any other smaller vein **(Fig. 9)**.

9. The further steps of central line insertion are like routine central line insertion with dilatation of tissue over the guidewire using the dilators followed by central line insertion over the guidewire **(Figs. 10 and 11)**.
10. A check X-ray is obtained for any complication and confirmation of the tip of the catheter **(Fig. 12)**.

The same steps can be used for insertion of central line in other vessels like femoral vein, EJV, and subclavian vein.

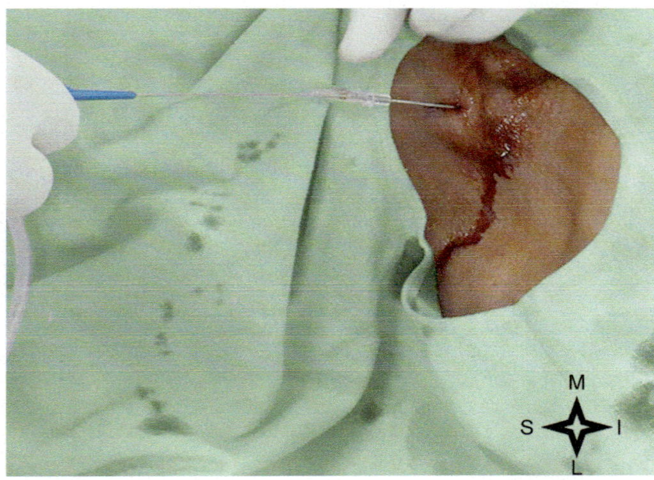

Fig. 6: Guidewire passed through the introducer needle.

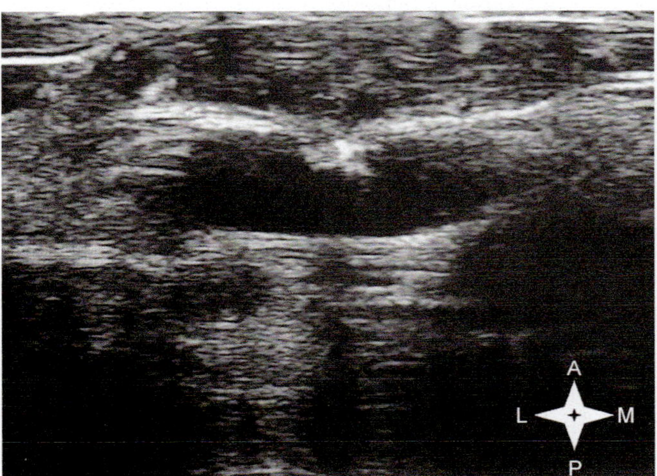

Fig. 4: Tenting of the anterior wall of the internal jugular vein (IJV) by the introducer needle.

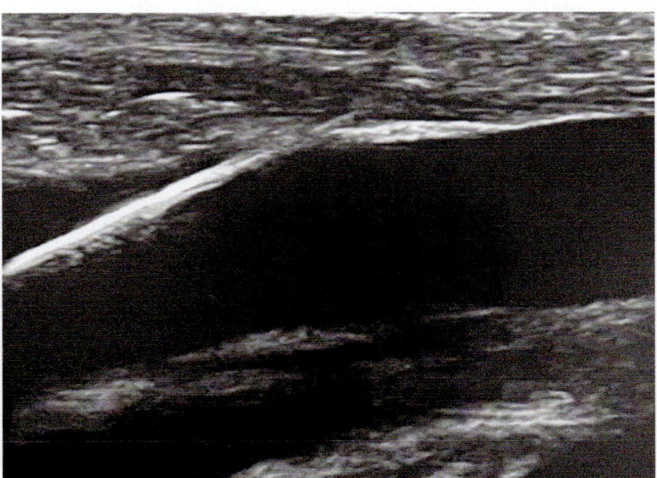

Fig. 7: Right internal jugular vein (IJV) with guidewire seen in it (longitudinal view).

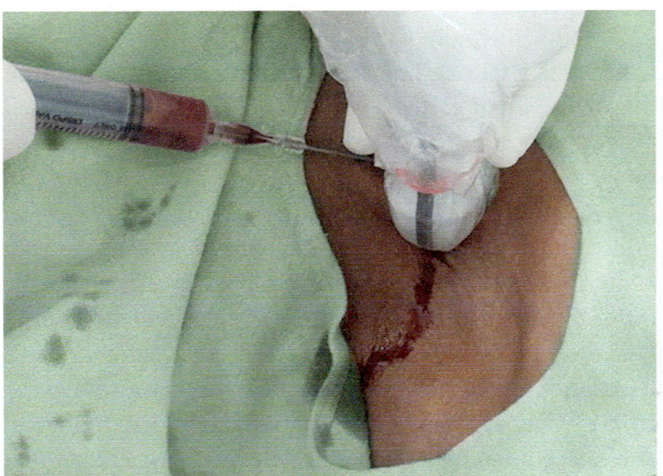

Fig. 5: Confirmation of intravascular position of the needle by dark red blood in the syringe.

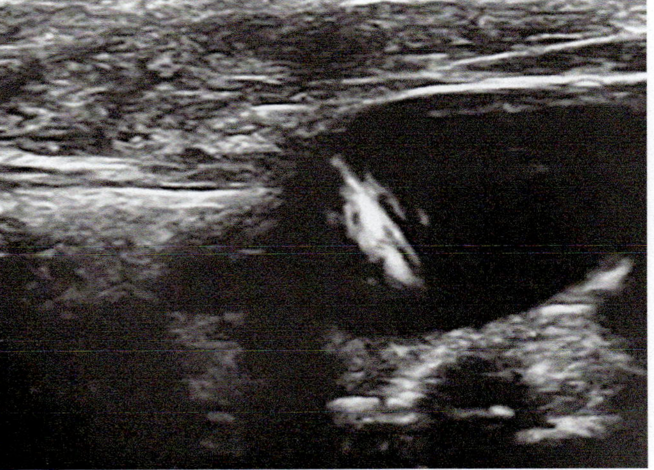

Fig. 8: Right internal jugular vein (IJV) with guidewire seen inside lumen (transverse view).

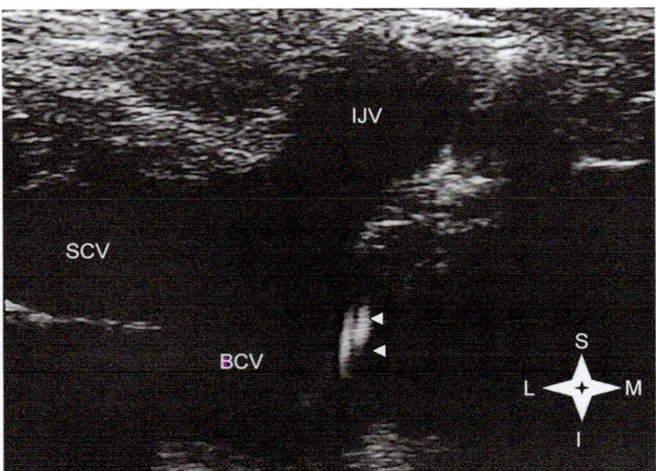

Fig. 9: Guidewire in the innominate vein. (BCV: brachiocephalic vein; IJV: internal jugular vein; SCV: subclavian vein)

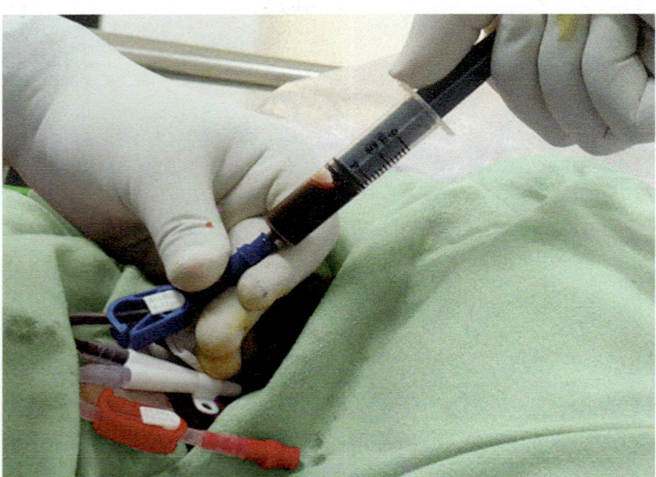

Fig. 10: Good flow checked through the venous lumen of the catheter.

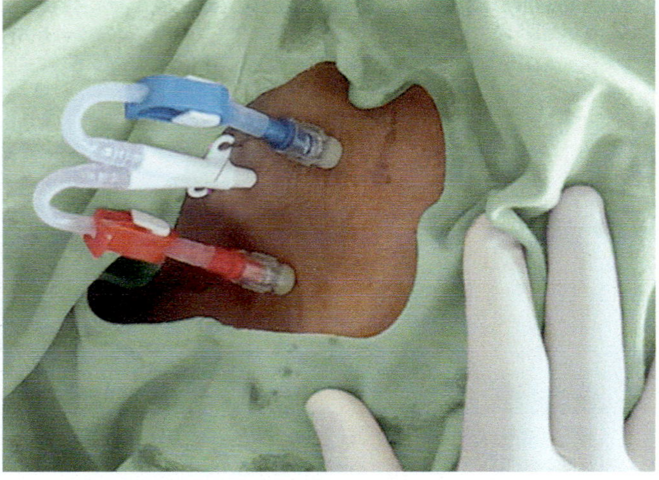

Fig. 11: Final position of the catheter over the neck.

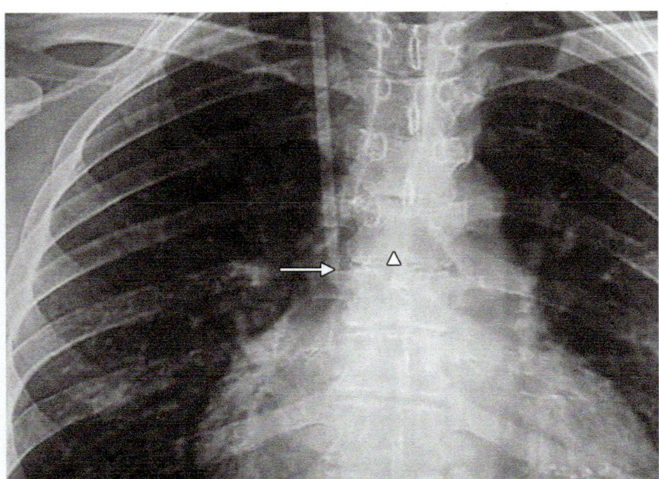

Fig. 12: X-ray chest after catheter insertion. The arrowhead indicates the carina, a radiological landmark for the cavoatrial junction placement of the catheter tip (white arrow).

INSERTION OF NONTUNNELED DIALYSIS CATHETER USING ANATOMICAL LANDMARKS IN THE INTERNAL JUGULAR VEIN

Proficiency with the insertion of NTDC without USG guidance is essential because USG machines may be unavailable in all the healthcare facilities in India for legal and financial reasons.

Steps 3 and 4 remain the same as under POCUS guidance. The skin and subcutaneous tissue should be infiltrated generously with 2% Xylocaine. The targeted puncture site for venous cannulation is at the apex of the lesser supraclavicular triangle. The needle should be directed 45 to the skin and toward the ipsilateral nipple. A pilot/finder needle is used to assess the depth and direction of the path of the introducer needle. This is done with a 22/26 G needle. Any advertent arterial puncture by such a small caliber needle can easily be controlled by applying manual pressure locally. Once the vein is localized, an introducer needle attached to a saline-filled syringe is advanced slowly keeping in mind the direction and depth of the finder/pilot needle. If the vein is not punctured despite inserting the introducer needle more than the expected depth, then the needle should be withdrawn slowly, and the vein may be located. Once dark blood comes into the syringe without any jet flow, it confirms venous puncture. The syringe is disconnected, and the guidewire is advanced through the introducer needle to the appropriate length as described in step 7. The rest of the steps are the same as in a POCUS-guided procedure.

Video 1 showing stepwise procedure of non-tunneled catheter insertion is available at the end of the chapter.

CATHETER COMPLICATIONS

Nontunneled catheters are recommended for short duration mainly because of high complication rates. Complications can be infectious such as CRBSI and catheter site infections. Patients present with fever, chills, hypotension, or weakness, especially during or after dialysis. Infected catheters can lead to infective endocarditis, septic embolism, or metastatic infections such as vertebral bone infections. Infections secondary to catheters are estimated to be 10 times higher as compared to AVF. The incidence of CRBSI is 0.6–6.5 episodes per 1,000 catheter days.[12] The management includes removal of catheter and appropriate antibiotics.

Acute mechanical complications occurring peri procedure include local hematoma, bleeding, pneumothorax, hemothorax, arterial puncture, cardiac arrythmia, air embolism, and catheter malposition. Arterial puncture is noted in 3.7–12% of all central venous access procedures.[13] It can lead to life-threatening neck hematomas which can compress the airways. These complications can be reduced by catheter insertion under ultrasound guidance.

Central venous obstruction is a dreaded complication of catheter insertion. Stiff NTDC use can lead to vessel injury that, upon healing, leads to an area of fibrotic stenosis. Points within the vessel that are repeatedly injured by the catheter may also be injured and subsequently stenosis and thrombosis. HD additionally creates turbulent blood flow at the catheter tip leading to endothelial injury and venous thrombosis. The incidence of central venous stenosis in patients with CVC is 20–40%[14] which increase with longer catheter time, recurrent episodes of infection, and choice of catheter site for, e.g., left-sided IJV and subclavian vein. Other long-term complications include catheter malposition, atrial thrombosis, and catheter dysfunction.

CONCLUSION

It is necessary to acquire the skill of nontunneled catheter insertion as it is most useful for urgent HD. However, its limitations and complications should be kept in mind and every effort should be made to change the vascular access to an AVF or a tunneled catheter at the earliest.

REFERENCES

1. Drew DA, Lok CE, Cohen JT, Wagner M, Tangri N, Weiner DE. Vascular access choice in incident hemodialysis patients: a decision analysis. J Am Soc Nephrol. 2015;26(1):183-91.
2. Ramachandran R, Bhargava V, Jasuja S, Gallieni M, Jha V, Sahay M, et al. Interventional nephrology and vascular access practice: A perspective from South and Southeast Asia. J Vasc Access. 2022;23(6):849-60.
3. Parienti JJ, Thirion M, Megarbane B, Souweine B, Ouchikhe A, Polito A, et al. Femoral vs jugular venous catheterization and risk of nosocomial events in adults requiring acute renal replacement therapy: a randomized controlled trial. JAMA. 2008;299(20):2413-22.
4. Sohail MA, Vachharajani TJ, Anvari E. Central Venous Catheters for Hemodialysis-the Myth and the Evidence. Kidney Int Rep. 2021;6(12):2958-68.
5. Choi YH, Cheon JE, Shin SH, Shin SM, Lee SM, Cho HH, et al. Optimal insertion lengths of right and left internal jugular central venous catheters in children. Pediatr Radiol. 2015;45(8):1206-11.
6. Clinical practice recommendation 8: vascular access in pediatric patients. Am J Kidney Dis. 2006;48 Suppl 1: S274-6.
7. Andropoulos DB, Bent ST, Skjonsby B, Stayer SA. The optimal length of insertion of central venous catheters for pediatric patients. Anesth Analg. 2001;93(4):883-6.
8. "AMECACTH." Amecathgroup.com, 2023, www.amecathgroup.com/products/20-uniqath-dual-lumen-catheter. [Last accessed 19 June 2025].
9. Caridi JG, Hawkins IF Jr, Wiechmann BN, Pevarski DJ, Tonkin JC. Sonographic guidance when using the right internal jugular vein for central vein access. Am J Roentgenol. 1998;171(5):1259-63.
10. McGee DC, Gould MK. Preventing complications of central venous catheterization. N Engl J Med. 2003;348:1123-33.
11. O'Grady NP, Alexander M, Burns LA, Dellinger EP, Garland J, Heard SO, et al. Summary of Recommendations: Guidelines for the Prevention of Intravascular Catheter-related Infections. Clin Infect Dis. 2011;52(9):1087-99.
12. Lok CE, Mokrzycki MH. Prevention and management of catheter-related infection in hemodialysis patients. Kidney Int. 2011;79(6):587-98.
13. Teja B, Bosch NA, Diep C, Pereira TV, Mauricio P, Sklar MC, et al. Complication Rates of Central Venous Catheters: A Systematic Review and Meta-Analysis. JAMA Intern Med. 2024 1;184(5):474-82. [Erratum in: JAMA Intern Med. 2024;184(6):707]
14. McFall RG, Lu T. Application of intravascular ultrasound in end-stage renal patients with central venous occlusive disease. Methodist Debakey CardioVasc J. 2018;14:196-9.

SECTION

4 Postoperative Care and Follow-up of Vascular Access

CHAPTER 14

Monitoring and Surveillance of Vascular Access

Lalathaksha Kumbar, Manish Lalwani

CASE STUDY

A 58-year-old male patient with a *right cephalic arteriovenous fistula (RCF)* has been on a *maintenance hemodialysis (MHD) three times per week* at a community dialysis center. Over the past month, the patient's *Kt/V was noted to be decreasing. The dialysis team initially increased both blood and dialysate flow rates,* after which Kt/V improved temporarily. Routine *monthly access flow monitoring showed stable flow values* with no significant drop compared to previous months. However, *venous pressure readings during dialysis were progressively increasing*. There were no clinical signs of access dysfunction, such as prolonged bleeding or loss of thrill/bruit.

The patient presented with high venous pressures, normal flow, and decreased Kt/V. Upon examination, a poststenotic thrill was detected. Doppler screening revealed anatomical outflow stenosis. This was addressed through a fistulogram and a fistuloplasty performed in the same session. This case highlights the critical importance of monitoring surveillance and the role of training dialysis technicians and vascular nurses in recognizing and addressing such complications effectively.

INTRODUCTION

Chronic, life-sustaining hemodialysis requires durable access to the circulatory system to support the extracorporeal circuit. An optimal dialysis requires properly functioning vascular access with sufficient blood flow to meet the dialysis prescription. Access dysfunction restricts the effective dose of dialysis, significantly impacting both the biological and economic health of the patient and the healthcare system. The high prevalence of chronic lifestyle-related diseases in end-stage renal disease patients requiring dialysis increases their risk of inefficient arteriovenous (AV) access.[1] Once an access point is functional, maintaining its patency becomes the primary focus. Access surveillance and monitoring are critical components in the management of patients undergoing hemodialysis. Proper surveillance methods ensure timely detection of complications such as stenosis, thrombosis, or access failure, which can lead to loss of patency, significant morbidity, and necessitate surgical intervention. By combining physical examinations, imaging techniques, pressure measurements, and flow assessments, healthcare providers can enhance patient safety, improve the longevity of vascular access, and reduce the need for surgical interventions. This comprehensive approach promotes a better quality of life for patients and optimizes the overall efficacy of hemodialysis treatment.

DEFINITIONS: MONITORING AND SURVEILLANCE

Monitoring

According to the National Kidney Foundation (NKF) Kidney Disease Outcomes Quality Initiative (KDOQI) guidelines, redefined access flow dysfunction as clinically significant abnormalities in AV access [arteriovenous fistula (AVF) or arteriovenous graft (AVG)] flow or patency due to underlying stenosis, thrombosis, or related pathology. The two commonly used words associated with access flow dysfunction are monitoring and surveillance. The monitoring encompasses combination of clinical symptoms and physical examination (inspection, palpation, and auscultation) of the vascular access to detect signs of dysfunction. The common symptoms of flow dysfunction include but not limited to the following:

- *Prolonged bleeding* after needle withdrawal
- *Inadequate dialysis delivery*
- *Documented recirculation*
- *Elevated dynamic venous pressures (DVP),* though definitions vary by center
- *Other clinical clues* indicating access issues

In AVFs, sequential monitoring of parameters such as urea reduction ratio (URR) or Kt/V may help detect correctible stenosis, while these measures are less reliable for AVG. The physical examination is described in another chapter.

These monitoring activities are considered as an integral part of comprehensive care of hemodialysis treatments. Newly created accesses are monitored by vascular access management team comprising multidisciplinary specialties such as nephrologist, vascular surgeon, interventionalist (radiology or nephrology), and experienced dialysis nurses.

Surveillance

Surveillance involves periodic evaluations using specialized tests to assess critical parameters such as access flow, resistance, intra-access pressure (IAP), and recirculation. Unlike monitoring, these tests require specialized instruments and may involve dedicated staff to ensure accuracy and consistency. Stenosis-centric fluid mechanics underpin surveillance methodologies. The relationship between reduced luminal diameter, increased blood flow resistance, elevated prestenotic pressure, and decreased flow is well established in hemodialysis access physiology. Stenosis in the vascular access leads to increased resistance, causing elevated pressure upstream (prestenotic) and reduced blood flow downstream. This hemodynamic alteration can result in blood recirculating through the dialysis circuit, forming the basis for recirculation-based surveillance methods. Additionally, studies have shown that poor blood flow in vascular access causes recirculation, which reduces treatment efficiency. Monitoring parameters such as the resistance index (RI) can help evaluate the state of vascular access and predict recirculation rates.[2] Commonly employed surveillance methods include the following **(Fig. 1)**:

- *Access flow measurements* to evaluate the efficiency of blood flow through the access
- *Access pressure measurements* to detect potential blockages or changes in the vascular access
- *Direct recirculation measurements* to quantify the backflow of blood and identify dysfunctions.

Surveillance tests require additional staff time and resources, and in some circumstances, dedicated technicians or nurses are needed to yield consistent results. Blood flow measurements obtained through indicator dilution techniques and pressure measurements provide indirect evidence of stenosis-driven access dysfunction. The direct visualization of blood vessel access can be achieved through angiography and Doppler duplex ultrasound (DDU). DDU is particularly useful as it can measure flow and visualize stenosis severity **(Table 1)**.

Imaging Techniques

Duplex ultrasound: This is a noninvasive technique that provides real-time images of blood flow and anatomical structures. It enables the assessment of blood flow velocity and direction, as well as the identification of abnormalities such as stenosis. However, the accuracy of this method depends on the operator's skill and the angle of insonation, which can introduce variability in measurements. Furthermore, the optimal site for measurement, whether the access or feeding artery, is debated. In any case, serial measurements should be conducted at the same site.

- *Probe requirements:* High-frequency linear probes (7.5–13 MHz) are used, particularly for superficial AVF vessels.
- *Examination areas:* These include arterial inflow, anastomotic chamber, and venous outflow.
- *Examination findings:* Visible narrowing on gray-scale image; draining vein peak systolic velocity ratio >2:1 suggests >50% stenosis.[3]

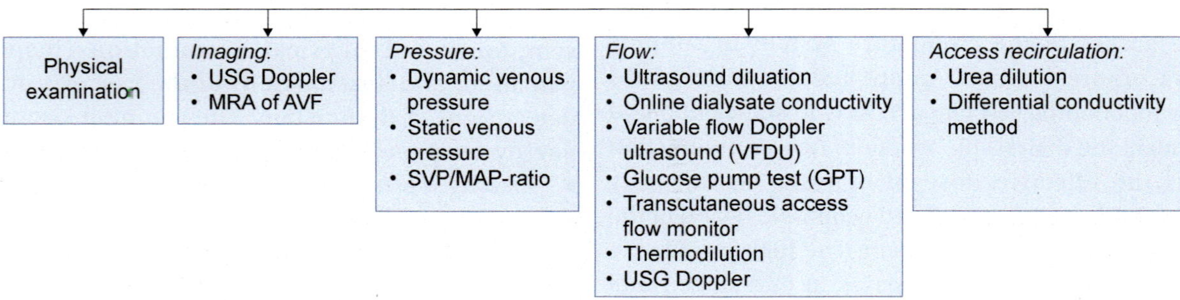

Fig. 1: Monitoring and surveillance methods. (AVF: arteriovenous fistula; MRA: magnetic resonance angiography)

TABLE 1: Differences between monitoring and surveillance.

Feature	Monitoring	Surveillance
Tools	Clinical examination, dialysis adequacy	Ultrasound, pressure transducers
Performed by	Dialysis staff	Trained technician/ interventionist
Frequency	Every session	Weekly to monthly
Cost	Minimal	Higher
Purpose	Detect dysfunction via symptoms	Detect dysfunction early, even without symptoms
Interventions Prompted	Confirm clinical suspicion	Preventive or early elective intervention

- *Recommended monitoring:* Regular physical examinations and monthly flow assessments are advised, with optimal flow rates ranging from 700 to 1,300 mL/min.

Criteria for AVF functionality:
- *NKF criteria:*
  - AVF outflow vein lumen diameter ≥6 mm
  - Blood flow ≥600 mL/min
- *University of Alabama at Birmingham (UAB) criteria:*[3]
  - AVF outflow vein lumen diameter ≥4 mm
  - Blood flow ≥500 mL/min

The *UAB criteria* show higher sensitivity (89% vs. 68%) but lower specificity (42% vs. 70%) compared to the *NKF criteria* for predicting unassisted AVF use.

Once an AVF is functional and in use, a Doppler ultrasound can be utilized for surveillance to measure blood flow and identify anatomical stenosis.

Practice point: Surveillance measurements should not be taken during dialysis or immediately after dialysis.[2]

Magnetic resonance angiography (MRA): This provides high-resolution images of vascular structures, offering superior detail for detecting stenoses compared to duplex ultrasound. However, despite its diagnostic benefits, MRA is time-consuming and costly, which limits its practicality for use during routine dialysis sessions.

Intra-access Pressure-based Surveillance Methods

Pressure measurement techniques evaluate the relationship between access flow and pressure, enabling the prediction of impending access failure. The primary methods are given in the following text.

Direct venous pressure: Direct venous pressure (DVP) is measured at the onset of dialysis, providing a snapshot of venous pressure. Although useful, DVP measurements can be influenced by factors such as needle size and blood flow rate. The KDOQI guidelines caution against using unstandardized DVP as a sole indicator of access stenosis. It is considered to be supplementary to clinical monitoring.

Static pressure measurement: These measurements are performed prior to dialysis, avoiding the influence of extracorporeal blood flow. The IAP is normalized against mean arterial pressure (MAP) to calculate arterial and venous pressure ratios, aiding in the identification of stenosis.

Static pressure measurements are critical for detecting *outflow stenosis* and predicting thrombosis in vascular accesses.

- *Measuring IAP* **(Figs. 2A and B)**:
  - Use a pressure transducer or a catheter-based system to measure the IAP at the site of the AVF, usually near the anastomosis (where the artery and vein are joined).
  - The transducer is connected to the venous line of the dialysis access.
  - This pressure measurement reflects the resistance within the access and can be influenced by any stenosis or narrowing that may be present.
- *Calculate the static pressure ratio*:
  - The static pressure ratio is calculated by comparing the *intra-access systolic pressure* to the *arterial systolic pressure.*
  - *Formula:* A ratio closer to *0.45* or *0.55* indicates a significant stenosis. Higher values typically signal more severe obstruction, which may require intervention.
- *Interpreting results:*
  - If the static pressure ratio exceeds the threshold (e.g., 0.55), it may suggest significant stenosis, indicating that intervention (such as percutaneous transluminal angioplasty or PTA) may be required to restore adequate flow and prevent thrombosis. IAP normalized to MAP as a ratio of 0.5 has a sensitivity of 81% and specificity of 80% in detecting a stenosis of >50%.
  - Lower ratios may suggest good access flow with minimal stenosis. The *original static pressure measurement* used inline pressure transducers, which were expensive and required careful calibration, leading to challenges in routine clinical use.

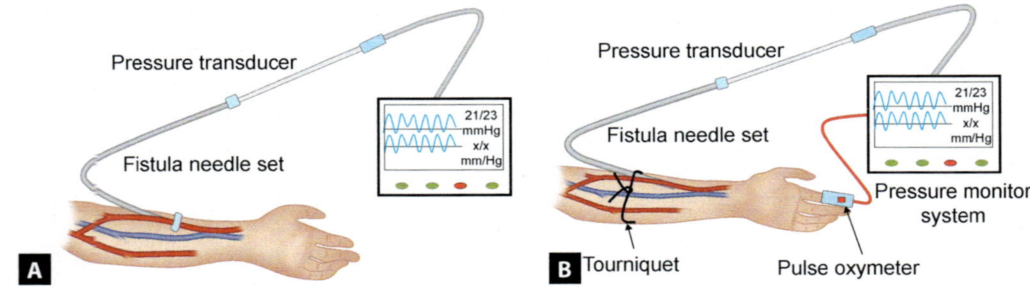

Figs. 2A and B: Intra-access pressure measurement. (A) Static pressure measurement; (B) Total pressure measurement.

- A computerized method was developed to address these issues, using pressure readings taken throughout dialysis sessions. This method factors in variables like *chair height, blood pump flow,* and *hematocrit. VascAlert*®, a computerized tool, has been successfully used to monitor static pressure ratios and assess hemodynamic changes in both *AVF* and *AVG*.

Flow Measurements

Intra-access flow measurements are essential for assessing the adequacy of vascular access during dialysis.

Flow measurements remain essential for *inflow stenosis*, but combining both flow and pressure methods offers a more complete understanding of the access function. In *grafts*, flow *measurements* alone may not always correlate with the location or severity of stenosis. This suggests that measuring flow and static pressure provides a more comprehensive evaluation of the access function.

All flow measurements are based on the principle of induced recirculation, where the arterial and venous bloodlines are reversed. A signal is generated by infusing a substance (such as saline or glucose), altering the ultrafiltration rate (which changes hematocrit levels), or adding sodium (which affects conductance) to the venous return line. This introduced signal mixes with the incoming arterial blood at the needle site, altering the signal's magnitude. The modified signal is then detected by a sensor placed on the arterial line; the access blood flow is calculated by multiplying the area under the curve by the measured arterial blood pump flow **(Fig. 3)**.

In the case of the injection of saline indicator (as shown by the syringe) using the ultrasound dilution method, the signal is the change in velocity of sound through blood and saline and measured as the time-area under the curve (AUC) that is detected by independent sensors on the arterial and venous lines. Access flow (Q_A) can be determined because blood pump flow (Q_{bpf}) is accurately measured using the same ultrasound transducers. The ratio of the arterial flow to the total flow between the needles is given by the injected into the venous line; the ratio of the arterial and venous dilution curves is also R. Solving the equation for R to determine Q_A yields the equation:

$$Q_A = Q_{bpf}\,[1/R - 1].$$

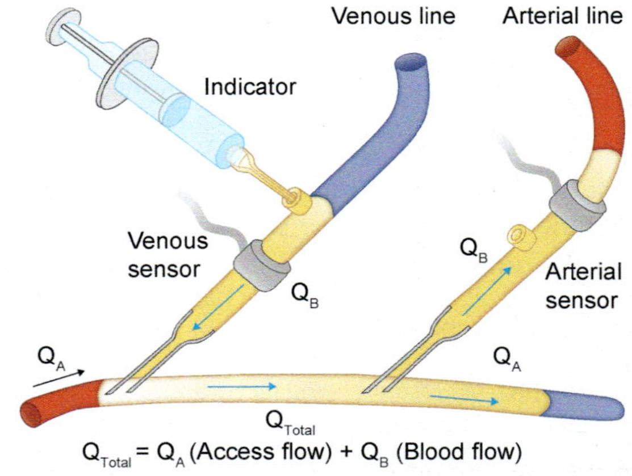

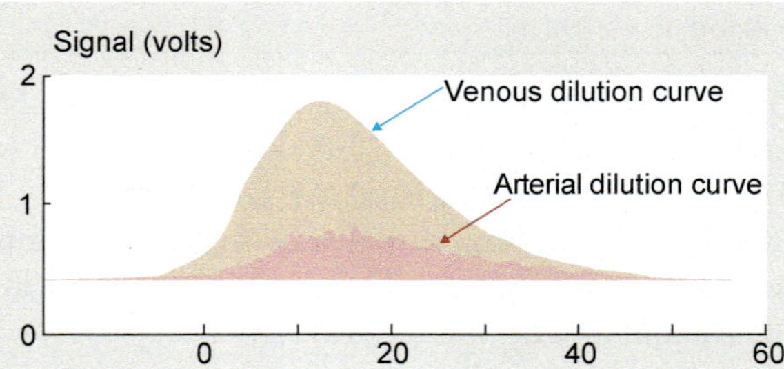

Fig. 3: Principles of access flow measurement through induced recirculation. Top panel shows a segment of access that is cannulated with needles. A signal that can be measured is generated in many ways (see the text). Note that the venous needle is upstream of the arterial needle through deliberate reversal of the bloodlines. Blood that has gone through the dialyzer and contains the "signal indicator" now returns into the access and mixes with arterial blood diluting the indicator. This is deliberately induced recirculation (*R*).

Accuracy: The earlier studies have highlighted significant variability in the measurement of access flow (QA) and MAP during hemodialysis sessions, which can impact the accuracy of surveillance for vascular access dysfunction.[4] Factors such as needle orientation, higher flow rates in elbow-level AVFs, hydration status, MAP, and hematocrit influenced QA by up to 30% week-to-week. These findings highlight the need for consistent monitoring and techniques to ensure accurate assessment and timely intervention for access dysfunction and its author's suggestion not to take single reading into account but rather the trend.

Ultrasound dilution: The ultrasound dilution method, also known as the Krivitski method, involves injecting a saline bolus and measuring the resulting dilution to calculate access flow rates. This method is widely used but requires careful calibration and can be affected by cardiopulmonary recirculation.

Online dialysate conductivity: This real-time method measures dialysate sodium conductivity to estimate blood flow, leveraging the correlation between sodium and urea diffusion across the dialyzer membrane. Access blood flow can be inferred without reversing dialysis lines by measuring conductivity changes.

Variable flow Doppler ultrasound (VFDU): This employs Doppler technology to assess blood flow without the need to reverse dialysis lines. It measures the Doppler signal at varying pump speeds, providing a more accurate assessment of access flow rates by adjusting for beam angle and cross-sectional area variability.

Glucose pump test (GPT): This is a rapid, noninvasive method that calculates access blood flow by infusing a constant glucose bolus into the arterial line and measuring blood glucose changes before and after infusion.

Transcutaneous access flow monitor: This noninvasive technique utilizes an optical sensor placed over the access site to monitor hematocrit concentration changes in response to saline injected into the venous line. The resulting changes in hematocrit allow for the calculation of intra-access blood flow.

Thermodilution: The thermodilution technique assesses intra-access blood flow by measuring changes in blood temperature after introducing a cold injectate into the access. Temperature-sensitive sensors detect the thermal gradient, allowing for flow calculations based on the mean blood temperature and transit duration.

Practice point: Arteriovenous fistula Doppler, even when the patient is not on dialysis, is a common surveillance method to monitor access flow. High Qa diagnosis relies on accurate measurement, best achieved with Doppler ultrasound. Flow should be measured from *the brachial artery at least 5 cm proximal to the anastomosis, regardless of fistula type.* In cases of high brachial artery bifurcation, measure proximal to the bifurcation. Access site measurements are unreliable due to variable diameter and compressibility. Brachial artery flow offers a consistent method for detecting high or low-flow fistulas.

Access Recirculation

Urea dilution method:

- *Principle:* This method measures the difference in urea concentration between arterial and venous lines. By temporarily reversing blood flow and observing the dilution of urea, clinicians can estimate access blood flow and recirculation percentages.
- *Limitations:* Although commonly used, this method is prone to sampling errors and is a late indicator of access dysfunction. It is more effective in detecting issues in AVF than in AVG.

Differential conductivity method:

- *Principle:* This technique involves injecting a hypertonic saline solution and measuring changes in conductivity between arterial and venous lines. Variations in conductivity indicate the level of recirculation, helping to quantify access abnormalities.
- *Advantages:* This technique provides a more immediate assessment compared to urea-based methods and is less prone to sampling errors.

Issues with Monitoring and Surveillance

Importance of Accurate Prediction

Effective monitoring and surveillance is crucial for early detection of AVF dysfunction, allowing for timely intervention to prevent underdialysis. Addressing anatomical stenosis promptly can prevent severe complications. Evidence shows that proactive monitoring and surveillance to detect stenosis reduces access failure and thrombosis rates, especially in AVGs. Regular surveillance enables earlier interventions such as percutaneous transluminal angioplasty (PTA), which can preserve access function

Patient Concerns

- Nearly 60% of hemodialysis patients fear access thrombosis, second only to concerns about pain.

- Loss of access patency affects not just patients but also disrupts the workflow of dialysis staff.

Outcomes of Elective Percutaneous Transluminal Angioplasty

Research by Lilly et al.[5] found that grafts treated electively with PTA maintain longer patency compared to those treated after thrombosis. An access loss from thrombosis increases catheter usage increasing risk of morbidity and mortality.

Factors Affecting Patency

The duration of access patency post-PTA is inversely related to the degree of residual stenosis and static venous pressure after the procedure. Restoration of access flow postintervention is a better predictor of long-term patency than simply reducing the degree of stenosis. Interventions in AVFs generally show better durability compared to AVGs; however, there is a lack of robust comparative studies on this topic. However, postprocedure, 30% stenosis is considered as acceptable anatomical success. Postintervention pressure reduction of <30% was associated with a 62% higher risk of access failure requiring further intervention.[4]

Intervention Versus Thrombosis

While surveillance can reduce thrombosis rates, studies indicate it may not decrease the overall number of interventions (thrombosis treatment or elective PTA). Still, early intervention is preferred because treating thrombosis is more time-consuming and costly than performing elective interventions.

Clinical Implications

Ensuring effective treatment of stenotic lesions is essential to avoid thrombosis and reduce the reliance on catheters, which carry higher health risks.

CONCLUSION

Effective surveillance and monitoring of vascular access are crucial for the optimal management of patients undergoing hemodialysis. A comprehensive approach that combines imaging techniques, pressure measurements, and flow assessments can help detect and address complications related to vascular access. By employing these methods, healthcare providers can ensure timely interventions, improving patient outcomes and enhancing hemodialysis treatment's overall effectiveness.

Practice point: Dr Hoon Suk Park, often emphasized: "Each institution should tailor its AVF monitoring and surveillance plan according to its specific resources, expertise, equipment, and patient load. Every patient requires comprehensive monitoring of Kt/V, access flow, and venous pressure. In both low- and high-volume centers, static venous pressure is preferred for its reliability; however, tracking dynamic venous pressure trends can still offer valuable insights."

Regarding flow monitoring, monthly Doppler ultrasounds of the brachial artery flow are recommended in low-volume centers. In *high-volume centers,* vascular nurses should record monthly flow measurements using a *transonic machine,* ensuring recirculation is documented during each assessment. The Transonic measurements serve as a screening tool, with further confirmation provided by *brachial artery Doppler* to verify the flow. A *flow decrease >20%* or an *increasing trend in venous pressure* should raise clinical suspicion of stenosis, prompting further evaluation.

Regular surveillance not only increases patient safety but also extends the lifespan of vascular access, thereby reducing the need for surgical interventions and promoting a better quality of life for patients. When surveillance is conducted intelligently—using repeated measurements and physiological principles—it can effectively reduce clot formation without raising the rates of false-positive diagnoses, subsequently leading to fewer PTA procedures.

REFERENCES

1. Conjeevaram A, Anupama YJ, Vincent L, Sastry NB, Siddini V, Revanasiddappa M, et al. Clinico-epidemiological profile of dialysis services in Karnataka, India - A multicentric exploratory study. Indian J Nephrol. 2022;32(3):223-32.
2. Umei K, Toda N, Izumi J, Umeda Y. Relationship between resistance index and recirculation rate in vascular access. Ren Replace Ther. 2022;8:56.
3. Robbin ML, Oser RF, Allon M, Clements MW, Dockery J, Weber TM, et al. Hemodialysis access graft stenosis: US detection. Radiology. 1998;208(3):655-61.
4. Kumbar L, Peterson E, Zaborowicz M, Besarab A, Yee J, Zasuwa G. Sentinel vascular access monitoring after endovascular intervention predicts access outcome. J Vasc Access. 2019;20(4):409-16.
5. Lilly RZ, Carlton D, Barker J, Saddekni S, Hamrick K, Oser R, et al. Predictors of arteriovenous graft patency after radiologic intervention in hemodialysis patients. Am J Kidney Dis. 2001;37(5):945-53.

CHAPTER 15

Access Maintenance and Cannulation Techniques

Aakash Kirit Shingada, Vivek Goel, Neil Saldanha

INTRODUCTION

Hemodialysis remains the most widespread modality of renal replacement therapy[1] and vascular access remains the most integral part of dialysis patients. The functioning and quality of access is the biggest determinant of the longevity on dialysis. The ideal hemodialysis vascular access should be suitable to patient, reliable, and complications free to provide prescribed dialysis. The 2019 Kidney Disease Outcomes Quality Initiative (KDOQI) clinical practice guidelines for vascular access emphasize a more patient-focused approach and recommend the development of an end-stage kidney disease (ESKD) life-plan, taking each patient's needs and preferences into consideration when choosing an access. The focus moves away from the prior "Fistula First" approach.

FIRST ARTERIOVENOUS FISTULA CANNULATION

After the respective nephrologist orders to cannulate, the qualified staff who has ample experience in cannulating new arteriovenous fistulas (AVFs) should take the task at hand considering the patient's anxiety is also maximum. For all vascular accesses, an aseptic technique should be used for all cannulation and catheter accession procedures. Despite the general acceptance of the importance of standard precautions for hand washing and glove changes, these simple acts to minimize transmission of disease are frequently skipped. Strict hand washing, sterile gloves, and masks are a mandate. A primary fistula should be mature, ready for cannulation with minimal risk for infiltration, and able to deliver the prescribed blood flow throughout the dialysis procedure. The vessel wall should be firm and tough to touch and no prominent collaterals should be present. It is preferable but to monitor fistula development using Doppler ultrasonography. Fistulas are more likely to be useable when they meet the rule of 6s: Flow >600 mL/min, diameter of at least 0.6 cm, no more than 0.6 cm deep and discernible margins.

The steps of AVF cannulation include the following **(Video 1: Steps of Cannulation)**:

1. Skin preparation includes washing the access site with antibacterial soap and water and then cleansing the skin with 2% chlorhexidine gluconate (30 seconds) or 70% isopropyl alcohol (30 seconds) or 10% povidone iodine (2 minutes). The skin is to be left to dry and not wiped off. Clean gloves are to be worn by the staff for each cannulation.
2. Reassuring the patient during the first cannulation wins the confidence of the patient and ensures more compliance. After skin preparation, apply a tourniquet high up in the arm to increase the venous pressure and pull skin taut in a direction opposite to cannulation. For an easily palpated vessel, cannulate at a 25° angle with bevel up. Arterial needle can be placed antegrade or retrograde, but the venous needle should always be in the same direction of the blood flow.
3. Using a smaller gauge needle like the 17-gauge when cannulating for the first time is advisable. One may use a single needle, preferably arterial needle, during the first cannulation. Only when the arterial needle functions without bleeding, infiltration, hematoma, or prolonged post-hemodialysis bleeding, and with adequate blood flow rate (BFR) for two to six treatments should one advance to two needles. When both needles function adequately, one should gradually advance the needle gauge size.
4. Once the vessel has been penetrated, advance the needle slowly with the cutting-edge facing top of the vessel and without rotating the access. The needle removal is also to be done at the same angle and pressure is never to be applied before the needle is totally out.

Mild infiltration injury can occur in as frequently as >50% of all AVF cannulations and major infiltrations of 5–7%.[2] Thus, it is critical to ensure that cannulators have received adequate training and mentoring to facilitate and achieve successful cannulation. A successful cannulation is one where two needles of adequate size are inserted into the arteriovenous (AV) access at the right depth and angle to facilitate prescribed dialysis and in which this is achieved with minimal pain or no complications. Successful cannulation requires skilled cannulators who have received adequate initial and ongoing training and who continue close monitoring of the AV access. Needle selection for the initial cannulation is critical. One method used to select the appropriate needle size is a visual and tactile examination. This examination allows the cannulator to determine which needle gauge would be most appropriate, based on the size of the vessels in the fistula. The use of smaller-gauge and Teflon needles should be considered when cannulating smaller and more fragile vessels.

Needle Size Selection

When choosing the needle size, follow the 2:1 rule—arterial and venous pressure should not exceed 50% of the pump speed, e.g., 400 mL/min blood flow rate (BFR), arterial and venous pressure should be –200/200 mm Hg, respectively. Arterial and venous pressure should not exceed –250 or 250 mm Hg to avoid damage to the access

General needle gauge guidelines and maximum BFR:

- 17-gauge needle = 200–250 BFR
- 16-gauge needle = 250–350 BFR
- 15-gauge needle = 350–450 BFR
- 14-gauge needle = >450 BFR

Needle Site Selection

- 4–5 cm (1.5–2 inches) apart, hub to hub, if needles in the same direction
- 2.5 cm (1 inch) apart, hub to hub, if needles in opposite direction
- Insertion site or needle tip once inserted, 4 cm (1.5 inches) away from the anastomosis

Troubleshooting Needle Placement and Increased Venous and/or Arterial Pressures

In a dialysis unit, a common challenge is poor flow in the arterial needle or increased venous pressure, which may be a result of incorrect cannulation. In such cases, the fistula should be assessed for presence of thrill and bruit and checked for infiltration. Access limb should be carefully repositioned and a small gauze can be placed under the needle wings and the tapes may be carefully readjusted (as needed), while closely monitoring venous and arterial pressures. If successful, the needle should be secure in position with tape while monitoring venous and arterial pressures. If unsuccessful, recirculate patient's blood and recheck needle position with portable ultrasound (if available) and if repositioning is unsuccessful, fistula needle should be removed.

Poor flows or increased venous pressures may occur because of inappropriate blood pump speed for the needle gauge used and may correct by decreasing blood pump speed. In case the needle placement and the needle gauge are correct, the fistula my need assessment with a Doppler to rule out inflow or outflow stenosis. Blood pressure should be checked ensuring the patient is not hypotensive; reviewing previous clinical records is necessary to determine baseline blood pressure, venous and arterial pressures, and BFR. Worsening numbers may suggest impending fistula failure and will merit early vascular surgery referral. It is always recommended to avoid repeated cannulations without further information.

Securing of Needles

Fistula needles should be secured at the same angle of insertion to avoid change in needle position and minimize risk of infiltration. It also should be secured during treatment to avoid accidental malposition or dislodgment of needles. Access limb and connections should be visible at all times and should not be covered with blankets. Taping styles also influence needle security and chevron and butterfly taping styles are associated with lesser risk of needle dislodgement.[3]

Needle Removal (Video 2: Steps of Decannulation)

Needle removal is as important if not more as cannulation to ensure maintenance of AVF. Needles should be removed one at a time. Needles should be removed at the same angle as angle of insertion. Compression should not be applied before complete needle removal. Once the needle is completely removed, use a two-digit technique (one finger at the skin level and one at the vein level) for maximum hemostasis. The cannulation site should be compressed for at least 10 minutes following which bandage should be applied. While applying pressure, ensure a thrill can be felt in the access, if the thrill cannot be felt, release the pressure slowly till thrill is felt. In case of prolonged bleeding, it is important to rule out venous stenosis and merits vascular surgery referral.

ARTERIOVENOUS FISTULA CANNULATION TECHNIQUES

Guidelines describe three possible ways to cannulate an AVF: (1) Rope ladder (RL), (2) area puncture (AP), and (3) buttonhole (BH):

- *RL technique:* We create a new puncture site each time, where the puncture site is placed 0.5 cm from the last puncture site. The whole length of the AVF is utilized in RL technique.
- *AP:* Cannulators using AP also create new puncture sites each time, but all sites are placed in the same area, the diameter of cannulation rarely surpassing 2–3 cm.
- *BH:* When BH is used, the needle is placed in exactly the same cannulation tract, using the same angle each time. Sharp needles are used to create a tunnel tract. When the tract is formed, blunt needles may be used for cannulation. Even though blunt needles are most common using BH, sharp needles might be a long-time solution.[1] Long-time use with sharp needles is referred to as buttonhole sharp (BHs) and the cannulation technique using blunt needles as buttonhole blunt (BHb).

The different cannulation techniques are used to varying extents worldwide. In the US, RL is the most common technique,[4] whereas in Europe, AP is most frequently used (66% vs. RL 30% and BH 6%).[5] Both the American and European guidelines conclude majorly that with AP the risk of complications such as aneurysms and hemorrhage is imminent, so it is better to be avoided.[6,7] Opinions differ when it comes to RL and BH. RL leads to more infiltrations and aneurysms, but the risk of infection is lesser compared to BH.[8] A systematic literature review showed that compared to RL, BH led to fewer interventions related to thromboses and stenosis. Aneurysms are also fewer with BH.[9] On the contrary, the risk of infections is higher with BH.[8] Studies comparing BHb versus BHs have not reported any significant difference in the incidence of stenosis. The KDOQI guidelines recommend rope ladder cannulation as the preferred cannulation technique for AVFs. It also considers reasonable to limit AV access BH cannulation only to special circumstances given the associated increased risks of infection and related adverse consequences.[10] Circumstances where BL cannulation may be acceptable are: AVFs having only a short segment for cannulation, enlarging aneurysm to prevent its further expansion or failure of RL cannulation for cannulators (e.g., home hemodialysis) who have established excellent hygiene and cannulation technique.

CANNULATION COMPLICATIONS

Cannulation complications range from minor hematomas to acute bleeding from pseudoaneurysms that required emergency surgical procedures. These complications can occur during needle placement, during hemodialysis or post needle removal.

Infiltration Injury

Infiltration of the vein can occur when a needling an AVF which is too small, not mature enough, or very mobile, leading to extravasation, the needle thus, may inadvertently pierce through the side or back wall of the fistula. This can result in some degree of swelling, bruising, and pain. Infiltration injury can be categorized as follows:

- *Minor cannulation injury:* An injury that causes infiltration and swelling that can be managed with conservative measures and in which cannulation can be reattempted for the next dialysis session.
- *Major cannulation injury:* An injury that results in significant bleeding infiltration and swelling that necessitates rest for the fistula for >7 days.
- *Severe cannulation injury:* An injury that results in significant bleeding complications needing blood transfusion and endovascular or surgical intervention.

Prevention and Treatment

An AV access assessment prior to cannulation is essential. The use of bedside ultrasound can lead to improved cannulation outcomes.[10] Experienced cannulators should be used for AV accesses at risk of complications. If a cannulator is unsuccessful cannulating an AV access, a maximum of two attempts should be done before seeking expert advice. Smaller-gauge and Teflon needles scan be used when needling smaller and more fragile vessels.[10]

Hematomas

Hematomas occur as a consequence of an infiltration of the vein or due to leaking of blood around the puncture site during cannulation or after removal of a needle at the end of dialysis. The size of hematomas varies, from a diffuse area to a large, firm mass that can leading to compression of the vessel, resulting in clotting of the AV access. Management of cannulation complications such as infiltration and resulting hematoma is dependent on the extent of swelling, pain, and patient anxiety. Apply ice for a minimum of 10 minutes in all cases. If the infiltration is moderate, the needle should be withdrawn and manual pressure held over the infiltration site. Appropriate rest to the fistula with bridging with a hemodialysis catheter must be done in case of a large hematoma formation.

Needle Dislodgement

Needle dislodgement can be identified by pressure alarms on the machine, bleeding from needle entry site, excessive pain, swelling, and bruising. It can be resolved by adjusting the needle or by removing the needle and recannulation.

Delayed Hemostasis

Delayed hemostasis is one of the most common complications following dialysis. The common causes include not turning off the heparin infusion soon enough, using too much heparin, inadequate pressure being applied on site of cannulation, or pressure being taken off too soon following needle removal. If over-heparinization is suspected, protamine may be administered. A very important cause of delayed hemostasis is venous stenosis and patients with repeated events of delayed hemostasis merit evaluation of the access by a Doppler and deserve early referral to vascular surgeon.

DELAYED CANNULATION COMPLICATIONS

Aneurysm and Pseudoaneurysms

Another complication of frequent cannulation of a fistula is aneurysm development. The hemodynamic changes resulting from an AV access creation are likely exacerbated by the repeated cannulations and injury to the vein which can lead to pseudoaneurysms or aneurysms. The incidence of true aneurysm formation that involves all three layers of the venous wall is reported at 5–7%.[11] The potential complications of an aneurysm include ischemic skin overlying the aneurysm, with potential for spontaneous rupture and exsanguination. The management of aneurysms should be individualized, with options that include various surgical revisions and endovascular stent placements. AVF aneurysm rupture can be a catastrophic event, in which blood loss can lead to hemorrhagic shock and hemodynamic compromise. An urgent vascular surgery intervention is required to ligate the bleeding vessel.

Arteriovenous Fistula Infections

The incidence of AVF infections can be modified by cannulation techniques with BH cannulation putting AVF at greater risk of infection. Skin organisms, *Staphylococcus aureus* and *S. epidermidis*, account for 70–90% of AV access infections.[12] Patients with AV access infections require timely detection, diagnosis, and treatment with antibiotics to prevent poor outcomes. Rarely, there may be abscesses, which require surgical excision and drainage.

Fistula Thrombosis

Difficulties in access cannulation can also lead to fistula thrombosis presenting as absence of thrill/bruit at site of AVF, this necessitates early intervention with thrombectomy or catheter-directed thrombolysis, where thrombectomy is not feasible.

Thus, vascular access cannulation can lead to a myriad of issues, regular assessment of the puncture site and proper precautions are essential to prevent loss of vascular access.

Successful AV fistula access cannulation is fundamental to ensuring effective dialysis and promoting long-term vascular access viability. Proper technique, early identification of complications, and regular monitoring are the key to minimizing issues such as infection, thrombosis, and stenosis. Additionally, patient education and individualized care plans play a crucial role in optimizing cannulation outcomes. By emphasizing careful and skilled cannulation practices, healthcare providers can significantly improve the quality of life for dialysis patients, supporting both the longevity of the AV fistula and the overall effectiveness of the dialysis process.

CONCLUSION

Effective arteriovenous access cannulation is central to sustaining reliable hemodialysis and preserving vascular access over time. By adhering to meticulous aseptic technique, selecting appropriate needle size and site, and applying evidence-based cannulation methods, clinicians can greatly reduce the risk of complications such as infiltration, hematoma, infection, and thrombosis.

Continuous training, careful monitoring, and timely intervention when problems arise are vital to maintaining access function. Ultimately, combining skilled practice with patient-centered planning supports better dialysis outcomes and enhances the long-term quality-of-life for individuals dependent on vascular access.

REFERENCES

1. Staaf K, Uhlin F. Cannulation with sharp or blunt needles for haemodialysis: the importance of cannulation technique for the patient's lifeline. J Vasc Access. 2019;20(2):161-8.
2. Lee T, Barker J, Allon M. Needle infiltration of arteriovenous fistulae in hemodialysis: risk factors and consequences. Am J Kidney Dis. 2006;47(6):1020-6.
3. Chan YFC, Dobson S, Barber T. Hemodialysis taping styles and their effect on reducing the chance of venous needle dislodgement. Semin Dial. 2021;34(3):218-223.
4. Lyman M, Nguyen DB, Shugart A, Gruhler H, Lines C, Patel PR. Risk of vascular access infection associated with buttonhole cannulation of fistulas: data from the National Healthcare Safety Network. Am J Kidney Dis. 2020; 76(1):82-9.
5. Parisotto MT, Schoder VU, Miriunis C, Grassmann AH, Scatizzi LP, Kaufmann P, et al. Cannulation technique influences arteriovenous fistula and graft survival. Kidney Int. 2014;86(4):790-7.
6. Parisotto MT, Pancirova J. Vascular access cannulation and care: A nursing best practice guide for arteriovenous fistula. Lucerne, Switzerland; European Dialysis and Transplant Nurses Association/European Renal Care Association (EDTNA/ERCA); 2014.
7. Almehmi A, Wang S. Partial aneurysmectomy is effective in managing aneurysm-associated complications of arteriovenous fistulae for hemodialysis: case series and literature review. Semin Dial. 2012;25(3):357-64.
8. Wong B, Muneer M, Wiebe N, Storie D, Shurraw S, Pannu N, et al. Buttonhole versus rope-ladder cannulation of arteriovenous fistulas for hemodialysis: a systematic review. Am J Kidney Dis. 2014;64(6):918-36.
9. Grudzinski A, Mendelssohn D, Pierratos A, Nesrallah G. A systematic review of buttonhole cannulation practices and outcomes. Semin Dial. 2013;26(4):465-75.
10. Lok CE, Huber TS, Lee T, Shenoy S, Yevzlin AS, Abreo K, et al. KDOQI Clinical Practice Guideline for Vascular Access: 2019 Update. Am J Kidney Dis. 2020;75(4)(suppl 2):S1-164.
11. Pasklinsky G, Meisner RJ, Labropoulos N, Leon L, Gasparis AP, Landau D, Tassiopoulos AK, Pappas PJ. Management of true aneurysms of hemodialysis access fistulas. Journal of vascular surgery. 2011;53(5):1291-7.
12. Lafrance J-P, Rahme E, Lelorier J, Iqbal S. Vascular access-related infections: definitions, incidence rates, and risk factors. American journal of kidney diseases. 2008;52(5):982-93.

CHAPTER 16

Pathophysiology of Vascular Access Dysfunction

Dinesh Khullar, Lalathaksha Kumbar, Anish Kumar Gupta

INTRODUCTION

Vascular access serves as the cornerstone for hemodialysis, a life-saving therapy for patients with end-stage renal disease (ESRD). It enables repeated and effective removal of metabolic waste products, excess fluids and toxins from the bloodstream. However, the functionality of vascular access can deteriorate due to various complications, including stenosis, thrombosis, and infections. These complications lead to increased patient morbidity, frequent hospitalizations, and elevated healthcare costs. A profound understanding of the pathophysiological mechanisms underlying vascular access dysfunction is crucial to improving patient outcomes and developing preventive and therapeutic strategies.[1] In this chapter, we explore the pathophysiology of vascular access dysfunction and provide a comprehensive discussion on associated factors and underlying causes.

ANATOMY AND TYPES OF VASCULAR ACCESS

Arteriovenous Fistulas

An arteriovenous fistula (AVF) is a surgically established connection between an artery and a vein, usually located in the forearm or upper arm. This procedure enables the vein to undergo arterialization, which enhances its size and wall strength to handle the elevated blood flow necessary for hemodialysis. AVFs are considered the preferred vascular access method due to their longevity, lower infection rates, and better patency compared to alternative options. However, they are susceptible to primary failure, often resulting from inadequate venous maturation or the development of stenosis caused by intimal hyperplasia.[2]

Arteriovenous Grafts

Arteriovenous grafts (AVGs) involve the use of synthetic materials, typically polytetrafluoroethylene (PTFE), to create a connection between an artery and a vein. These grafts are used when the patient's native vessels are unsuitable for AVF creation. While AVGs can be utilized relatively soon after placement and are simpler to construct surgically, they are more prone to complications such as thrombosis, infection, and neointimal hyperplasia at the graft–vein junction, a key factor contributing to graft failure.[3]

Central Venous Catheters

Central venous catheters (CVCs) are inserted into large central veins, such as the internal jugular or subclavian veins, and are commonly used in short-term or emergency scenarios. While offering the advantage of immediate usability, CVCs are associated with significant risks, including bloodstream infections, thrombosis, and central vein stenosis. Prolonged usage may lead to endothelial irritation, increasing the risk of luminal narrowing and catheter dysfunction.[4]

MATURATION OF VASCULAR ACCESS

The maturation of an AVF is a multifaceted process, characterized by the enlargement of both arterial and venous diameters after the creation of an arteriovenous (AV) connection. This connection results in increased blood flow, pressure, and shear stress, exposing the vein to a high-oxygen environment. This exposure initiates vascular remodeling, vasodilation, and thickening of the vessel wall. Critical adaptive mechanisms involved in this process include the production of nitric oxide (NO), the activation of growth factors that facilitate the migration and proliferation of smooth muscle cells, the upregulation of enzymes such as matrix metalloproteinases, and the breakdown of the extracellular matrix. Maturation typically occurs within 4–6 weeks, with physical and ultrasound evaluations after 4 weeks helping to assess adequacy and identify issues such as insufficient venous diameter (<4 mm) or blood flow (<500 mL/min), which can hinder maturation. As per 2005 Kidney Disease Outcomes Quality Initiative (KDOQI) guidelines, by 6 weeks, a mature AVF should have a venous diameter ≥6 mm, blood flow ≥600 mL/min, skin depth < 6 mm, and a straight segment of ≥6 cm for cannulation.[4,5] The definition of a mature fistula has evolved beyond the traditional anatomical perspective. Recently, a mature fistula is described as physiologically or functionally mature. According to the latest KDOQI guidelines, a mature fistula is one that can reliably support dialysis with two needles for more than two thirds of dialysis sessions over a 4-week period. The two-thirds criterion is used to encompass studies mentioned in these guidelines. However, it is important to note that a truly mature AV access should provide consistent and reliable dialysis most of the time, assuming expert cannulation techniques are employed and there are no cannulation or other technical complications.[4]

PATHOPHYSIOLOGY OF VASCULAR ACCESS DYSFUNCTION

There are two primary causes of AVF failure: (1) Failure to mature and (2) subsequent venous stenosis, which can lead to thrombosis. The exact pathophysiology of nonfunctioning of vascular access is unclear. *Juxta-anastomotic stenosis* is a common complication noted in AVF; this can lead to low flow or vascular thrombosis. However, it is unclear whether the primary cause of this stenosis is venous neointimal hyperplasia or secondary to surgical creation injury. Stenoses typically develop near the anastomotic site (in wrist fistulas) and in the proximal vein (in elbow fistulas).[6] The evidence has shown the high incidence of Inflow arterial stenosis.[7]

Vascular access failure has been characterized as a process involving upstream and downstream factors **(Fig. 1)**. These lead to venous neointimal hyperplasia (NIH) or inadequate outward remodeling. *Upstream factors* include: (1) Surgical trauma at the time of AV surgery; (2) hemodynamic shear stress at the vein-artery or vein-graft anastomosis (as a result of low shear stress, turbulence, and compliance mismatch between artery and veins);[8] (3) graft bioincompatibility;[9] (3) vessel injury from needle cannulations (most relevant in the setting of intragraft stenoses) or angioplasty;[10] and (5) uremia, which is shown to exacerbate endothelial dysfunction and predispose to venous NIH.[11] Downstream events are a reaction to injury in endothelial and smooth muscle cells caused by upstream factors. *Downstream factors* involve oxidative stress, inflammation, and the migration and proliferation of fibroblasts, smooth muscle cells, and myofibroblasts **(Figs. 2 and 3)**.

Intimal Hyperplasia

Intimal hyperplasia is the thickening of the intimal layer of blood vessels and is the primary pathological process leading to stenosis in AVFs and AVGs. It is initiated by endothelial injury caused by surgical manipulation, altered shear stress, or hypoxia at the anastomotic site. This injury triggers an inflammatory response characterized by the recruitment of macrophages, platelets, and other immune cells. Cytokines and growth factors such as platelet-derived growth factor (PDGF) and transforming growth factor-β (TGF-β) are released, promoting the migration and proliferation of smooth muscle cells (SMCs) from the medial layer to the intima. Additionally, SMCs produce extracellular matrix (ECM) components such as collagen and elastin, leading to vessel wall thickening and luminal narrowing. Molecular pathways such as nuclear factor kappa B (NF-κB) signaling play a central role in perpetuating inflammation and SMC activation.[12]

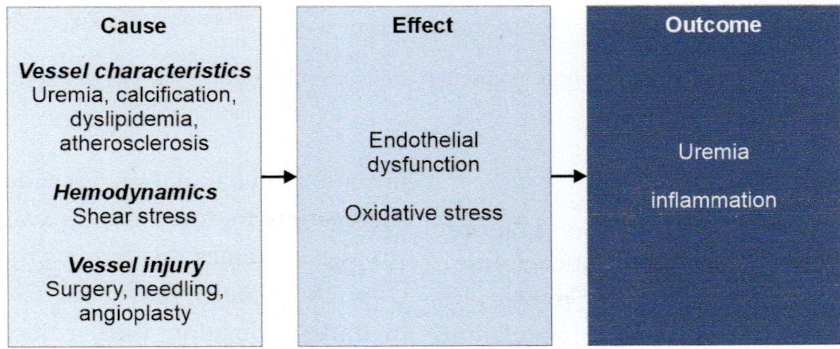

Fig. 1: Risk factors associated with vascular access dysfunction.

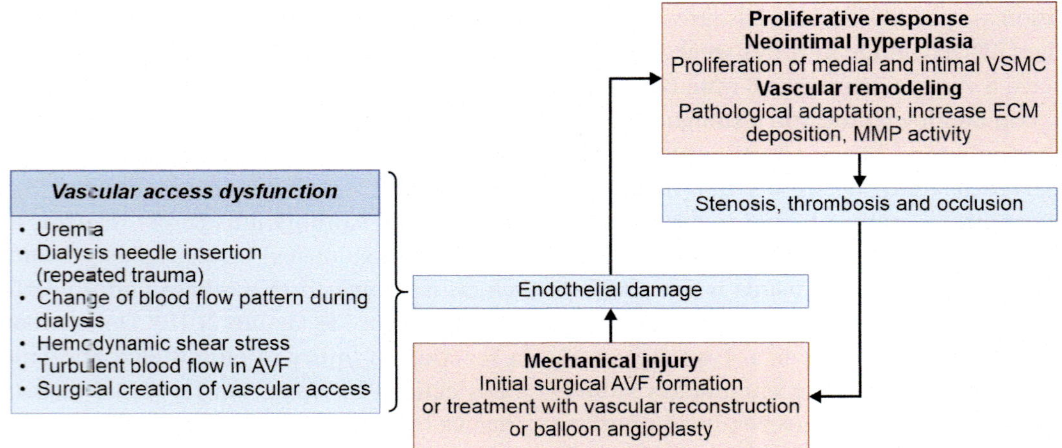

Fig. 2: Pathophysiology of vascular access dysfunction. (AVF: arteriovenous fistula; ECM: extracellular matrix; MMP: matrix metalloproteinase; VSMC: vascular smooth muscle cells)

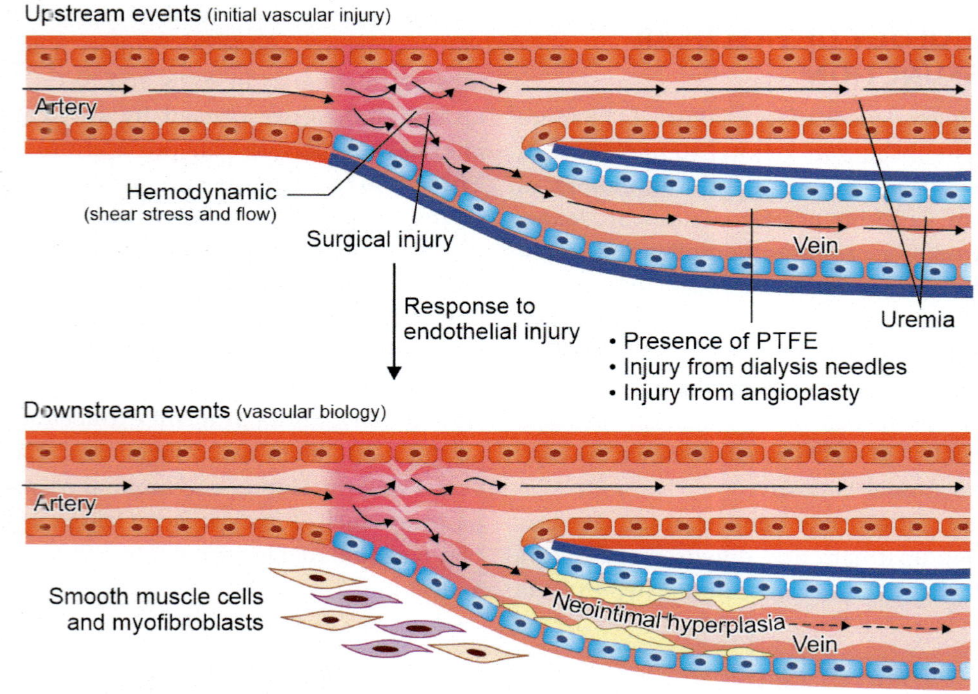

Fig. 3 Upstream and downstream events in vascular access dysfunction. (PTFE: polytetrafluoroethylene)

Thrombosis

Thrombosis is a major cause of vascular access failure, often secondary to stenosis. The prothrombotic environment within the vascular access site is driven by endothelial dysfunction, which leads to the upregulation of tissue factor and von Willebrand factor. These molecules initiate the coagulation cascade and promote platelet aggregation. Reduced NO bioavailability due to oxidative stress exacerbates this process by increasing vasoconstriction and platelet activation. The thrombus is stabilized by fibrin deposition, further obstructing blood flow and compromising the functionality of the vascular access.[1]

Inflammation and Oxidative Stress

Chronic systemic inflammation and oxidative stress are pervasive in dialysis patients and significantly contribute to vascular access dysfunction. The repeated needling of AVFs or AVGs, combined with bioincompatible dialysis membranes, perpetuates local and systemic inflammatory responses. Reactive oxygen species (ROS) generated during oxidative stress damage endothelial cells, reducing NO production and impairing vascular relaxation. This environment favors vasoconstriction, thrombosis, and intimal hyperplasia, creating a vicious cycle of vascular injury.[13,14]

Hemodynamic Contributions to Dysfunction

Shear Stress

Shear stress plays a critical role in maintaining vascular homeostasis. Under normal physiological conditions, laminar shear stress promotes endothelial health by stimulating NO release, which has anti-inflammatory and antithrombotic properties. However, vascular access creation alters shear stress patterns. High-shear stress at the arterial anastomosis can lead to endothelial cell activation and subsequent inflammation, while low-shear stress in other segments encourages intimal hyperplasia and thrombosis.[1,14,15]

Turbulent Flow

Creating an anastomosis introduces turbulent flow patterns, particularly at the arterial-venous junction. Turbulence exacerbates endothelial dysfunction by increasing the deposition of proinflammatory molecules and mechanical stress on the vessel wall. This abnormal flow environment accelerates neointimal hyperplasia and contributes to early and recurrent stenosis.[14]

Central Venous Catheter-related Dysfunction

Fibrin Sheath Formation

Fibrin sheaths form around central venous catheters (CVCs) due to endothelial irritation and thrombin generation. These sheaths consist of fibrin, platelets, and trapped leukocytes adhering to the catheter surface. Fibrin sheaths impede blood flow and create a nidus for bacterial colonization, increasing the risk of infection and functional failure.[16]

Central Vein Stenosis

Central vein stenosis is a common complication of prolonged CVC use. Endothelial damage caused by catheter placement and chronic irritation leads to inflammation and fibrosis. Over time, the accumulation of fibrotic tissue reduces the luminal diameter of the central veins, resulting in impaired venous drainage and reduced dialysis efficiency. Chronic inflammation perpetuates the cycle of injury and repair, worsening the stenosis.

Systemic Influences on Access Dysfunction

Uremia

Uremic toxins impair vascular endothelial function by disrupting NO production and enhancing oxidative stress. The accumulation of these toxins also dysregulates matrix metalloproteinases (MMPs), which are involved in ECM remodeling. This dysregulation contributes to abnormal vascular remodeling, intimal hyperplasia, and access dysfunction.[1]

Comorbidities

- *Diabetes mellitus:* Hyperglycemia accelerates vascular injury through oxidative stress and the formation of advanced glycation end-products (AGEs). These factors impair endothelial repair mechanisms and promote fibrosis.[3]
- *Hypertension:* Elevated blood pressure exacerbates endothelial injury, leading to increased vascular remodeling and a heightened risk of access dysfunction.

Preoperative Artery and Vein Characteristics

The role of preoperative vessel characteristics in AVF failure is increasingly recognized. Ultrasound mapping reveals that vessel diameter and distensibility affect AVF maturation and patency. CKD-associated dyslipidemia, cardiovascular risk, and secondary hyperparathyroidism contribute to vascular calcification, while vasculopathy involves accelerated atherosclerosis, thickening, and calcification, impairing vessel remodeling.[17-19] Noninvasive tests, such as flow-mediated dilation, correlate with postoperative AVF measurements. Preoperative arterial medial fibrosis is linked to better AVF maturation, while arterial calcification shows no clear association with dysfunction. Preoperative venous intimal hyperplasia of the target vein is noted in up to 88% of patients undergoing

AVF creation. While it is logical to assume a relationship with AVF maturation failure, the Hemodialysis Fistula Maturation Failure study failed to demonstrate this.[20] Patient characteristics, including advanced age, hypertension, smoking, hypomagnesemia, and coronary artery disease negatively impact AVF outcomes.[14] Thrombophilia and coagulation abnormalities further contribute to AVF failure, highlighting the complexity of its prognosis.

Novel Concepts in the Pathophysiology of Vascular Access Dysfunction

Importance of Vascular Remodeling

The functional determinant of hemodialysis vascular access dysfunction is the luminal cross-sectional area at the site of stenosis, influenced by both neointimal hyperplasia and vascular remodeling (vasoconstriction or vasodilation).[21] Adverse remodeling factors are still unclear, though adventitial angiogenesis and fibroblast scar formation are thought to play a role. Thus, ideal therapy should target both adverse vascular constriction and neointimal hyperplasia.

Adventitia-derived and Bone Marrow-derived Neointimal Cells: A Role for Fibroblasts and Myofibroblasts

Recent research highlights alternative origins for neointimal cells, including adventitial fibroblasts and bone marrow-derived cells. After vascular injury, fibroblasts from the adventitia migrate into the intima, acquiring a myofibroblast phenotype and contributing to neointimal hyperplasia. Studies have shown that in PTFE dialysis grafts, nearly 50% of neointimal cells are fibroblasts or myofibroblasts, not smooth muscle cells.[22] This suggests that the adventitia is actively involved in the pathogenesis of neointimal hyperplasia, making it a target for therapeutic interventions focusing on multiple cell types.

Endothelial Progenitor Cells and Vascular Repair

Endothelial progenitor cells (EPCs), derived from the bone marrow, play a crucial role in vascular repair and the reduction of neointimal hyperplasia by promoting endothelialization. EPC mobilization can be enhanced by agents such as statins and granulocyte colony-stimulating factor (GCSF), which aid in vascular repair and reduce smooth muscle proliferation. This new understanding indicates that therapies aimed at modifying adventitial responses and enhancing the balance between smooth muscle progenitor cells and endothelial progenitor cells may provide the most effective approach for preventing neointimal hyperplasia and vascular stenosis. Traditional therapies focused only on smooth muscle cell migration may be less effective due to the involvement of alternative pathogenic pathways.[1,23]

CONCLUSION

Vascular access dysfunction is a multifactorial process involving complex interactions between mechanical forces, biological responses, and systemic factors. Understanding the maturation process of AVFs and the pathophysiology of vascular access dysfunction is crucial in improving patient outcomes. Complications such as stenosis and thrombosis can jeopardize access longevity, highlighting the need for ongoing research and improved strategies. By elucidating the underlying mechanisms, clinicians and researchers can better predict, prevent, and manage these complications, ultimately improving the quality of life for dialysis patients. Advances in diagnostic tools, pharmacological therapies, and innovative materials hold great promise for the future of vascular access care.

REFERENCES

1. Roy-Chaudhury P, Sukhatme VP, Cheung AK. Hemodialysis vascular access dysfunction: A cellular and molecular viewpoint. J Am Soc Nephrol. 2006;17(4):1112-27.
2. Rooijens PPGM, Tordoir JHM, Stijnen T, Burgmans JPJ, Smet de AAEA, Yo TI. Radio-cephalic wrist arteriovenous fistula for hemodialysis: Meta-analysis indicates a high primary failure rate. Eur J Vasc Endovasc Surg. 2004;28(6):583-9.
3. Lok CE, Foley R. Vascular access morbidity and mortality: Trends of the last decade. Clin J Am Soc Nephrol. 2013; 8(7):1213-9.
4. Lok CE, Huber TS, Lee T, Shenoy S, Yevzlin AS, Abreo K, et al. KDOQI Clinical Practice Guideline for Vascular Access: 2019 Update. Am J Kidney Dis. 2020;75(4):S1-64.
5. Vascular Access 2006 Work Group. Clinical practice guidelines for vascular access. Am J Kidney Dis. 2006;48 Suppl 1:S176-247.
6. Turmel-Rodrigues L, Pengloan J, Baudin S, Testou D, Abaza M, Dahdah G, et al. Treatment of stenosis and thrombosis in haemodialysis fistulas and grafts by interventional radiology. Nephrol Dial Transplant. 2000;15:2029-36.
7. Asif A, Gadalean FN, Merrill D, Cherla G, Cipleu CD, Epstein DL, et al. Inflow stenosis in arteriovenous fistulas and grafts: A multicenter, prospective study. Kidney Int 2005;67:1986 -992.

8. Remuzzi A, Ene-Iordache B, Mosconi L, Bruno S, Anghileri A, Antiga L, et al. Radial artery wall shear stress evaluation in patients with arteriovenous fistula for hemodialysis access. Biorheology. 2003;40:423-30.
9. Roy-Chaudhury P, Kelly BS, Miller MA, Reaves A, Armstrong J, Nanayakkara N, et al. Venous neointimal hyperplasia in polytetrafluoroethylene dialysis grafts. Kidney Int. 2001;59:2325-34.
10. Miller PE, Tolwani A, Luscy CP, Deierhoi MH, Bailey R, Redden DT, et al. Predictors of adequacy of arterio-venous fistulas in hemodialysis patients. Kidney Int. 1999;56:275-80.
11. Mezzano D, Pais EO, Aranda E, Panes O, Downey P, Ortiz M, et al. Inflammation, not hyperhomocysteinemia, is related to oxidative stress and hemostatic and endothelial dysfunction in uremia. Kidney Int. 2001;60:1844-50.
12. Lee T, Roy-Chaudhury P. Advances and new frontiers in the pathophysiology of venous neointimal hyperplasia and dialysis access stenosis. Adv Chronic Kidney Dis. 2009;16(5):329-38.
13. Kaygin MA, Halici U, Aydin A, Dag O, Binici DN, Limandal HK, et al. The relationship between arteriovenous fistula success and inflammation. Ren Fail. 2013;35(8):1085-8.
14. Gameiro J, Ibeas J. Factors affecting arteriovenous fistula dysfunction: A narrative review. J Vasc Access. 2020;21(2): 134-47.
15. Fitts MK, Pike DB, Anderson K, Shiu YT. Hemodynamic shear stress and endothelial dysfunction in hemodialysis access. Open Urol Nephrol J. 2014;7(Suppl 1 M5):33-44.
16. Santilli J. Fibrin sheaths and central venous catheter occlusions: Diagnosis and management. Tech Vasc Interv Radiol. 2002;5(2):89-94.
17. Wahl P, Ducasa GM, Fornoni A. Systemic and renal lipids in kidney disease development and progression. Am J Physiol Renal Physiol. 2016;310(6):F433-45.
18. Hruska KA, Seifert M, Sugatani T. Pathophysiology of the chronic kidney disease-mineral bone disorder. Curr Opin Nephrol Hyper. 2015;24(4):303-9.
19. Lee T, Safdar N, Mistry MJ, Wang Y, Chauhan V, Campos B, et al. Preexisting venous calcification prior to dialysis vascular access surgery. Semin Dial. 2012;25(5):592-5.
20. Cheung AK, Imrey PB, Alpers CE, Robbin ML, Radeva M, Larive B, et al.; Hemodialysis Fistula Maturation Study Group. Intimal hyperplasia, stenosis, and arterio-venous fistula maturation failure in the Hemodialysis Fistula Maturation Study. J Am Soc Nephrol. 2017;28(10): 3005-13.
21. Libby P, Tanaka H. The molecular bases of restenosis. Prog Cardiovasc Dis. 1997;40:97-106.
22. Roy-Chaudhury P, McKee L, Miller M, Reaves A, Armstrong J, Nanayakkara N, et al. Adventitial fibroblasts contribute to venous neointimal hyperplasia in PTFE dialysis grafts [Abstract]. J Am Soc Nephrol. 2001;12:301.
23. Urbich C, Dimmeler S. Endothelial progenitor cells: Characterization and role in vascular biology. Circ Res. 2004;95:343-53.

CHAPTER 17

Diagnosis of Vascular Access Dysfunction

Bharat Sachdeva, Ruhani Sachdeva

INTRODUCTION

Dialysis vascular access is the lifeline for hemodialysis patients, as it allows repeated access to the bloodstream for adequate clearance of waste products and excess fluids. Functional access is crucial for optimal dialysis efficiency and patient outcomes.[1] Dialysis access is associated with frequent complications and requires close monitoring and surveillance (Chapter 14) to diagnose signs of dysfunction **(Table 1)**.

Proper functioning of the vascular access is essential to ensure adequate hemodialysis treatment. Dysfunction can lead to reduced dialysis efficiency as well as vascular complications and increased morbidity or mortality.

PATHOPHYSIOLOGY AND COMMON CAUSES OF ACCESS DYSFUNCTION

Stenosis and thrombosis are the primary causes of arteriovenous (AV) access dysfunction. Progressive vessel lumen narrowing, often at the anastomosis or venous outflow region, due to neointimal hyperplasia (NIH) is a common culprit. Endothelial injury (arterial or venous) during access creation, repeated injury with needles at the cannulation segment (CS), and turbulent blood flow exacerbate the vessel wall thickness. Stenosis often precedes clot formation due to reduced blood flow and turbulence.

TABLE 1: Common complications associated with dialysis vascular access.

Access type	*Infection risk*	*Common complications*
AVF	Low	Stenosis, delayed maturation, aneurysms, high flow
AVG	Moderate	Thrombosis, infection, stenosis
CVC-T	High	Infection, fibrin sheath, poor flow

(AVF: arterial venous fistula; AVG: arterial venous graft; CVC-T: central venous catheter tunneled)

The insertion of a central venous catheter (CVC), whether tunneled or nontunneled, can initiate the formation of fibrin sheaths or intraluminal blood clots within hours. Repeated catheter placements may further damage the vessel wall, promoting fibrosis and vascular narrowing. In addition, biofilm formation on the catheter surface significantly increases the risk of catheter-related bloodstream infections (CRBSIs).

Biology and risk factors associated with central venous stenosis are discussed in Chapter 16.

CLINICAL PRESENTATION AND HISTORY-TAKING

A comprehensive historical assessment of dialysis access is essential prior to any intervention. A detailed history helps identify risk factors, previous complications, and potential underlying causes of the current access dysfunction **(Table 2)**. It is crucial to ascertain the type of access [arteriovenous fistula (AVF), arteriovenous graft (AVG) or CVC], its anatomical location, and the duration of its usage.[2] Document the onset and progression of symptoms, such as swelling and pain, as well as any deterioration in dialysis efficiency, as indicated by low Kt/V or urea reduction ratio (URR).

The history of delayed maturation of AVFs or recurrent access failures should be investigated. Collect comprehensive data related to all previous medical interventions. This includes inquiries into earlier procedures such as angioplasty, thrombectomy, or other surgical interventions. Document any access-related infections or thrombosis, along with records of catheter placements.

Review the dialysis parameters, concentrating on trends in blood flow rates, venous pressures, alarms

TABLE 2: Common signs of vascular dialysis access dysfunction.

Problem with dialysis access	*Comments*
• Poor blood flow • Elevated venous pressures • Elevated (negative) arterial pressure • Altered thrill or bruit in AV access • Swelling of extremity • Inadequate dialysis clearance (Kt/V) • Pain or discomfort over the access site • Signs of Infection • Changes in extremity veins appearance • Difficulty cannulation • Prolonged bleeding	• Common for AVF, AVG, and CVC • Can be seen with all access, including CVC • Suggests poor flow of blood into pump • Found on routine monitoring of AV access • Suggests high venous pressures • Suboptimal clearance of uremic toxins • May be due to stenosis, thrombus, or infection • Redness, warmth, or drainage from access site • Suggestive of proximal venous stenosis • Sign of poor flow and or stenosis • Suggestive of high venous pressures

(AV: arteriovenous; AVF: arterial venous fistula; AVG: arterial venous graft; CVC: central venous catheter)

related to access, and occurrences of prolonged bleeding or aneurysm formation.

A comprehensive account of the patient's medication history is also crucial, particularly concerning anticoagulants or antiplatelet therapies. These medications significantly impact vascular health and access functionality, as they influence clotting mechanisms and the risk of hemorrhage. Diabetes, atherosclerosis, and peripheral vascular disease (PVD) can also significantly impact vascular biology.

PHYSICAL EXAMINATION

A structured physical examination of dialysis access is essential for the early detection of dysfunction. Inspection, palpation, and auscultation to evaluate the inflow, body, and outflow (IBO) access segments should precede any intervention.[3] An exam aids in understanding the underlying causes of dysfunction and devising the most effective management strategy.[3,4]

Visual Inspection

Visual inspection provides key clues about vascular access dysfunction. The inflow segment extends from anastomosis to the start of the access CS. Skin changes, discoloration, erythema, or swelling may indicate poor perfusion, infection, or thrombosis. Arterial steal syndrome presents with signs of ischemia in the distal hand (e.g., pale or cool fingers).

TABLE 3: Inspection of dialysis access for signs of dysfunction.

Observation	*Possible cause*
Redness, warmth, or pus	Infection of skin or artery/vein/graft
Bulging or pulsatile mass	Aneurysm/pseudoaneurysm
Swelling in the arm	Venous outflow obstruction, central vein stenosis
Pale, cool fingers	Distal arterial hypoperfusion syndrome (steal)

The body of access is the CS. Inspect for bruising, hematomas, or scarring. Aneurysms will have bulging areas on the access. Look for signs of infection (redness, warmth, swelling, or pus).

Proximal to CS is the outflow segment. Inspect for edema or swelling. This would suggest venous stenosis in the outflow segment of access or a central vein obstruction. Collateral veins show as prominent veins over the chest, neck, or shoulder and may indicate central vein stenosis **(Table 3)**.

Palpation

Palpation should start at the site of anastomosis/inflow of the access and track the access across the entire body and outflow of access. A palpable vibration (thrill) over the access site is caused by turbulent blood flow. A normal thrill is continuous, most substantial at the anastomosis, and decreases distally. Weak thrill suggests thrombosis or severe stenosis. Strong thrill at one spot but absent elsewhere indicates a stenosis distal to the palpable site. Tenderness along the access may indicate infection, thrombosis, or inflammation.

Auscultation of the Access

Auscultation of the access is performed to evaluate blood flow quality through the fistula or graft. The audible blood flow sound caused by turbulence within the access generates bruit. A continuous low-pitched "machinery-like" sound that is loudest near the anastomosis and decreases distally is typical. A systolic-only bruit indicates severe stenosis or reduced blood flow. High-pitched bruit suggests significant narrowing (stenosis) at the auscultated site, while its absence indicates complete thrombosis or occlusion.

The augmentation and arm raise test are two key assessments that utilize a combination of inspection and palpation skills to evaluate the inflow and outflow. An AVF uses natural veins as a blood conduit; these veins are elastic and expand or collapse with changes in luminal pressure. In contrast, an AVG made of synthetic polymers has a stiff wall and may not expand or collapse with changes in intravascular pressure.

The augmentation test is a clinical bedside maneuver used to assess the adequacy of arterial inflow in the access. Begin the test by palpating the fistula close to arterial anastomosis to detect the baseline thrill. Next, compress the body of the fistula proximal to the arterial anastomosis **(Figs. 1 and 2)** using your fingers.

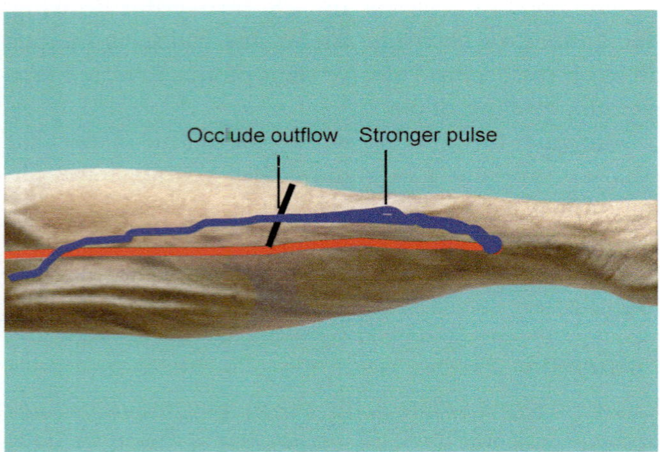

Fig. 1: *Augmentation:* Palpation begins at the site of the radial artery anastomosis in this radial artery to cephalic vein fistula. As you progress by impeding the outflow of blood in the cephalic vein, a bounding pulse is felt near the anastomosis when there is no stenosis.

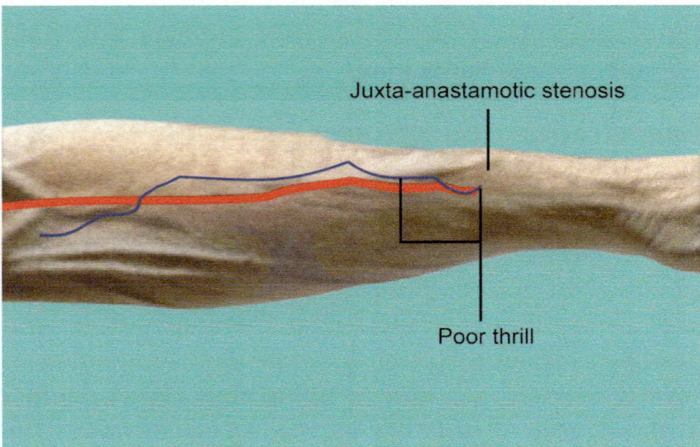

Fig. 2: *Poor augmentation:* When there is a stenosis in the inflow artery or at the venous segment adjacent to the anastomosis (juxta-anastomosis), the outflow occlusion does not result in significant flow augmentation.

While maintaining compression of the fistula, palpate the thrill near the anastomosis. Increased bounding pulsation indicates adequate arterial inflow. No change in thrill or minimal augmentation after compression of the outflow suggests compromised arterial inflow.

This test is subjective, relying on the clinician's skill to identify changes in thrill upon occlusion of the AVF outflow via palpation. The augmentation test may miss mild proximal stenosis in the artery or juxta-anastomosis segment of the fistula. When there is dual stenosis in the access circuit (inflow and outflow), outflow stenosis may mask the change in pulsation **(Table 4)**.

The arm raise test is used to evaluate venous outflow in an AVF. To assess for venous outflow obstruction in an AVF, observe the behavior of the fistula veins when the arm is elevated. Ask the patient to stand comfortably with the arm hanging free. Inspect the fistula and surrounding veins while the arm is dependent (below the heart). Note the size and distension of the veins. Prominent veins are a normal finding due to the gravitational force on blood when the arm is dependent.

Instruct the patient to extend and elevate the arm above heart level (approximately 90–180°). This position helps reduce hydrostatic gravitational pressure and allows venous blood to flow toward the central circulation. Without outflow stenosis, veins collapse when the arm is raised, but remain engorged, dilated, or prominent even with arm elevation in the distal segment of the fistula **(Fig. 3)**. This indicates venous stenosis that restricts blood flow in the AV access from the CS and fails to collapse to the central vein, which hinders proper outflow.

NONINVASIVE DIAGNOSTIC TECHNIQUES

Ultrasound is beneficial for assessing AVF and AVG function. It enables real-time evaluation of blood flow and vessel anatomy as well as the identification of dysfunctions such as stenosis, thrombosis, or other complications. Ultrasound is a versatile tool with several modalities useful in examining AV access.[5-7]

B-Mode Ultrasound (Gray Scale)

B-mode ultrasound is a fundamental imaging technique for detecting structural abnormalities in arteriovenous (AV) access. It provides critical anatomic details to identify and localize stenosis.

Transverse views should be used to assess vessel lumen diameter and wall thickness. Measure vessel diameters and

TABLE 4: Inflow and outflow stenosis of arterial venous access (fistula/graft), clinical examination, and angiographic findings.

	Inflow stenosis	*Outflow stenosis*
Location of stenosis (fistula/graft)	At the inflow artery or at the distal anastomosis of vein/graft	Venous outflow/anastomosis (graft) within or proximal to the cannulation zone to central veins
Pulse at inflow (fistula/graft)	Weak at the inflow segment	Strong pulse at inflow segment
Pulse augmentation test (fistula)	Minimal or no augmentation with arm elevation or compression of the outflow	Normal or increased augmentation
Thrill (fistula/graft)	Weak or absent thrill over the access site	Normal to strong thrill near anastomosis, but diminished or absent more distally
Bruit (fistula/graft)	Soft or absent bruit at the inflow segment	Loud, continuous bruit over the stenotic area
Arm elevation test (fistula)	Rapid collapse of fistula	Delayed to no collapse and fistula remains engorged
Venous distention (fistula)	Decreased venous filling	Prominent venous engorgement upstream of stenosis
Swelling (fistula/graft)	Rare extremity swelling	None to severe swelling especially if the stenosis is in central vessels
Dialysis parameters (fistula/graft)	Poor arterial flow, negative arterial pressures, difficult cannulation	Poor venous return, elevated venous pressures
Angiogram requirements (fistula/graft)	Requires inflow assessment with retrograde access into the inflow artery or direct cannulation of the artery	Antegrade cannulation of the access with study of cannulation zone and outflow vein
Angiographic findings (fistula/graft)	Stenosis of the inflow artery (rare) or the juxta-anastomosis segment of the fistula (common), arterial anastomosis of graft	Stenosis of the venous/intragraft segment at or proximal to cannulation zone with or without collaterals

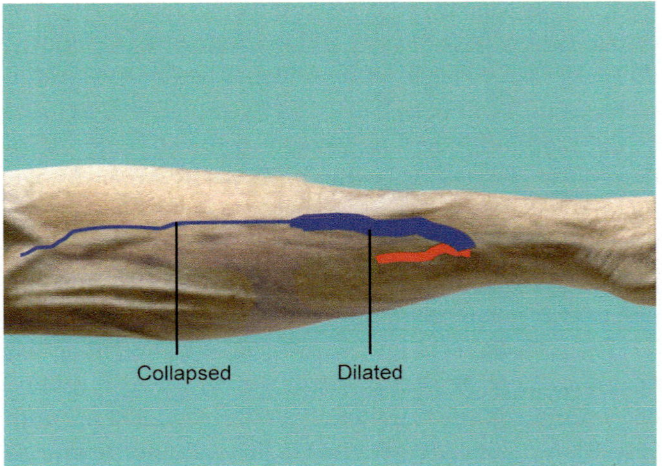

Fig. 3: *Arm raise test:* The veins collapse near the midarm but remain engorged, dilated, or prominent even with arm elevation in the distal segment of the fistula. This suggests venous stenosis, and the test can help estimate the location of the stenosis.

compare the stenotic segment diameter to the prestenotic segment. Longitudinal views provide an overview of the stenotic segment length and structural changes.

Examine the entire accessible segment of the AV access and check for thrombus, calcifications, or fibrotic changes that may contribute to stenosis. Additionally, evaluate for dilated segments within the circuit and aneurysms.

B-mode visualizes the degree of vessel narrowing, identifying focal stenotic segments. Stenosis appears as a concentric or eccentric narrowing of the vessel wall. Fibrotic segments may appear as echogenic (bright) areas within the vessel wall, decreasing lumen diameter. Accessory veins can be seen as branches of the main AVF vessel **(Fig. 4)**. These vessels may divert significant blood flow from the main channel, reducing total blood flow through the CS of the fistula. Significant accessory veins have a diameter of >30% of the fistula's body. The depth of the vein from the skin surface can be measured in the CS. A depth >10 mm poses challenges for cannulation **(Fig. 5)**.

Stenosis may involve a thrombus, which appears as hyperechoic (bright) material within the lumen. Chronic thrombus is often heterogeneous, exhibiting mixed echogenicity, and can be seen as luminal narrowing without complete flow occlusion or as a complete occlusive disease with total flow cessation (clotted access). Calcifications are seen as bright hyperechoic foci accompanied by posterior acoustic shadowing. These are often observed in chronic AV access with prolonged use for dialysis and dystrophic

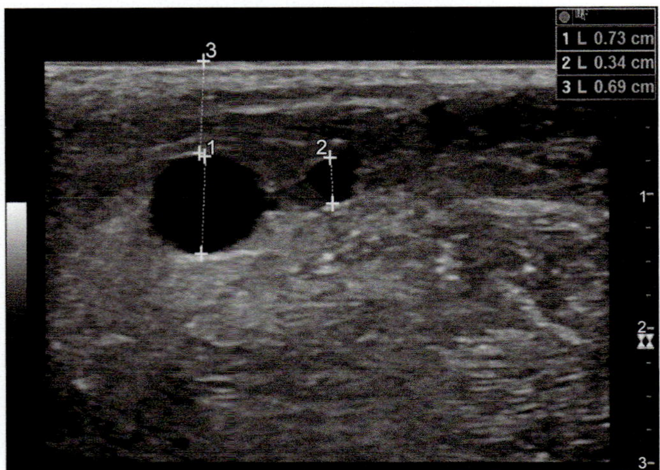

Fig. 4: B-mode transverse view ultrasound reveals the primary fistula (1) with a diameter of 0.73 cm and a significant accessory vein (2) measuring over 40% of the body of the arteriovenous fistula (AVF).

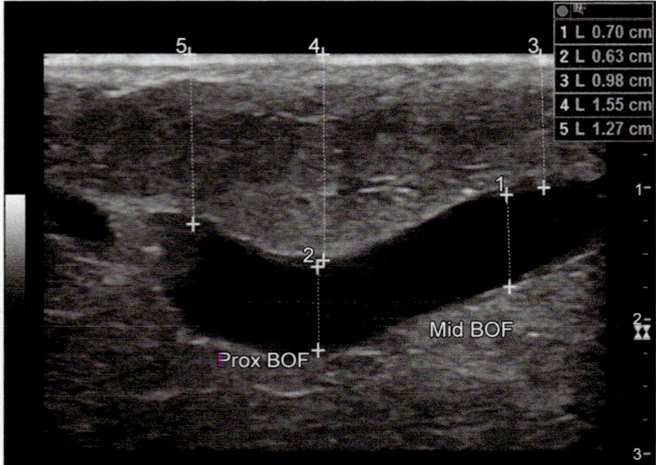

Fig. 5: B-mode longitudinal view ultrasound provides clarity on the arteriovenous fistula's (AVF) depth. While the fistula in the cannulation zone or body of fistula (BOF) has a diameter of 7 mm, its deepest point is located 15 mm beneath the skin, complicating the cannulation process.

calcification of the vessel wall. Stenosis can open collateral veins to bypass the occluded segment.

Color Doppler Ultrasound

The color overlay provided by Doppler imaging illustrates the direction and velocity of blood flow within the AV access. Normal flow in an AV access presents as a laminar, uniform color flow pattern (blue or red, depending on the direction of the flow).

Stenotic segments may exhibit aliasing, which is marked by abrupt changes in color flow and turbulent, high-velocity blood flow. Aliasing occurs when blood flow velocity exceeds the Nyquist limit (the Nyquist limit is half the sampling rate of a signal, named after engineer Harry Nyquist), represented as a mosaic or turbulent color flow pattern (a mixture of red and blue). Proximal to the stenosis, the flow may be dampened or show reduced velocities. At the stenotic site, blood flow accelerates, generating turbulent, aliasing flow on color Doppler.

Thrombosed segments show absent color flow or very slow flow. The thrombus may appear as an echogenic structure on B-mode ultrasound. Aneurysms appear as pulsatile cystic structures with swirling blood flow ("yin-yang" sign).

Spectral Doppler Ultrasound (Pulse Wave)

This technique quantifies blood flow velocities (peak systolic and diastolic) and provides waveforms to assess the rate of change in flow velocity during the systolic and diastolic cycles of the heart.

The average velocity of flow through a segment of laminar flow in a vessel can be used to calculate total flow in access by considering the diameter of the vessel. Peak systolic velocity (PSV) is noted as an increase in flow velocity at the stenotic site and is a hallmark of stenosis. PSV >400 cm/s suggests hemodynamically substantial stenosis in AV access. The velocity ratio (VR), defined as the ratio of blood flow velocity at the stenotic site to that at the prestenotic segment, serves as a measure for quantifying the severity of stenosis. VR is calculated using the formula VR = PSV at the stenotic segment/PSV at the prestenotic segment. A VR exceeding 2.0 indicates the presence of greater than 50% stenosis.

The total flow volume is assessed at a straight access segment. Typical access flow rates in an AVF exceed 600 mL/min, while those in an AVG exceed 800 mL/min **(Fig. 6)**. A significant reduction in flow volume, defined as <500 mL/min, may indicate critical stenosis.

Complete ultrasound examination of an AV access should follow a structured approach:

- *Evaluate arterial inflow:* Assess the feeding artery for adequate flow. Look for stenosis, wall thickening, or aliasing near the anastomosis.
- *Assess anastomotic site:* Carefully evaluate the AV connection point for narrowing, turbulent flow, or aliasing.

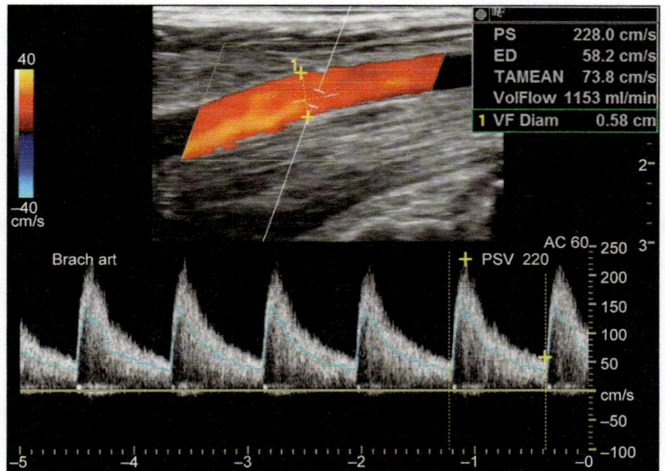

Fig. 6: Doppler color flow of brachial artery flow 5 cm above the anastomosis. Peak systolic velocity (PSV) of 220 m/s is noted, with an arterial flow of 1,153 mL/min. Flow in an access should be checked in a straight segment without any dilations and turbulence. Arterial flow is the preferred way to calculate access flow.

- *Examine the body of the access:* Check for focal stenosis, thrombus, or irregular flow within the graft or fistula body.
- *Assess venous outflow:* Examine draining veins for stenosis or obstruction. Look for turbulent flow, velocity changes, or aliasing in the draining segment.
- *Document access flow pattern:* Measure blood flow velocities (using spectral Doppler) and confirm laminar flow with Color Doppler.
- *Identify collateral vessels:* Look for evidence of collaterals, which indicate significant obstruction or central venous stenosis.

Invasive Diagnostic Techniques

Angiography, the gold standard for detecting access dysfunction in AV access, is crucial for accurate diagnosis and treatment planning. This methodology provides precise localization and assessment of the severity of lesions. Furthermore, it may be integrated with therapeutic interventions, such as angioplasty. Advanced techniques, including intravascular ultrasound and pressure monitoring across the stenosis, are also indispensable tools that contribute to a comprehensive understanding of the physiological implications of stenosis on vascular function. These techniques will be discussed in Chapter 20.

CONCLUSION

The effective assessment of dialysis access dysfunction requires a comprehensive approach that combines clinical evaluation with suitable diagnostic techniques. Noninvasive methods, including duplex ultrasound and Doppler studies, serve as valuable first-line tools for initial evaluation due to their safety, accessibility, and capacity to provide functional and anatomical insights. Invasive techniques such as angiography still remain essential for confirming diagnoses. By integrating these modalities, healthcare providers can ensure timely and accurate diagnosis, optimize patient outcomes, and extend the functional lifespan of dialysis access.

REFERENCES

1. Lok CE, Huber TS, Lee T, Shenoy S, Yevzlin AS, Abreo K, et al. National Kidney Foundation, et al. 2019 Update. Am J Kidney Dis. 2020;75:S1-164. [Erratum in: Am J Kidney Dis. 2021;77:551].
2. Quencer KB, Kidd J, Kinney T. Preprocedure Evaluation of a Dysfunctional Dialysis Access. Tech Vasc Interv Radiol. 2017;20:20-30.
3. Abreo K, Amin BM, Abreo AP. Physical examination of the hemodialysis arteriovenous fistula to detect early dysfunction. J Vasc Access. 2019;20(1):7-11.
4. Raksasuk S, Naweera W, Rojwatcharapibarn S, Srithongkul T. Comparing non-invasive diagnostic methods for arteriovenous fistula stenosis: a prospective study. J Ultrasound. 2023;26(3):687-93.
5. Pietryga JA, Little MD, Robbin ML. Sonography of Arteriovenous Fistulas and Grafts. Semin Dial. 2017;30:309-18.
6. Wiese P, Nonnast-Daniel B. Colour Doppler ultrasound in dialysis access. Nephrol Dial Transplant. 2004;19:1956-63.
7. AIUM Practice Parameter for the Performance of Vascular Ultrasound Examinations for Postoperative Assessment of Hemodialysis Access. J Ultrasound Med. 2020;39:E39-48.

CHAPTER 18

Maintenance of Tunneled Cuffed Catheters

Prashant C Dheerendra, Karthikeyan Balasubramanian, Denis Dawle Tirkey

CASE SCENARIO

Mrs ABC has been on maintenance hemodialysis through a right internal jugular vein (IJV) tunneled cuffed catheter (TCC) for 6 months. A recently created left radiocephalic fistula is yet to mature. The technician reports high venous pressures and frequent need to reverse the dialysis lines over the last 2 weeks. The patient feels more fatigued of late. Do any steps need to be taken?

INTRODUCTION

Proper maintenance of TCCs is essential to ensure safe and effective hemodialysis, prevent infections, maintain catheter patency, and improve patient quality of life. Following aseptic technique, routine site inspection, flushing protocols, and regular staff training ensure better outcomes and minimize complications.

KEY PRACTICES

- Inspect the catheter site before each dialysis for signs of infection, bleeding, cuff extrusion, and integrity of the catheter.
- A transparent dressing is preferred at the exit site which must be changed at least weekly or when it becomes wet, soiled, or blood stained.
- Perform proper exit-site cleaning with special attention to the recommended contact time and compatibility with the catheter material as per the manufacturer's instructions. Chlorhexidine-based and iodine-based solutions are generally used.

CATHETER CONNECTION AND DISCONNECTION

The important steps for catheter connection and disconnection as advised by the Centers for Disease Control and Prevention (CDC) are as follows:[1]

Connection steps:

1. Hand hygiene and gloves
2. Clamp catheter before cap removal
3. Disinfect each hub with individual antiseptic pad
4. Flush with sterile syringe
5. Connect bloodlines aseptically

Disconnection steps:

1. Clamp catheter
2. Disinfect each hub.
3. Replace sterile caps.
4. Avoid contact with nonsterile surfaces.
5. Hand hygiene after glove removal.

Locking Solutions

Tunneled cuffed catheter lumens should be "locked" with the recommended volume of a lock solution after each session of dialysis to prevent thrombosis. In specific situations, an antibiotic lock solution can be considered. The usual lock solutions and their pros and cons are listed in **Table 1**.[2]

Tunneled Cuffed Catheter Dysfunction

Tunneled cuffed catheter dysfunction is defined as inability to attain and maintain a blood flow rate sufficient

TABLE 1: Usual lock solutions and their pros and cons.

Solution	*Pros*	*Cautions*
Heparin (1,000–5,000 IU/mL)	Effective anticoagulant	Risk of bleeding, HIT
Citrate (<5%)	Anticoagulant + mild antimicrobial	Safer systemic profile
Antibiotic locks	For recurrent infections only	Should be guided by infectious disease team

(HIT: heparin-induced thrombocytopenia)

to perform hemodialysis without significantly lengthening the hemodialysis treatment.

Signs of TCC dysfunction:

- High arterial pressures (<–250 mm Hg)
- High venous pressures (>250 mm Hg)
- High pressure alarms
- Decreased blood flow rates
- Inability to withdraw and/or flush catheter lumens
- Need to reverse lines
- Reduced urea clearance (Kt/V <1.2 or urea reduction ratio <65%)

If these signs are progressive in consecutive dialysis sessions, catheter dysfunction is highly likely.[3]

Catheter Dysfunction: Causes

The causes of TCC dysfunction can be classified into early and late.

Early TCC dysfunction is related to technical problems with catheter placement or positioning. Technical problems include insertion into the wrong vessel, an improperly positioned catheter or a kinked one.

Late TCC dysfunction can be due to:

- Thrombosis
- Fibrin sheath

MANAGEMENT OF DYSFUNCTIONAL TUNNELED CUFFED CATHETER DUE TO THROMBUS

Intraluminal recombinant tissue plasminogen activator (rtPA) has primarily been used in the treatment of dysfunctional TCC due to thrombosis. Alteplase, Reteplase, and Tenecteplase are the available forms of rt-PA.

The Kidney Disease Outcomes Quality Initiative (KDOQI) recommends use of alteplase as intraluminal lock solution for dysfunctional TCC due to thrombus.[2] The recommended dose of alteplase is 2 mg in each lumen with dwell time of 30 minutes to 2 hours and it can be repeated if the first attempt fails. Several trials have found that alteplase administered as lock solution with a dwell time of 1-4 hours produced catheter clearance rates of 85–95%.[4,5] A "low-dose" protocol using 1 mg per lumen has also been described.[6]

Reteplase is a variant of recombinant TPA which differs from alteplase in lacking several structural domains. These alterations lead to a weaker binding to the clot allowing increased diffusion, increased half-life, and thrombus penetration. Studies analyzing the efficacy of reteplase indicate catheter clearance of 67–74% after 30–40 minutes with overall clearance rates ranging from 80 to 95%. Reteplase at the dose of 0.5–1.0 U in each lumen is usually used for TCCs.[7,8]

Tenecteplase at a dose of 2 mg in each lumen with a dwell time of 1 hour is associated with improvement in blood flow rate of TCC compared to placebo in a randomized trial.[9]

Various protocols with urokinase have also been described, but the availability of urokinase has declined over the years.[10-13]

Fibrin Sheath

In patients undergoing hemodialysis, TCC dysfunction caused by fibrin sheath is reported to be between 13 and 57%.[14] The fibrin sheath starts from the catheter entry site into the vessel. It is composed of smooth muscle, endothelial cells, and thrombus. The sheath becomes more collagen based and eventually becomes an endothelium indistinguishable from vessel wall.[15] Fibrin sheaths are colonized with bacteria. Therefore, fibrin sheath development will determine the long-term performance of the catheter.[16]

Catheter malfunction in TCC occurs when fibrin sheath covers side holes and tip and becomes adherent to vessel wall. The typical sign of fibrin sheath in TCC is the ability to flush the catheter but not be able to aspirate (ball valve effect).[17]

Catheter venography in the setting of fibrin sheath shows an abnormal flow jet from the TCC endhole, where the contrast stream may be disrupted, turbulent, or refluxed along the length of the catheter under the fibrin sheath before it diffuses into the vein.[18]

Fibrin sheath is managed by either stripping the sheath using a snare or disrupting the sheath using a large-sized balloon followed by guidewire exchange of the catheter. Balloon disruption is the preferred method and results in durable improvement in catheter blood flows.[19,20] Catheter removal and reinsertion at a different site should be the last resort after the above measures have failed.[2]

CONCLUSION

Tunneled cuffed catheter insertion is a fundamental procedure for nephrologists and they need to be proficient in routine performance of the same. Attention to detail and safety are important. Developing competence with the procedure translates into better outcomes for the patients over the long term.

REFERENCES

1. O'Grady NP, Alexander M, Burns LA, Dellinger EP, Garland J, Heard SO, et al. Guidelines for the prevention of intravascular catheter-related infections. Clin Infect Dis. 2011;52(9):e162-93.
2. Lok CE, Huber TS, Lee T, Shenoy S, Yevzlin AS, Abreo K, et al. KDOQI Clinical Practice Guideline for Vascular Access: 2019 Update. Am J Kidney Dis. 2020;75(4):S1-164.
3. Besarab A, Pandey R. Catheter management in hemodialysis patients: Delivering adequate flow. Clin J Am Soc Nephrol. 2011;6(1):227-34.
4. Little MA, Walshe JJ. A longitudinal study of the repeated use of alteplase as therapy for tunneled hemodialysis catheter dysfunction. Am J Kidney Dis. 2002;39(1):86-91.
5. Mendes ML, Castro JH, Silva TN, Barretti P, Ponce D. Effective use of alteplase for occluded tunneled venous catheter in hemodialysis patients. Artif Organs. 2014;38(5):399-403.
6. Haymond J, Shalansky K, Jastrzebski J. Efficacy of low-dose alteplase for treatment of hemodialysis catheter occlusions. J Vasc Access. 2005;6(2):76-82.
7. Hyman G, England M, Kibede S, Lee P, Willets G. The efficacy and safety of reteplase for thrombolysis of hemodialysis catheters at a community and academic regional medical center. Nephron Clin Pract. 2004;96(2):c39-42.
8. Hilleman DE, Dunlay RW, Packard KA. Reteplase for dysfunctional hemodialysis catheter clearance. Pharmacotherapy. 2003;23(2):137-41.
9. Tumlin J, Goldman J, Spiegel DM, Roer D, Ntoso KA, Blaney M, et al. A phase III, randomized, double-blind, placebo-controlled study of tenecteplase for improvement of hemodialysis catheter function: TROPICS 3. Clin J Am Soc Nephrol. 2010;5(4):631-6.
10. Van Hulle F, Bonkain F, De Clerck D, Aerden D, Vanwijn I, Tielemans C, et al. Efficacy of urokinase lock to treat thrombotic dysfunction of tunneled hemodialysis catheters: A retrospective cohort study. J Vasc Access. 2019;20(1):60-9.
11. Deng J, Luo W, Zhang W, Xiong S, Wang L. Efficacy of urokinase in maintaining patency of hemodialysis catheters: A meta-analysis. Clin Nephrol. 2024;102(4): 212-22.
12. Shavit L, Lifschitz M, Plaksin J, Grenader T, Slotki I. High dose urokinase for restoration of patency of occluded permanent central venous catheters in hemodialysis patients. Clin Nephrol. 2010;74(4):297-302.
13. Donati G, Colì L, Cianciolo G, La Manna G, Cuna V, Montanari M, et al. Thrombosis of tunneled-cuffed hemodialysis catheters: treatment with high-dose urokinase lock therapy. Artif Organs. 2012;36(1):21-8.
14. Santilli J. Fibrin sheaths and central venous catheter occlusions: diagnosis and management. Tech Vasc Interv Radiol. 2002;5(2):89-94.
15. Forauer AR, Theoharis CGA, Dasika NL. Jugular vein catheter placement: histologic features and development of catheter-related (fibrin) sheaths in a swine model. Radiology. 2006;240(2):427-34.
16. Lucas TC, Tessarolo F, Veniero P, Caola I, Piccoli F, Haase A, et al. Hemodialysis catheter thrombi: visualization and quantification of microstructures and cellular composition. J Vasc Access. 2013;14(3):257-63.
17. Beathard GA. Dysfunction of new catheters by old fibrin sheaths. Semin Dial. 2004;17(3):243-4.
18. Crain MR, Horton MG, Mewissen MW. Fibrin sheaths complicating central venous catheters. Am J Roentgenol. 1998;171(2):341-6.
19. Shanaah A, Brier M, Dwyer A. Fibrin sheath and its relation to subsequent events after tunneled dialysis catheter exchange. Semin Dial. 2013;26(6):733-7.
20. Oliver MJ, Mendelssohn DC, Quinn RR, Richardson EP, Rajan DK, Pugash RA, et al. Catheter patency and function after catheter sheath disruption: a pilot study. Clin J Am Soc Nephrol. 2007;2(6):1201-6.

SECTION 5

Interventional Cath Lab Techniques

CHAPTER 19

Hardware Requirements for Cath Laboratory Interventions by Nephrologists

J Balasubramaniam, Karthik Balasubramaniam

INTRODUCTION

Cath laboratories rely on specialized tools to perform lifesaving interventions with precision and efficiency. This chapter provides a practical overview of the critical hardware used in cath laboratory procedures, focusing on equipment essential for nephrologists performing interventions such as AV fistula maintenance and vascular access management.

In recent years, nephrologists have increasingly taken an active role in performing interventions within catheterization laboratories—traditionally the domain of cardiologists and interventional radiologists. Mastering cath laboratory hardware not only enhances procedural safety and efficiency but also empowers nephrologists to perform these interventions independently.

This chapter outlines the basic, cost-effective tools used in day-to-day practice. While individual operator preferences may evolve, the following inventory remains fundamental for achieving consistent and successful outcomes:

- *Vascular access devices:* Needles and sheaths
- *Navigation aids:* Guidewires and catheters
- *Imaging systems:* Fluoroscopy and ultrasound
- *Interventional tools:* Angioplasty balloons, stents, and ancillary equipment

By the end of this chapter, readers will have a solid foundation in selecting and utilizing cath laboratory hardware, enabling them to manage complications and refine their procedural techniques.

IMAGING TOOLS

Fluoroscopy

- *Function:* Provides real-time X-ray guidance for accurate navigation and placement.
- *Systems:* Options range from a simple mobile C-arm (ideal for beginners) to advanced cath laboratory systems offering enhanced clarity, additional features, and reduced radiation exposure.

Ultrasound

- *Function:* It assists in guiding procedures while reducing radiation exposure.
- *Use:* It can be used to complement, and in some cases replace, fluoroscopy for certain interventions.

Intravascular Ultrasound

- *Function:* Delivers cross-sectional imaging of vessel interiors for precise assessments.
- *Note:* Currently regarded as an advanced tool rather than a necessity in routine practice.

IODINATED CONTRAST MEDIUM (FIG. 1)

Iodinated contrast agents enhance vessel visualization during angiographic procedures. Two commonly used agents are: (1) Omnipaque (Iohexol) and (2) visipaque (Iodixanol).

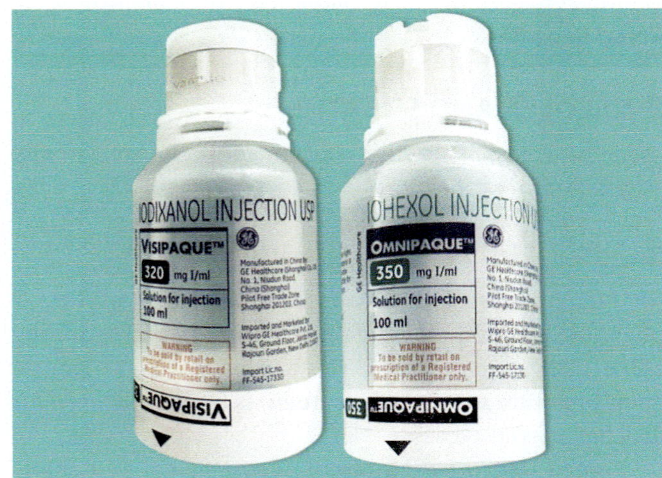

Fig. 1: Iodinated contrasts.

Omnipaque (Iohexol)

- *Type:* Nonionic, low osmolar contrast medium (LOCM)
- *Concentrations:* 140, 240, 300, and 350 mg I/mL with osmolalities of 322, 520, 672, and 844 mOsm/kg water, respectively.
- *Usage:* Typically, Omnipaque 300 or 350 is used for AV access angioplasty.
    - *Administration:* Generally, 40–50 mL of undiluted contrast is needed per procedure; each angiogram run uses 4–6 mL of diluted contrast (dilutions of 1:1 or 1:2).
    - *Packaging:* Available in 50 and 100 mL bottles
    - *Cost:* Approximately INR 2,400 per 100 mL bottle

Visipaque (Iodixanol)

- *Type:* Nonionic, iso-osmolar contrast medium (IOCM)
- *Concentrations:* Available in 270 and 320 mg I/mL with an osmolality of 290 mOsm/kg water.
- *Usage:* Visipaque 320 is generally used for AV access angioplasty; dilution and volume requirements are similar to Omnipaque.
- *Benefits:* Lower risk of contrast-induced acute kidney injury (CI-AKI).
- *Cost:* Approximately INR 4,000 per 100 mL bottle.

CONTRAST INJECTORS

Automated contrast injectors enhance the efficiency of contrast delivery during angiography, particularly for flush studies. However, in many cases, manual syringe injection remains sufficient for nephrologists. Aortic flush study to identify renal arteries is one situation where nephrologists would need these.

NEEDLES AND SHEATHS

Vascular access is the first and most crucial step in any cath laboratory procedure.

Needles (Fig. 2)

Needles are essential for vascular puncture, and their selection is based on gauge size and the corresponding color-coding system. For example, a 21-gauge micropuncture needle (often green) is frequently used for delicate arterial access.

Figure 1 shows example of needle gauge and color-coding scheme.

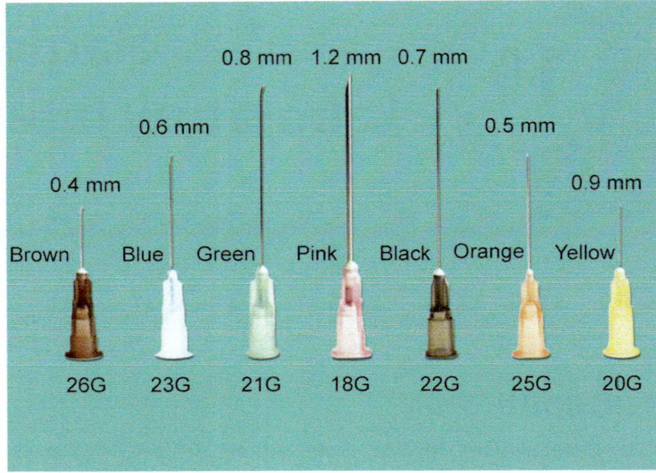

Fig. 2: Hypodermic sterile needle size chart.

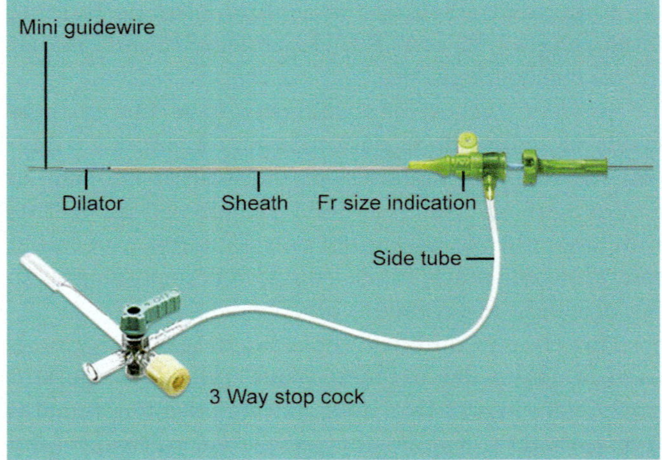

Fig. 3: Radifocus introducer kit.

Types

- *Access needles:* Typically range from 18G to 21G. Smaller gauges (i.e., higher numbers) are used for delicate vessels.
- *Micropuncture needles:* Usually, 21G, these are used for precision in small or calcified vessels, minimizing trauma.
- *Trocar systems:* Feature a blunt outer cannula with a sharp, three-sided inner needle for precise vessel entry.

Sheaths (Fig. 3)

Introducer sheaths provide a secure gateway into the vascular system, often equipped with one-way valves to prevent blood backflow.

- *Specifications:*
  - *Length:* Commonly available in 5 cm and 7 cm lengths
  - *Diameter:* Ranges from 4F to 7F (inner diameter measurements)
  - *Design features:*
    - Radio-opaque construction
    - Cross-cut valve for hemostasis
    - Side tube with a three-way stopcock
    - Color-coded systems [e.g., 4F (red), 5F (gray), 6F (green), 7F (orange)]
- *Included accessories:* Typically supplied with a matching dilator and a mini guidewire (e.g., 0.025 in, 45 cm).

Figure 2 shows radifocus introducer II transradial kit (Terumo Interventional Systems).

Figure 4 shows prelude sheath introducer kit (Merit Medical)—showing sheath and guidewire options.

Figure 5 shows detailed view of sheath components and color-coding for size identification.

Practical Tips

- Always insert the sheath with its dilator in place to minimize vessel trauma.
- Verify compatibility between the sheath, guidewire, and other devices.

GUIDEWIRES (FIGS. 6 TO 11)

Guidewires are the navigational tools that enable the precise movement of catheters and other devices through the vasculature.

Key Properties

- *Torquability:* Ability to transmit rotational force from the proximal end to the tip.
- *Flexibility:* Critical for trackability while maintaining tip strength.
- *Shapeability and shape retention:* Allows customization of the distal tip for difficult anatomies; nitinol wires often excel in shape retention.

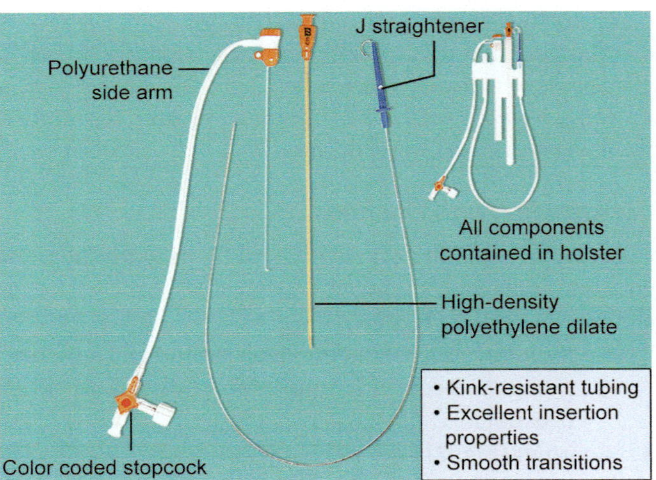

Fig. 4: Prelude sheath.

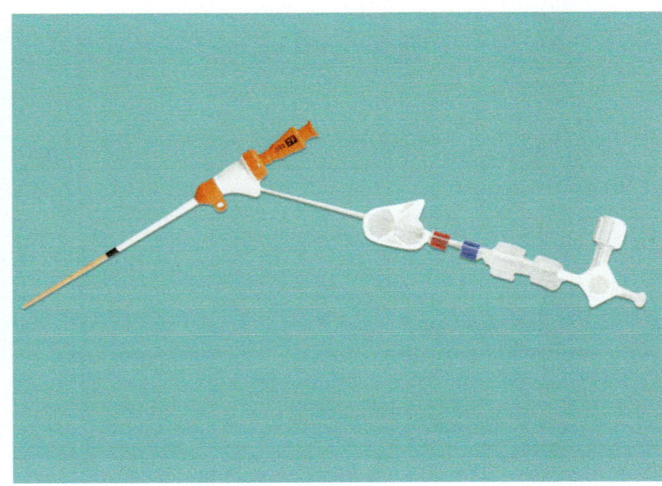

Fig. 5: Sheath components and color-coding for size identification.

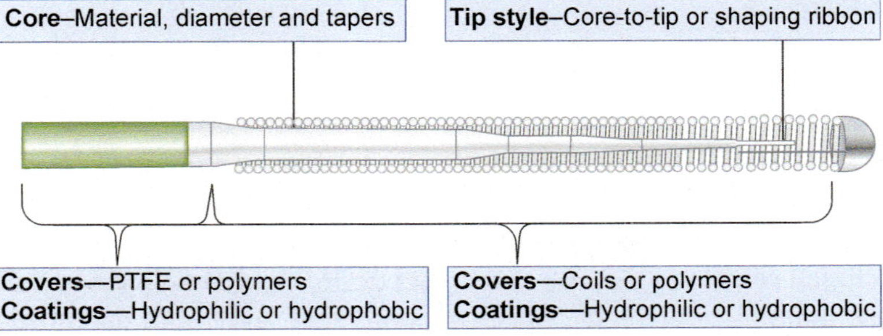

Fig. 6: Parts of a guidewire.

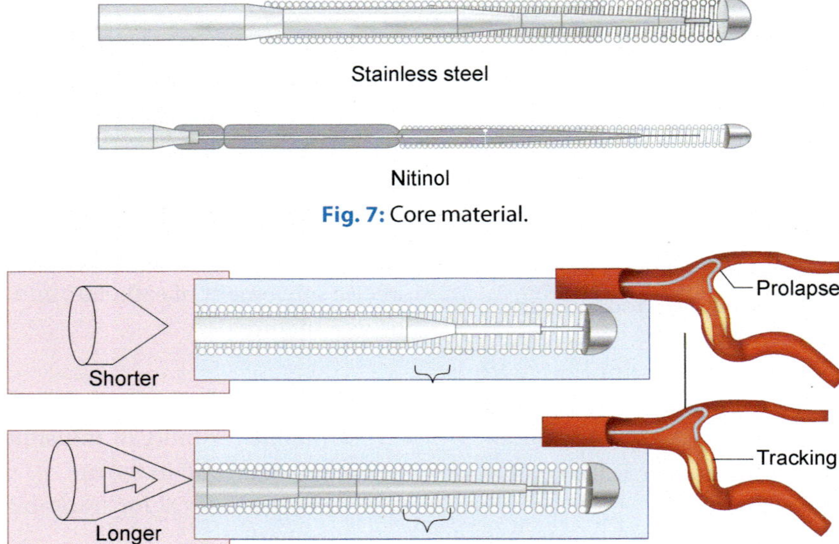

Fig. 7: Core material.

Fig. 8: Core taper.

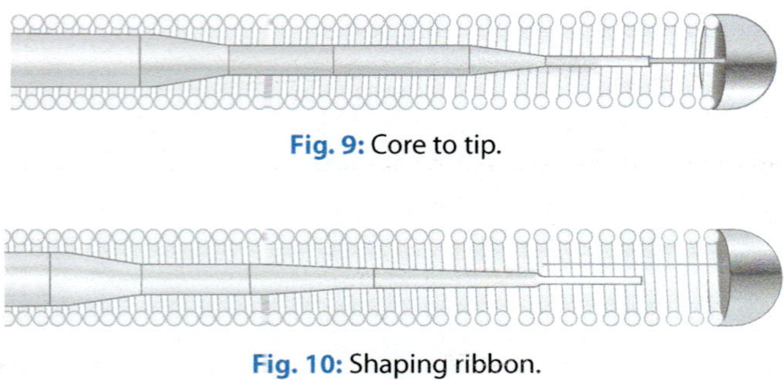

Fig. 9: Core to tip.

Fig. 10: Shaping ribbon.

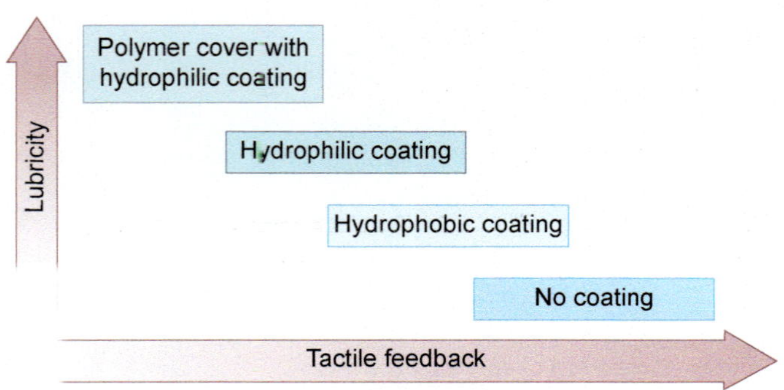

Fig. 11: Classification of guidewires according to use.

- *Tactile feedback:* Physical sensations transmitted through the wire aid in procedural navigation.
- *Trackability:* The ease with which the wire advances through stenotic or occluded vessels.
- *Tip load and support:* Balance between crossing resistant lesions and ensuring a safe, atraumatic tip.

Categories of Guidewires

- *Access wires:* Primarily used for initial vascular entry; typically feature a hydrophilic coating.
- *Maneuvering wires:* Designed for navigating tortuous vessels with a soft, shaped tip.
- *Support wires (rail wires):* Stiffer wires used to stabilize devices during interventions.

Construction and Coatings

Guidewires come in various constructions, with different core materials and coatings:

- *Core materials* ***(Fig. 6)****:*
  - *Stainless steel:* Offers excellent torque and support.
  - *Nitinol:* Provides super-elasticity and kink resistance.
- *Coatings* ***(Fig. 7)****:*
  - *Hydrophilic:* Reduce friction for smoother navigation.
  - *Hydrophobic:* Enhance tactile feedback and control.
- *Design variants:*
  - **Figure 8** shows *guidewire core taper illustration—demonstrating the length of taper and its effect on torque transmission.*
  - **Figure 9** shows *key features of guidewires, including coating types, diameters, and tip design.*

CATHETERS (FIGS. 12 AND 13)

Catheters serve both diagnostic and therapeutic roles by delivering contrast media, medications, and devices.

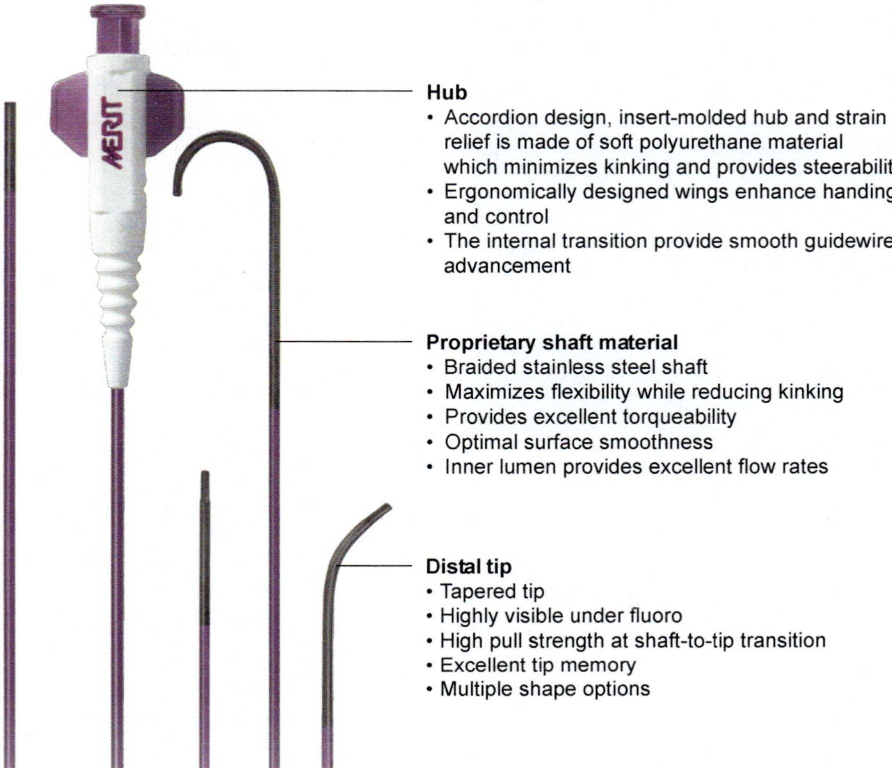

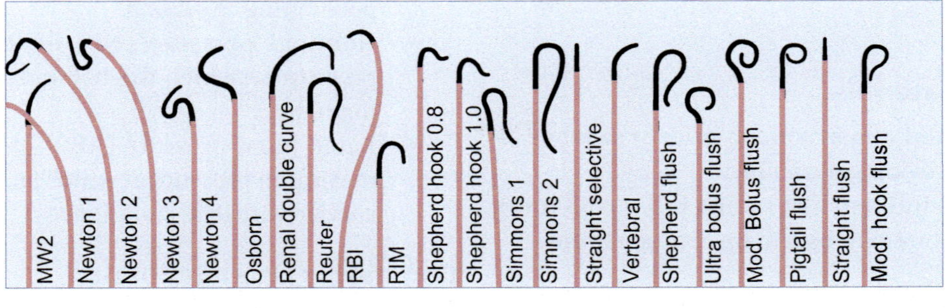

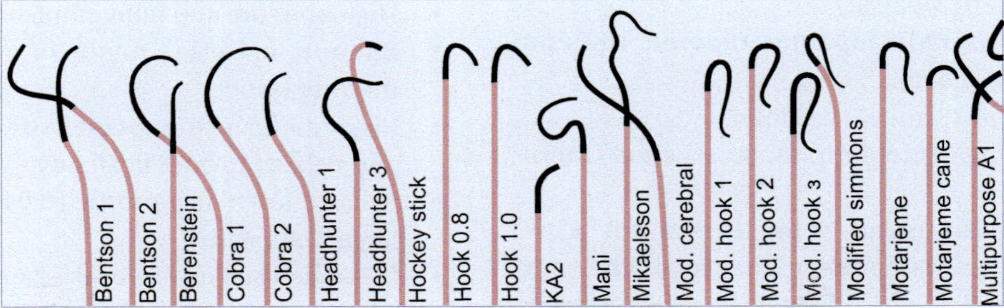

Fig. 12: Performa diagnostic peripheral catheters (Merit Medical).

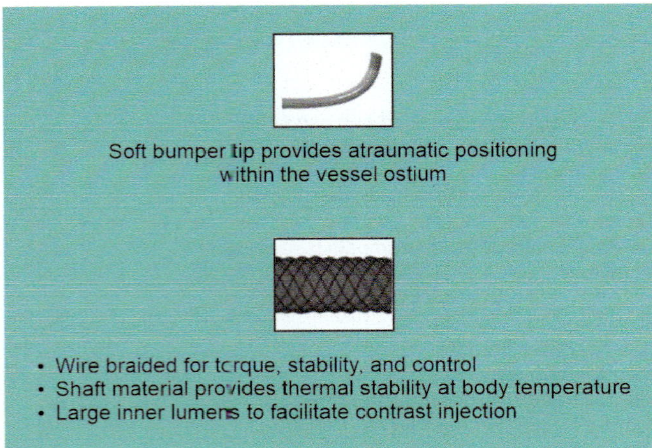

Fig. 13: Peripheral angiographic catheters.

Types of Catheters

- *Diagnostic catheters:* Such as pigtail and multipurpose angiographic (MPA) catheters, used for imaging, and pressure measurements
- *Guiding catheters:* Shaped to facilitate device delivery and support guidewire advancement.
- *Specialized catheters:* There are number of catheters available to facilitate cannulation of different interventions, examples include Judkins and Cobra head catheters.

Features and Materials

- *Material:* Braided constructions offer resistance to kinking while providing durability.
- *Size:* Measured in French (F) units (1F = 0.33 mm); available in various lengths and tip configurations.
- *Examples:*
  - Impress peripheral hydrophilic angiographic catheters (Merit Medical):
    - Features a radio-opaque tapered tip and hydrophilic coating
    - Available in 4F and 5F versions
  - Performa diagnostic peripheral catheters (Merit Medical):
    - Constructed from Nylon-Pebax for kink resistance and enhanced maneuverability
    - Offered in 4F, 5F, and 6F sizes

ANGIOPLASTY BALLOONS

Angioplasty balloons are essential for restoring blood flow in stenotic vessels.

Balloon Types

- *Compliant balloons:* Adapt to vessel contours and are typically used for initial dilations.
- *Noncompliant balloons:* Maintain their shape under high pressure, ideal for calcified or fibrotic lesions.
- *Cutting balloons:* Equipped with microblades to score and dilate fibrotic lesions.
- *Drug-coated balloons:* Deliver medications (e.g., paclitaxel) to reduce the risk of restenosis.

Pressure Resistance

- *Two types of balloons:* High pressure balloons and low pressure balloons
  - High pressure balloons are made up of Nybax or Pebax or Nylon or polyethylene terephthalate (PET). They have high tensile strength and can maintain its design shape and size within the rated pressure range. Its main function is to expand the blood vessel under the action of high-pressure fluid.
  - Low pressure balloons are mostly made of compliant materials such as PVC, latex, or silicone rubber. Such balloons are easily deformed under internal pressure. The size under pressure may be several times the design size. Mainly used for positioning or sealing.
  - Nominal pressure (NP) of the balloon is the pressure at which the balloon reaches its labeled diameter.
  - Rated burst pressure (RBP) of the balloon is the maximum pressure at which 99.9% of balloons can survive with 95% confidence.

Commonly Used Balloons

- *Mustang PTA balloon dilatation catheters* **(Fig. 14)***:*
  - High pressure and noncompliant balloon
  - Balloon material made of Nylon and Pebax thermoplastic
  - Elastomer. Nylon provides strength for High RBP and Pebax provides flexibility.
  - It has a low entry profile (0.040 inch): Only 15% larger than wire
  - It can be used in 1 F lower sized sheath compared to Conquest-40 and Chameleon PTA balloon dilatation catheters of same diameters.
  - It has a rapid Inflation and deflation time (6-mm balloon deflates in 4 seconds)
  - It is compatible with 0.035 inch guidewire only

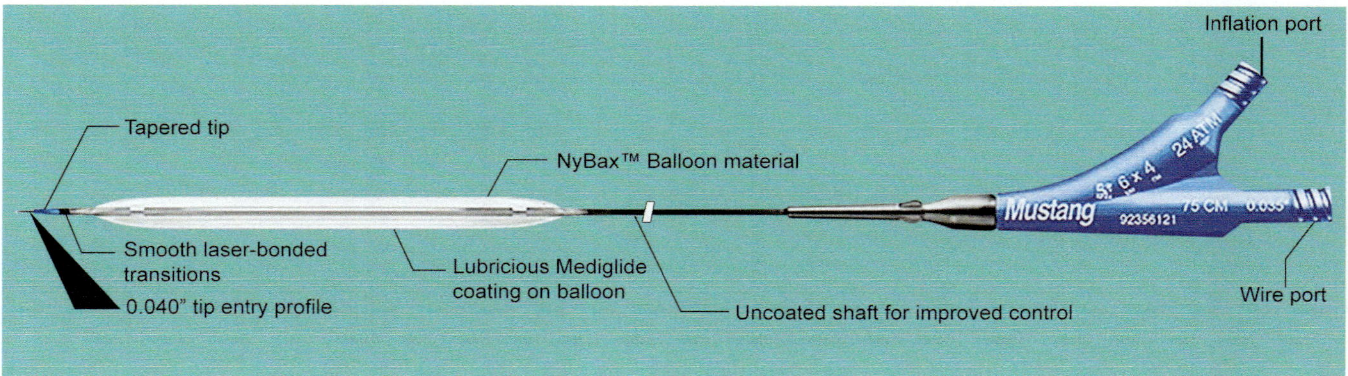

Fig. 14: Mustang.

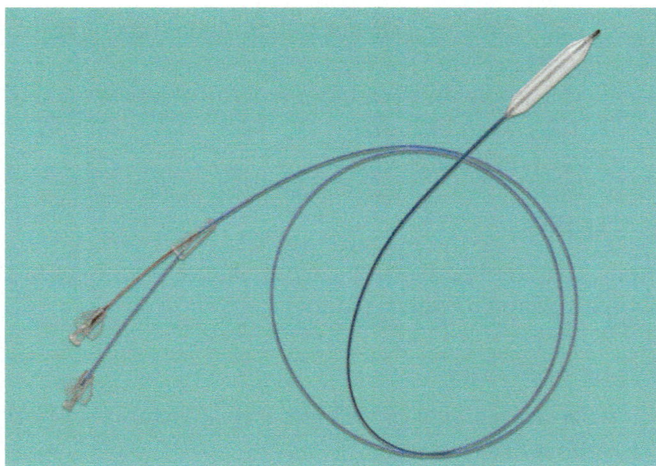

Fig. 15: Conquest.

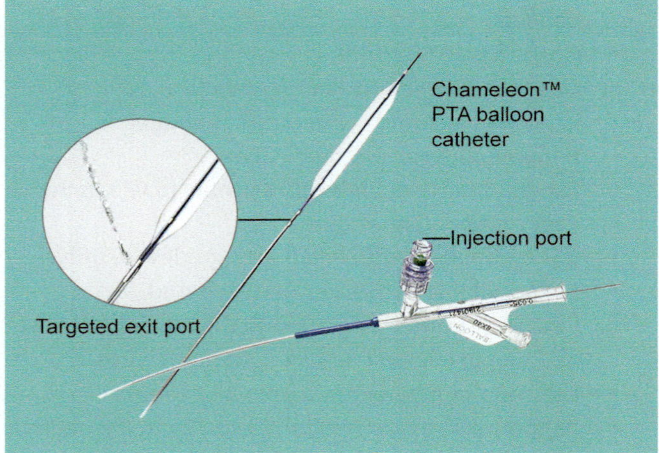

Fig. 16: Chameleon—is a new type balloons with specific advantages.

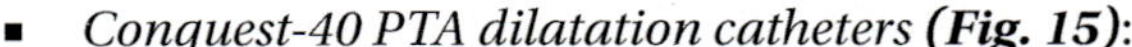

- *Conquest-40 PTA dilatation catheters* ***(Fig. 15)***:
  - Ultrahigh pressure and ultra-noncompliant balloon
  - Balloon has a three-layered design—the inner layer is constructed of noncompliant PET material. Ultrahigh-molecular-weight PE fibers are wrapped circumferentially and longitudinally around the inner PET layer.
  - The PE fibers are affixed to the inner PET material by an extremely thin covering layer of polyether block amide (Pebax) material.
  - The balloon is relatively puncture resistant and does not cause vessel overexpansion.
  - It is compatible with 0.035 inch guidewire only.
- *Chameleon PTA balloon catheter* ***(Figs. 16 and 17)***:
  - High pressure and noncompliant balloon
  - Almost similar to mustang PTA balloon dilatation catheter
  - But compared to mustang, it has a higher entry profile and needs sheath diameter almost similar to Conquest-40
  - Dilatation catheters
  - The added advantage of Chameleon PTA balloon catheter is that it doubles up as diagnostic catheter due to presence of a third port which enables proximal injection of contrast medium enabling hands-free reflux angiography thereby minimizing radiation exposure
  - It is compatible with 0.035 inch guidewire only.
  - Balloon length 4 cm for all balloon diameters
  - Balloon catheter shaft length available in 75 cm
  - NP of 14 ATM for balloon diameter 5–8 mm and 12 ATM for balloon diameter 10–12 mm
  - RBP of 25 ATM for balloon diameters 5–6 mm, 22 ATM for balloon diameters 7–8 mm and 14 ATM for balloon diameters 10–12 mm

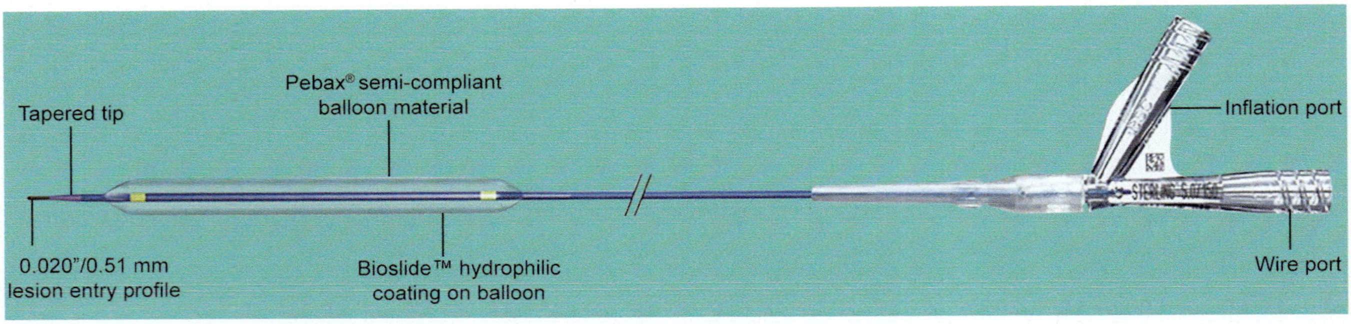

Fig. 17: Chameleon—is a new type balloons with specific advantages.

- Compatible sheath diameters: 6F for 5–8 mm balloon, 7F for 10 mm balloon and 8F for 12 mm balloon
- Cost: INR 30.500/unit

- *Sterling PTA balloon dilatation catheters:*
  - High pressure and semicompliant balloon
  - Balloon material made of Pebax
  - Exceptionally very low entry profile (0.020 inch)
  - Very rapid deflation time
  - It is compatible with 0.018 inch guidewire only.
  - Also available in Mono-rail with Rapid
  - Exchange guidewire port with the advantage of not needing to use exchange length guidewires
  - Balloon diameters range from 2 to 10 mm
  - Balloon length ranges from 2 to 22 cm for balloon diameters 2 mm–7 mm and 2 cm to 8 cm for balloon diameters 8 mm to 10 mm
  - Balloon catheter shaft length available in 40 cm, 80/90 cm, 135 cm, and 150 cm
  - NP of 6 ATM for all balloon size
  - RBP of 14 ATM for balloon diameters 2 mm–7 mm, 12 ATM for balloon diameter 8 mm and 10 ATM for balloon diameter 10 mm
  - Compatible sheath diameters (for up to 4 cm balloon length): 4F for 2–8 mm balloon, 5F for 10 mm balloon
  - Cost: INR 13,500/unit
- *Performa diagnostic peripheral catheters:*
  - Made of Nylon-Pebax material shaft which is kink resistant and smooth.
  - It also has a wire braided design for greater torque, greater longitudinal stability, high degree of maneuverability, and pushability.
  - Almost all tip shape choices available as with impress peripheral angiographic catheters.
  - It has a polycarbonate hub.
  - The tip has good memory and also available in soft bumper tip in 4F catheters.
  - It is available in inner lumen diameters of 4F, 5F, and 6F.
  - It is available in catheter lengths of 40 cm, 65 cm, 100 cm, and 125 cm
  - *Cost:* INR 2,000/unit

STENTS

Stents are deployed when angioplasty alone does not suffice to maintain vessel patency.

Types of Stents

- *Bare-metal stents (BMS):* Provide structural support without drug coating.
- *Drug-eluting stents (DES):* Coated with antiproliferative agents to reduce restenosis.
- *Covered stents:* Used to seal vessel tears or aneurysms.

Deployment Considerations

- *Indications:* Typically reserved for cases with significant elastic recoil or recurrent stenosis.
- *Selection:* Stent flexibility and radial strength are critical for long-term success.

INFLATION DEVICES

Presto Inflation Device (Fig. 18)

- Inflates to ultrahigh atmospheric pressures of 40 ATM
- To inflate the balloon with the lever in the up position, turn the handle clockwise to inflate the balloon to the desired pressure.
- To deflate the balloon, rotate the handle counter-clockwise to 0 ATM prior to pressing the lever. Once 0 ATM has been reached, press the lever and pull back on the handle to evacuate the balloon entirely.

- Maximum volume of contrast that can be filled is 30 cc.
- *Cost:* INR 7,500/unit

ANCILLARY EQUIPMENT (FIGS. 19 AND 20)

In addition to the primary devices, several ancillary tools support cath laboratory interventions:

- *Thrombectomy devices:* Employed for fistula thrombosis with a heavy thrombus load.
- *Snares:* Used for foreign body retrieval and fibrin sheath disruption.
    - *Types:* Ensnare and Gooseneck snares
- *Atherectomy devices:* Considered in cases of severe calcified lesions

CASE STUDIES

Case 1: Juxta-Anastomotic Stenosis in a Radiocephalic Fistula

Objective: Restore adequate flow in an AV fistula compromised by neointimal hyperplasia near the anastomosis.

Procedure:

- *Patient preparation:*
    - *Position:* Supine with the arm extended
    - *Anesthesia:* Local (1% lidocaine)
    - *Access:*
        - Prefer antegrade venous puncture in the cephalic vein
        - If needed, use retrograde puncture; arterial access via the radial artery is an alternative in complex cases.
- *Device selection:*
    - *Sheath:* 5F or 6F short introducer sheath.
    - *Guidewire:* Start with a 0.035" hydrophilic guidewire; switch to a 0.018" stiff wire (or a 0.014" PTCA floppy guidewire for very tight lesions).
    - *Diagnostic catheter*: Multipurpose angiographic (MPA1/MPA2) catheter
- *Balloon angioplasty:*
    - *Predilatation:* Use a 4–6 mm balloon (40–60 mm length) for initial dilatation
    - *High pressure balloon:* If residual stenosis > 30%, consider a high-pressure balloon (6–8 mm) at 10–20 ATM.
- *Postangioplasty:*
    - *Angiography:* Repeat contrast injection to assess for residual stenosis.

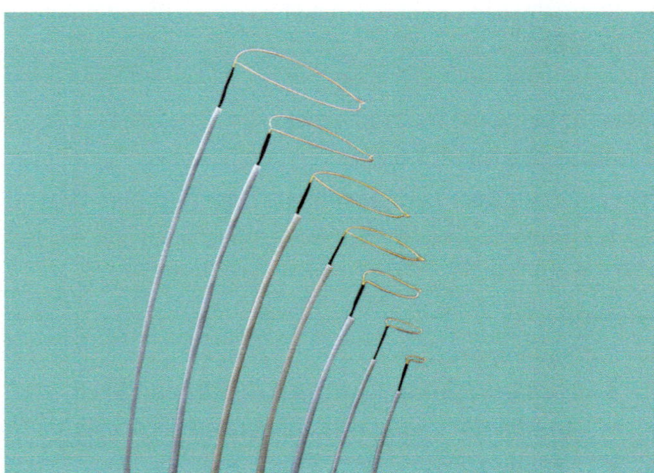

Fig. 19: Snare—single loop.

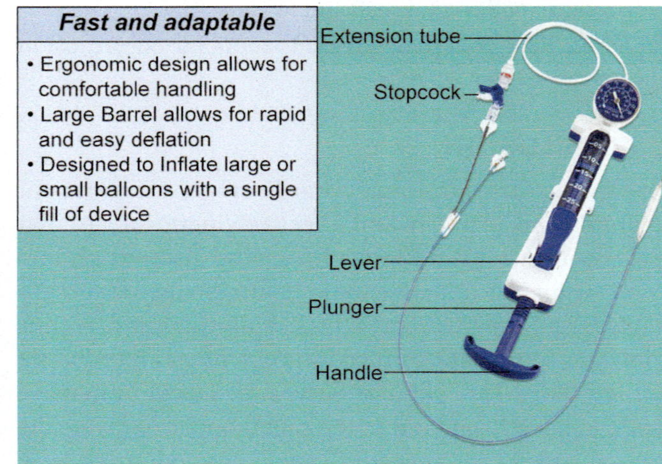

Fig. 18: Inflator device.

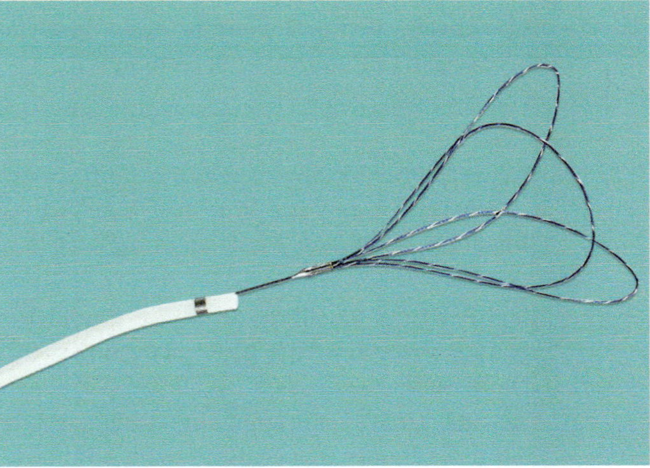

Fig. 20: Snare—multiple loops.

- *Stent placement:* Rarely required unless significant recoil is observed.
- *Hemostasis and postprocedural care:*
  - *Sheath removal:* Manual compression (5–10 minutes; longer for arterial access)
  - *Follow-up:* Duplex ultrasound in 4–6 weeks; consider antiplatelet therapy (e.g., aspirin ± clopidogrel).

Key equipment summary:

- *Sheath:* 5F–6F introducer sheath
- *Guidewire:* 0.035" hydrophilic guidewire, with an option for a 0.018" stiff wire
- *Diagnostic catheter:* 4F–5F multipurpose catheter
- *Balloon catheter:* 4–6 mm standard balloon; 6–8 mm high pressure balloon (if required)
- *Stent:* Covered stent reserved for recurrent or refractory lesions

Case 2: Central Vein Stenosis in the Left Brachiocephalic Vein

Objective: Address central vein stenosis in a patient with a left elbow AV fistula to restore adequate outflow and prevent complications such as arm swelling.

Procedure:

- *Patient preparation:*
  - *Position:* Supine, with arms slightly abducted
  - *Anesthesia:* Local (1% lidocaine) at access sites
  - *Venous access:*
    - *Primary:* Left basilic or cephalic vein (retrograde access).
    - *Alternative:* Femoral vein or right internal jugular vein (for pull-through technique).
- *Hardware selection:*
  - *Sheaths:*
    - Use a 6F–8F introducer sheath; a short sheath (11 cm) for antegrade arm access or a long sheath (25–45 cm) for jugular/femoral access.
  - *Guidewires:*
    - Begin with a 0.035" hydrophilic guidewire; upgrade to a stiff wire (e.g., Amplatz Super Stiff) if necessary.
    - Consider a 0.018" wire for highly resistant lesions and use a buddy wire technique for additional support
  - *Diagnostic catheters:*
    - MPA1/MPA2 or selective catheters (JR 4, Cobra) for contrast injection and mapping.
- *Angioplasty:*
  - *Predilatation:* Perform angiography to visualize the lesion.
  - *Balloon selection:*
    - *Standard:* 10–14 mm balloon (40–60 mm length)
    - *High-pressure:* For resistant lesions, up to 20 ATM if necessary.
  - *Stenting:*
    - Indicated in cases of severe elastic recoil or if PTA fails.
    - *Stent options:* Self-expanding BMS (e.g., Wallstent and SMART) or covered stents (e.g., Viabahn and Fluency).
- *Postprocedure:*
  - *Hemostasis:* Manual compression for 10–15 minutes (or use closure devices for jugular/femoral access)
  - *Poststenting assessment:* Ensure optimal stent expansion and restored thrill/bruit.
  - *Follow-up:* Duplex ultrasound in 4–6 weeks; antiplatelet therapy as indicated.

Key equipment summary:

- *Sheath:* 6F–8F introducer sheath
- *Guidewire:* 0.035" hydrophilic guidewire, with escalation to a stiff guidewire as needed
- *Diagnostic catheter:* 4F–5F multipurpose or selective catheter (JR 4, Cobra)
- *Balloon catheter:* 10–14 mm standard balloon; high pressure balloon for resistant lesions
- *Stent:* Bare-metal or covered stents based on lesion characteristics

CONCLUSION

Mastering cath laboratory hardware is essential for nephrologists to safely and effectively perform vascular interventions. By understanding the properties and applications of imaging tools, contrast media, access devices, guidewires, catheters, balloons, and stents, clinicians can optimize procedural outcomes and enhance patient care. This chapter serves as a comprehensive guide to the critical tools in the cath laboratory, laying the groundwork for improved independence and expertise in interventional nephrology.

ACKNOWLEDGMENTS

Special thanks to Dr Hemant Kumar and Dr Manish Lalwani.

SUGGESTED READING

1. Catheters Fundamentals You Should Know Cherian 1 (Transcription): Discusses the construction, types, and applications of catheters used in cathlab interventions. https://youtu.be/LhWFolNMHF0?si=P68Uw4whZTR_7Lec
2. FDA. (2023). Drug-Coated Balloons: Overview and Indications. [online] Available from https://www.fda.gov [Last accessed July, 2025].
3. Interventional Radiology Series Part 2: Needles, Catheters, Wires, Sheaths (Transcription): Provides a comprehensive review of essential hardware in interventional radiology. https://www.youtube.com/live/kz2EUIVLyWY?si=zwcBkoo_s-IhHn9X
4. Mayo Clinic. (2023). Cardiac Catheterization: What You Need to Know. [online] Available from https://www.mayoclinic.org/tests-procedures/cardiac-catheterization/about/pac-20384695 [Last accessed July, 2025].
5. Radiographics. (2023). Understanding Interventional Radiology Equipment. [online] Available from https://pubs.rsna.org [Last accessed July, 2025].

CHAPTER 20

Angioplasty/Stenting

Rajendran Vilvendan, Ayush Thomas

INTRODUCTION

Arteriovenous fistulas (AVFs) and arteriovenous grafts (AVGs) serve as the primary modes of vascular access for these patients, functioning as a critical component of their ongoing care. While both AVFs and AVGs facilitate hemodialysis, AVFs are generally favored due to their demonstrated superior long-term patency rates and a lower propensity for complications such as thrombosis and infection.[3] The emphasis on AVF creation was initially driven by the "Fistula First" initiative; however, contemporary guidelines have evolved to a more patient-centered approach that prioritizes "the right access, in the right patient, at the right time".[4] This evolution acknowledges the complexities inherent in vascular access management and the necessity of tailoring strategies to individual patient needs and vascular anatomy.

Despite the preference for AVFs, both access types are susceptible to dysfunction, primarily due to stenosis, which often results from neointimal hyperplasia.[4] Thrombosis frequently occurs as a secondary complication of stenosis or due to other predisposing factors.[1] Additional complications such as recoil after angioplasty,[5] contrast extravasation,[2] aneurysms,[1] and central venous stenosis[3] further contribute to access failure and necessitate intervention. The high incidence of stenosis and thrombosis underscores the critical need for effective surveillance and intervention strategies to maintain the patency of these vital vascular accesses.

Percutaneous transluminal angioplasty (PTA) has emerged as the primary endovascular technique employed in interventional radiology for the treatment of AV access stenosis and the subsequent improvement of blood flow.[1] PTA is frequently performed on an outpatient basis under image guidance.[6] While PTA demonstrates high initial technical success rates, its long-term effectiveness is often limited by the recurrence of stenosis, necessitating the exploration and application of adjunctive techniques and technologies such as drug-coated balloons and stents.[4] This chapter aims to provide a comprehensive and evidence-based review of angioplasty techniques in the setting of AV access dysfunction. It will delve into specific technical aspects, procedural outcomes, and the role of adjunctive therapies, offering a valuable resource for interventional radiologists engaged in the management of hemodialysis access.

TECHNICAL CONSIDERATIONS IN CATHETERIZATION LABORATORY

Preprocedural Evaluation

A comprehensive preprocedural assessment guides the procedural strategy, including determining the optimal approach for preparation and the type and number of access sites required.

Clinical and Laboratory Assessment

The initial evaluation begins with a thorough review of relevant labs, such as coagulation profiles, and a clear understanding of the indication for the procedure (e.g., access dysfunction, thrombosis, surveillance findings). A focused clinical examination is performed to assess for signs of central venous stenosis (ipsilateral arm swelling, facial edema, or prominent collaterals in the chest wall) **(Fig. 1)**, fistula characteristics such as a hyperpulsatile fistula (indicating a downstream stenosis), weak or absent thrill (inflow stenosis), and the presence of aneurysm or overlying skin changes (signs of infection, skin defect).

Preprocedural Ultrasound Examination

Whenever feasible, a point-of-care ultrasound (POCUS) or a formal duplex ultrasound examination should be performed prior to transferring the patient to the

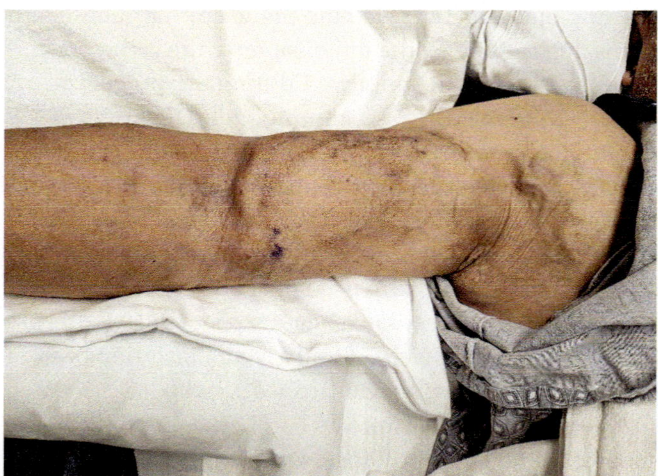

Fig. 1: Initial clinical examination showed a hyperpulsatile arteriovenous fistula with collateral veins in the right shoulder region. Clinical findings are suspicious for central venous stenosis/occlusion.

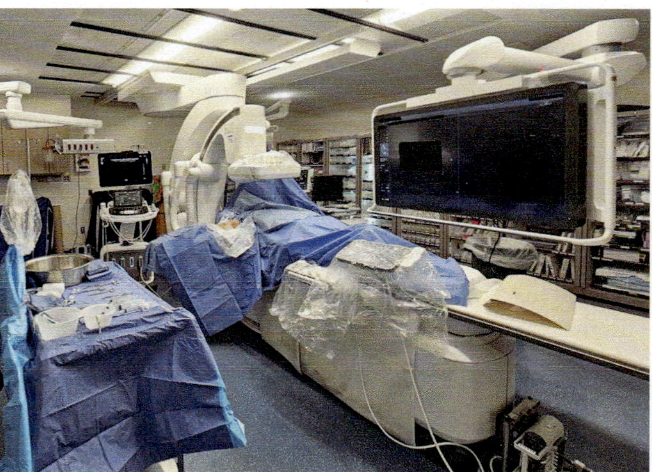

Fig. 2: Patient in supine position in the cath lab table. The right upper extremity extended and prepared for sterile access. The C-arm imaging system is positioned cephalad, allowing for comprehensive fluoroscopic coverage from the wrist to the thorax.

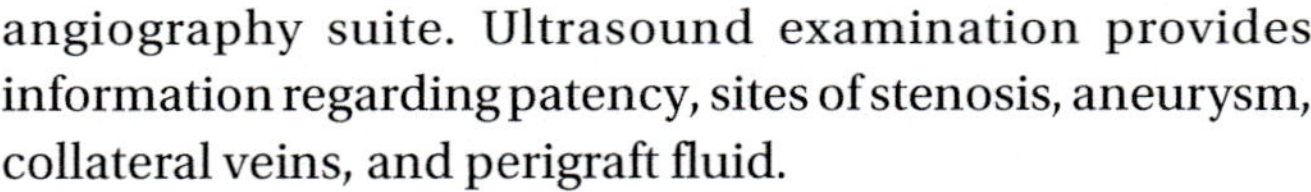

angiography suite. Ultrasound examination provides information regarding patency, sites of stenosis, aneurysm, collateral veins, and perigraft fluid.

Informed Consent

Obtaining detailed, written informed consent is a mandatory prerequisite. The discussion with the patient (and family, if appropriate) must encompass the nature and purpose of the proposed procedure, potential benefits and alternatives (including conservative management or surgical revision), specific risks, including but not limited to bleeding or hematoma formation at the access site(s), infection, with particular emphasis on the higher susceptibility in AVGs, venous rupture or dissection, which may necessitate the deployment of bare metal or covered stents for management, allergic reactions to contrast media or medications, and the potential for access failure or thrombosis. Consent should also be explicitly obtained for the possible placement of a tunneled dialysis catheter should the AVF/AVG intervention be unsuccessful or result in access failure.

Patient Preparation in the Angiography Suite

The patient is placed in the supine position on the angiography table. The arm with dialysis access is typically abducted to approximately 90° and supported comfortably. The C-arm (fluoroscopy unit) must be positioned to permit fluoroscopic visualization from the wrist (or relevant inflow) extending proximally to the chest, encompassing the entire dialysis access circuit and its drainage into the central veins **(Fig. 2)**. The arm is often rested on a dedicated arm board or extender. The wrist may be gently secured with tape to the extender to maintain position and prevent inadvertent movement.

The skin overlying the intended puncture site(s) and the broader procedural field is meticulously prepped. A combination of chlorhexidine gluconate and alcohol is commonly used. In instances of open wounds or known chlorhexidine allergy, povidone-iodine may be substituted. For open wounds, cleansing should be performed with povidone-iodine alone, avoiding alcohol. The antiseptic solution must be allowed to air dry completely before draping to ensure efficacy and reduce the risk of skin irritation or fire (if electrocautery is anticipated, though rare in these procedures). The operative field is then isolated with sterile drapes, ensuring that the margins of the area of interest are adequately covered.

Sedation and analgesia: Conscious sedation is routinely administered at the authors' institution to enhance patient comfort and cooperation. Titrated intravenous doses of a benzodiazepine (e.g., midazolam) and an opioid analgesic (e.g., fentanyl) are typically used. The dosage is carefully adjusted based on the anticipated complexity and duration of the procedure, as well as the individual patient's tolerance, comorbidities, and response to medication. Continuous monitoring of vital signs, oxygen saturation, and level of consciousness is essential throughout the procedure.

Antibiotic prophylaxis: The routine use of prophylactic antibiotics prior to fistulography or intervention is generally not recommended for native AVFs. However, practice may vary, and specific guidelines or institutional protocols should be consulted, particularly for procedures involving AVGs or when there is a heightened risk of infection (e.g., recent bacteremia, known skin colonization with resistant organisms).[1]

Intraprocedural Considerations

Anticoagulation

Routine anticoagulation is generally not administered during angioplasty for AVFs. Systemic heparin may be used during the procedure, often at lower doses such as 1,000–2,000 units. The focus of the procedure is typically on the local mechanical dilation of the stenosis rather than systemic anticoagulation for preventing thrombus formation during the intervention itself. However, in selected cases where significant recoil occurs after the initial angioplasty, anticoagulation can be considered prior to prolonged balloon angioplasty. This selective use is predicated on the rationale of preventing acute thrombosis in a vessel with a compromised lumen and potential wall injury due to recoil, especially when extended balloon inflation is planned to address the recoil. Research on anticoagulation treatments in hemodialysis patients has shown that unfractionated heparin is the most common anticoagulant used in AVF patients, although not specifically in the setting of postangioplasty recoil.[3] The decision to administer anticoagulation in cases of recoil is therefore highly individualized, likely depending on the severity of the recoil, the anticipated duration of prolonged balloon inflation, and the patient's specific risk profile for both thrombosis and bleeding.

Vascular Access Technique and Sheath Selection

At the authors' institution, ultrasound is routinely used for obtaining vascular access. The direction of access is pointed toward the arteriovenous (AV) anastomosis if juxta-anastomotic stenosis is suspected and away from the anastomosis if outflow stenosis is suspected. Multiple accesses can be performed depending on the complexity and extent of stenosis. Vascular access for angioplasty typically involves the use of introducer sheaths, starting from 5 French (F) upward, with 7 F being a common size for AVF angioplasty.[7] The selection of the appropriate sheath size is determined by the dimensions of the catheters and balloons that will be employed during the procedure.[7] A 7 F sheath is capable of accommodating a variety of 7 F guiding catheters and balloons.[8] However, for certain situations such as central venous angioplasty or when inserting a stent graft, larger sheaths may be required. High-pressure balloons, particularly those with diameters ranging from 12 to 20 mm used in central venous stenosis treatment, may necessitate sheath sizes of 8–10 F or even larger for proper delivery.[9] Similarly, the insertion of stent grafts often requires introducer sheaths with larger French sizes, typically ranging from 10 F to 12 F, depending on the specific characteristics of the device being used.[10]

Initial Fistulogram

The initial fistulogram for AV access procedures should include comprehensive visualization from the arterial anastomosis to the central veins **(Fig. 3)**. This complete assessment is essential for identifying all potential sites of stenosis or obstruction throughout the entire AV access circuit, including the central veins, which may not be evident through clinical examination alone. The imaging is typically performed by retrograde or antegrade puncture of the fistula or graft, followed by the injection of contrast media under fluoroscopic guidance. If antegrade access is performed, then pressure is applied distal to the tip of the sheath and evaluation of the arterial anastomosis is then performed using fistulography with reflux of contrast into the AV anastomosis **(Fig. 4)**. In upper extremity accesses, the visualization should extend to encompass the subclavian vein, brachiocephalic vein, and superior vena cava. Digital subtraction angiography (DSA) is a commonly employed technique for visualizing blood flow and detecting stenoses. Often, multiple imaging views and projections are necessary to thoroughly characterize the lesion and accurately assess its severity. Road mapping techniques can also be utilized to facilitate the guidance of catheters and wires to the target lesion.

DIAGNOSIS AND MANAGEMENT OF STENOSIS

Diagnosis of Stenosis

Stenosis is diagnosed angiographically when there is more than 50% narrowing in the lumen of the fistula or graft and/or by the presence of significant collateral veins bypassing the stenotic segment. It is important to note

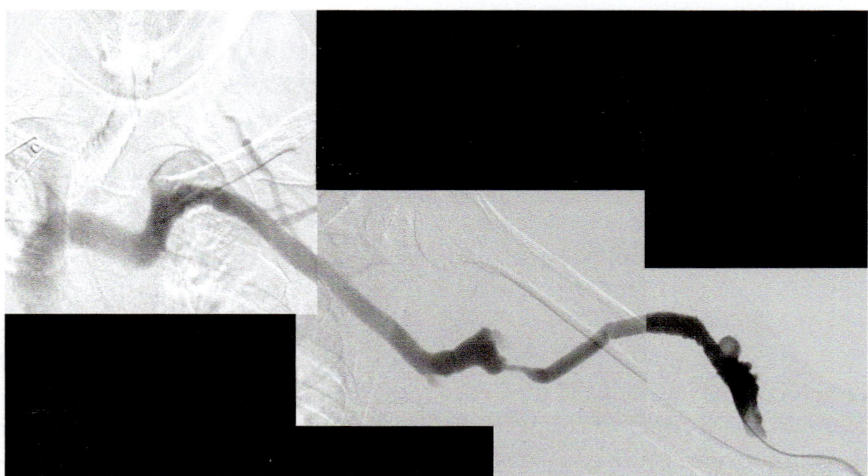

Fig. 3: Fistulogram should extend from the access site to the central vein. In this patient with left arm brachioaxillary arteriovenous graft show severe stenosis at the venous anastomosis. Central veins are patent without any evidence of stenosis.

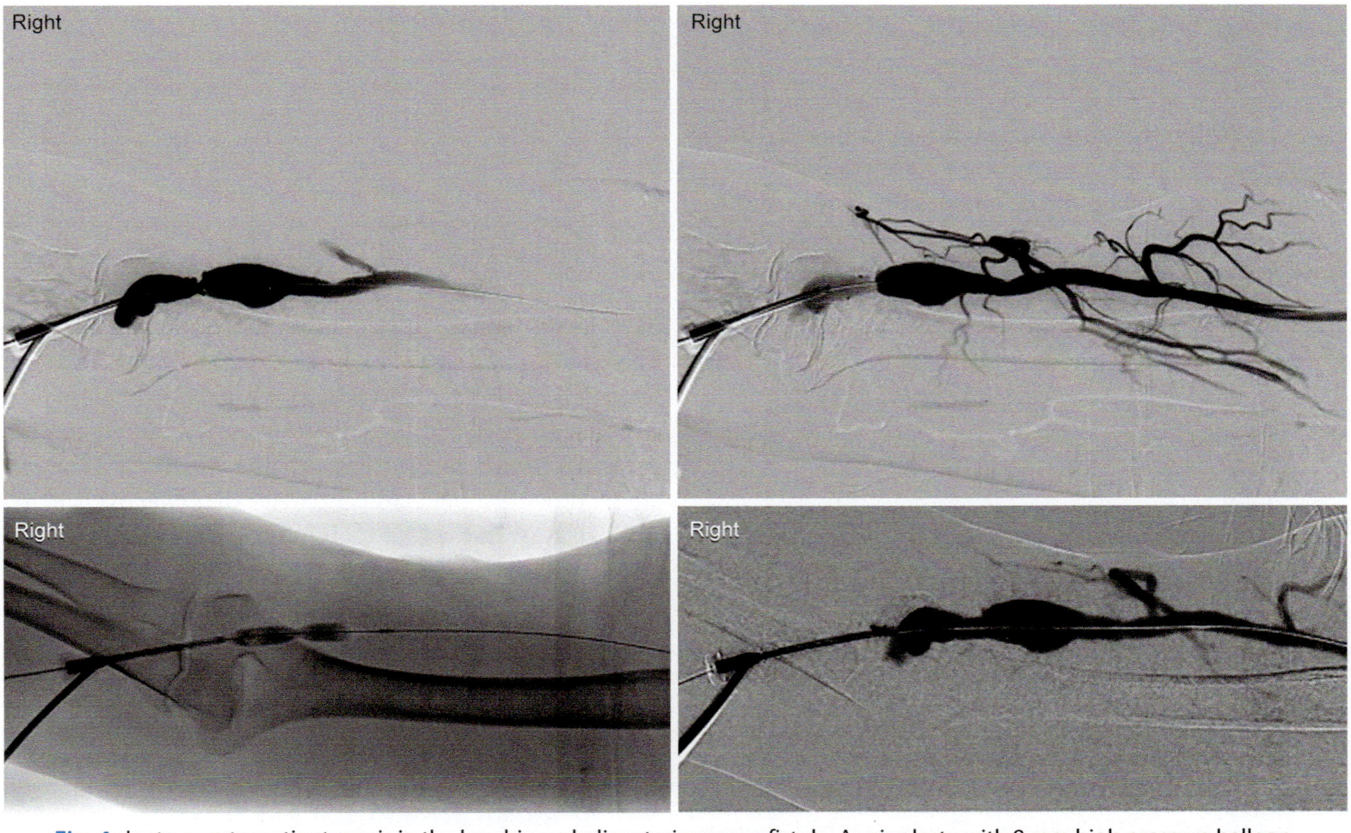

Fig. 4: Juxta-anastomotic stenosis in the brachiocephalic arteriovenous fistula. Angioplasty with 8 mm high pressure balloon. Post-angioplasty venogram showed significant improvement to the stenosis.

that asymptomatic central venous stenosis is not usually treated, as intervention may lead to an increased incidence of recurrent stenosis and potentially necessitate multiple future interventions.[11]

Balloon Angioplasty and Sizing

Balloon angioplasty is the primary treatment for stenotic lesions. Standard balloon sizing in AV access angioplasty generally recommends using a balloon with a diameter approximately 1 mm larger than the native vein diameter, measured proximal and distal to the stenosis. This slight oversizing is intended to ensure adequate dilation of the stenosis and to counteract the elastic recoil of the vessel wall that can lead to early restenosis. Ideally, the balloon diameter should closely match the reference vessel diameter in a 1:1 ratio. However, when dealing with aneurysmal veins, balloon sizing requires particular caution due to the inherent weakness of the vessel walls and the increased risk of rupture. In such cases, the balloon diameter should be carefully selected to match the diameter of the nonaneurysmal segment of the vein to avoid overdilation of the aneurysmal portion.[12] For stenoses associated with aneurysms, the use of stent grafts might be considered to provide additional structural support to the weakened vessel.

Use of High-Pressure Balloons

High-pressure balloons play a significant role in AV access angioplasty, particularly when there is a significant recoil after the initial dilation with standard balloons. These balloons are capable of exerting greater radial force to maintain the patency of the vessel. Balloons rated for pressures exceeding 14 atmospheres (atm) are generally classified as high-pressure balloons, while ultra-high-pressure balloons, capable of pressures >20 atm, may be employed for highly resistant lesions.[13] In the author's institute, the routine practice is to use high-pressure balloons as the initial choice for treating AV access stenosis. This approach may be based on institutional experience indicating improved immediate outcomes and potentially better long-term patency compared to standard pressure balloons. Studies have reported high technical success rates, ranging from 90 to 95%, with the use of high or ultra-high-pressure PTA.[14,15]

Management of Resistant Stenosis (Persistent Waist)

When a persistent waist (indentation on the inflated balloon) is observed at the time of maximal balloon dilation, it indicates a resistant stenosis. The initial management strategy involves the sequential use of larger-sized balloons, followed by high-pressure balloons, to overcome the resistance. A larger ratio of the balloon diameter to the minimal luminal diameter at the stenotic waist has been associated with procedural success when using ultra-high-pressure balloon angioplasty.[16] If these measures fail to eliminate the persistent waist, cutting balloons can be utilized. Cutting balloons are equipped with microsurgical atherotomes (blades) that create longitudinal incisions in the stenotic plaque and vessel wall during inflation. This mechanism can facilitate dilation at lower pressures and potentially reduce the incidence of vessel recoil. However, cutting balloons have limitations in terms of available sizes and can typically only be inflated once. The standard technique involves using the cutting balloon after a failed angioplasty with standard balloons, followed by dilation with a high-pressure balloon. If angioplasty is unsuccessful even after employing a cutting balloon, proceeding with stent placement is generally not recommended, and surgical revision should be considered instead.

MANAGEMENT OF COMPLICATIONS

Contrast Extravasation

For small, focal contrast extravasation observed after angioplasty, the recommended management involves performing prolonged balloon inflation (e.g., 5–10 minutes) at low pressure at the site of the leak. This prolonged inflation helps to tamponade the bleeding and seal the vessel perforation. Following the prolonged inflation, an angiographic study should be repeated to confirm the resolution of the contrast extravasation. It is also essential to clinically palpate the site of extravasation and evaluate for the presence and expansion of a hematoma. In cases where an expanding hematoma is noted after angioplasty, the placement of a covered stent is warranted to seal the perforation and prevent further bleeding. Covered stents provide a mechanical barrier that effectively stops the extravasation while maintaining the patency of the vessel. Multifocal sites of contrast extravasation are often encountered in the setting of chronic long-segment stenosis or occlusion. In these situations, the use of long-length covered stents is typically indicated to address the diffuse vessel wall compromise and seal the multiple sites of leakage.

Elastic Recoil after Initial Angioplasty

Elastic recoil is defined as luminal narrowing of >50%, 15 minutes after initial angioplasty. It is seen in approximately 16% of PTA and is more common in cephalic arch stenosis and central venous stenosis. This occurrence does not influence the access primary patency after PTA.[17] A common strategy to address the elastic recoil is the use of ultra-high-pressure balloons, prolonged balloon angioplasty, or the use of cutting balloons.

Central Venous Stenosis

Central venous stenosis **(Fig. 5)** is a common complication that can arise after catheter placement, particularly with prolonged insertion in hemodialysis patients.[18] Patients with central venous stenosis are prone to developing multiple collateral vessels as a compensatory mechanism.[9] Treatment for central venous stenosis is typically indicated only when patients are symptomatic, presenting with issues such as nonmaturation of an AVF, prolonged bleeding after dialysis, arm swelling, or cerebral symptoms related to the stenosis.[9] When treatment is deemed necessary, it often involves the use of high-pressure balloons with diameters ranging from 12 to 20 mm, depending on the size of the vein being treated.[9] The balloon diameter should ideally be 1–2 mm larger than the diameter of the adjacent normal vein, as assessed on venography.[19] However, angioplasty for central venous stenosis, particularly in the superior vena cava, carries a risk of vessel rupture and subsequent pericardial tamponade, although this is a rare occurrence.[6]

Balloon-assisted maturation (BAM) angioplasty plays a role in maturation assistance for AVFs, particularly those created with small-caliber veins.[20] This is often termed balloon-assisted maturation.[21] The procedure can be performed via arterial access or through direct puncture of the fistula.[7] It is typically initiated at least 4 weeks after the creation of the fistula.[20] Initially, a 4 mm balloon is often used, with subsequent dilation using larger-sized balloons approximately a week later.[22] The balloon diameter is often set about 1 mm larger than the native vein size and incrementally increased in subsequent procedures to facilitate maturation.[23]

DRUG-COATED BALLOONS

Drug-coated balloons improve the primary patency rate after 6 months when compared to standard balloons.[24] There are at least three drug-coated balloons available in the US market, Adminal (Meditronic), Lutonix (Bard Peripheral Vascular Inc), and a high-pressure balloon, Aperto (Cardionovum GmbH). In some markets, the Lutonix balloon is available up to 12 mm in diameter and can be used in central venous stenosis. Drug-coated balloons are designed to deliver paclitaxel at a predetermined dose to the angioplasty zone to prevent neointimal hyperplasia. When a drug-coated balloon is considered, angioplasty of the site of stenosis is performed initially with a standard balloon to achieve venous patency. Then, the site is dilated with the drug-coated balloon and is left in place for a few minutes as per manufacturers' recommendations. In a randomized controlled trial, drug-coated balloons improve primary patency from 59.5 to 82.2% at 6 months when compared to the standard balloons.[25] There is no universally accepted standard for routine use of antiplatelet after drug-coated balloon.

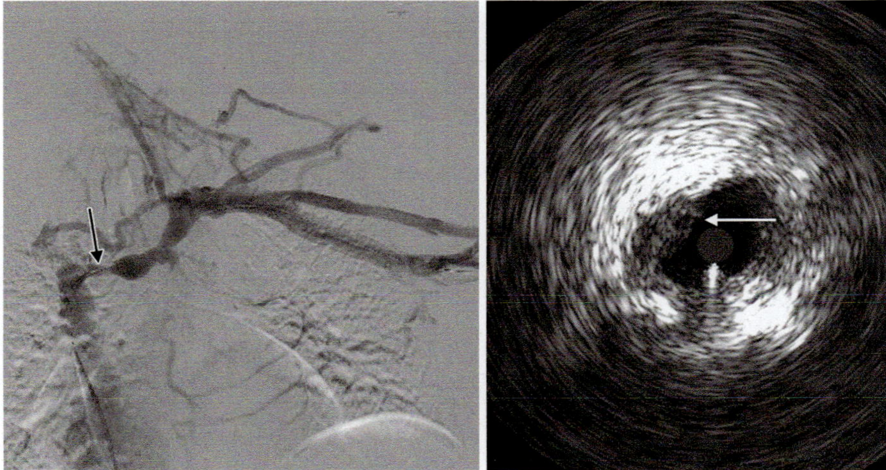

Fig. 5: Patient with left arm brachiocephalic AV fistula, presenting with arm swelling and high pressure during dialysis. Fistulogram show moderate-to-severe stenosis in the left brachiocephalic vein with collateral veins in the neck and intercostal veins. IVUS images show neointimal thickening at the site of stenosis.

CHRONIC TOTAL VENOUS OCCLUSION

Chronic total venous occlusion commonly arises from prior use of central venous catheters or previous or current cardiac leads, leading to chronic thrombosis and scar formation. Four types of chronic total occlusions have been described: Type 1 (single internal jugular or subclavian vein obstruction), type 2 (unilateral brachiocephalic vein obstruction or equivalent), type 3 (bilateral brachiocephalic venous occlusion with patent superior vena cava), and type 4 (any superior vena cava occlusion).[26]

The success of recanalization for chronic total occlusion depends on the length of the occlusion, its chronicity, and the morphological characteristics of the vein just proximal to the occlusion. Recanalization can be achieved through several methods: Traditional endovascular techniques utilizing hydrophilic guidewires or 0.018-inch wires with weighted tips (similar to those used for crossing chronic total occlusions in peripheral arterial disease); sharp recanalization techniques employing 20–22 gauge long Chiba needles, transseptal needles, or Colapinto needles [as used in transjugular intrahepatic portosystemic shunt (TIPSS) procedures] **(Fig. 6)**; or radiofrequency-assisted recanalization using RF wires. Once the total occlusion is crossed, PTA of the occluded segment is performed. Stenting with bare metal or covered stents is typically performed for significant recoil or contrast extravasation. Data are lacking regarding the routine use of anticoagulation or antiplatelet therapy after PTA/stenting for chronic total venous occlusion.

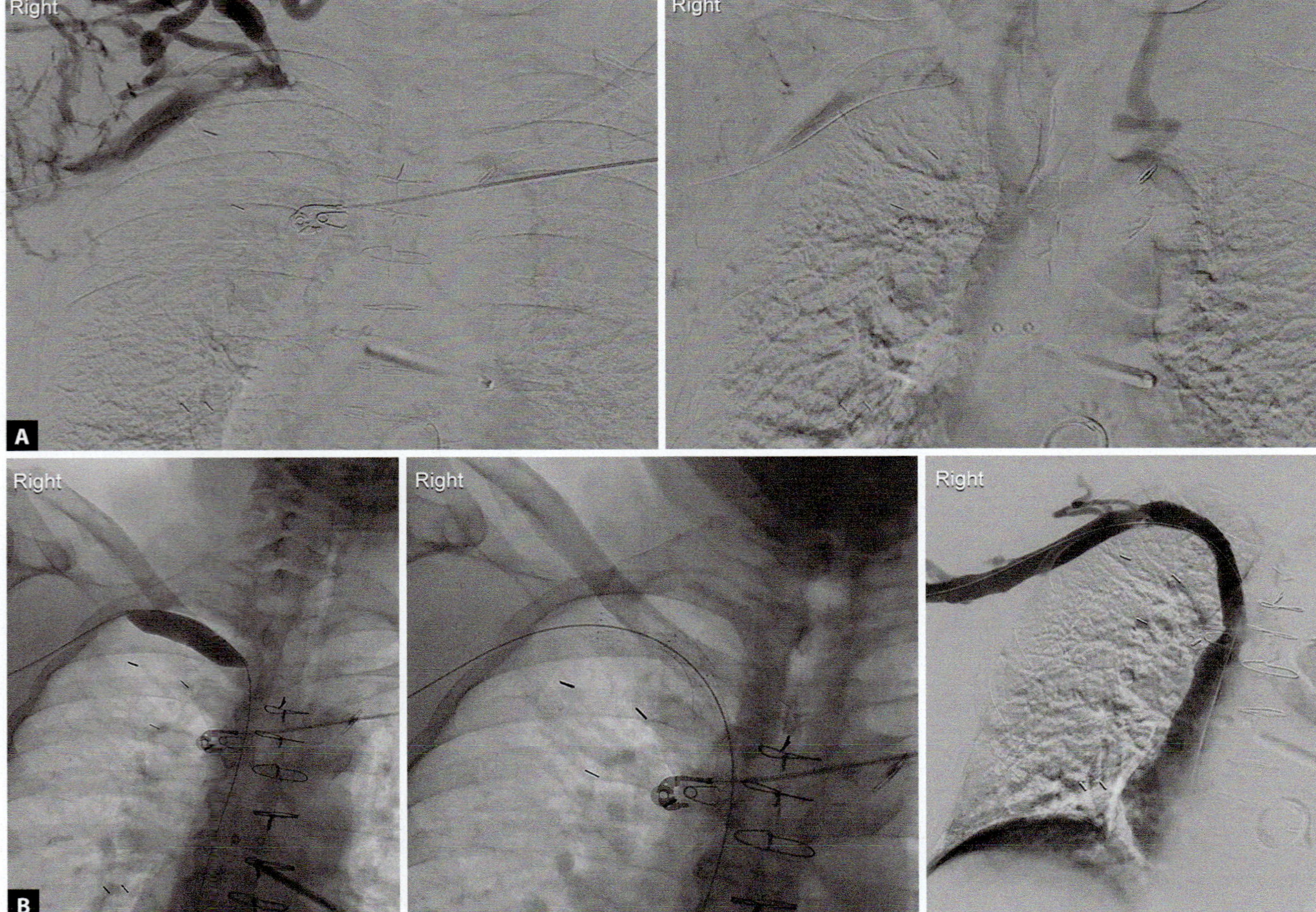

Figs. 6A and B: (A) Early and delayed images of the central veins show short segment occlusion at the right subclavian: Brachiocephalic vein junction; (B) After sharp recanalization of the occluded segment, angioplasty and stenting was performed. Final fistulogram showed patent central veins with brisk flow.

SHEATH REMOVAL AND POSTPROCEDURE OBSERVATIONS

The sheath is removed after the completion of the procedure and manual pressure is applied for 5–10 minutes depending on the fistula type, sheath size, and anticoagulation status. Some institutions use purse-string sutures at the site of the fistula. The technique of purse-string suture involves placing subcutaneous sutures around the puncture site. A tourniquet, created from segments of the sheath introducer's side tube, was positioned under the suture before it was tightened. While an assistant applied pressure and held the tourniquet, they removed the sheath introducer, allowing the operator to secure the suture with three knots **(Fig. 7 and Video)**.[27] Sutures can be removed after 20 minutes in the recovery unit or at the time of dialysis if performed within 24 hours. Patients are routinely monitored for 2 hours in the observation unit prior to the discharge.

OUTCOMES OF ANGIOPLASTY

The immediate technical success rate of angioplasty for AVF stenosis is generally high, reported between 89.5 and 97%.[13] Specific studies have documented success rates of 91%,[7] 95.8%,[28] 98.4%,[29] and 86.67%,[23] often defined as achieving less than 30% residual stenosis.[13] Clinical success, typically defined as at least one successful dialysis session using the treated access, also demonstrates high rates, including 98%,[7] 95.8%,[28] 98.0%,[5] and 81.5%.[30] The restoration of a palpable thrill in the access can also indicate clinical success.[13] However, the long-term outcome of angioplasty is often limited by restenosis. Primary patency rates at 6 months range from 42 to 63%[31] and at 1 year from 40 to 60%.[32] Various studies have reported a range of primary patency rates at 6 and 12 months.[30]

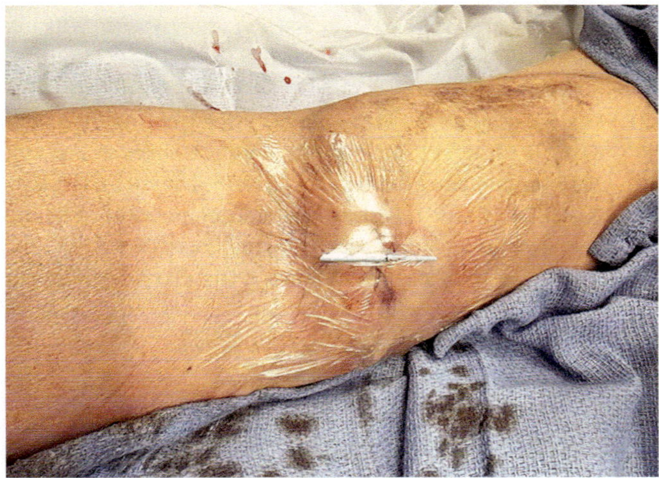

Fig. 7: Access site closure with modified purse string technique. Suture and the plastic were removed after 2 hours.

OUTCOMES AFTER STENTING

Stenting in AV access can be considered as primary stenting or salvage stenting. Increasing evidence suggests improved long-term patency of grafts and fistulas with primary stenting.[33] However, bare metal stents have demonstrated significantly lower patency compared to covered stents.[34] Long-term patency of cephalic arch stenosis has been reported with covered stents.[35] Salvage stenting is typically indicated for significant recoiling or contrast extravasation following angioplasty. The immediate outcome of stenting shows high technical success rates, with one study reporting 97% technical success in juxta-anastomotic stenting.[10] Clinical success, defined as successful dialysis after the procedure, is also high, with a rate of 92% reported in one study.[36] Long-term outcomes of stenting vary. One study reported primary patency rates of 92%, 81%, 31%, and 31% at 3, 6, 12, and 24 months, respectively, with secondary patency of 92% at 3 months and 82% at 6, 12, and 24 months.[36] Another study on central venous stenosis treated with stenting showed primary patency rates of 81%, 52%, 47%, 41%, and 41% at 12, 24, 36, 48, and 60 months, respectively, and assisted patency rates of 98%, 98%, 82%, 82%, and 82% at the same time points.[37] Routine antiplatelet therapy after bare metal or covered stent placement for fistula is generally not required. However, some centers may administer dual antiplatelet therapy for a limited period after covered stent placement.[38] Complications of stenting can include re-occlusion, stent migration (especially in central venous stenting), and device fracture (particularly in stents placed across joints).[39]

CONCLUSION

Angioplasty remains a cornerstone in the management of AV access dysfunction, offering high immediate technical and clinical success rates. However, the challenge of long-term patency due to restenosis necessitates a comprehensive approach that includes meticulous technical execution, judicious use of adjunctive therapies such as high-pressure and cutting balloons, and selective application of stenting. The management of complications like recoil and contrast extravasation requires prompt recognition and tailored interventions. While routine anticoagulation is not typically administered, its selective use in cases of significant recoil may be beneficial. The choice of sheath size and balloon diameter should be guided by the specific clinical scenario and vessel characteristics. A thorough initial fistulogram is crucial for identifying all relevant lesions within the AV access circuit. Angioplasty for maturation assistance in low-caliber veins is a valuable technique to improve the usability of AVFs. Stenting, particularly with covered stents, shows promise in improving long-term patency in certain indications, such as cephalic arch stenosis and salvage of angioplasty failures. However, potential complications of stenting, including re-occlusion, migration, and fracture, must be carefully considered. Continued research and refinement of these techniques are essential to optimize outcomes and prolong the functional lifespan of hemodialysis vascular access.

REFERENCES

1. National Kidney Foundation. KDOQI Clinical Practice Guideline for Vascular Access: 2019 Update. Am J Kidney Dis. 2019;75(4 Suppl 2):S1-S164.
2. Haskal ZJ. Heparin-bonded stent-grafts for treatment of hemodialysis access outflow stenosis and aneurysm: technical feasibility and single-center experience. Cardiovasc Intervent Radiol. 2012;35(5):1098-1104.
3. MacRae JM, Ahmed SB, Hemmelgarn BR, Moist LM, Peacock N, Clemens KK. Anticoagulation for hemodialysis in patients with arteriovenous fistulas. Kidney Int. 2019;95(1):175-84.
4. Kiemeneij F, Laarman GJ, Slagboom T, Stella PR, Ammerer M, Cornelis K. The distal transradial approach for coronary angiography and intervention: a series of 1000 patients. Catheter Cardiovasc Interv. 2014;83(3):E172-6.
5. Shah B, Agarwal A, Munjal M, Mittal K, Aggarwal D. Percutaneous transluminal angioplasty for dialysis access dysfunction: a single-center experience. Indian J Radiol Imaging. 2016;26(1):66-70.
6. Clark TWI, Kurian G, Guben J, Clark TW. Percardial tamponade from central venous angioplasty: A rare but potentially fatal complication. J Vasc Interv Radiol. 2008;19(3):447-9.
7. Clark TW, Cohen R, Kwok-Keung S, Lau J. Performed angioplasty of hemodialysis access grafts: early and late results. J Vasc Interv Radiol. 2002;13(9 Pt 1):891-8.
8. Patel MV, Mehta AB, Shah D, Goyal RC, Parikh P. Feasibility and safety of 7 Fr guiding catheters and balloons for percutaneous coronary intervention. J Invasive Cardiol. 2007;19(11):464-8.
9. Girsowicz E, Ascher E, Marks N, Levi M, Jacob T, Rubenzik L, et al. Treatment of central venous stenosis in hemodialysis patients with transluminal angioplasty and stenting. J Vasc Surg. 2005;42(5):940-7.
10. Kundu S, Modanlou KA, Jafar MZ, Smith TP. Use of covered stents in hemodialysis access. Tech Vasc Interv Radiol. 2010;13(4):259-66.
11. Rajan DK, Clark T. Treatment of asymptomatic central venous stenosis: a critical review. Semin Intervent Radiol. 2010;27(1):64-9.
12. Vesely TM. Use of cutting balloons in hemodialysis fistulas and grafts. Tech Vasc Interv Radiol. 2010;13(4):248-52.
13. Saad TF. Outcomes of percutaneous transluminal angioplasty of hemodialysis access fistulas and grafts using high-pressure balloons. J Vasc Interv Radiol. 2008;19(3):337-42.
14. Girsowicz E, Ascher E, Marks N, Levi M, Jacob T, Rubenzik L, et al. Use of high-pressure angioplasty balloons for the treatment of hemodialysis access stenoses. J Vasc Surg. 2004;39(3):614-9.
15. Funaki B, Shlansky-Goldberg RD, Van Praet VE, Lorenz JM, Leef JA, Zivin S. Percutaneous treatment of hemodialysis access dysfunction: utility of ultra-high-pressure balloons. J Vasc Interv Radiol. 2006;17(5):789-95.
16. Funaki B, Rosenblum JD, Leef JA, Lorenz JM, Zivin S. Ultra-high-pressure balloon angioplasty for hemodialysis access stenoses: experience in 100 patients. J Vasc Interv Radiol. 2003;14(12):1509-13.
17. Rajan DK, Clark T. Does elastic recoil influence access primary patency after percutaneous transluminal angioplasty of hemodialysis fistulas and grafts? J Vasc Interv Radiol. 2007;18(1):51-7.
18. Konner K. Vascular access for hemodialysis: An update. J Am Soc Nephrol. 2005;16(5):1567-77.
19. Vesely TM. Central venous stenosis in hemodialysis patients. Tech Vasc Interv Radiol. 2003;6(4):207-11.
20. Robbin ML, Chamberlain NE, Lockhart ME, Gallichio MH, Sanyal S, Mathis JM, et al. Hemodialysis access fistula maturation: prognostic features from US evaluation. Radiology. 2002;225(1):59-64.
21. Lok CE, Rajan DK, Trerotola SO, Moist LM, Robbin ML. KDOQI Clinical Practice Guideline for Vascular Access: 2019 Update. Am J Kidney Dis. 2019;75(4 Suppl 2):S1-S164.
22. Rajan DK, Clark T. Balloon-assisted maturation of failing arteriovenous fistulas. J Vasc Interv Radiol. 2005;16(7):993-8.
23. Shintani Y, Nishikawa M, Nishiya T, Okazaki K, Shimada K. Balloon-assisted maturation for autogenous arteriovenous fistulas in hemodialysis patients. Ther Apher Dial. 2007;11(6):448-52.
24. Swinnen J, Heye S, Koolen M, Van Loon R, Van Craenenbroeck AH, Vermassen F, et al. Drug-coated balloons for the treatment of dysfunctional hemodialysis arteriovenous fistulas and grafts: a systematic review and meta-analysis. J Vasc Access. 2019;20(5):501-10.

25. Lookstein RA, Haruguchi H, Ouriel K, Weinberg I, Lei L, Cihlar S, et al. Drug-Coated Balloons for Dysfunctional Dialysis Arteriovenous Fistulas. N Engl J Med. 2020;383(8): 733-42.
26. Dolmatch BL, Gurley JC, Baskin KM, Angle JF, Davidson CJ, D'Othee BJ, et al. Society of Interventional Radiology reporting standards for thoracic central vein obstruction: endorsed by the American Society of Diagnostic and Interventional Nephrology (ASDIN), British Society of Interventional Radiology (BSIR), Canadian Interventional Radiology Association (CIRA), Heart Rhythm Society (HRS), Indian Society of Vascular and Interventional Radiology (ISVIR), Vascular Access Society of the Americas (VASA), and Vascular Access Society of Britain and Ireland (VASBI). J Vasc Interv Radiol. 2018;29:454-60.e3.
27. Kim D, Kim BK, Kim YH, Na DJ, Oh KS, Won JY, et al. Purse-string suture for hemostasis after percutaneous intervention for arteriovenous fistulas. Korean J Radiol. 2015;16(4):866-71.
28. Matsuoka S, Ohki T, Usui Y, Kawamura M, Mineta T, Matsubara T, et al. Percutaneous transluminal angioplasty for hemodialysis access dysfunction: efficacy and complications. Ann Vasc Dis. 2014;7(2):128-32.
29. Turmel-Rodrigues L, Peng CT, Liou CC, Shan DD, Hsieh MY, Chou CC, et al. Percutaneous treatment of stenotic lesions in hemodialysis fistulas and grafts: a multicenter experience. J Vasc Interv Radiol. 2006;17(5):811-20.
30. Manninen H, Karjalainen P, Kiviniemi V, Rasanen HT. Percutaneous transluminal angioplasty in failing and thrombosed hemodialysis shunts. Acta Radiol. 2000;41(1): 59-64.
31. Shin SW, Do YS, Kim DI, Park KB, Choo SW, Kim SY, et al. Long-term patency of percutaneous transluminal angioplasty for hemodialysis access stenosis. J Vasc Interv Radiol. 2006;17(11):1733-8.
32. Dolmatch BL, Gray RJ, Bleicher J, Miller DL, Peden EK, Sicard GA, et al. Percutaneous transluminal angioplasty of arteriovenous fistulas and grafts for hemodialysis: results of a multicenter clinical trial. J Vasc Interv Radiol. 2004;15(12):1275-82.
33. Dukkipati R, Shenoy S. Covered stents vs. bare metal stents for dialysis access stenosis: a systematic review and meta-analysis. J Vasc Access. 2018;19(1):1-10.
34. Sheahan MG, Ross JR, Davis J, Al-Baldawi M, D'Amico M, Shah T. Covered versus bare metal stents for hemodialysis access stenosis: a systematic review and meta-analysis. J Vasc Surg. 2017;66(6):1878-87.
35. Rajan DK, Rajan M, Clark T. Stent grafts for cephalic arch stenosis in hemodialysis fistulas. J Vasc Interv Radiol. 2010;21(3):343-8.
36. Vesely TM, Sicard GA, Windus DW, Brown C, Juergens M, Lessne ML. Covered stents for the treatment of hemodialysis access graft stenosis. J Vasc Interv Radiol. 2004;15(11):1227-34.
37. Vesely TM. Long-term results of stent placement for central venous obstruction in hemodialysis patients. J Vasc Interv Radiol. 2010;21(6):838-42.
38. KDOQI Vascular Access Work Group. KDOQI Clinical Practice Guidelines for Vascular Access: 2006. Am J Kidney Dis. 2006;48 Suppl 1:S176-322.
39. Nassar GM, Talley JD. Complications of hemodialysis access interventions. Semin Intervent Radiol. 2010;27(1):70-6.

CHAPTER 21

Thrombolysis Techniques

Jia Shen-Goh, Rauri A Clerk, Saeed Ahmed, Shalabh Srivastava

CASE SCENARIO

A 70-year-old man with a background of previous complicated intra-abdominal surgery resulting from a motor vehicle accident and end-stage renal disease (ESRD) secondary to type 2 diabetes mellitus, currently undergoing regular hemodialysis (HD), has been observed to have poor blood flow during dialysis. A subsequent fistulogram revealed thrombosis. How should a clinician proceed in this situation? Given his medical history, transitioning to peritoneal dialysis would be challenging, making the preservation of fistula access critically important.

INTRODUCTION

The prevalence of chronic kidney disease (CKD) and subsequent end-stage renal disease has been rising annually, contributing to the global burden of disease. Currently, hemodialysis is the most common modality of long-term renal replacement therapy worldwide. It is best performed using an arteriovenous fistula (AVF) or an arteriovenous graft (AVG) rather than central venous line as the latter has a higher risk of complications such as catheter-related bloodstream infections. However, long-term vascular access often necessitates frequent interventions to maintain access patency, which places a significant strain on healthcare resources and adversely affects patients' quality of life, with implications for both morbidity and mortality.

Thrombosis is the primary cause of access loss in AVF and AVG, accounting for 65–85% of cases, primarily due to progressive narrowing caused by neointimal hyperplasia and repeated trauma from cannulation. If left untreated, thrombosis can lead to permanent loss of access. Additional risk factors for access thrombosis include hypercoagulability, low ejection fraction, hypotension, and hemoconcentration. Therefore, with the limited number of possible access sites in mind, the immediate declotting of thrombosed vascular accesses is essential for ensuring effective hemodialysis. Current methods of treatment for AVF or AVG thrombosis can be divided into endovascular thrombolysis, pharmacomechanical thrombolysis (PMT), percutaneous thrombectomy (rheolytic and mechanical), aspiration thrombectomy, and surgical thrombectomy **(Box 1)**.

ENDOVASCULAR THROMBOLYSIS

Endovascular thrombolysis originated in 1984 when Hunter et al.[1] demonstrated that thrombosed fistulas could be treated with percutaneous infusion of streptokinase. Several studies in the 1990s also demonstrated that infusion thrombolysis for thrombosed AVG had a technical success rate of 60–80% with a 6-month patency rate of 13–80%. These studies showed that patency rates were improved when stenoses were corrected immediately by angioplasty or surgery.

Up to date, we have two methods of endovascular thrombolysis:

1. CDT
2. Pulsed-spray thrombolysis

Fibrinolytic agents, including streptokinase, urokinase, and tissue plasminogen activator (tPA), have been shown to be effective for acutely formed thrombi. Currently, commonly used recombinant tPA agents include alteplase, reteplase, and tenecteplase.

BOX 1: Types of thrombolysis and thrombectomy.

Thrombolysis:
- Endovascular thrombolysis
- Catheter-directed thrombolysis (CDT)
- Pulse-spray thrombolysis
- Pharmacomechanical thrombolysis

Thrombectomy:
- Percutaneous thrombectomy
- Rheolytic thrombectomy
- Mechanical thrombectomy
- Aspiration thrombectomy
- Surgical thrombectomy

As with any procedure, before we start, we must always ensure that the patient has no contraindications for the procedure. Contraindications include allergies to recombinant tPA (rTPA) and bleeding diathesis.

Catheter-directed Thrombolysis

This procedure should be performed in an intensive care or high-dependency setting to allow for close monitoring of vital signs, including the Glasgow Coma Scale. Yeo et al.[2] described this technique starting with accessing the AVF either antegrade or retrograde using an ultrasound-guided percutaneous puncture to insert a 6 Fr sheath. After navigating the thrombosed AVF with a hydrophilic wire, we position the multilevel infusion catheter under fluoroscopy guidance. Commonly used catheters include Fountain thrombolysis infusion catheters and Cragg-McNamara catheters. Next, we secure the sheath to the skin with stitches and stabilize the CDT catheters with light gauze and dressing to prevent dislodgement. An initial pulsed dose of rtPA, e.g., 15 mg alteplase, is administered, followed by a continuous infusion of 0.5 mg/h of rtPA over the next 24 hours via the catheter. To maintain sheath patency, we infuse saline and administer intravenous heparin at 200 IU/h through the side port of the 6 Fr sheath. Additional methods to enhance thrombolysis include using rotating angled or pigtail catheters to macerate the clot or performing manual graft massage. A check angiogram is performed the following day, and if the clot burden is significantly reduced, we proceed with balloon maceration and fistuloplasty to treat the culprit lesion. Prolonged CDT may be considered based on clinical judgment if the clot burden remains heavy, but it should not continue beyond 48 hours. All patients should undergo angioplasty for the culprit lesion after CDT, as studies show a higher patency rate when stenoses are corrected immediately by angioplasty or surgery.

Pulsed-spray Thrombolysis

Pulsed-spray thrombolysis utilizes a pulse injector to deliver high-pressure pulses of concentrated fibrinolytic agents directly into the clot via multi-sidehole catheters. The procedure is similar to CDT. According to Valji et al.,[3] instead of starting with an initial pulsed dose of rtPA followed by a continuous rtPA infusion over 24–48 hours, we administer 25,000 IU/mL of urokinase mixed with heparin directly into the clot using a high-pressure pulse spray for 15–20 minutes. Several studies have reported technical success rates of 85–94%, with approximately 1 hour required for lysis using this method. The primary advantage of pulsed-spray thrombolysis is its shorter lysis time compared to conventional thrombolysis techniques, which typically necessitate overnight stays in the intensive care unit for infusion. The currently available pulse injector is the Pulse Spray Injector system, which can deliver 2 mg of tPA through a multi-sidehole infusion catheter for thrombolysis.

Pharmacomechanical Thrombolysis

The PMT technique employs balloon catheters and tPA, with or without specialized thrombectomy devices, achieving high technical and clinical success rates of 95%, along with primary patency rates of 45% and 22% at 12 and 24 months, respectively, without major complications as documented by Wu et al.[4] The procedure begins with accessing the AVF or AVG antegradely using a micropuncture access system under ultrasound guidance, which is then upsized to a 6 or 7 Fr short vascular sheath. Next, a 5 Fr angled catheter and a 0.035" hydrophilic guidewire are used to navigate across the clotted venous outflow into the central veins. A venogram of the central veins is performed to check for any stenosis in the superior vena cava and brachiocephalic and subclavian veins. A "pull-back" venogram is conducted by injecting contrast material through the catheter while retracting it from the central veins to the AVF or AVG, revealing the thrombus burden in the venous outflow and any significant stenosis. Then, 2–6 mg of tPA (e.g., alteplase) is administered directly into the thrombus for thrombolysis, unless contraindications are present, along with intravenous heparin at 50–60 units/kg body weight. Early balloon maceration of the clot in the venous outflow is performed to create a channel for blood flow, as studies recommend removing venous outflow clots first to minimize the risk of clot fragments embolizing into the forearm artery. Retrograde access is then obtained using a micropuncture access system, upsized to a 5 or 6 Fr short vascular sheath. A 5 Fr angled catheter and 0.035" hydrophilic guidewire are used to navigate through the AVF or AVG across the arterial anastomosis into the upstream artery. Contrast material is injected into the artery to assess the extent of arterial thrombus and downstream artery patency. An over-the-wire Fogarty thrombectomy catheter is introduced through the sheath to perform sweeps for removing the arterial plug and restoring arterial inflow; this maneuver must be done gently to avoid dislodging thrombi into the arterial system. Restoration of pulsatility in the AVF or AVG indicates that inflow patency has been achieved. If stenosis is present near the arterial anastomosis, we treat it with balloon angioplasty. Subsequently, balloon maceration is performed throughout the clot. Once flow is established postmaceration, manual aspiration through the side ports of the vascular sheaths may be attempted to remove the clot. After reducing the clot burden, additional angioplasty is performed on any hemodynamically significant stenoses using appropriately sized balloons. Declotting is considered complete when satisfactory antegrade blood flow is observed on completion angiograms and thrill is restored upon physical examination. Finally, vascular sheaths are removed after achieving hemostasis with purse-string sutures.

PERCUTANEOUS THROMBECTOMY

A variety of dedicated advanced thrombectomy devices are available for percutaneous thrombectomy and can also serve as endovascular adjuncts to PMT as mentioned by Wu et al.[4] In PMT, these devices are utilized toward the end of the procedure to address any residual thrombus and clear the remaining clot. The goal of using these devices is to minimize surgical exposure, reduce costs, shorten treatment times, and decrease the length of stay in the intensive care unit compared to surgical thrombectomy. These devices operate using different mechanisms, which can be broadly categorized into two groups:

1. *Hydrodynamic recirculation devices for rheolytic thrombectomy:* The mechanism relies on the Venturi effect generated by high-speed saline jets, which draw the thrombus into the device and break it down. The resulting debris is then expelled through an exhaust lumen within the device. An example of this is the angiojet rheolytic system.
2. *Rotational recirculation devices for mechanical thrombectomy:* For these devices, the clot is broken down by generating a hydrodynamic vortex produced by a high-speed rotating impeller or basket. Examples include the Arrow–Trerotola percutaneous thrombectomy device and the Cleaner XT™ Rotational Thrombectomy System.

RHEOLYTIC THROMBECTOMY

Rheolytic thrombectomy is a flow-based thrombectomy system that utilizes a high-velocity saline jet, generated by a pump and drive unit, to create a negative pressure gradient (Venturi effect) at the catheter tip. This process fragments the thrombus near the catheter tip and evacuates the fragments through the inflow port into a collection bag. The AngioJet Rheolytic System is a modern version of such a device. The AngioJet, combined with a Fogarty balloon, is often used for cases that do not respond to conventional balloon maceration and thrombectomy. Once wire access is established across the clotted segments of the arteriovenous (AV) circuit, the AngioJet catheter is advanced over the wire and approximately 4 mg of tPA is delivered into the clot using the Power-Pulse Delivery mode. After allowing the lytic agent to act for about 10–20 minutes, the mode is switched to thrombectomy and the clot is evacuated into the catheter. Typically, three to four passes are made with the AngioJet catheter across the clotted segments. In comparison to the Cleaner XT™ Rotational Thrombectomy System (mechanical), AngioJet thrombectomy is performed over a wire, which helps preserve wire access. It is important to note that the use of AngioJet is associated with transient bradyarrhythmias, which usually resolve after the device is turned off. A recent study comparing AngioJet with surgical thrombectomy for clotted AV access found no significant differences in success rates or primary and secondary patency rates at 12 months. Additionally, the percutaneous technique was linked to a lower risk of bleeding compared to surgical thrombectomy in this study.

An accessory known as the ClotHunter has recently been developed for the AngioJet system. The ClotHunter is attached to a helical wire that fits into the guidewire lumen of the ZelanteDVT catheter. A dial on the ClotHunter hand-held system generates a rotary helical motion for the ZelanteDVT catheter during thrombectomy, expanding the treatment area within the vessel. However, further studies are needed to assess the effectiveness of this accessory, particularly in patients with AV access thrombosis.

MECHANICAL THROMBECTOMY

A wide range of mechanical thrombectomy devices is currently available for treating clotted AV access. Examples include the Arrow-Trerotola Percutaneous Thrombolytic Device (PTD) and the Cleaner XT™ Rotational Thrombectomy System.

The Arrow-Trerotola PTD is a spinning nitinol basket specifically designed for macerating clots in thrombosed AV access. The device is connected to a hand-held rotator drive unit and an introducer sheath. The nitinol basket adapts to the vessel wall to maximize contact with the clot during the procedure.

The Cleaner XT™ Rotational Thrombectomy System features a rotating sinusoidal wire connected to a battery-powered hand-held controller, designed for macerating clots in thrombosed vessels. While it is approved by the Food and Drug Administration for treating deep vein thrombosis, it is also commonly used for clotted AV access **(Videos 1 to 4)**. Huan et al.[5] showed that by using the Cleaner XT™ device in conjunction with thrombolytics in treating clotted AVG and AVF, they were able to achieve technical and clinical success rates of 88% resulting in 65% 1-month and 47% 3-month primary patency rates **(Video 5)**. The width of the sinusoidal wire adjusts to the vessel diameter, maximizing contact with the clot. Additionally, it includes a built-in side port for administering thrombolytics. One important consideration is that the Cleaner XT™ device cannot advance over a wire. It is advisable to position the tip of the vascular sheath close to the treatment site before introducing the Cleaner XT™ device. Since the guidewire may need to be removed for this introduction, there is a risk of losing access, particularly in cases of severe venous stenosis or total venous occlusion.

ASPIRATION THROMBECTOMY

Aspiration thrombectomy using the Indigo system is employed for patients with contraindications to thrombolysis.[4] The Indigo thrombectomy system is a vacuum-assisted device that facilitates continuous thrombus aspiration through end-hole catheters of various sizes. The CATD Indigo system features an 8 Fr suction catheter specifically designed for AV access thrombectomy, with a shorter length of 90 cm. The newly released Lightning system is compatible with the CAT12 12 Fr catheter, which is designed for enhanced venous clot retrieval. To minimize blood loss while using the larger CAT12 catheter, the Lightning system includes a sensor that adjusts the suction power based on blood flow. Given its effectiveness in removing clots, the Indigo system is also utilized in patients with low pulmonary reserve, who are at an increased risk of decompensation if pulmonary embolism (PE) occurs during the declotting procedure.

SURGICAL THROMBECTOMY

Surgery is a well-established method for salvaging a thrombosed AV access. The surgical technique employs a Fogarty thrombectomy catheter for retrograde manual clot removal. The benefits of surgical thrombectomy include a lower risk of thrombus dislocation, minimal use of thrombolytics, and the ability to repair any ruptured access or pseudoaneurysm during the same procedure. In cases of large aneurysmal fistulas, surgical thrombectomy is preferred for removing chronic wall-adherent thrombus, with the option to revise the aneurysm simultaneously. While endovascular treatments may offer advantages over surgical thrombectomy—such as reduced surgical exposure, lower costs, and shorter treatment times—it is important to remember that endovascular approaches tend to have higher technical failure rates compared to surgical options.

CONCLUSION

Thrombosis of arteriovenous access presents a major challenge to maintaining effective hemodialysis in patients with end-stage renal disease, potentially compromising both access durability and overall clinical outcomes. In the case of the 70-year-old patient with a complex medical and surgical background, and few viable alternatives to hemodialysis, swift and appropriate management is essential. A range of therapeutic options—including catheter-directed, pulsed-spray, pharmacomechanical, mechanical and aspiration thrombectomy—allow for customized treatment based on clot characteristics and patient condition. While endovascular approaches are generally less invasive and more resource-efficient, surgical thrombectomy remains an important option in certain scenarios. Ultimately, the timely preservation of vascular access through individualized intervention is crucial to ensuring ongoing dialysis and maintaining patient well-being.

REFERENCES

1. Hunter DW, Castaneda-Zuniga WR, Coleman CC, Young AT, Salomonowitz E, Mercado S, et al. Failing Arteriovenous Dialysis Fistulas: Evaluation and Treatment. Radiology. 1984;152:631-5.
2. Yeo CB, Yong E, Hong Q, Kwan J, Quek LHH, Pua U, et al. Outcomes Of Catheter-Directed Thrombolysis For Arteriovenous Fistula Thrombosis In Singapore: Is It Still Relevant Today? Ann Vasc Dis. 2021;14:5-10.
3. Valji K, Bookstein JJ, Roberts AC, Oglevie SB, Pittman C, O'neill MP. Pulse-Spray Pharmacomechanical Thrombolysis Of Thrombosed Hemodialysis Access Grafts: Long-Term Experience And Comparison Of Original And Current Techniques. AJR Am J Roentgenol. 1995;164:1495-500; Discussion 1501-3.
4. Wu V, Kalva SP, Cui J. Thrombectomy Approach For Access Maintenance In The End Stage Renal Disease Population: A Narrative Review. Cardiovasc Diagn Ther. 2023;13:265-80.
5. Huan K, Tan CS, Chua D, Yap CJQ, Tan RY, Chong TT, et al. The Cleaner Xt Device As An Endovascular Adjunct For Pharmacomechanical Thrombolysis Of Thrombosed Arteriovenous Fistulas And Grafts. Ann Vasc Dis. 2020;13:390-6.

CHAPTER

22 Renal Artery Angioembolization

Hardik B Patel, Rozil Jayesh Gandhi

INTRODUCTION

Renal artery angioembolization (RAE) is a lifesaving procedure for many postprocedure complications and for treatment of variety of conditions. In this chapter, we will cover indications and techniques for RAE. RAE offers significant benefits, such as hemorrhage control and tumor reduction, often serving as a viable alternative to surgery, particularly in preserving renal function. While effective, the procedure is not without complications, which should be closely monitored during postprocedural care.

ANATOMY

The basics of renal anatomy should be known before the procedure. Both renal arteries arise from abdominal aorta at the level of L1 and L2 vertebrae. Near the hilum, the artery divides into anterior and posterior branch, which in turn divides into upper, middle, and lower segmental branches. Subsequently, this artery divides into segmental and arcuate arteries. There are anatomical variations also, which are mainly of two types. One type is early branching, which may not be of great concern for RAE and the second variation is extrarenal arteries or accessory renal arteries, which are seen in up to 30% of patients. Identification of accessory renal arteries is important for RAE because it may be a source of bleeding or the supplying artery to the lesion. The origin of accessory artery can be variable, so it is important to delineate these arteries before the procedure with CT angiography whenever possible **(Fig. 1)**.

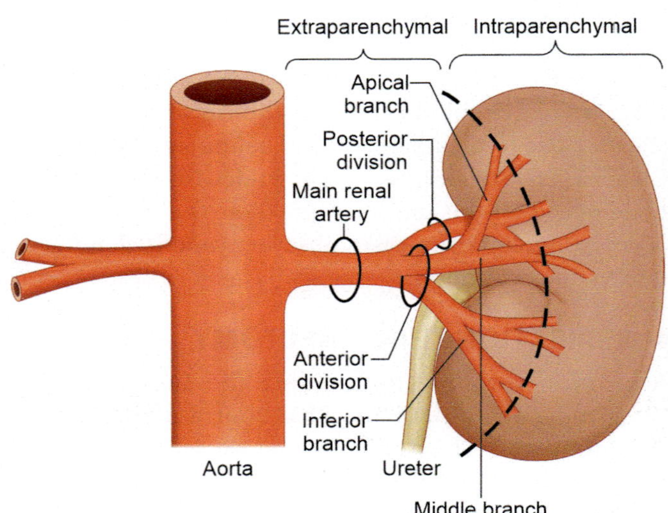

Fig. 1: Anatomy of renal artery.

INDICATIONS

Malignant Renal Tumors

Renal artery angioembolization is generally used for reduction in tumor size and vascularity before surgery. Also, it is used for palliative care for reducing bleeding from unresectable renal mass or in a patient who are poor candidates for surgical resection. RAE should be performed before 48–72 hours before planned surgery for better result. Feeding artery or main renal artery can be occluded with the help of ethanol mixed with lipiodol, polyvinyl alcohol (PVA) particle or gelfoam slurry, and coil embolization. It is important to leave residual renal stump to allow surgical clamping and ligation during nephrectomy. Superselective embolization is preferred in patients planned for radiofrequency ablation (RFA) and cryoablation.[1]

Although long-term survival benefit is questionable as only one study shows survival advantage for a patient who underwent RAE before surgery compared to patients who underwent surgery alone (62% vs. 35%).[2]

Renal Angiomyolipoma

Renal angiomyolipoma of size >4 cm are at a greater than 50% risk of rupture and hemorrhage.[3] Embolic agents typically used are microcoils, nonresorbable particles, and N butyl-2-cyanoacrylate. Considering highly vascular nature of lesion, a technical success of 80–90% has been reported with long-term follow-up showing recurrence of 30% with higher recurrence of tuberous sclerosis patients.[4] The patient should be counseled before the procedure regarding the risk of recurrence and sometimes incomplete nature of cure.

Traumatic Renal Bleeding

Renal injuries following blunt abdominal trauma are not uncommon. Hematuria and perinephric hematoma are presenting complaints most of the time. Majority of renal artery injuries are minor, which can be managed conservatively. In 10% of patients, injuries are of serious nature that are amenable to renal artery embolization.[5] Early diagnosis and treatment are the key to preserving renal function because prolonged renal ischemia leads to permanent loss of function, and large perinephric hematoma prevents superselective embolization.

Narrow tract injuries by assaults, biopsies, and nephrostomy tube placements lead to false aneurysms with or without arteriovenous fistulas (AVF). The exact location of bleeding can be assessed by CT angiography, but direct angiography is more definitive and therapeutic at the same time. Most of the renal injuries after biopsy of nephrostomy are self-limiting but if hematuria persists for longer than 3 days, angiographic intervention and embolization are needed.[6,7] A patient with hemodynamic instability should undergo immediate angiography and treatment. Most of the times, the agent used is microcoil. Superselective embolization with good technical success rate results in preservation of renal function.

Arteriovenous Fistulas

Arteriovenous fistulas often results from biopsy, partial nephrectomy, nephrostomy, or penetrating trauma. Although 70% AVF resolve within 2 years, embolization is reserved for symptomatic patients.[8,9] One of the diagnostic features of AVF is early opacification of vein during arteriogram. Large high-flowing AVF have been treated successfully with RAE, without significant loss of renal function. Superselective catheter with coaxial systems to embolize fistula tract with microcoil has a good technical success rate. Particles should be avoided as they pose a risk of migration to pulmonary circulation from arteriovenous connection. In cases of large communication, high-flow temporary occlusion of vein with the help of balloon is needed to prevent coil migration into systemic circulation.[10]

Renal Artery Pseudoaneurysm

Renal artery pseudoaneurysms are uncommon, usually occurring after renal biopsy or partial nephrectomy. Most of the lesions are small and tend to undergo spontaneous thrombosis; only selected patients with mass effect, bleeding, and renal dysfunction due to shunting or compression need treatment. Most of the small lesions are managed well with coils; an aneurysm arising from the main renal artery needs covered stents to exclude the pseudoaneurysm with preservation of renal flow **(Figs. 2A to C)**.[11]

Arteriovenous Malformations

Arteriovenous malformations (AVMs) are rare, and they can be congenital or acquired. Congenital malformations are small and asymptomatic. Acquired AVMs have a complex course. They can present with hematuria, hypertension, and high-output cardiac failure. Due to complexity of lesion, treatment is difficult and the goal of treatment should be symptomatic rather than curative. Patients should be counseled for need for repeat procedures in case of reappearance of symptoms. The goal of optimal treatment is to ablate the nidus of the AVM, which is the epicenter of the abnormal vessels. For this reason, sclerosant agents are preferred over coil, gelfoam. Balloon occlusion catheter may be needed in high-flow situation, so a sclerosant agent can dwell into nidus and not pass through AVM.

Renal Artery Aneurysm

Renal artery aneurysms are rare lesions with a prevalence of 0.7% based on CT imaging of general population,[12] connective tissue disorder and atherosclerosis being most common risk factors. There are no definite indications for treating asymptomatic patients; treatment is reserved for symptomatic patients, size of 1.5–2.0 cm in diameter, women of childbearing age group, and patient with polyarteritis nodosa. Location and morphology of lesion decide the technique. Main artery lesions are more amenable to stent graft. Stent graft placement also needs at least 1.5-mm distance from ostium and bifurcation for suitable placement. Distal lesion can be managed with coils alone. Lesion with wide neck needs combination technique like stent graft or balloon occlusive device with coils **(Figs. 3A and B)**.[13]

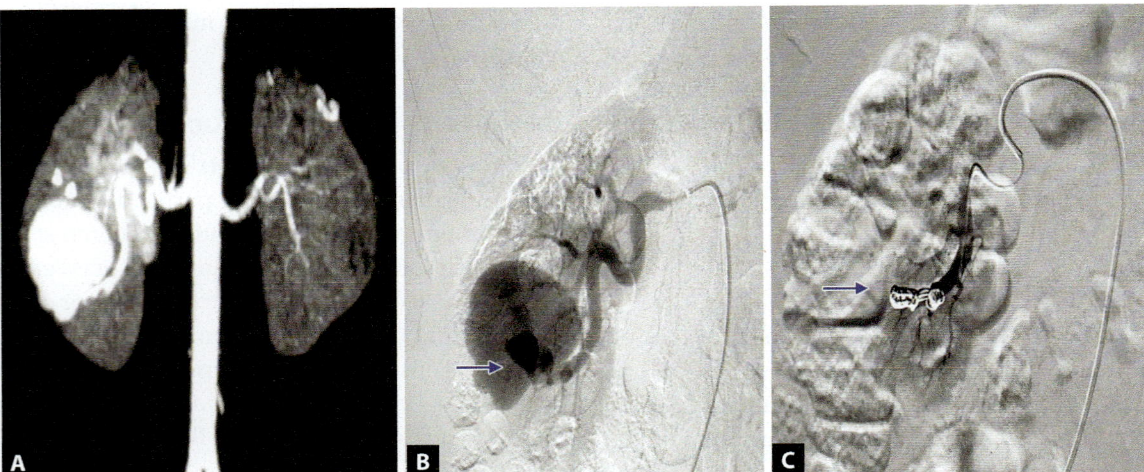

Figs. 2A to C: (A) Computerized tomography angiogram image showing single right renal artery with aneurysm arising from lower polar branch; (B) Right renal artery angiogram–digital subtraction angiography image showing a large aneurysm (blue arrow) with fistula from the lower polar branch; (C) Postembolization, right lower polar angiogram from microcatheter (blue arrow) showing no filling of aneurysm after coil occlusion (blue arrow).

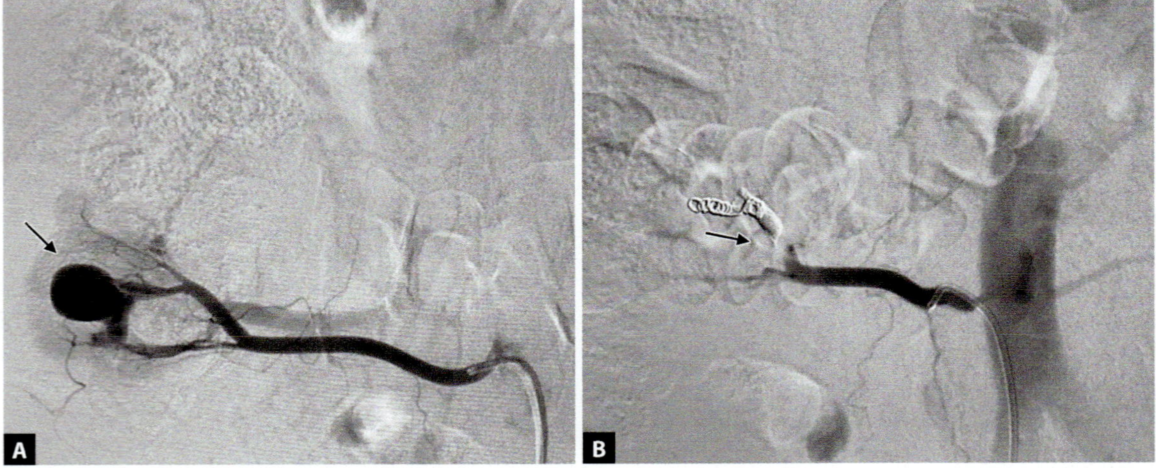

Figs. 3A and B: (A) Right accessory renal artery angiogram–digital subtraction angiography image showing large pseudoaneurysm (black arrow) with fistula; (B) Postembolization, right lower polar angiogram showing no filling of aneurysm because of occlusion by coils (black arrow).

Chronic Renal Parenchymal Diseases

End-stage renal failure with severe nephrotic syndrome, resistant hypertension, hematuria, urinary leak, and irreversible transplant rejection has been a reported indication for complete renal artery embolization in patients who may be poor candidates for surgical nephrectomy.[14-16] The treatment goal is to eliminate renal function and reduce morbidity. Technical success can be achieved using a liquid agent or large coils. The end-stage kidney has small caliber of renal artery, so it is important to use a balloon occlusion catheter to prevent migration of coil into aorta.

TECHNIQUES AND MATERIALS

The process of renal artery embolization involves accessing the renal arteries, identifying the vessels contributing to pathology, and selectively occluding them with embolic agents. The following details the techniques and materials commonly used in RAE.

Embolic Agents

- *Polyvinyl alcohol particles:* These embolic agents come in various sizes and are effective for occluding both small and larger vessels. They are frequently used due to their ability to obstruct blood flow in both fine and larger arteries.

- *Coils:* These are mechanical embolic devices that help block larger arteries. Coils are deployed through a catheter and cause thrombosis, leading to occlusion of the targeted blood vessels.
- *Gelatin sponge:* A temporary embolic material often used in acute hemorrhage control, gelatin sponge can be resorbed over time, making it suitable for cases where permanent occlusion is not desired.
- *Microspheres/embolization beads:* These spherical agents are commonly used in tumor embolization, including for AMLs, as they provide both mechanical and chemical occlusion. They are well suited for managing tumors due to their ability to reduce vascularity and cause tumor shrinkage.

Procedure Steps

- *Access and catheterization:* The procedure typically begins with the patient being sedated and the femoral artery being accessed. Typically, a 5- or 6-Fr angiographic sheath is introduced in the femoral artery. A catheter is introduced over the wire and guided to the renal artery using fluoroscopic imaging along with anatomical bony landmark.
- *Selective embolization:* Once in position, a microcatheter (Progret®) is passed through an angiographic catheter (typically renal double curve or multipurpose catheter) and it is manipulated with the help of guidewire to selectively target the feeding vessels of the renal lesion or hemorrhage. Embolic agents are then injected through the microcatheter to block blood flow to the targeted area, effectively treating the pathology. Postembolization, it is advisable to wait for 7–10 minutes to make sure that target vessel occlusion is achieved.
- *Postprocedure monitoring:* Patients are closely monitored after the procedure for complications such as postembolization syndrome (PES) or changes in renal function. Follow-up imaging may be conducted to assess the success of the embolization and to ensure that there are no residual issues.

Complications

Renal artery angioembolization, while effective, can lead to certain complications:

- *Postembolization syndrome:* A common side effect characterized by fever, pain, and fatigue. These symptoms typically resolve within a few days.
- *Renal dysfunction:* In cases of nonselective embolization or excessive embolization, renal damage can occur, potentially leading to renal insufficiency or failure.
- *Infection:* As with any catheter-based procedure, there is a risk of infection at the puncture site or within the kidney.
- *Ureteral obstruction:* In rare cases, embolization near the renal pelvis may lead to obstruction, requiring additional interventions.

CONCLUSION

Renal artery embolization is a highly effective treatment for a wide array of renal conditions, particularly in cases of trauma, tumors, and vascular malformations. It is especially beneficial in the management of renal angiomyolipomas, where it offers a safe, minimally invasive alternative to surgery, effectively reducing tumor size and controlling hemorrhage. While the procedure generally has excellent outcomes, the potential for complications underscores the importance of careful technique and patient monitoring. Ongoing advances in embolic materials and methods will continue to enhance the efficacy and safety of RAE in clinical practice.

REFERENCES

1. Yamakado K, Nakatsuka A, Kobayashi S, Akeboshi M, Takaki H, Kariya Z, et al. Radiofrequency ablation combined with renal arterial embolization for the treatment of unresectable renal cell carcinoma larger than 3.5 cm: initial experience. Cardiovasc Intervent Radiol. 2006;29(3):38994.
2. Zielinski H, Szmigielski S, Petrovich Z. Comparison of preoperative embolization followed by radical nephrectomy with radical nephrectomy alone for renal cell carcinoma. Am J Clin Oncol. 2000;23(1):6-12.
3. Rimon U, Duvdevani M, Garniek A, Golan G, Bensaid P, Ramon J, et al. Large renal angiomyolipomas: digital subtraction angiographic grading and presentation with bleeding. Clin Radiol. 2006;61(6):520-6.
4. Kothary N, Soulen MC, Clark TW, Wein AJ, Shlansky-Goldberg RD, Crino PB, et al. Renal angiomyolipoma: Long-term results after arterial embolization. J Vasc Interv Radiol. 2005;16(1):45-50.
5. Fisher RG, Ben-menachem Y. Angiography and embolization in renal trauma. In: Baum S (Ed). Abram's Angiography: Vascular and Interventional Radiology, 4th edition. Boston: Little, Brown and Company; 1997:1230-43.
6. Fisher RG, Ben-Menachem Y, Whigham C. Stab wounds of the renal artery branches: angiographic diagnosis and treatment by embolization. Am J Roentgenol. 1989;152(6):1231-5.

7. Cope C, Zeit RM. Pseudoaneurysms after nephrostomy. Am J Roentgenol. 1982;139(2):255-61.
8. Maleux G, Messiaen T, Stockx L, Vanrenterghem Y, Wilms G. Transcatheter embolization of biopsy-related vascular injuries in renal allografts. Long-term technical, clinical and biochemical results. Acta Radiol. 2003;44(1):13-7.
9. Dorffner R, Thurnher S, Prokesch R, Bankier A, Turetschek K, Schmidt A, et al. Embolization of iatrogenic vascular injuries of renal transplants: immediate and follow-up results. Cardiovasc Intervent Radiol. 1998;21(2):129-34.
10. Nakatani T, Uchida J, Han YS, Iwai T, Nakamura K, Kawashima H, et al. Renal allograft arteriovenous fistula and large pseudoaneurysm. Clin Transplant. 2003;17(1):9-12.
11. Horwitz MD, Hanbury DC, King CM. Renal artery pseudoaneurysm following partial nephrectomy treated with stent-graft. Br J Radiol. 2005;78(926):161-3.
12. Zhang LJ, Yang GF, Qi J, Shen W. Renal artery aneurysm: Diagnosis and surveillance with multidetector-row computed tomography. Acta Radiol. 2007;48(3):274-9.
13. Abath C, Andrade G, Cavalcanti D, Brito N, Marques R. Complex renal artery aneurysms: liquids or coils. Tech Vasc Interv Radiol. 2007;10(4):299-307.
14. Millard FC, Hemingway AP, Cumberland DC, Brown CB. Renal embolization for ablation of function in renal failure and hypertension. Postgrad Med J. 1989;65(768):729-34.
15. Keller FS, Coyle M, Rosch J, Dotter CT. Percutaneous renal ablation in patients with end-stage renal disease: alternative to surgical nephrectomy. Radiology. 1986;159(2):447-51.
16. Hahn ST, Park SH, Lee JM, Kim CY, Chang YS. Renal artery embolization controls intractable pain in a patient with polycystic kidney disease. Cardiovasc Intervent Radiol. 1999;22(5):422-4.

SECTION

6

Vascular Access Related Complications and Management

CHAPTER 23

Tunneled Cuffed Catheter Access Dysfunction and Salvage

Hemant J Mehta, Wasiyeeullah Z Shaikh

INTRODUCTION

Meaning of salvage is "to save something valuable from damage, destruction, or losses". The use of tunneled cuffed hemodialysis catheters (TCCs) across the globe is high due to various reasons, but mainly because of not having arteriovenous fistula (AVF) in place at appropriate time. These TCCs have complications that can be either infective or noninfective. This chapter will deal with salvaging the TCC due to noninfectious complications. This could be salvaging the same catheter or salvaging the site with a new TCC. The site needs to be salvaged because there are multiple levels of central vein stenosis and the patient's hemodialysis (HD) is dependent on TCC. The problems can occur during insertion or maintenance of the TCC.

The parts of a TCC are a catheter hub, a segment of subcutaneous tunnel, Dacron cuff, the subcutaneous portion of the TCC including the curve, and the intravenous portion of the TCC and the tip. The TCC can develop mechanical complication, summarized in **Table 1**. These can occur due to TCC related issues (tip configuration, TCC size, or length), technical issues (not using USG and fluoroscopic guidance, central vein stenosis, and abnormal anatomy) or personnel issue (awareness about the need for vascular access for HD, training, and expertise).

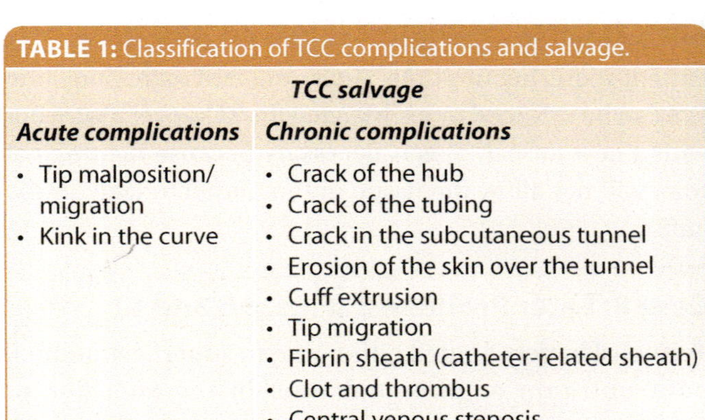

TABLE 1: Classification of TCC complications and salvage.

TCC salvage	
Acute complications	***Chronic complications***
• Tip malposition/ migration • Kink in the curve	• Crack of the hub • Crack of the tubing • Crack in the subcutaneous tunnel • Erosion of the skin over the tunnel • Cuff extrusion • Tip migration • Fibrin sheath (catheter-related sheath) • Clot and thrombus • Central venous stenosis

CASE SCENARIOS

Several among these situations are described here.

Case 1: Always Document Postprocedure Image (Fig. 1)

Chest X-ray should be done mandatorily after TCC placement and documented for the tip position. For example, the patient had this TCC inserted 15 days ago and presented with poor flow, had no documentation of the procedure. The X-ray revealed malpositioning and kink in the TCC.

Problems: Wrong length, low exit site, tip is at the level of carina and this is likely due to superior vena cava (SVC) stenosis related to prior right internal jugular vein (IJV) TCC three times.

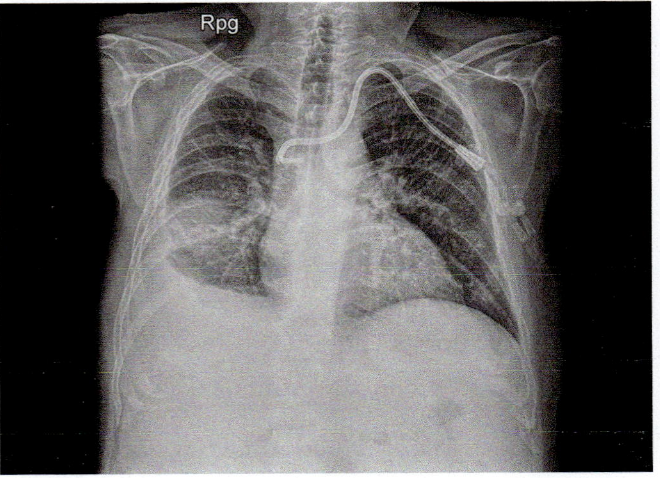

Fig. 1: Immediate postprocedure X-ray shows wrong tip position and kink in the TCC.

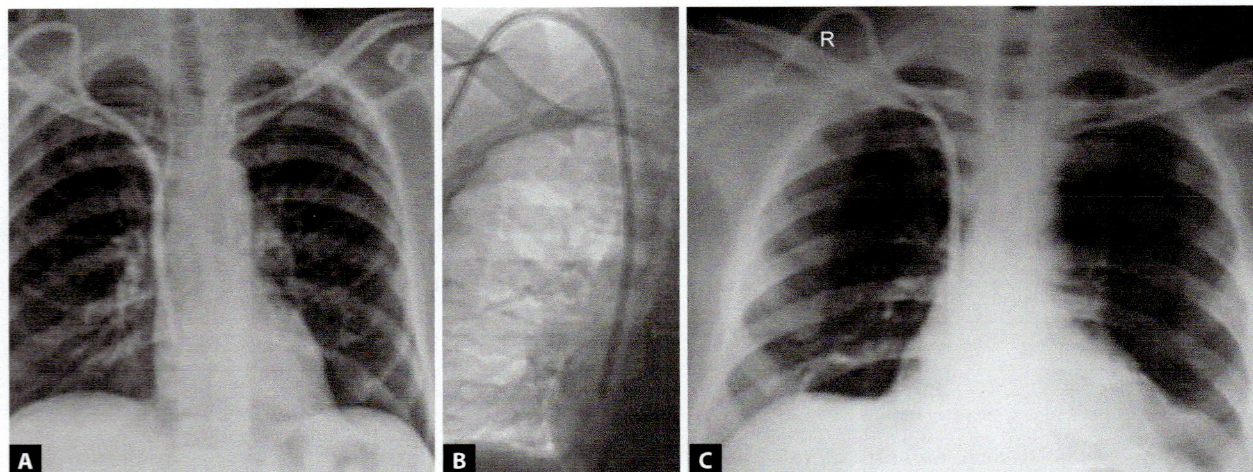

Figs. 2A to C: (A) Kink of TCC; (B) Repair under vision; (C) Final position of TCC.

Case 2: Immediate Problem After Insertion of TCC: 1 (Figs. 2A to C)

Formation of a kink while inserting is a common problem, especially for external jugular vein (EJV) catheters. This is because of EJV is superficial and the TCC has to traverse from superficial to deeper vein. Many a times, a pull on the TCC from exit site solves the problem, but sometimes, one needs surgical revision.

Case 3: Immediate Problem After Insertion of TCC: 2 (Figs. 3A to E)

The catheters in all these cases were salvaged with exchange over a wire.

Case 4: Immediate Problem After Insertion of TCC: 3 (Figs. 4A to D)

It is not unusual to get an image on frontal view which raises the doubt about kink, curve and tip position. Always take different view for clarity on TCC position.

Case 5: Immediate Problem After Insertion of TCC: 4 (Figs. 5A to C)

How was the salvage carried out?

Catheter repositioning was under taken with a new puncture in the right IJV, higher up and a glidewire was passed. A 5F sheath was inserted and a check angiogram confirmed the position to be in the right atrium and IVC. Taking this wire as a guide, another puncture was made in the right IJV lower down and another glidewire was passed parallel to the first wire and a check angiogram was performed. Previous wire was pulled out. The previously inserted TCC was exposed with a small dissection in the neck and pulled back. Pressure was applied over the incision to ensure no air would gush in. After confirming absence of air in the pleura or mediastinum under fluoroscope, the catheter was inserted over the wire, after serial dilatation of the track and inserting pull apart sheath. Catheter tip position, flow, and curve were checked and found perfect.

Case 6: Later Problem 1 (Figs. 6A and B)

Co-existence of 2 problems is a common problem, tip malposition and TCC infection. The wrong tip position leads to thrombus formation at the tip, which in turn gets infected.

Case 7: Later Problem 2 (Figs. 7A and B)

Patient requiring multiple TCCs, and cuff extrusion—the site can be salvaged by exchanging the TCC over a wire but with a new tunnel. This is necessary because the original tract will not allow the tissue in the tunnel to take on the cuff.

Case 8: Later Problem 3 (Figs. 8A and B)

Tunnel skin gets eroded either due to superficial tunnel, poor nutrition or prior radiation in the area due to carcinoma of breast.

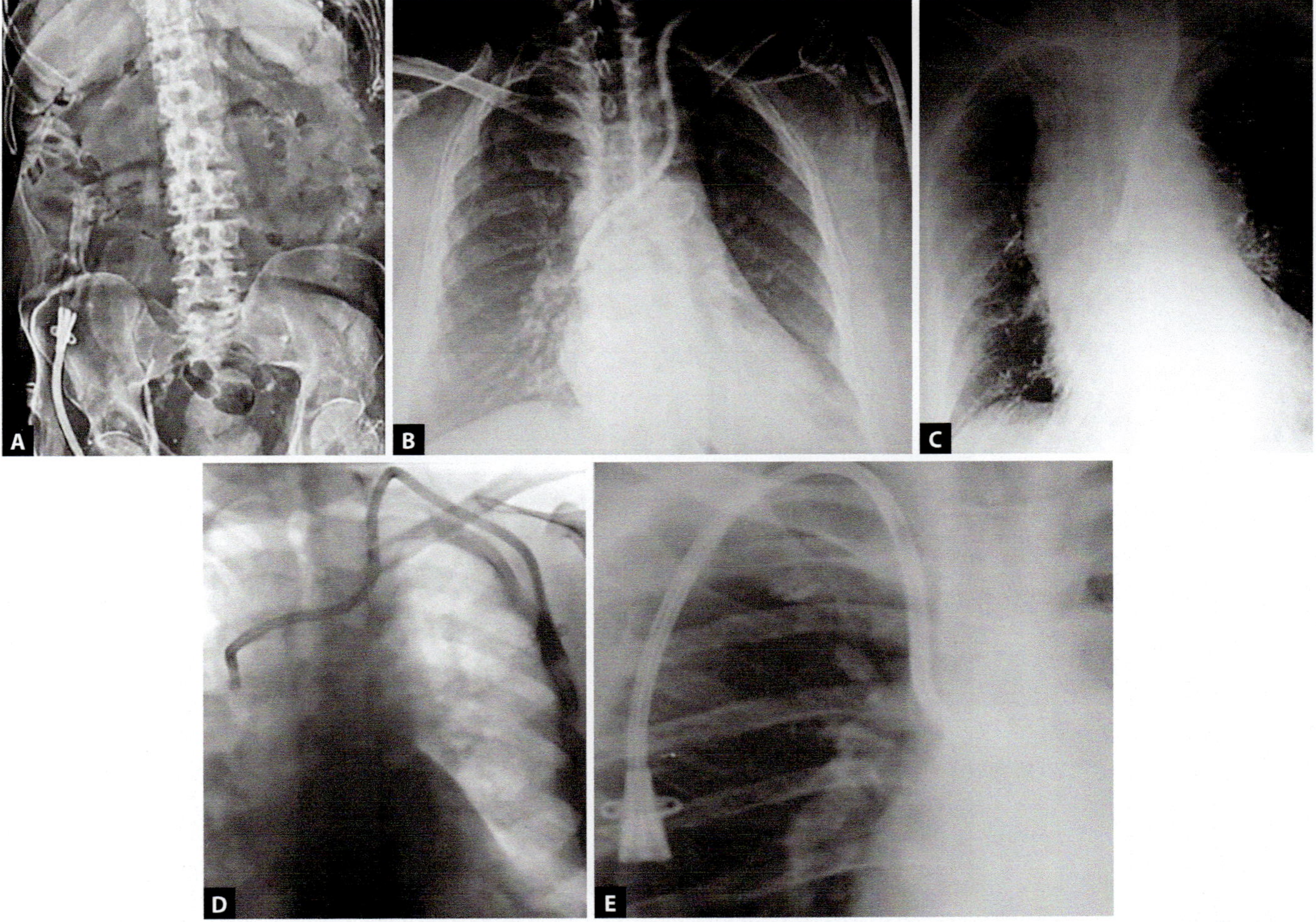

Figs. 3A to E: Case 3: Tip misplacement (A) femoral TCC, wrong length, tip has not reached inferior vena cava (IVC); (B) TCC in SVC, very large curve and long tunnel, wasting the insertion length; (C) Blind insertion of left IJV TCC, kink at the tip and probable passage in the left superior intercostal—accessory hemiazygos vein; (D) Tip in internal thoracic (mammary) vein, part of azygos venous system; and (E) Tip in azygos vein. (IJV: internal jugular vein; SVC: superior vena cava; TCC: tunneled cuffed hemodialysis catheter)

Case 9: Later Problem 4 (Figs. 9A to D)

Clots can occur due to TCC, which could be intra or extra luminal and cause partial or complete lumen occlusion.

Case 10: Later Problem 5 (Figs. 10A and B)

The TCC tip migration can occur in a well-functioning catheter after several months.

Case 11: Later Problem 6 (Figs. 11A and B)

Cracks can happen after several years of TCC in place, e.g., this particular case, who presented with blood leak from exit site during dialysis, after 10 years of TCC. It was confirmed after the TCC removal, where there was a small crack in the TCC, around the subcutaneous cuff. The cracks need not be in the extra-corporeal portion of TCC, they can occur in the subcutaneous portions of TCC also.

Case 12: Later Problem 7 (Figs. 12A and B)

Why would this happen after 3 years of left IJV TCC? Patient presented with a complaint of ballooning of venous arm of TCC while flushing, though the flow was normal. This can happen due to distal obstruction along the course of the TCC. Patient was taken up for TCC exchange **(Figs. 13A and B)**, fibrin sheath (CRS—catheter-related sheath) was documented. TCC exchange after balloon disruption of CRS was difficult **(Figs. 14A to E)** due to underlying stenosis at SVC-atrial junction. The TCC when threaded over super stiff wire, got stuck at the level of SVC-atrial junction, where stenosis was encountered. Through

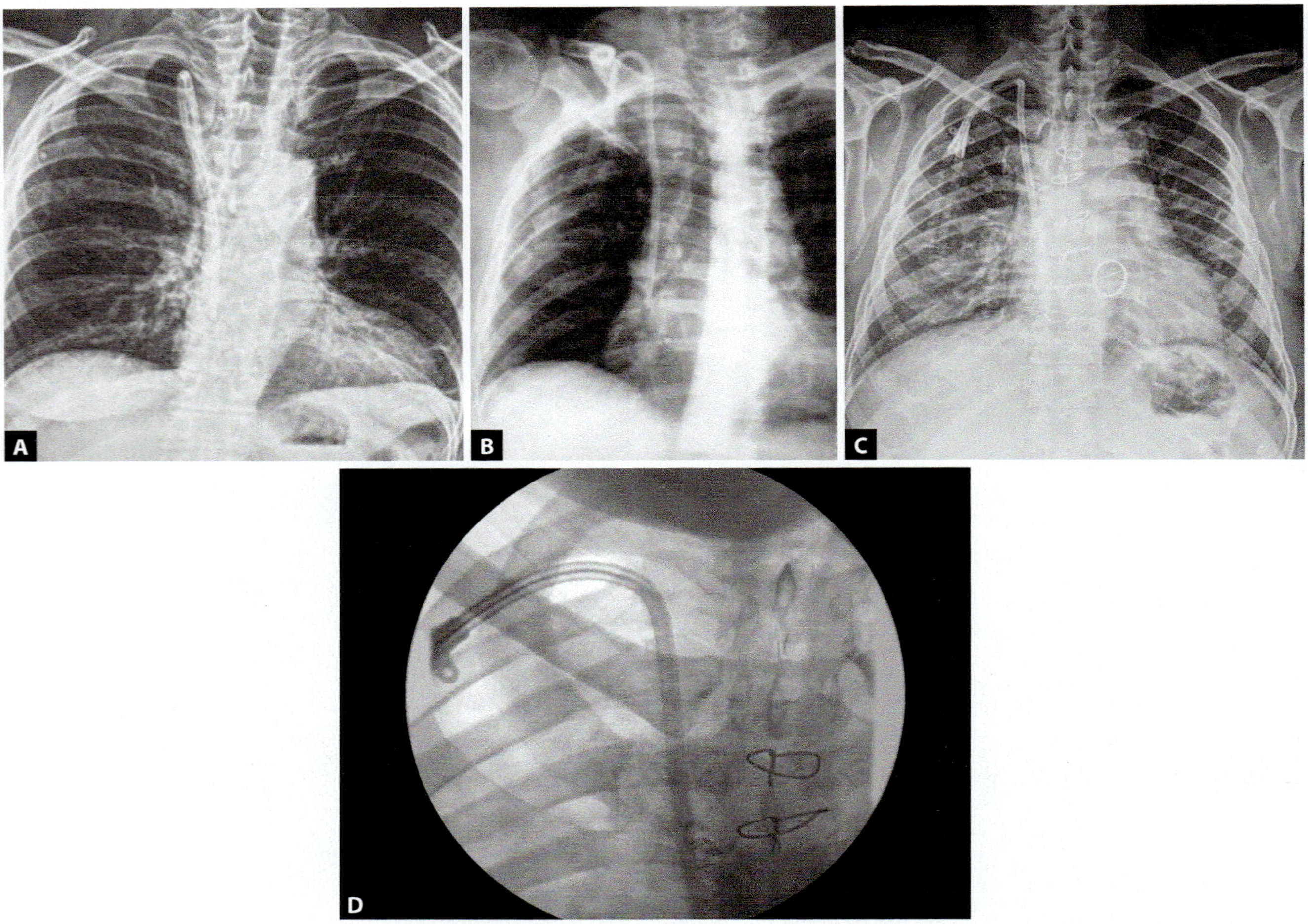

Figs. 4A to D: Case 4: Always take different views: (A) Appears kink; (B) There is no kink on oblique view. (C and D) On table views: (C) Appears to have kink with neck turned to left side, but good flow; and (D) Neck turned straight, no kink, and good flow.

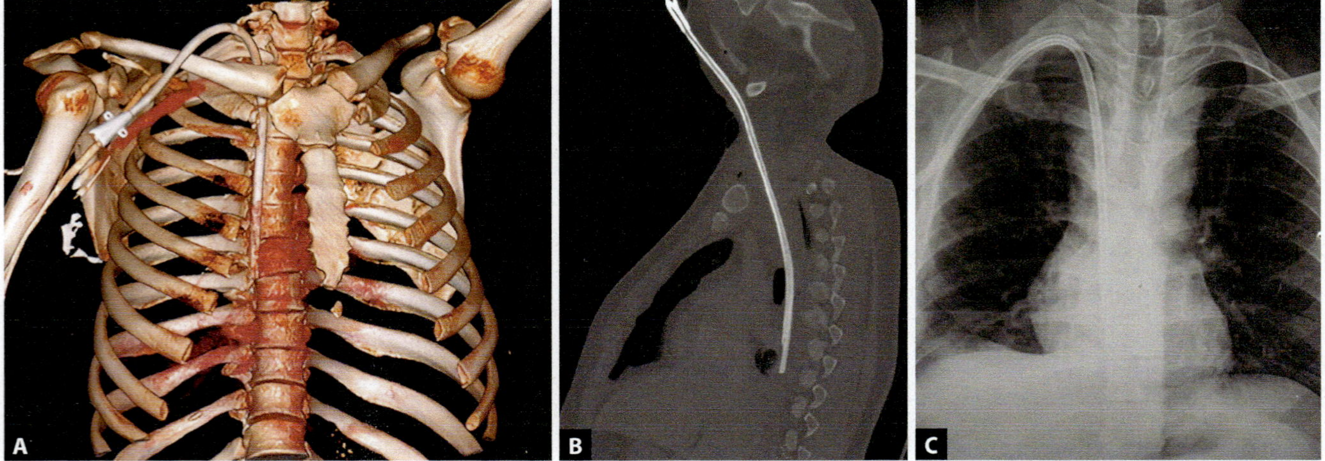

Figs. 5A to C: Case 5: On table TCC malfunction: Right IJV TCC insertion under fluoroscopic guidance, with IJV puncture under USG guidance was carried out. Right IJV had partial thrombus (No prior history of cannulation). TCC appeared to be in position but no flow, and patient had chest pain while flushing the TCC. Patient was shifted for CT chest. (A) CT showed proper position of TCC on AP projection, (B) on lateral view, TCC seen migrated to posterior mediastinum, and (C) same TCC salvaged. (CT: computed tomography; IJV: internal jugular vein; TCC: tunneled cuffed hemodialysis catheter; USG: ultrasonography)

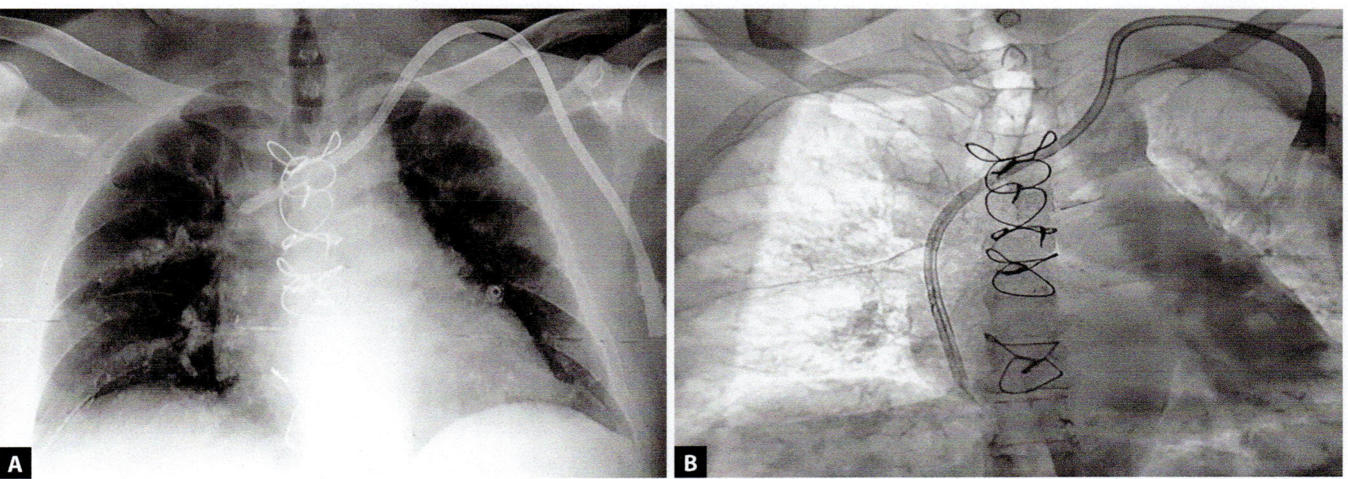

Figs. 6A and B: Case 6: (A) Malposition (and infected TCC with *Bacillus cereus*) and poor flow; (B) TCC replaced after controlling infection. (TCC: tunneled cuffed hemodialysis catheter)

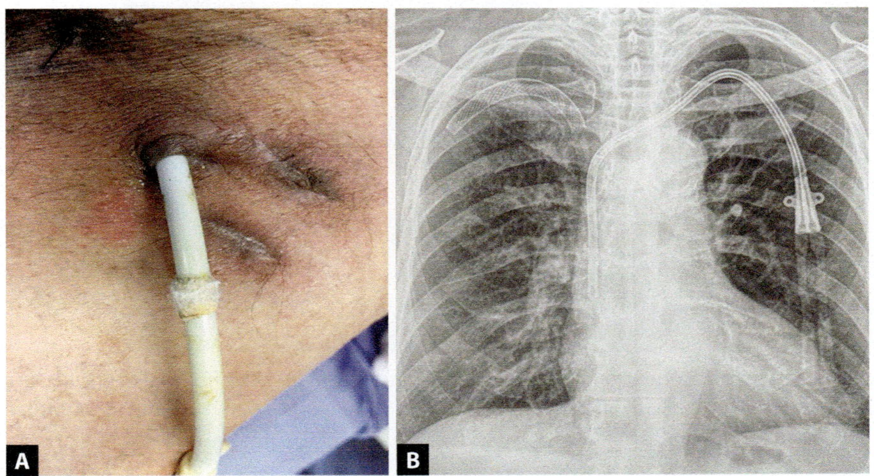

Figs. 7A and B: Case 7: (A) Cuff extrusion. Patient had multiple TCCs as evidenced by multiple scars; (B) TCC exchanged over a wire. (TCC: tunneled cuffed hemodialysis catheter)

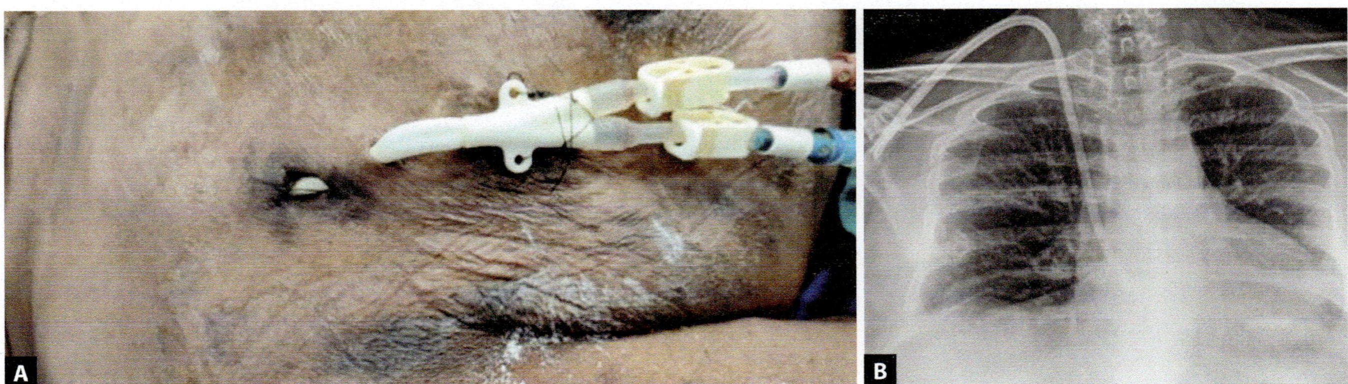

Figs. 8A and B: Case 8: (A) Erosion of skin over the tunnel; and (B) New TCC with lateral tunnel. (TCC: tunneled cuffed hemodialysis catheter)

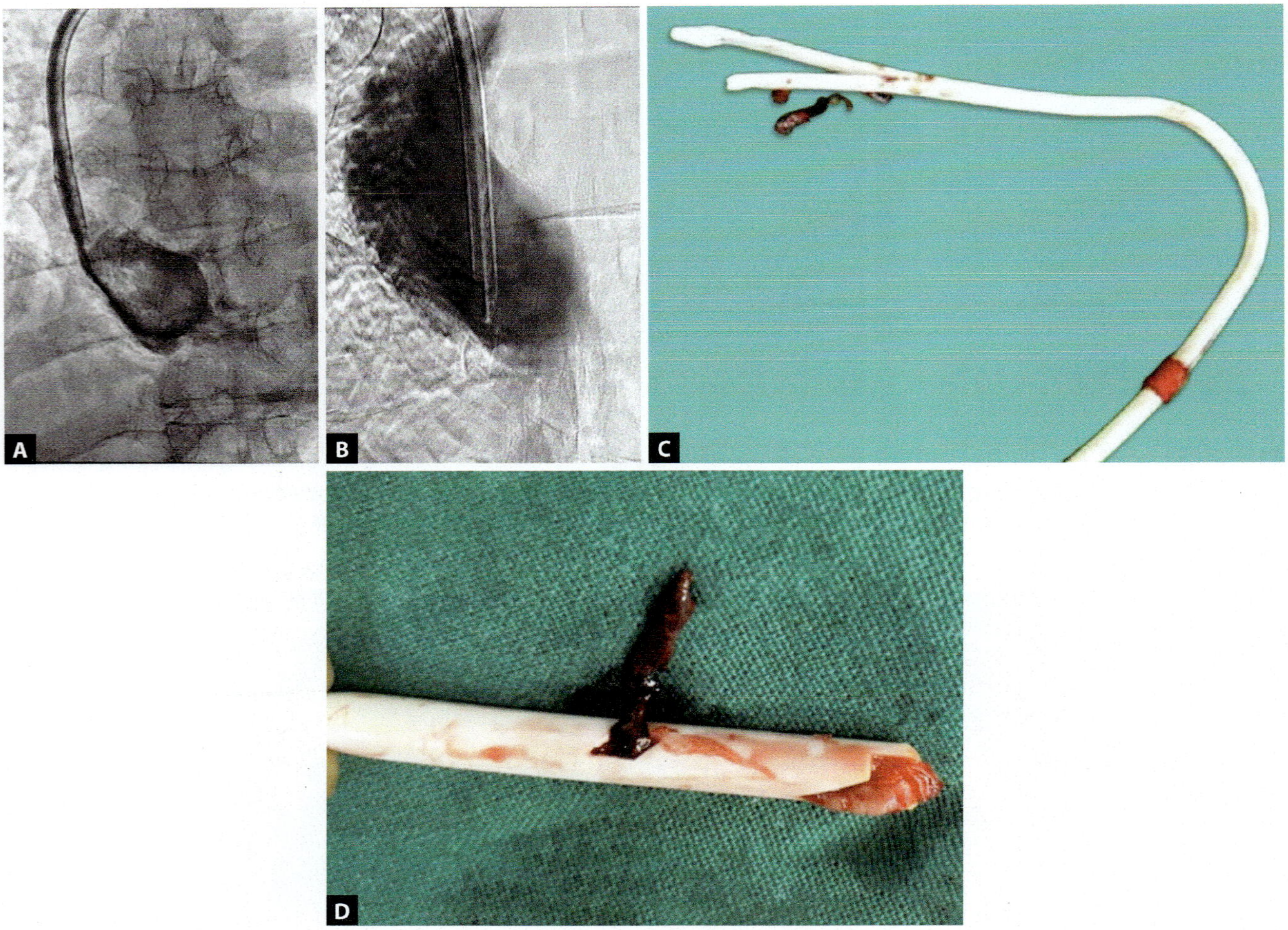

Figs. 9A to D: Case: (A) Reason for nonfunctioning of TCC—right atrial clot; (B) New TCC inserted with tip placed deep in RA; (C and D) Intraluminal clot and fibrin sheath. (TCC: tunneled cuffed hemodialysis catheter)

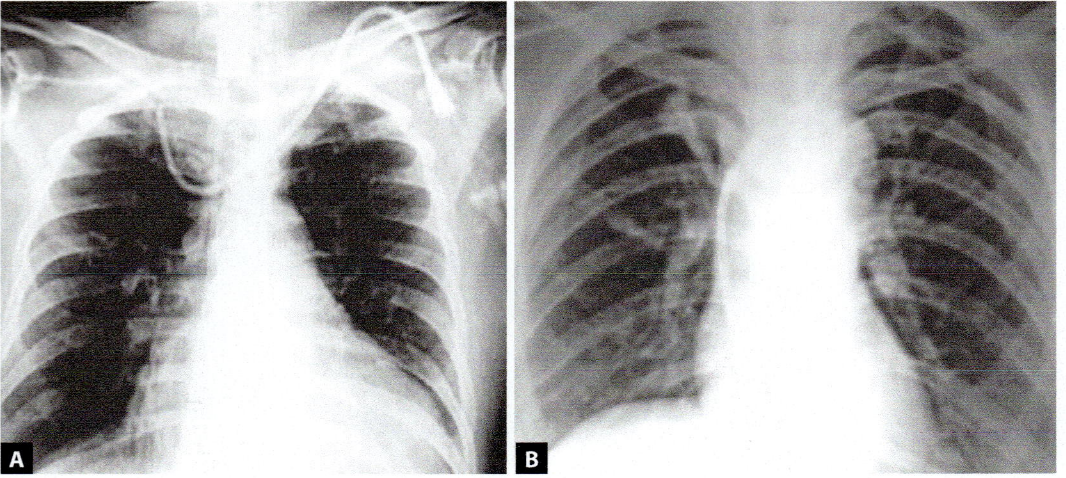

Figs. 10A and B: Case 5: (A) Spontaneous migration of TCC tip; (B) TCC repositioned over a guidewire. (TCC: tunneled cuffed hemodialysis catheter)

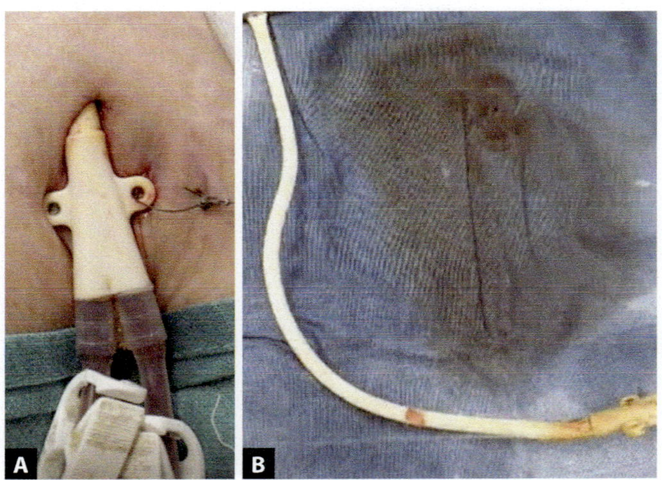

Figs. 11A and B: Case 11: TCC crack in the subcutaneous tunnel. (A) Blood leak observed during dialysis in 10 years old TCC; (B) The leak was confirmed after TCC removal.

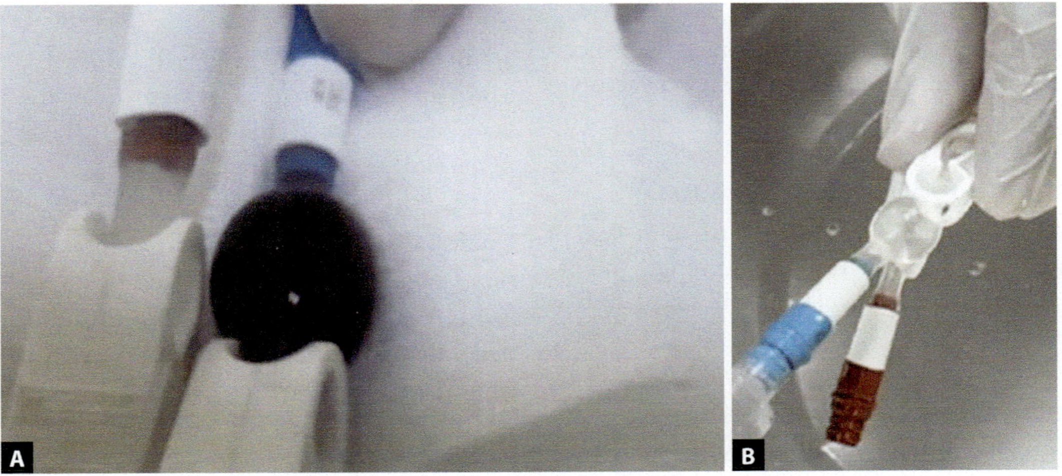

Figs. 12A and B: Venous limb of the TCC getting ballooned while flushing, with TCC in situ and confirmed after removing the TCC.

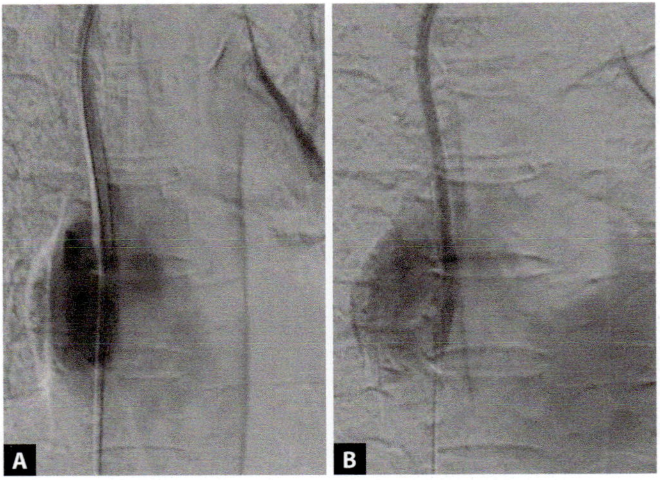

Figs. 13A and B: Fibrin sheath documented.

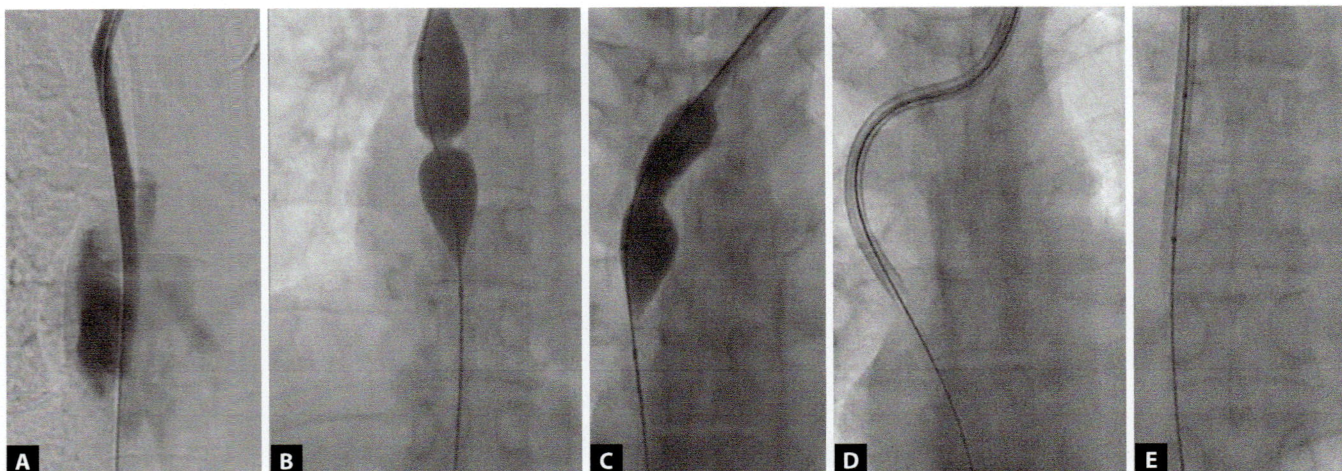

Figs. 14A to E: Balloon angioplasty for the fibrin sheath, also had cavo-atrial junction narrowing, resulting in TCC tip getting stuck over the narrowing. The TCC tip was positioned in the RA by pulling it with a balloon inserted from femoral vein and inflating it inside the TCC lumen.

right femoral vein approach, 4-mm balloon was advanced in to the TCC, inflated and TCC pulled down to position in the RA.

Case 13: Later Problem 8 (Figs. 15A to D)

The exchange of external tubing is from the non TCC of the same brands. This problem can be overcome in ante grade TCCs, where external set of tubing and hub is available separately.

Case 14: Later Problem 9 (Fig. 16)

A 58-year-old male, on HD for 6 months through TCC, was found to have BP of 80–90 mm Hg systolic during routine outpatient visit. Suspecting cardiac cause, two-dimensional (2D) echo was ordered, which showed a 19-mm catheter-related atrial clot (CRAT). He was subjected to thrombolysis with recombinant tissue plasminogen activator (rTPA) alteplase, in increasing doses from 0.1 mg/kg/h over 6 hours, injected from the two lumens of TCC; and gradually going up to 0.25 mg/kg/h for 6 hours over 7 days. Daily coagulation parameters were monitored, and no bleeding occurred. Serial 2D echo showed clot size reduce to 12 mm. He was discharged on oral anticoagulant for 3 months. The serial 2D echo did not show further regression of the clot, and the oral anticoagulation was stopped. No untoward bleeding was noticed. He continues to be on HD through the same catheter, and is not willing for AV fistula at present.

Case 15: Later Problem 10 (Figs. 17A to G)

The kink in the TCC is present from the time of TCC insertion, and needs to replace the TCC with preservation of the site.

Case 16

Sudden dysfunction in 1-year-old TCC, no flow. A 35-year-old type I diabetic on HD, AVF thrombosed suddenly 3 months ago, not getting the next fistula constructed in the hope of getting a kidney transplant. He is taking dialysis at another center **(Figs. 18A to K)**.

Case 17: TCC Salvage

A 48-year-old female had end-stage renal disease (ESRD) secondary to lupus nephritis with antiphospholipid antibody positive and multiple failed AVFs, hence on long-term oral anticoagulation. She was on HD through right IJV TCC which was changed over the wire after 3 years due to malfunction.

After 18 months, patient developed facial edema and had episodes of breathlessness daily at 5 AM, followed by a bout of cough and bringing out blood-streaked sputum. She would need nasal oxygen at home. She had multiple dilated veins over her chest and abdominal wall. The episodes were not related to her level of BP and the chest was clear. Obstructive sleep apnea (OSA) was ruled out. She had pulmonary hypertension (pulmonary artery systolic pressure—PASP 52) and hepatosplenomegaly.

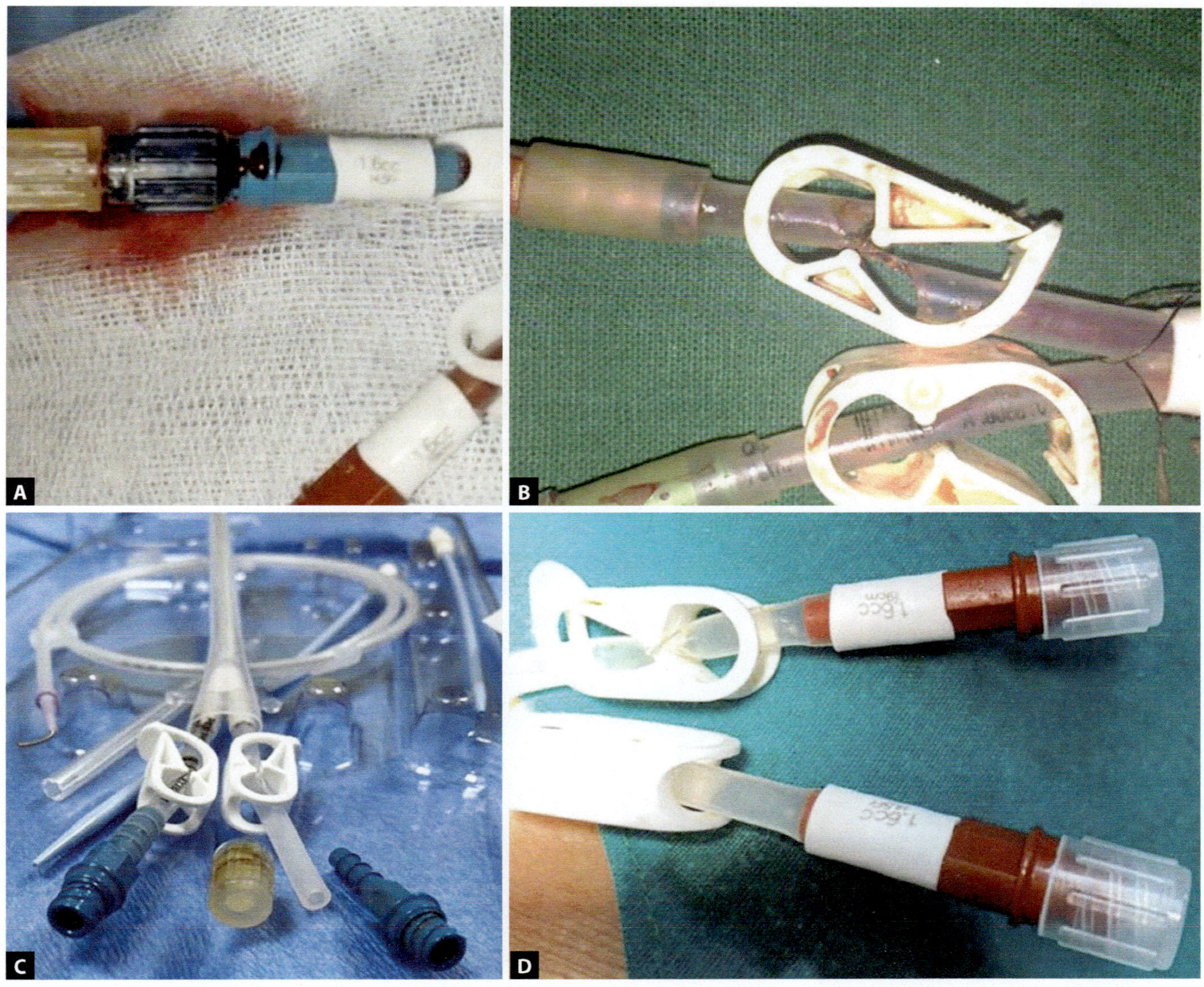

Figs. 15A to D: Cracked hub and tubing of TCC can be repaired using parts from new non-TCC catheter.

She was diagnosed to have SVC syndrome, related to the catheter.

Contrast CT angiogram showed a tight stenosis at the junction of SVC with right atrium (RA) and hardly any space between the catheter and the SVC **(Figs. 19A and B)**.

How was this TCC salvaged **(Figs. 20A to D)**?

Right femoral vein was punctured but the glidewire could not be negotiated across the stenosis at SVC-RA junction (A). Next, right cephalic vein was punctured which allowed the wire to cross the SVC occlusion (B and C). The wire was snared from the femoral vein (D). This is necessary because the large size balloon required for angioplasty cannot be accommodated from relatively smaller cephalic vein. Angiography showed complete obstruction of SVC with filling of azygos vein **(Figs. 21 A and B)**.

Angioplasty of SVC with TCC in situ **(Figs. 22A to D)**. The occluded segment was balloon dilated with OPTA-LP 12-mm diameter × 40-mm length (Cordis®) and MAXI-LD (14 mm × 40 mm) (Cordis®) used to dilate the stenosed junction. The free flow of blood from SVC to RA was confirmed. The cuffed tunneled catheter was left in situ. Following this, patient became asymptomatic, facial puffiness disappeared, hepatosplenomegaly regressed, and the pulmonary arterial pressure normalized. Open

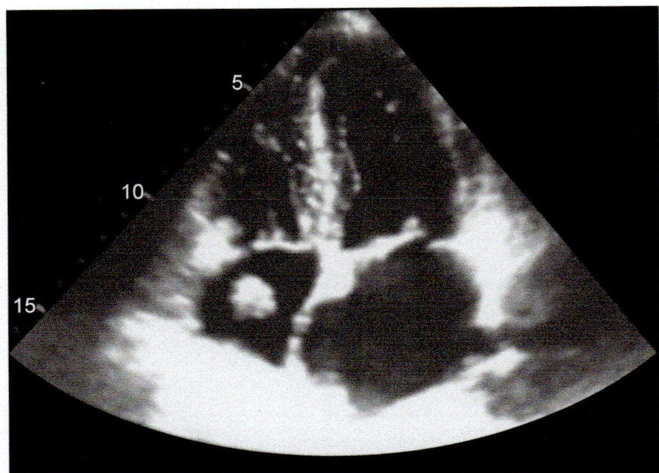

Fig. 16: Catheter-related atrial clot (CRAT) as seen on transthoracic echocardiography. It may be infected; a blood culture should be done.

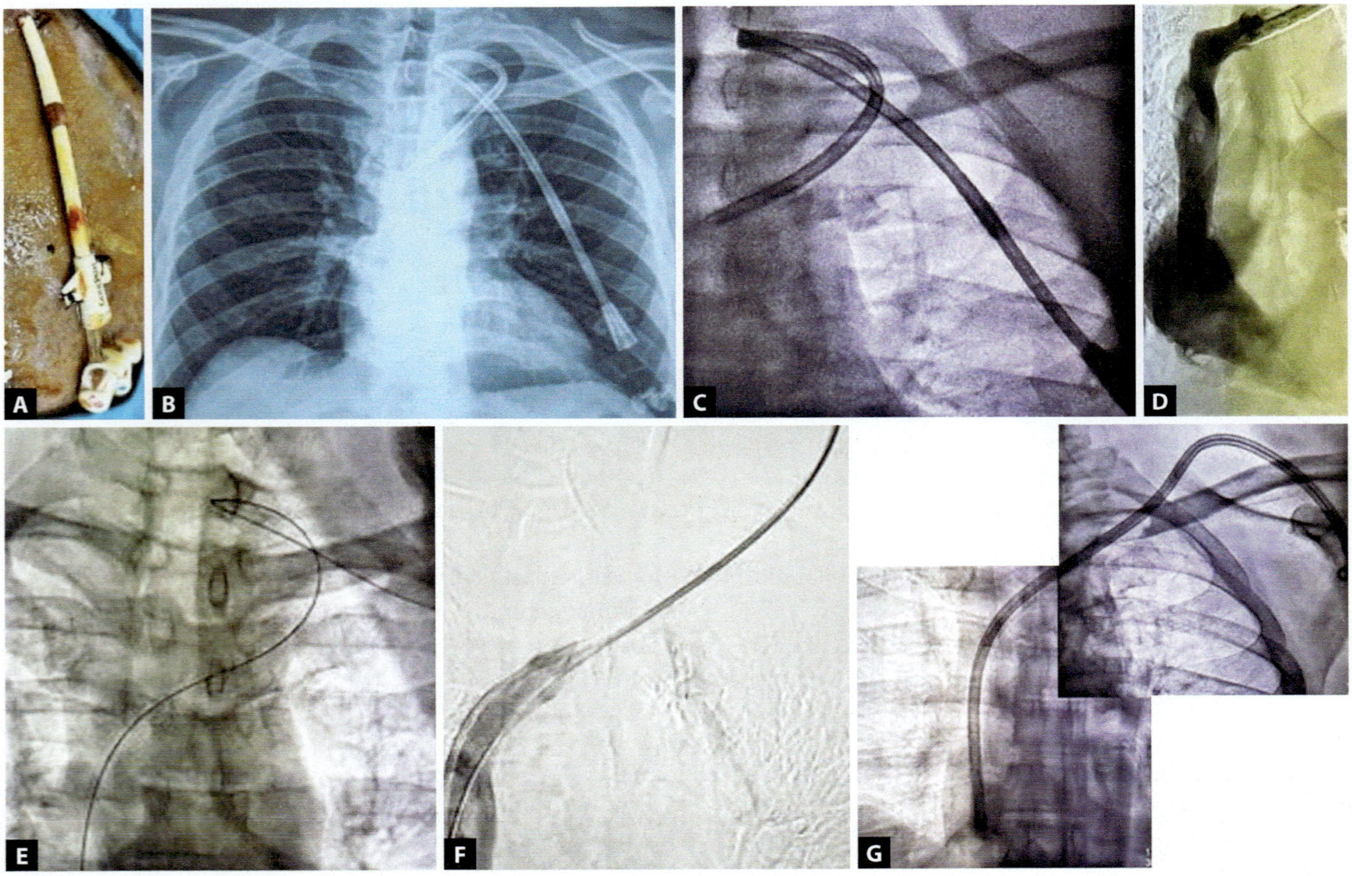

Figs. 17A to G: Case 14: (A) The TCC has been inserted in this fashion with cuff outside and sutures at the exit site. This was the chest X-ray (B) and image (C) in catheterization laboratory. (D) The angiogram through the TCC revealed patent SVC (why was the TCC tip bent mimicking HIV symbol?). Wire was passed (E), straightened (F), and a new TCC inserted (G). (SVC: superior vena cava; TCC: tunneled cuffed hemodialysis catheter)

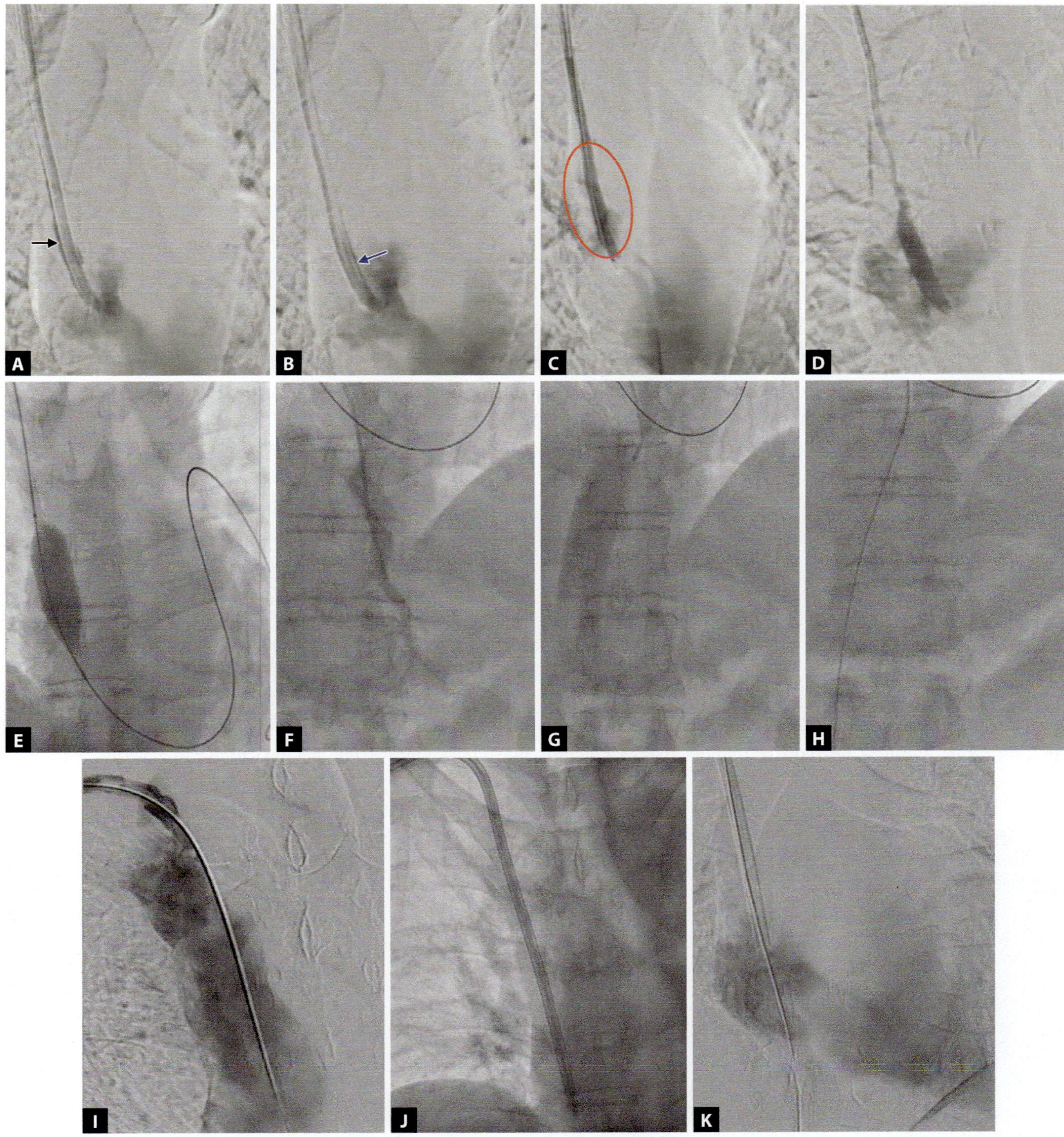

Figs. 18A to K: Case 15: (A) Angiogram through the TCC, venous lumen, shows a thin line (double shadow) around the tip on lateral side, suggestive of CRS (black arrow); (B) Similar finding after angiogram through arterial end, a thin line of double shadow seen on medial side (blue arrow). (C) CRS (red); (D) Similar CRS seen after injection from a diagnostic catheter; (E) The wire could not be parked in the IVC; hence it was pushed in the pulmonary circulation and balloon disruption of CRS was done; (F) The wire was going in the middle hepatic vein; (G and H) Wire manipulated in the IVC; (I) Opened up SVC; (J) New TCC inserted; (K) Tip confirmed in the RA. (CRS: catheter-related sheath; IVC: inferior vena cava; RA: right atrium; SVC: superior vena cava; TCC: tunneled cuffed hemodialysis catheter)

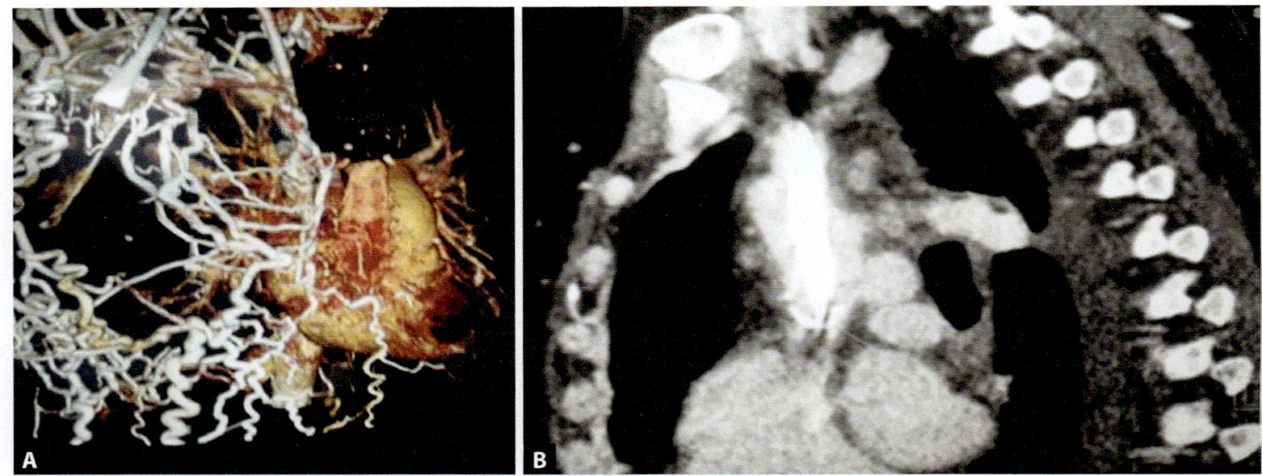

Figs. 19A and B: Contrast CT scan of chest showing superior vena cava stenosis, clot at the TCC tip and multiple chest collaterals confirming presence of chronic central vein stenosis.

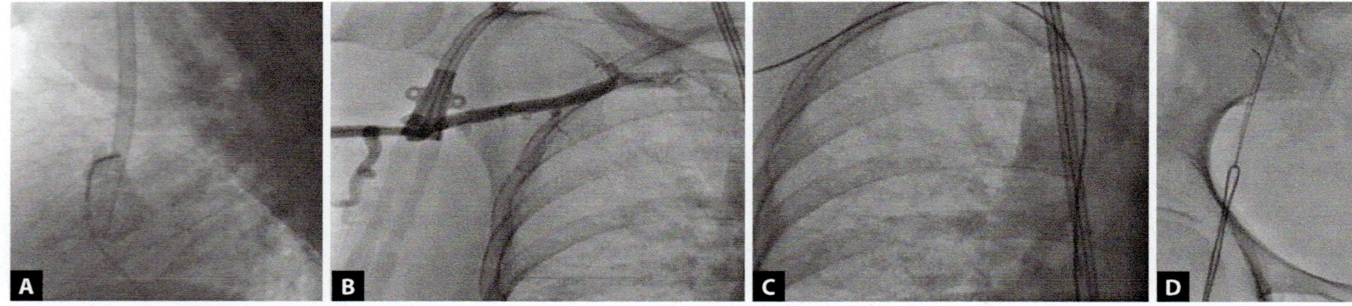

Figs. 20A to D: Crossing the superior vena cava stenosis from upper limb vein and snaring it from femoral vein.

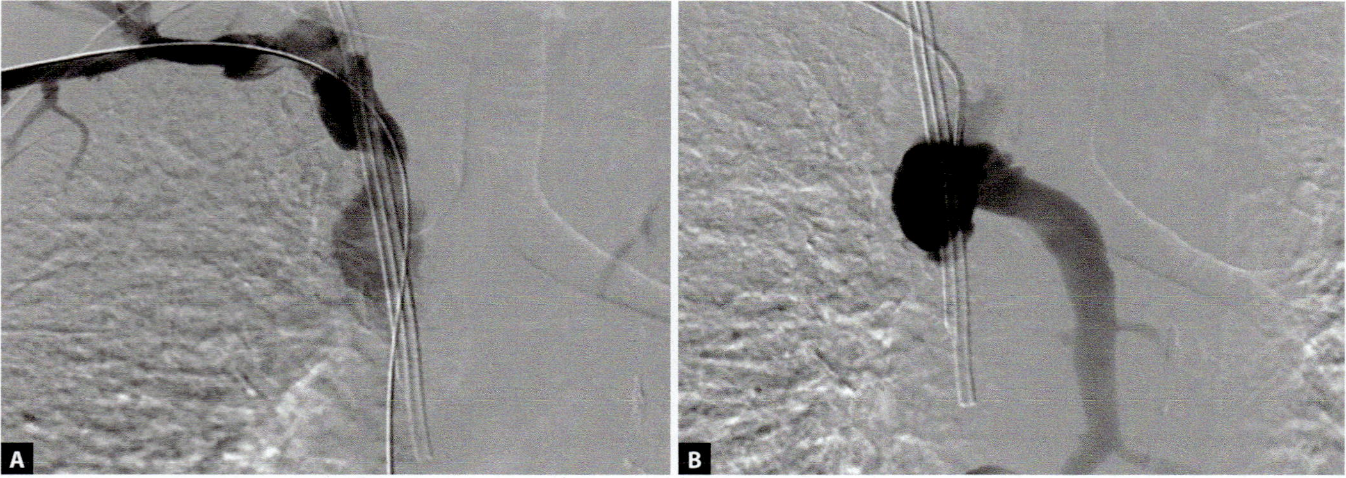

Figs. 21A and B: Filling of azygos vein is always suggestive of superior vena cava stenosis distally.

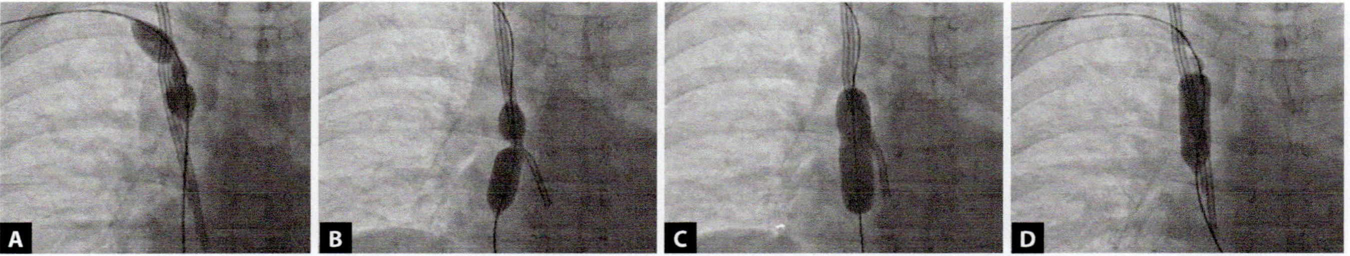

Figs. 22A to D: Angioplasty of superior vena cava can be done with TCC in situ.

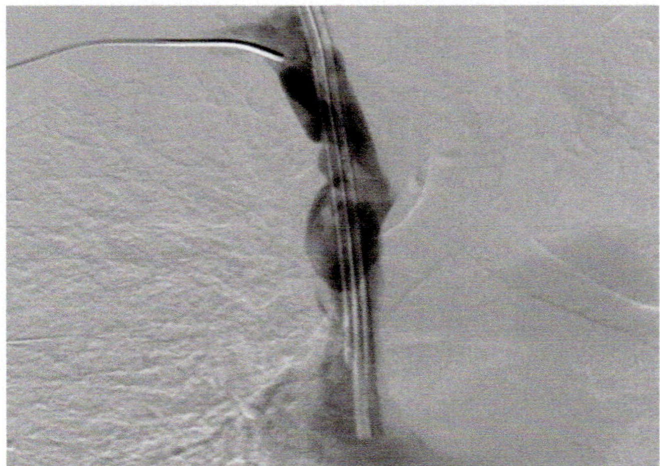

Fig. 23: Final status of superior vena cava after angioplasty, azygos vein filling has disappeared.

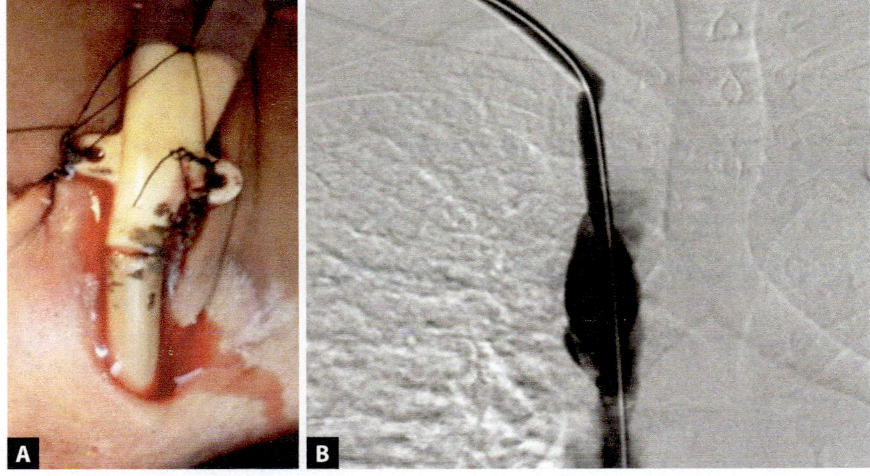

Figs. 24A and B: Tunneled cuffed hemodialysis catheter with silver ion sleeve developed a crack and also hadsuperior vena cava stenosis.

SVC with TCC in place is depicted in **(Fig. 23)**. She had immediate relief of symptoms.

However, after 5 months, a crack developed at the Y junction of TCC (with silver ion sleeve) **(Figs. 24A and B)**. She was subjected to TCC exchange. There was brachiocephalic vein (BCV) stenosis. A new TCC was inserted after angioplasty **(Figs. 25A to G)**.

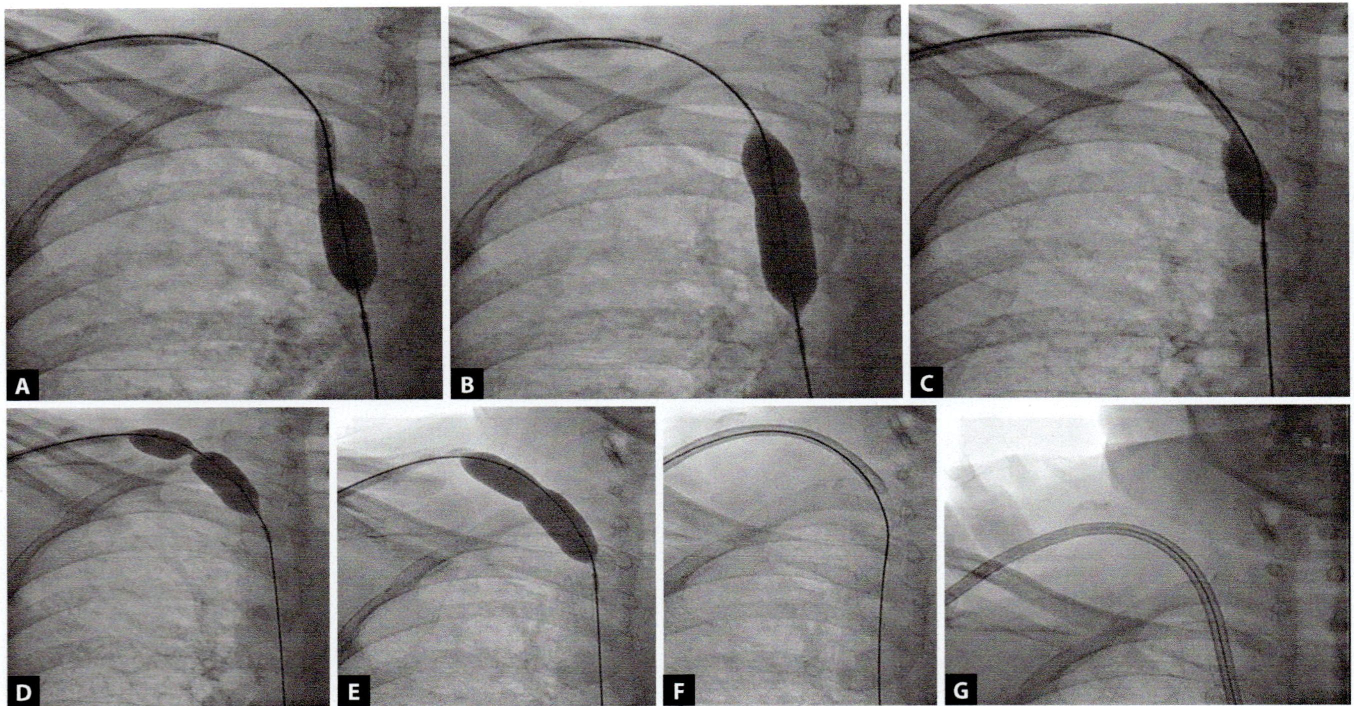

Figs. 25A to G: Angioplasty of entire vein from subclavian vein to superior vena cava and insertion of new TCC over the wire.

Case 18: What Happens to a Previously Perfect Positioned Catheter?

A 56-year-old female, HD × 12 years, seven-failed vascular access (VA) (6 AVFs, 1 graft). Right IJV TCC × 3 years, exchanged over a guidewire and new catheter working × 5 years. Till one day, poor flow, and chest X-ray revealed the tip migration **(Fig. 26)**. Contrast injected through the TCC shows obstruction of SVC with collateral veins **(Figs. 27A to C)**.

The SVC angioplasty was done, SVC opened, through which a new TCC was inserted **(Figs. 28A to C)**.

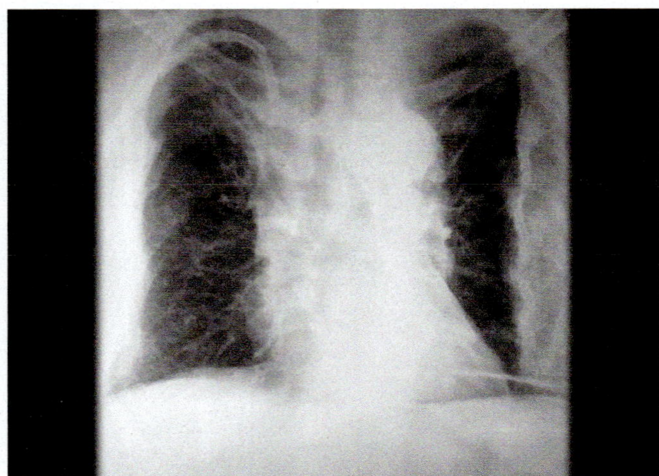

Fig. 26: Tip migration in long standing TCC.

Case 19: Salvaging the Site and the Tract (Figs. 29A to D)

Sometime, the same tract can be salvaged.

Case 20: Salvaging the Site versus TCC

A 65-year-old male, renal calculus disease, HD × 2 years. Initial access: Right IJV TCC, followed by left RC AVF which failed after 1.5 months (right IJV TCC was removed). Left IJV TCC was inserted (right IJV puncture could not be obtained), and left BC AVF was created. Soon, patient developed left upper limb (UL) severe swelling (the problem of TCC with ipsilateral AVF, seen very often, with associated central venous stenosis) **(Fig. 30)**. Two possible options were discussed. First: Insert right IJV TCC, remove left IJV TCC, do left subclavian and BCV angioplasty. By this option, AVF would be salvaged. Second: Keep left IJV TCC, do right BCV angioplasty, surgically ligate left BC AVF and create right UL AVF (there were adequate size vessels, confirmed on doppler). Patient opted for the first option.

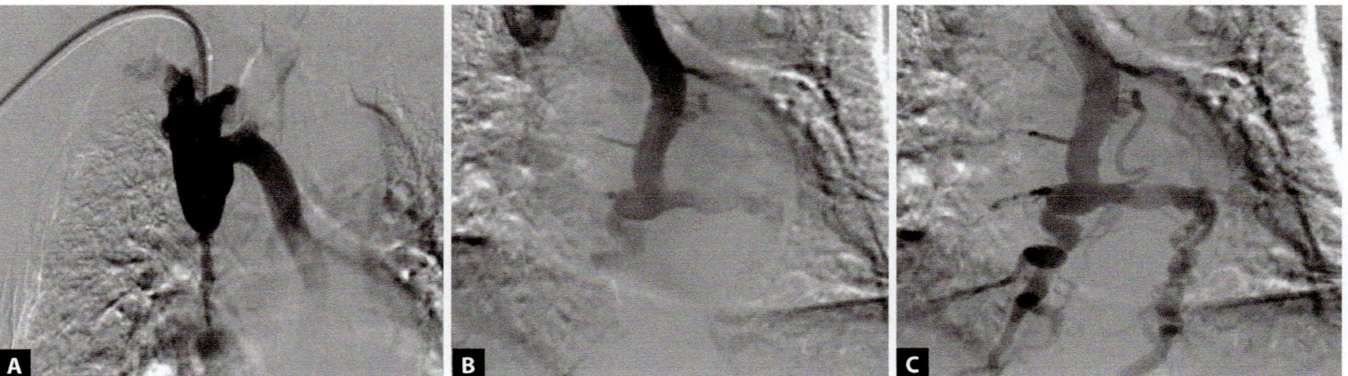

Figs. 27A to C: Superior vena cava angiogram, collateral veins and azygos vein visible.

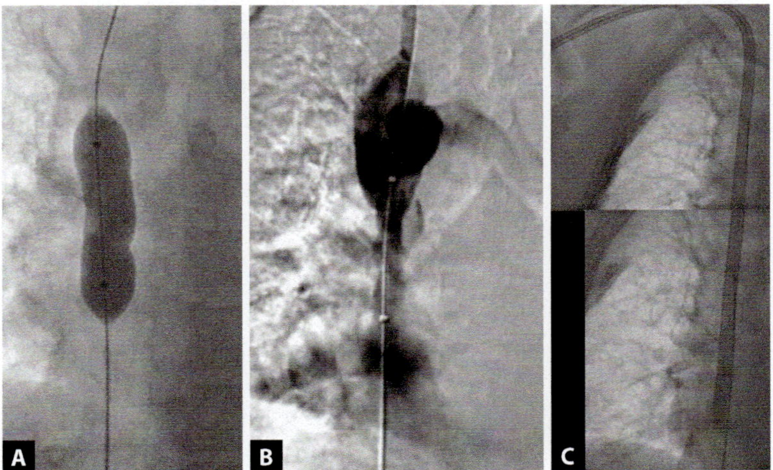

Figs. 28A to C: Superior vena cava angioplasty prior to insertion of new TCC.

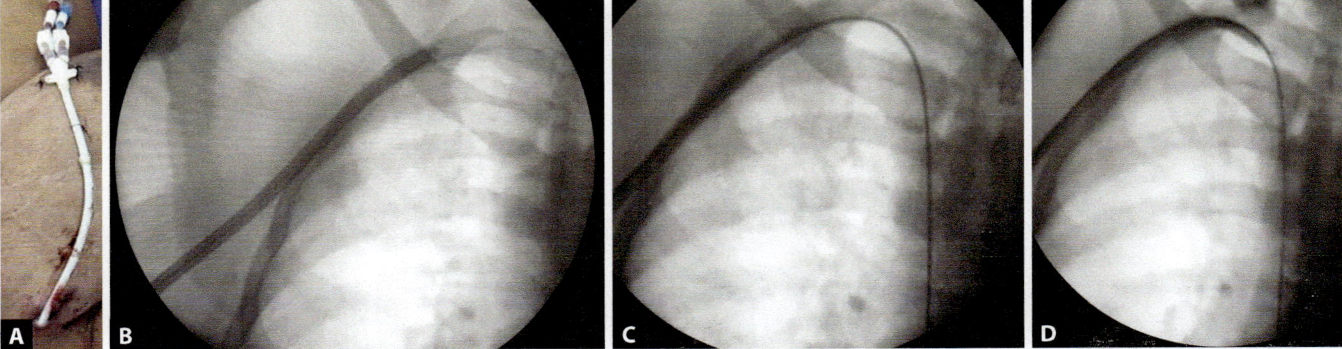

Figs. 29A to D: Case 18: A 42-year-old morbidly obese lady came after the weekend for HD and was found to have TCC having slipped out. (A) The tip of the catheter was barely inside the subcutaneous tunnel. Option was to either pull it out, make a fresh puncture for a new TCC OR explore the tract with a glidewire and see if it can reach the right atrium. Second option was attempted. The TCC in the subcutaneous tunnel; (B) The guidewire passed through the tract in the right atrium; (C) Angiogram confirms that the guidewire is in the heart; (D) New TCC was inserted over the wire.

Initial angiographic images showing left central vain stenosis (CVS) **(Figs. 31A and B)**.

On right IJV puncture, right BCV was patent, and right IJV TCC was inserted first **(Fig. 32)** (Do not remove left IJV TCC till right IJV TCC is secured). Next, successful attempt to cross the left BCV stenosis. It was difficult stenosis and required to use hard end of glidewire to create the tract, followed by crossing the lesion with soft end of the wire **(Figs. 33A and B)**. Left IJV TCC was removed, left BCV angioplasty was done, there was elastic recoil and stent was placed **(Figs. 34A to D)**.

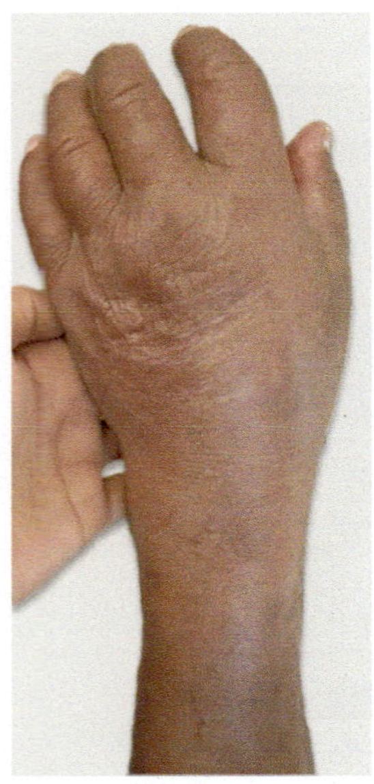

Fig. 30: Swollen arm with ipsilateral AVF and TCC.

Note: While inserting left BCV stent, ensure that SVC is not jailed. Hence right IJV TCC was inserted before inserting the left BCV stent.

Case 21 (Figs. 35A and B)

A 53-year-old male, diabetic kidney disease (DKD), ESRD. Left upper limb proximal AVF failed, infected, bleeding. Presented with swollen arm. Has right IJV non-TCC. In order to preserve right upper limb for AVF, TCC over left side of the neck will be preferable to avoid future swelling of right arm following right UL AVF. TCC preferable over acute catheters, as AVF is unlikely to mature soon.

Case 22: Salvaging the Site for Future AVF on Left UL and Getting TCC Through Right EJV (Figs. 36A to Q)

When a patient presents with a non-tunneled subclavian catheter, it implies that patient has a major vascular access problem, and very high possibility of central vein stenosis due to past multiple neck catheters for hemodialysis. Though the TCCs should be the last choice and AVF be the first choice, there are situations where one has to provide vascular access to these patients who are not willing for fistula creation. Salvaging the TCC and the site becomes extremely important in such situations.

Case 23: Using Inferior Vena Cava as an Access to Salvage the Dialysis Access (Fig. 37)

Diabetic, A 57-year-old female, on HD since 2 years. Presented with multiple neck and femoral catheters,

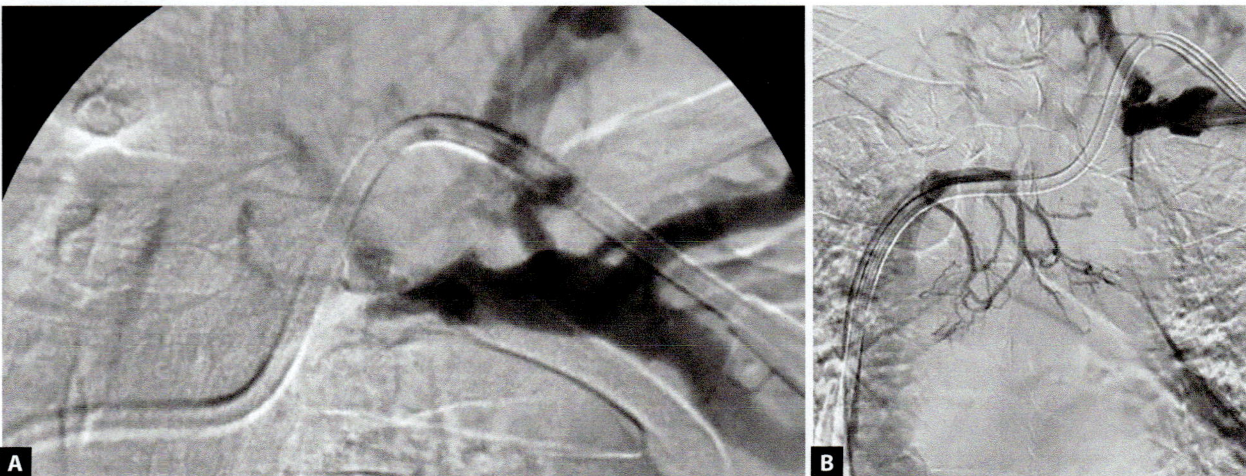

Figs. 31A and B: Central vein CTO.

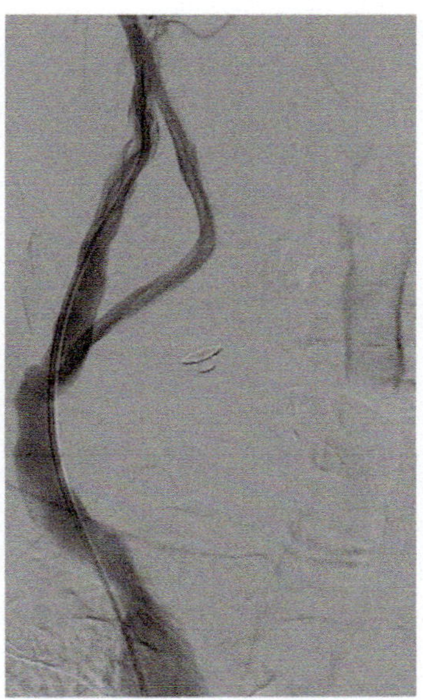

Fig. 32: Patent AVF.

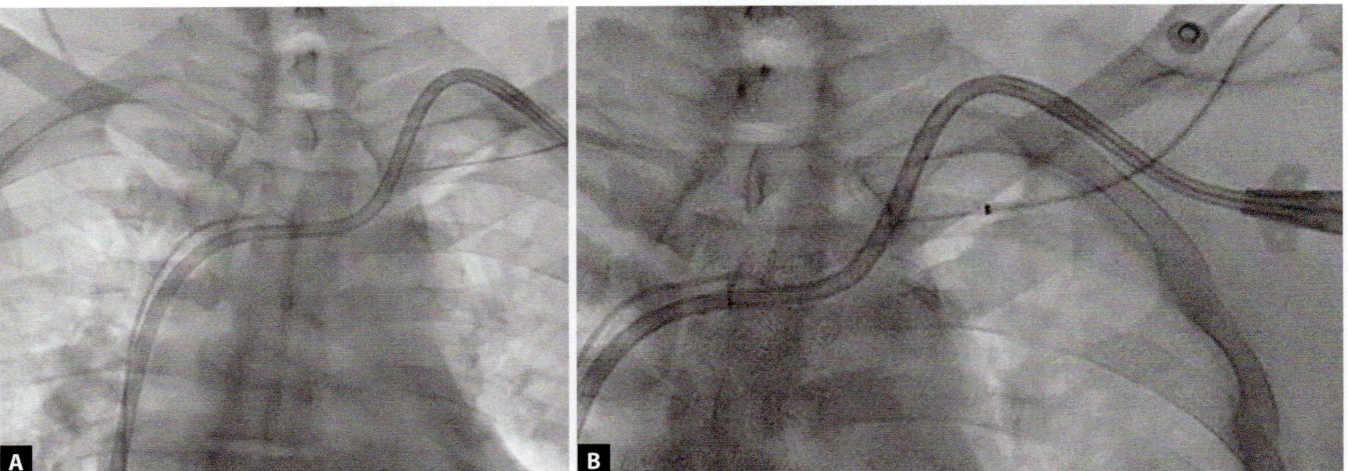

Figs. 33A and B: Crossing the CTO.

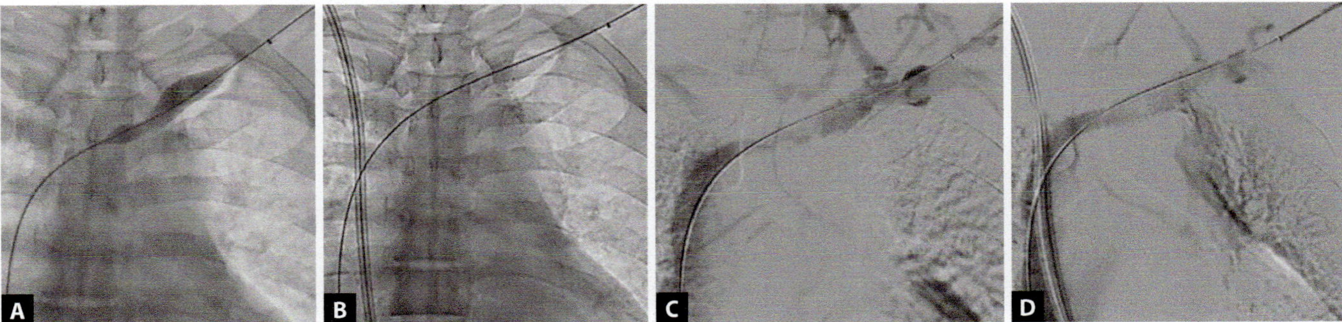

Figs. 34A to D: Brachiocephalic vein angioplasty and stenting.

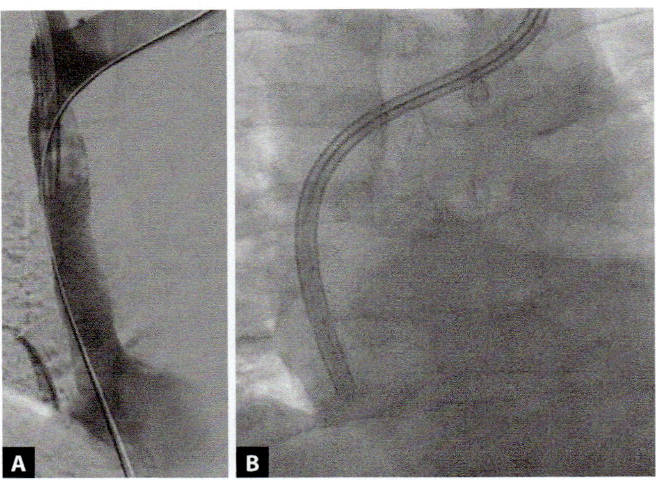

Figs. 35A and B: Removal of right non-TCC and insertion of left IJV TCC.

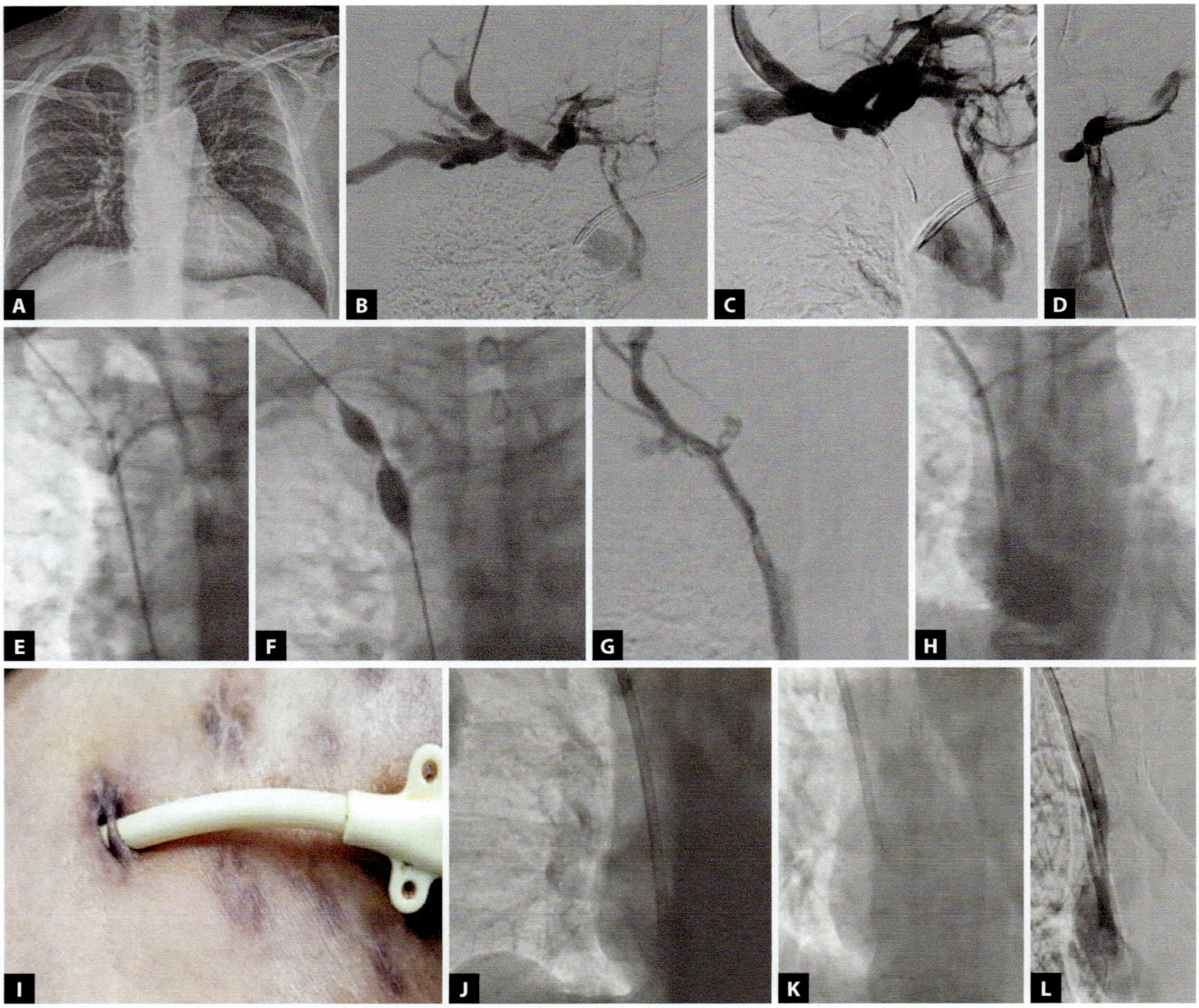

Figs. 36A to L

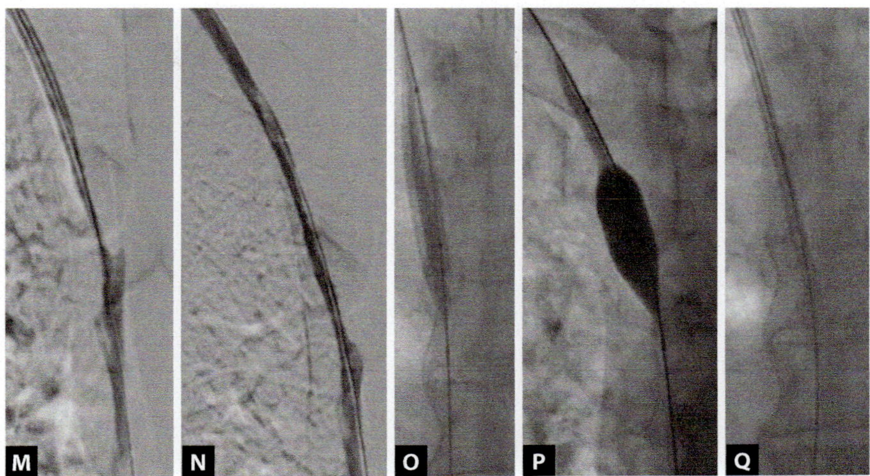

Figs. 36M to Q

Figs. 36A to Q: Multiple catheters in the neck and presenting with malfunctioning left subclavian vein non tunneled noncuffed catheter (A). The angiogram from right IJV (B). The angiogram from right external jugular vein (EJV) (C) and trying to explore the chronic thrombotic occlusion of the right BCV, and getting resistance. Approach from femoral vein, chronic total occlusion (CTO) confirmed (D), and a sharp needle cannulation (E) through this CTO to try and create a passage successfully. Balloon angioplasty of right BCV done (F) and patent EJV-BCV-SVC confirmed (G). The TCC inserted through right IJV (H). The patient did not undergo an AVF and presented 1 year later with no flow in the catheter, and was unable to undergo HD. On examination, the TCC has slipped out (I and K) compared to the previous tip position (J) and the reason was a fibrin sheath (L and M). The SVC and right BCV were narrowed (N). Balloon disruption of the fibrin sheath and angioplasty of right BCV was done (O and P), and a new TCC inserted (Q).

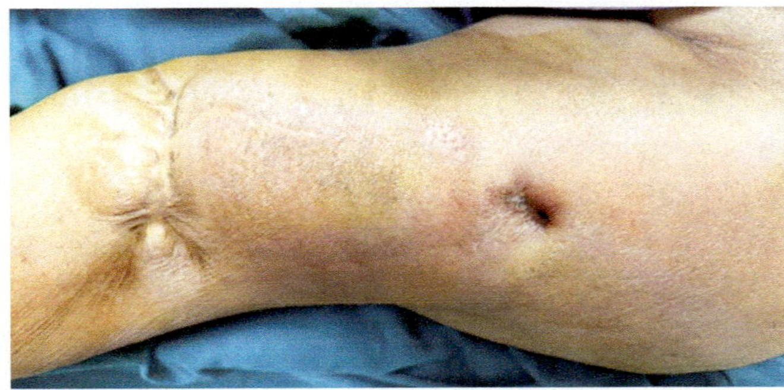

Fig. 37: The segment of cephalic vein subjected to repeated angioplasty, with sites of needle puncture.

multiple failed AVFs. She has a thrombosed left BC AVF which had undergone angioplasty 2 months back and repeated again 10 days back. She underwent 3 HD since last angioplasty before it thrombosed. Angioplasty was done for the cephalic vein in the arm and central veins were not studied. After the last thrombosis, she was subjected to CT venography, which showed narrowing of left BC vein and subclavian vein.

AVF angiography, obstruction of the outflow cephalic vein at the site of punctures **(Figs. 38 and 39)**.

This patient had a failed continuous ambulatory peritoneal dialysis (CAPD) after 2 months in the past. What options are there?

One can explore translumbar, transrenal, and transhepatic vein approaches. Hence, a CT angiogram was performed to look for patency of IVC which was confirmed **(Fig. 40A)**, and a TCC was inserted in the IVC from the level of L2 vertebra up to SVC level, image with patient in prone position **(Fig. 40B)**.

Case 24: Salvage the Site, Use Collateral Vein

A 67-year-old female, autosomal dominant polycystic kidney disease (ADPKD), with a H/O right IJV non-TCC 6 months ago, removed after 2 HD. Now ESRD, right neck doppler **(Figs. 41A and B)** shows an occluded right IJV and collateral veins. It was decided to pursue with a TCC on right side of neck, to keep left side free for AVF. Right IJV high puncture followed by low puncture once the collateral vein was visualized. A TCC was inserted, but developed a kink due to the position of the vein, hence the tunnel was modified on left side **(Figs. 41C to F)**.

DISCUSSION

Vascular access is a lifeline for HD patients. The types of VA are AVF, arteriovenous grafts (AVG), non-TCC, and TCC. Long-term HD catheters have various causes of catheter malfunction. One needs to study the cause of malfunction

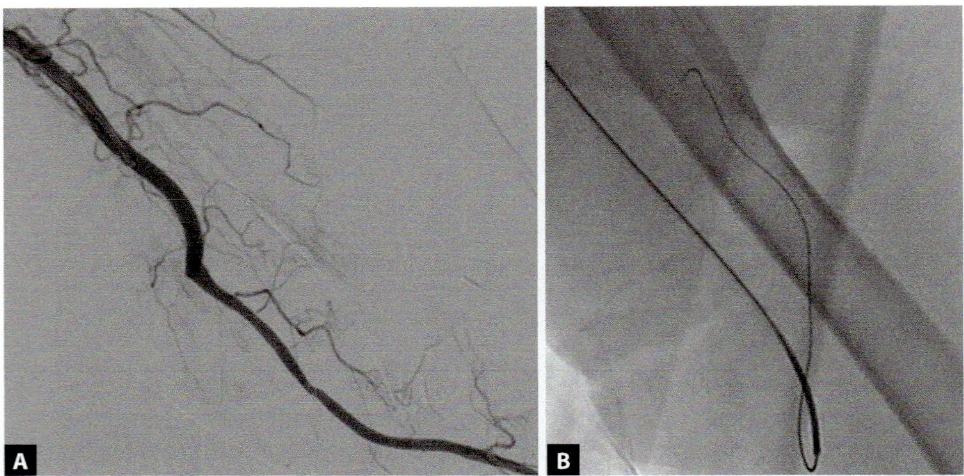

Figs. 38A and B: Thrombosed AVF, wire cannot be negotiated.

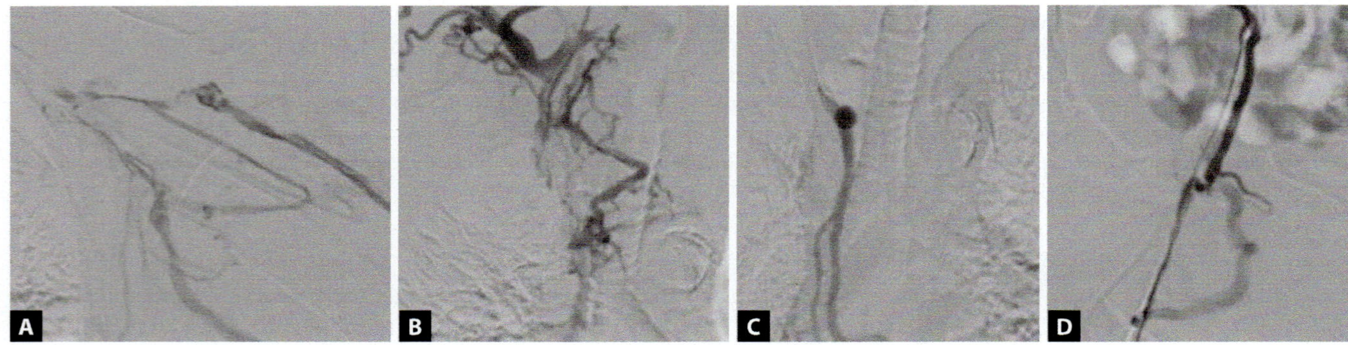

Figs. 39A to D: Central venous stenosis of upper and lower limb veins.

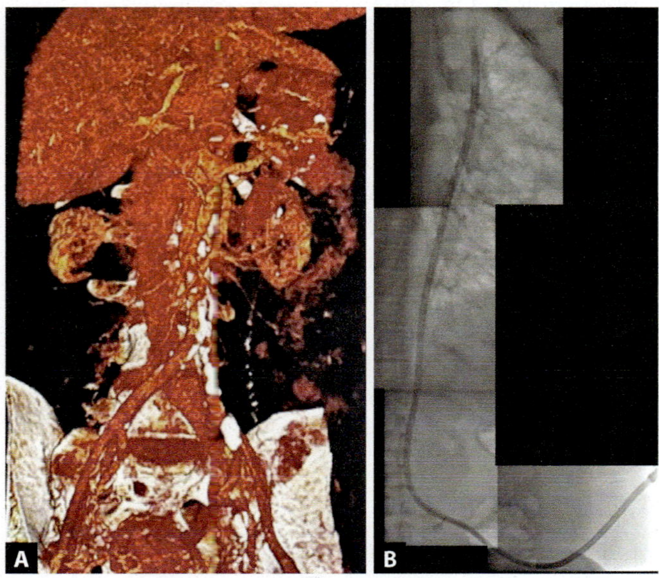

Figs. 40A and B: Patent IVC on CT angiography and insertion of trans-lumbar TCC, with tip in right atrium.

carefully so that further appropriate treatment can be planned.

Though AVF is considered superior to AVG and TCC, it may not be so for all the patients. For some patients, TCC may be an appropriate and a better or more so the only VA. What started as "Fistula first—catheter last" campaign,[1] has now been changed to the access choice as per end-stage kidney disease (ESKD) Life-Plan (PLAN—patient life-plan access needs) as per the latest kidney disease outcomes quality initiative (KDOQI) VA guidelines.[2] Hence the catheters conundrum continues where one hates to have the TCC but cannot live without it at times.[3] The TCCs are inserted in those who initiate the dialysis as emergency ("crash landers") where the opportunity was either missed or never available to plan the VA. The TCCs are also inserted as a bridge to transplant, for those whose AVF or AVG fail acutely and till there is restoration of original VA or those who have multiple VA failure and the TCC is the only life line for their survival. TCCs are also

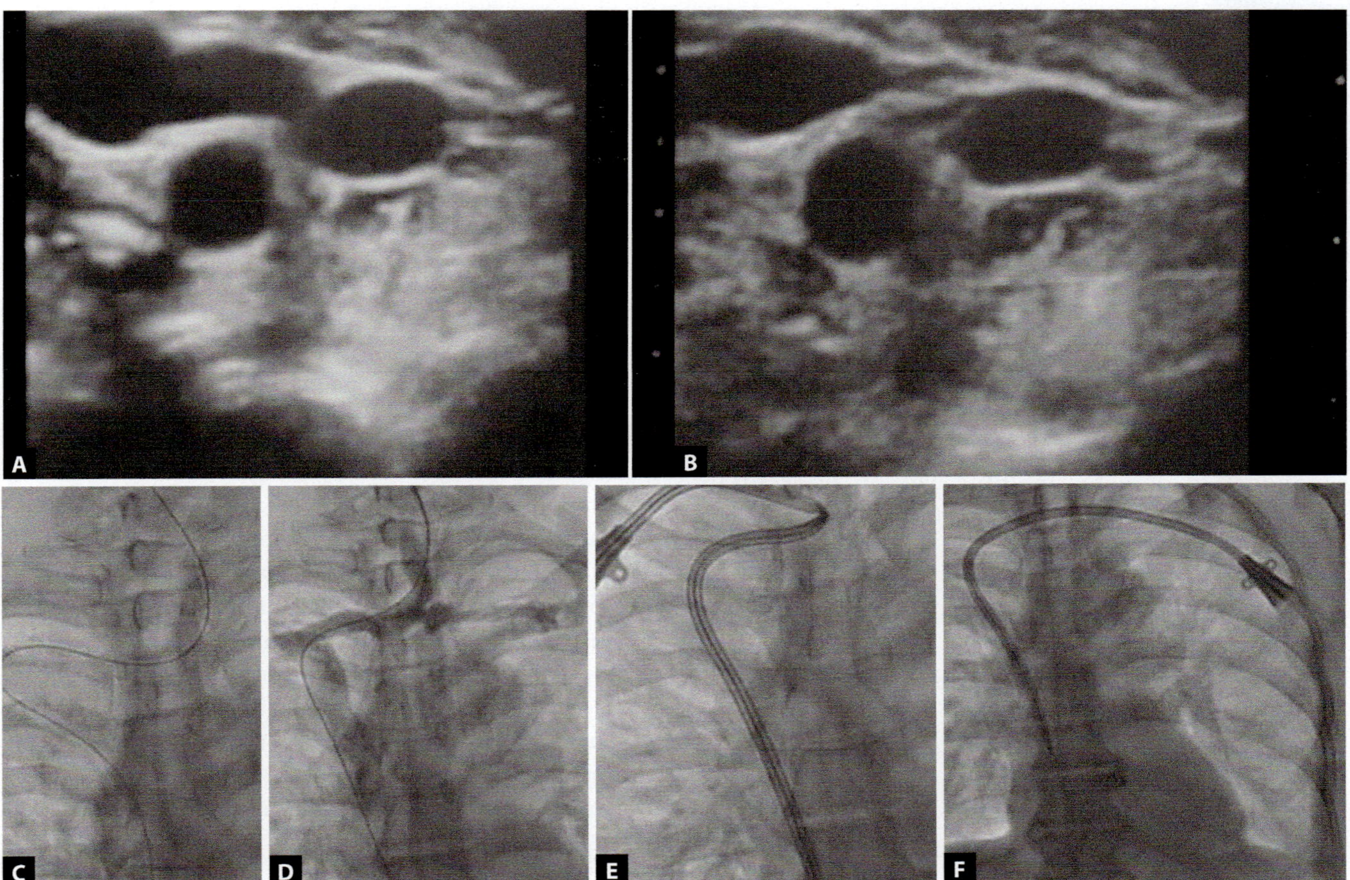

Figs. 41A to F: (A and B) Collateral veins in the neck, used for TCC insertion; (D to F) Changing the exit site to opposite side to overcome the kink.

considered as preferred modality for elderly, diabetics, hypertensive, and those having reduced left ventricular function or pulmonary hypertension.

The problem in the TCC can occur during the procedure of insertion or during its usage over short or long term requiring endovascular intervention to salvage the catheter or the site and ensure undisrupted HD. This is also a situation where surgical option is not feasible and the conservative approach is not an option because the TCC function restoration is a priority.

In the present chapter, many of the patients presented for solution of the problems which occurred outside our hospital. The complications of TCC malfunction, misplacement, clotting, crack or another mechanical defect in the catheter, etc., do occur and one has to solve it. Some of them may be preventable, some may just happen. If there is a problem, each patient should get appropriate quick and effective assessment to determine the cause of TCC-related problem, so that appropriate intervention can be done to have TCC back in working condition. Once salvaged, these catheters work well for long durations.

REFERENCES

1. Kalloo S, Blake PG, Wish J. A Patient-Centered Approach to Hemodialysis Vascular Access in the Era of Fistula First. Semin Dial. 2016;29(2):148-57.
2. Lok CE, Huber TS, Lee T, Shenoy S, Yevzlin AS, Abreo K, et al. KDOQI Clinical Practice Guideline for Vascular Access: 2019 Update. Am J Kidney Dis. 2020;75(4): S1-S164.
3. Schwab SJ, Beathard G. The hemodialysis catheter conundrum: hate living with them, but can't live without them. Kidney Int. 1999;56(1):1-17.

CHAPTER 24

Catheter-related Infections and its Prevention

Prem P Varma, Mehak Singla, Abhilasha Soni

CASE SCENARIO

A 70-year-old male with end-stage kidney disease secondary to diabetes mellitus was on intermittent hemodialysis (IHD) at our center for 3 years. He had a tunneled catheter for vascular access, which was placed at the time of initiation of dialysis. He presented to the emergency department with fever and confusion, ongoing for the past week.

The examination revealed a febrile drowsy patient with a temperature of 101°F, heart rate of 110/min, and blood pressure of 86/60 mm Hg. Catheter site was non-tender, with no discharge. No murmurs were audible.

The preliminary diagnosis was catheter-related bloodstream infection (CRBSI). Complete blood count, procalcitonin, and paired blood cultures were performed. The patient was started on broad-spectrum antibiotics. His blood counts showed hemoglobin of 11 g/dL, total leukocyte count of 18,900/cmm and procalcitonin of >100 µg/L. Blood cultures returned positive for *Pseudomonas aeruginosa*. The echocardiogram ruled out any valvular vegetation. In view of clinical profile of fever with chills, leukocytosis, and positive blood culture from two sites, the patient was diagnosed with CRBSI. Antibiotics were adjusted and catheter lock was given for 3 days. The patient showed clinical signs of recovery on the third day and was discharged after 6 days. Antibiotics were given for 3 weeks.

INTRODUCTION

Despite the recommendation of "fistula first" policy, majority of patients get started on intermittent hemodialysis (IHD) through temporary catheter or tunneled cuffed catheter (TCC). The United States Renal Data System (USRDS) 2024 data shows that 85% patients were initiated IHD with TCC.[1] In India, over 95% patients start IHD with catheters and 75% of them with temporary catheters.[2] The Kidney Disease Outcomes Quality Initiative (KDOQI) recommends TCC if catheter use of over 2 weeks is expected.[3] The European Best Practice guidelines (EBPG) also discourages use of temporary catheter for maintenance IHD.[4]

The preferable site for TCC placement is the right internal jugular vein. The subclavian vein is best avoided for fear of vascular stenosis. The femoral vein remains the least preferred site. Catheters offer immediate vascular access but are fraught with complications. Infections remain a dreadful complication of temporary or TCC. Compared to patients with arteriovenous fistula (AVF) or arteriovenous graft (AVG), patients with TCC have a 2–3-fold higher risk of hospitalization from infections and death.[5]

ETIOLOGY OF CATHETER-RELATED BLOODSTREAM INFECTION

Catheter-related bloodstream infection (CRBSI) remains the most important cause of catheter loss. The incidence of CRBSI is 0.7–5.5/1,000 catheter days for TCC and 7.5–23/1,000 for temporary catheters.[6] Incidence of 1.1/1,000 catheter days or below represents an excellent catheter care; incidence of 2.2/1,000 catheter days is acceptable but higher than this figure suggests poor catheter care and introspection.[7] India data shows a much higher rate of CRBSI. For temporary catheters, it is 7.5–23/1,000 catheter days and for TCC 1– 2.6/1,000 catheter days.[6] An AVF has a median infection complication rate of 0.11/1,000 days and positive blood culture rate of 0.08/1,000 days. Infections in AVGs have been reported in 1.6–35% of patients, with an overall incidence of positive blood cultures of 0.31/1,000 days.[8] Metastatic infectious complications of CRBSIs occur in 10–25% patients with *Staphylococcus* coagulase infections and include endocarditis, osteomyelitis, spinal epidural abscess, septic arthritis, brain abscess, and septic pulmonary emboli.[9]

CLINICAL PROFILE AND DIAGNOSIS

Catheter-related bloodstream infection generally presents with fever, chills, malaise, or hemodynamic compromise.

Data from north and south India suggests that fever with chills is the most common presentation and around 20% patients present with hemodynamic instability/shock.[10] A large Canadian study reported fever or chills as a presenting feature in 60–80% patients and 25% presented with hemodynamic instability, altered mental status, nausea, and vomiting. Leukocytosis (sometimes leukopenia) raised C-reactive protein (CRP) and procalcitonin are a common finding.[7] Patients with exit-site infection generally exhibit redness and induration within 2 cm of exit site and might have a purulent discharge. Those with tunnel infection have redness, induration, and tenderness >2 cm away from the exit site along the catheter tunnel. These patients may or may not have features of bacteremia. Pressure over the tunnel might express purulent discharge.[11]

As per the Infectious Diseases Society of America (IDSA) guidelines, for "definitive diagnosis", paired blood cultures (from catheter site and periphery) should grow the same organism. It is suggested that culture yield is better if blood is taken from blood circuit of dialysis machine rather than periphery. If culture positivity is from one site, diagnosis of "probable CRBSI" is made. Differential time to positivity (DTP) (organism growth 2 hours earlier from catheter than peripheral blood) and catheter tip culture growth >15 colonies per catheter segment are additional pointers to CRBSI.[11]

In patients who are persistently febrile or show signs of hemodynamic compromise, a thorough search for source of infection with suitable investigations and transesophageal echocardiography (TEE) should be considered.[10]

The KDOQI criteria for CRBSI are listed below:[3]

- *Definite:* Same organism growth from a semiquantitative culture of the catheter tip (>15 CFU/catheter segment) *and* from a blood culture in a symptomatic patient with no other apparent source of infection
- *Probable:* Defervescence of symptoms after antibiotic therapy with or without removal of the catheter, in the setting in which blood culture confirms infection, but catheter tip does not (or catheter tip does, but blood does not) in a symptomatic patient with no other apparent source of infection
- *Possible:* Defervescence of symptoms after antibiotic treatment or after removal of catheter in the absence of laboratory confirmation of bloodstream infection (BSI) in a symptomatic patient with no other apparent source of infection

MICROBIOLOGY

Most of the literature suggests that 40–80% of infections are due to gram-positive organisms. *Staphylococcus epidermidis, Staphylococcus aureus,* or *Enterococcus* are the common gram-positive organisms. Gram-negative organisms such as *Pseudomonas, Klebsiella,* or *Escherichia coli* account for 20–40% of CRBSI cases. In <10% cases, CRBSI may be polymicrobial and <5% are fungus related.[13]

However, Indian data suggests that gram-negative infections are equal and possibly more common than gram-positive organisms. Data from northern and southern India and our data suggest that gram-negative organisms are responsible for over 70% of CRBSI cases.[6,14] The reason for this difference in microbial spectrum is unclear. It is likely that injudicious use of antibiotics in our healthcare setting and higher prevalence of gram-negative organisms in the hospital environment account for this difference **(Table 1)**. Majority (70–90%) of AVF and AVG infections in upper extremity are due to skin-based organisms such as *S. aureus* and *S. epidermidis*, with a higher incidence of gram-negative organisms in lower-extremity AV accesses.[3]

TREATMENT

A patient with hemodynamic compromise or severe infection needs hospitalization.

In addition, admission for nonadherent patients should be considered.

Once CRBSI is suspected, broad-spectrum antibiotics covering gram-positive and gram-negative organisms, i.e., third-generation cephalosporins and intravenous vancomycin, are recommended as soon as samples for blood cultures are sent.

If there is a delay in collecting samples for blood cultures, antibiotic initiation should not be delayed. In addition, any discharge at the exit site or from tunnel should be swabbed and sent for culture.[12]

Antibiotic choice depends on the common organisms isolated and sensitivity pattern of the local hospital. Guidance from microbiology or infectious disease specialist can be sought. Once culture report is available, antibiotics should be tailored accordingly.

If a patient continues to be febrile despite 72 hours of intravenous antibiotics or develops hemodynamic instability at any stage, catheter removal is recommended.

TABLE 1: Microbiological spectrum of CRBSI.

Total number of patients	Episodes of CRBSI	Rate of CRBSI (per 1,000 catheter days)	Organisms (%)			
			GN	GP	Fungal	PM
81	34	1.3	++			
301	40	0.36	38	60	2	–
492	65	2.62	47	42	3	8
353	135	7.74	58	42	–	–
52	6		53	47	–	–
291	78	1.6	73	27	–	–
82	39		61	39	–	–
122	84	7.1	16	79	5	–
227	39	1.28	26	59	8	7

(CRBSI: catheter-related bloodstream infection; GN: gram-negative organism; GP: gram-positive organism; PM: polymicrobial)

In case it is not possible to remove the catheter because of challenging access, it can be exchanged over a guidewire once the patient becomes afebrile or CRP settles down.[12]

If isolate is *S. aureus*, *Pseudomonas,* or fungus, the IDSA recommends removal of catheter regardless of symptoms or antibiotic duration. The duration of antibiotics is 2–3 weeks depending on the organism isolated. For metastatic lesions such as endocarditis, osteomyelitis, and paraspinal abscesses, a 4–6-week course of antibiotics is recommended **(Flowchart 1)**.[12]

For any outpatient in the dialysis unit, exhibiting signs of systemic illness or suspected CRBSI, blood cultures and exit-site swabs, if relevant, should be sent promptly for diagnosis. Initial doses of broad-spectrum intravenous antibiotics should be administered while awaiting culture results. Following culture result, antibiotics can be tailored to the microbe and be continued for 2–3 weeks.[12]

For exit-site infections, shorter courses of intravenous antibiotics can be considered. In cases with tunnel infection, catheter removal is advocated.[12]

Besides systemic antibiotics, antibiotic catheter lock is recommended as part of CRBSI treatment, especially if catheter removal is not planned.[12]

A multicentric trial compared three arms of CRBSI patients for catheter outcome. In the first group, only systemic antibiotics were used; the second group used systemic antibiotics and antibiotic lock; while in the third group, besides antibiotics, catheter was changed over guidewire. Outcomes of second and third groups were similar, implying that antibiotics and antibiotic lock are as effective as catheter exchange.[15]

Personal Experience: Alcohol Lock versus Antibiotic Lock during CRBSI

We have been using 70% ethyl alcohol lock in place of antibiotic lock in cases of definite CRBSI since 2018, and our data suggests its superiority over antibiotic lock. We believe that alcohol breaks down the biofilm and has bactericidal effects.

1.5 mL of 70% ethyl alcohol is instilled in each port of the catheter. This is then aspirated out the next day and replaced with a fresh fill. This is repeated on 3 consecutive days. Of the 78 cases of definite CRBSI (57 gram negative and 21 gram positive), we used alcohol lock in 56 and antibiotic lock in 22 patients besides systemic antibiotics. Both groups were comparable. Catheter removal was required in 6/56 (10.7%) patients using alcohol lock and 15/22 (68%) cases using antibiotic lock ($p < 0.01$). With alcohol lock, we rarely required to remove the catheter despite the infecting organism being *Staphylococcus* or *Pseudomonas*.

There was initial concern that alcohol may damage the catheter material; however, our follow-up data of over 6 months did not show any catheter leak or damage.

We also used alcohol catheter lock in the subject case given above.[14,16,17]

PREVENTION

Hand hygiene while handling TCC remains the most important preventative strategy. Hand washing, use of antiseptic rub, and wearing sterile gloves remain the cornerstone for prevention. On occasion, two technicians

Flowchart 1: Approach to a case of CRBSI.

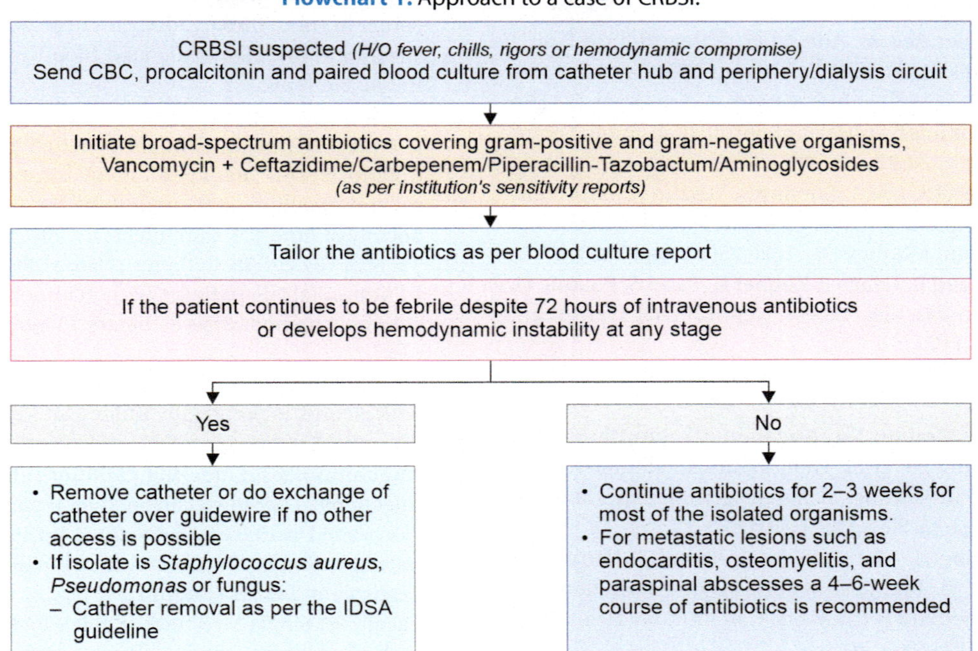

(CBC: complete blood count; CRBSI: catheter-related bloodstream infection; H/O: history of; IDSA: Infectious Diseases Society of America)

may be required to handle catheter connections. Proper handling may obviate the need for exit-site cream or catheter lock.[18]

At the time of the insertion of TCC, strict asepsis is needed. Use of gown, headwear, and sterile gloves is mandatory. Guidelines recommend daily use of antiseptic cream at the exit site till site heals well. After healing, antiseptic cream is optional. Catheter surveillance program is recommended by CDC for maintaining catheter diary and history, to pick up early infection and initiate timely treatment. Surveillance also sets goals on ways to reduce CRBSI rates.[18]

Local antiseptic cream application after each dialysis is being practiced by many centers with good results. However, for fear of antibiotic resistance, this has not turned to a formal recommendation. Medihoney application for prevention is as effective as mupirocin and comes with little fear of antibiotic resistance. The EBPG guidelines recommend antibiotic cream use after catheter insertion till complete local healing is achieved. However, routine antibiotic use at exit site is not recommended.[4]

Catheter Lock

There are several studies which suggest that routine antibiotic lock after each dialysis session lowers the risk of CRBSI. Antibiotic locks with aminoglycoside or cephalosporins can be used. Citrate, alcohol, or EDTA (ethylene diamine triacetic acid) locks possibly have additional advantage of breaking biofilm. High concentration of citrate (46.7% or 30%) can prove dangerous as its spillage in blood has been reported to cause fatal hypocalcemia and arrhythmias; therefore, a lower concentration citrate lock (4%) is most popular. Alcohol lock (60%) or sometimes 30% alcohol with 4% citrate has also been found to be promising. However, catheter manufacturer's recommendation on effect of these chemicals on catheter material should be kept in mind.[19]

CONCLUSION

Catheter-related bloodstream infection remains a dreaded complication in patients with TCC and is the leading cause of hospitalization and mortality in dialysis patients. Strict asepsis during catheter insertion and while handling is the key determinant for prevention. Exit-site antibiotic cream application and antibiotic lock seem to be beneficial, but their use has not been formalized in guidelines.

Once CRBSI is diagnosed, systemic antibiotics and antibiotic lock are the first line of treatment. Our personal experience suggests alcohol lock rather than antibiotic lock to be useful adjuncts to antibiotics for catheter salvage.

REFERENCES

1. USRDS. Vascular Access. Annual Data Report 2018. ESRD in United States: USA: USRDS; 2018. pp. 369-85.
2. Vachharajani T, Balasubramaniam J, Abraham G. The current state of interventional nephrology in India. Semin Dial. 2012;25(2):228-32.
3. Lok CE, Huber TS, Lee T, Shenoy S, Yevzlin AS, Abreo K, et al. KDOQI clinical practice guideline for vascular access: 2019 Update. Am J Kidney Dis. 2020;75(4 Suppl 2):S1-64.
4. Tordoir J, Canaud B, Haage P, Konner K, Basci A, Fouque D, et al. EBPG on Vascular Access. Nephrol Dial Transplant. 2007;22(2):88-117.
5. Ginley M, Owen A. Insertion of catheters. CARI Guidelines. 2012. pp. 1-14.
6. Bhojaraja MV, Prabhu RA, Nagaraju SP, Rao IR, Shenoy SV, Rangaswamy D, et al. Hemodialysis catheter-related bloodstream infections: A single-center experience. J Nephropharmacol. 2023;12(2):e10475.
7. Clark E, Kappel J, Mac Rae J, Dipchand C, Hiremath S, Kiaii M, et al. Practical aspects of non tunneled and tunneled hemodialysis catheters. Can J Kidney Health Dis. 2016;3:2054358116669128.
8. Al-Jaishi AA, Liu AR, Lok CE, Zhang JC, Moist LM. Complications of the arteriovenous fistula: a systematic review. J Am Soc Nephrol. 2017;28(6):1839-50.
9. Lisa M, Clark E, Dipchand C, Hiremath S, Kappel J, Kiaii M, et al. Hemodialysis Tunneled Catheter related Infections. Canadian Society of Nephrology. 2015;5:1-18.
10. Krishnan K, Kishan A, Sreedhara CG, Mythri S. Spectrum of hemodialysis catheter related blood stream infections: insights from a prospective Observational study at a tertiary center in south India. Kidney Int Rep. 2025;10(2):S720-1.
11. Treatment of Catheter-Related Bloodstream Infection. BC Renal. 2021. pp. 1-2.
12. Mermel LA, Allon M, Bouza E, Craven DE, Flynn P, O'Grady NP, et al. Clinical practice guidelines for the diagnosis and management of intravascular catheter-related infection: 2009 update by the Infectious Diseases Society of America. Clin Infect Dis. 2009;49(1):1-45.
13. Tal MG, Yevzlin AS. Catheter-related bloodstream infection in hemodialysis patients with symmetric tunneled non-side-hole hemodialysis catheters. J Vasc Access. 2023;24(4):614-9.
14. Varma P, Bajpai G. Improving catheter survival in CRBSI with alcohol lock catheter. Kidney Int Rep. 2021;6(4):273.
15. Almeida BM, Moreno DH, Vasconcelos V, Cacione DG. Interventions for treating catheter-related bloodstream infections in people receiving maintenance haemodialysis. Cochrane Database Syst Rev. 2022;4(4):CD013554.
16. Varma P, Singla M. Alcohol lock in CRBSI. Nephrol Dial Transplant. 2023;38(Suppl 1).
17. Varma PP, Singla M. Should alcohol lock replace antibiotic lock in catheter-related bloodstream infection (CRBSI) management? Kidney Week 2023; Abstract Fr-Po 482.
18. O'Grady NP, Alexander M, Burns LA, Dellinger EP, Garland J, Heard SO, et al. Healthcare Infection Control Practices Advisory Committee (HICPAC). Guidelines for the prevention of intravascular catheter-related infections. Clin Infect Dis. 2011;52(9):e162-93.
19. Inpatient antibiotic lock therapy adult guidelines. UCSF Health. 2024;1-4.

CHAPTER

25 High-flow Arteriovenous Fistula

Sneha Anna Joy, Manish Rathi

CASE SCENARIO

A 55-year-old man, a known case of chronic kidney disease (CKD) stage 5D, autosomal dominant polycystic kidney disease, on hemodialysis (HD) twice a week via left brachiocephalic arteriovenous fistula (AVF) presented to the outpatient department (OPD) with complaints of discoloration of extremities of the left upper limb, associated with symptoms of dull pain and paresthesias. Symptoms had developed slowly and progressively over many years. On examination, there was hyperpigmentation of the distal part of the left hand on both the dorsal and palmar aspects. The left brachiocephalic AVF was noted to have enlarged and tortuous veins with aneurysmal dilatation at places. The AVF thrill was felt all the way till the arm and also along veins which had developed in the forearm till the wrist. The left hand was warm to touch **(Figs. 1 and 2)**.

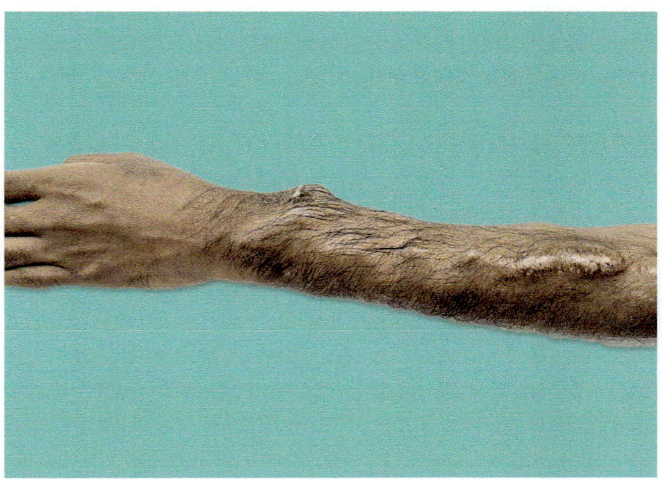

Fig. 1: Discoloration of extremities of the left upper limb.

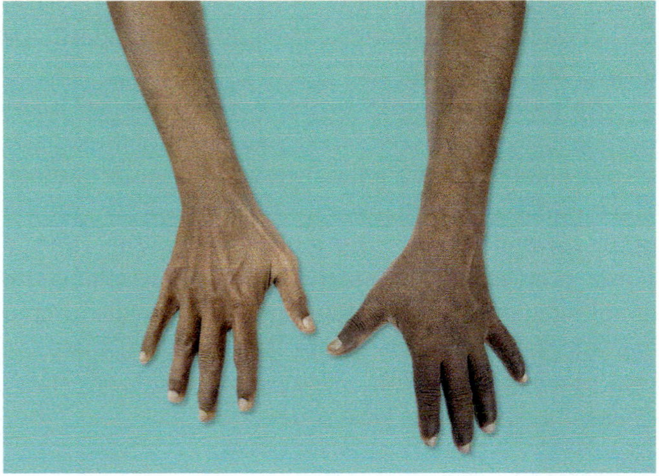

Fig. 2: Comparison between left upper limb and right upper limb.

Arteriovenous access for HD is the lifeline for any dialysis patient. However, some of these fistulas can be associated with certain complications, especially when there is increased blood flow in the AVF (Qa).[1] These complications include aneurysm formation, venous hypertension, peripheral steal phenomenon, and sometimes life-threatening complications such as cardiac failure.[2] In the above patient, based on the symptoms, the first diagnosis that we suspect is peripheral steal phenomenon with digital gangrene. But on examination, the hand is warm to touch. The discoloration was found to be due to venous eczema and he was noted to have venous hypertension secondary to a high-volume AVF. It is crucial to identify and intervene early in patients with high-volume vascular access to prevent adverse outcomes.

DEFINITION

A physiologically mature arteriovenous fistula (AVF) is defined by a blood flow in the AVF (Qa) of 500 mL/min or higher, which is the minimum required for efficient hemodialysis (HD) while maintaining arteriovenous (AV) access patency.[3] A high-volume or a high-flow AVF is a fistula with Qa greater than normal, often leading to complications. Studies have documented Qa ranging from 785 to 998 mL/min in radiocephalic AVFs and from 1,376 to 1,580 mL/min in brachial artery-based AVFs, with the latter consistently exhibiting higher Qa values than radial artery-based fistulas.[4,5] While there is no strict definition for high-flow AVFs, a Qa of 1,500 mL/min or greater, or a Qa that exceeds 20% of cardiac output, is generally accepted as a reasonable threshold.[6,7] However, certain patients with underlying comorbidities may develop symptoms at lower Qa levels, meaning that this threshold is not an absolute, and criteria should be individualized. An arbitrary guideline for blood flow ranges in typical dialysis includes low (600 mL/min), normal (600–1,500 mL/min), and high (1,500–4,000 mL/min).[8]

PATHOPHYSIOLOGY AND RISK FACTORS

Patients who have been on longstanding HD via AVFs develop fistula-related complications over time. Many of these patients develop stenotic segments at the cannulation sites and the perianastomotic areas. Some fistulas, however, become high-flow systems with arterial and venous hypertrophy. Cardiac output is the driving force, maintaining both flow and pressure within the fistula. High flow results in lumen sclerosis in some and lumen dilatation in others. Extremes of high flow will cause rapid dilation and formation of a "mega-fistula" **(Fig. 1)**. Aneurysmal dilation develops due to biologic factors, which induce outward wall remodeling, and physical factors such as wall tension, which is directly proportional to intra-access pressures.[8]

The pathophysiology of the development of high-volume AVFs thus involves the hypertrophy of the arterial system combined with a low-resistance venous outflow. The volume of flow across an AVF is dependent on the radius of the artery to the fourth power. Therefore, a 1-mm increase in lumen diameter will result in the doubling of the flow-carrying capacity. Once the arterial hypertrophy occurs, it is irreversible. Similarly, when the vein hypertrophies with aneurysmal dilation, it is also irreversible without surgical correction.[8]

CLINICAL EXAMINATION

The AVF is inspected for new or enlarging pseudoaneurysms or changes in the access topography (dips and curves) and palpated to further assess pseudoaneurysms, topography, and quality of the thrill or pulse. The fistula is auscultated for bruit and its uniformity throughout the access.[9] Some high-flow AVFs may develop into megafistulas which are identified by their dilated prominent veins.

The clinical examination will also elicit signs pertaining to the complications of these high-flow systems. High-flow AVFs sometimes lead to peripheral steal phenomenon, especially during dialysis. In these patients, the digits and the extremities on the fistula hand are colder to touch. Occasionally, some may even develop digital gangrene. If the patient has developed complications such as high output heart failure (HOHF) secondarily, clinical features pertaining to this will also be evident. If HOHF is suspected, look for elevated jugular venous pressure (JVP), evidence of fluid overload edema, lung crepitations, ascites, and S3 gallop rhythm on cardiac auscultation. The Nicoladoni–Israel–Branham sign is a finding of reflex bradycardia with fistula compression due to increased afterload.[10] It is the phenomenon in which temporary occlusion of the high-flow AVF may lead to a modest reduction in heart rate (~7 beats/min) via the vagus nerve-mediated baroreceptor reflex.

ULTRASOUND EXAMINATION

A duplex ultrasound (USG) is a noninvasive, inexpensive, and easy way to confirm the diagnosis of a high-volume AVF. The duplex USG demonstrates low-resistance flow in the feeding artery with turbulence and high-velocity flow at the anastomosis. Thickened walls and high-velocity flow are seen in the dilated draining veins of the AVF. A pseudoaneurysm, true aneurysm, or a dilated feeding artery may also be demonstrated on the USG examination.[11]

How do we examine the AVF using USG?

Use the vascular probe to map the AVF from the arterial limb, across the anastomosis and into the venous limb. The high-flow systems will often have dilated arterial and venous limbs. The diameter of the AVF at different points along its length can be measured using USG. Ensure that the probe is kept perpendicular to the blood flow in order to avoid errors. Calculate the flow using the M mode after identifying the point with maximum flow.

How do we calculate the flow volume across the AVF?

Step 1: Measure the diameter of the vein and calculate the radius **(Fig. 3)**.

Step 2: Calculate the area using the formula 3.14 × radius × radius ($A = \pi r^2$).

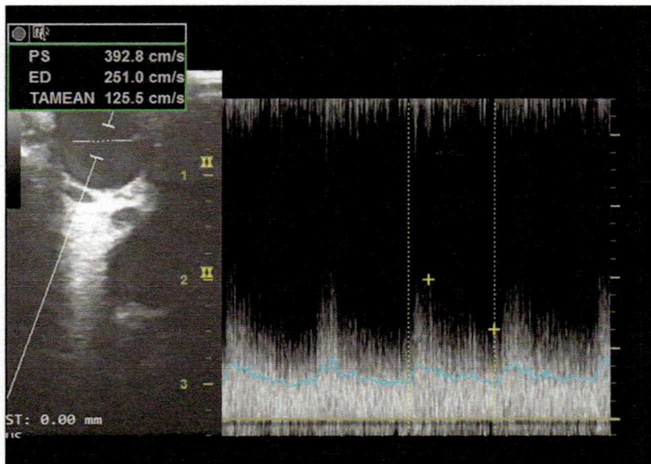

Fig. 3: Ultrasound.

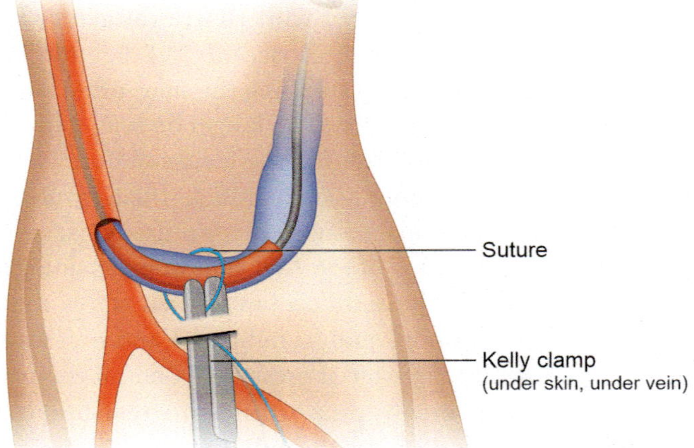

Fig. 4: MILLER (Minimally Invasive Limited Ligation Endoluminal-assisted Revision) banding.

Step 3: Using pulse-wave Doppler, measure the time average mean velocity of flow across the AVF **(Fig. 4)**. Ensure that the blood is flowing in a direction either toward or away from the USG wave. This can be done by adjusting the vascular probe to a slightly tilted angle and correction using shear angle.

Step 4: Calculate the flow volume across the AVF by multiplying the cross-sectional area with the measured time average mean velocity. This gives the flow volume per second as velocity is measured in cm/s.

Step 5: Multiply the value we get in step 4 by 60 in order to get the flow volume across the AVF in mL/min.

Flow volume (mL/min)
= Cross-sectional area (cm^2) × flow velocity (cm/s) × 60

DIAGNOSIS

Thus, a diagnosis of high-volume AVF is suspected based on the clinical examination and is confirmed with a duplex USG.

COMPLICATIONS

Cardiac Overload

Patients with high-flow AVFs can present with HOHF. Due to the short cut that the blood takes across the AVF, there is decreased peripheral resistance. To maintain blood pressure, the total circulating blood volume is increased, leading to heart failure. AVF duplex studies and flow measurements are always done at rest. With exertion, cardiac output can double or even triple. In these situations, the flow across the AVF could worsen to as much as 10–12 L/min, for example, after climbing a flight of stairs. This leads to easy precipitation of heart failure with minimal exertion.[8,12]

CARDIOPULMONARY RECIRCULATION

During dialysis treatment, fistula flow returns a high percentage of dialyzed blood to the right heart and pulmonary circulation. With the next stroke volume, a percentage of the freshly dialyzed blood will immediately be returned to the fistula. This percentage is higher in patients with high-flow AVFs and in patients with HOHF. Freshly dialyzed blood re-entering the fistula will be dialyzed again. Thus, the reduction in urea will not be as much as expected. Upper limb AVFs with Qa around 2,000 mL/min will return blood to the heart such that up to 30% of the next stroke volume and cardiac output represent already dialyzed blood. Therefore, a higher fistula flow will result in lower dialysis efficiency and a low urea reduction ratio (URR). Thus, a low URR in an otherwise "well-functioning fistula" can be indicative of a high-flow AVF.[8]

Aneurysm Growth

High flow results in dilation of the AVF lumen. When there is extreme high flow, this leads to rapid dilation and formation of a "mega-fistula" **(Fig. 1)** as described earlier. Biologic factors induce outward wall remodeling, along with physical factors such as wall tension, which in turn is determined by intra-access pressures. When a segment of the vascular wall is not exposed to needle injury, it dilates uniformly maintaining intact layers of vessel wall, namely the intima, media, and adventitia. These form true aneurysms. At points where there is repeated cannulation, there is a repeated cycle of tissue injury and healing. Frequent injury to the vascular wall replaces healthy tissue with scar formation. These points under hypervolemic pressure, undergo dilation to form pseudoaneurysms as they are unable to remodel and maintain wall thickness. Pseudoaneurysms are weak areas which are susceptible to rupture.[8]

Peripheral and Central Venous Stenosis

Pre-existing central and peripheral venous stenosis become symptomatic when high volume is introduced to the circulatory system. Over time, this may cause significant arm swelling and intra-access hypertension. Earlier, central stenoses were thought to result from previous subclavian catheters or jugular catheters. However, we now know that even in the absence of previous catheterization, stenosis can form due to the presence of hypervolemic, turbulent fistula flow near the cephalic arch. In some cases, the central stenosis may develop after many years on dialysis. This is because the high flow within the venous outflow of a high-flow AVF leads to intimal hyperplasia, which is triggered by intimal injury due to turbulent flow secondary to the high-flow volume. Such a trigger for intimal hyperplasia can be mitigated by reducing flow within the AVF.[8]

Peripheral Steal

High-flow AVFs will cause significant shunting of blood from the artery. The blood flow to the extremity distal to the AVF will thus be compromised especially during dialysis treatment. The patient will have symptoms of cold extremities, bluish discoloration of digits, neuropathy, muscle cramps, and wasting. In rare cases, distal digital gangrene may develop.[13]

Venous Hypertension

High-volume AVF may in certain patients cause venous hypertension of the involved limb, especially when there is an absolute or relative stenosis at the cephalic arch. This may cause edema of the limb and symptoms of venous congestion. Venous eczema may also develop.

MANAGEMENT

Medical Management

Medical management involves strict control of blood pressure and optimization of cardiac medications in order to improve heart failure. Management is similar to that in other end-stage kidney disease patients with heart failure.

Surgical Management

Although some high-volume AVFs are asymptomatic, eventually they may lead to complications such as heart failure, aneurysms, central vein stenosis, and peripheral steal syndrome. The decision for surgical intervention should be made after careful medical optimization, especially in patients with high output cardiopulmonary compromise.[6] Right heart catheterization can be used to evaluate cardiac hemodynamics at rest and with the occlusion of the AVF to evaluate volume status, pulmonary artery pressures, and cardiac output to guide the management.[12]

There are two major approaches to surgically treating AVFs, especially if associated with HOHF refractory to diuretics: Ligation and flow restriction. AVF ligation or closure involves completely stopping the flow, often with excision of the AVF. The AVF will no longer be available for further dialysis, and so this is not the ideal solution. Flow restriction is most commonly via banding, which involves the creation of a surgical stenosis within the AV access site to reduce the radius of the AVF. Banding physiology is best explained by Poiseuille's law, which states that fluid flow (Q) is proportional to radius (r) and pressure across a gradient (ΔP) (Arterial pressure – Central venous pressure) and inversely proportional to resistances. Banding techniques decrease the radius at a specific point, thus decreasing the flow.[8] The challenge is to achieve the correct diameter which ensures adequate dialysis while correcting the high flow simultaneously, ensuring that the bands are not too tight. Tight bands lead to poor dialysis efficiency, and stenosis and thrombosis of the AVF.

Different Methods of Flow Restriction

The *Minimally Invasive Limited Ligation Endoluminal-assisted Revision* (MILLER) banding procedure **(Fig. 4)** is a flow-restrictive banding which uses a balloon to achieve the precise amount of narrowing.[12] It overcomes the inherent difficulties of sizing by using a 3- or 4-mm diameter intraluminal balloon as a sizing dowel. With the inflated appropriately sized balloon in the vessel, subcutaneous 2-0 Prolene sutures are tied around the outside of the vessel. The intraluminal balloon ensures that the end-lumen diameter is precise and predictable. If finally the bands are too tight, they can be stretched or

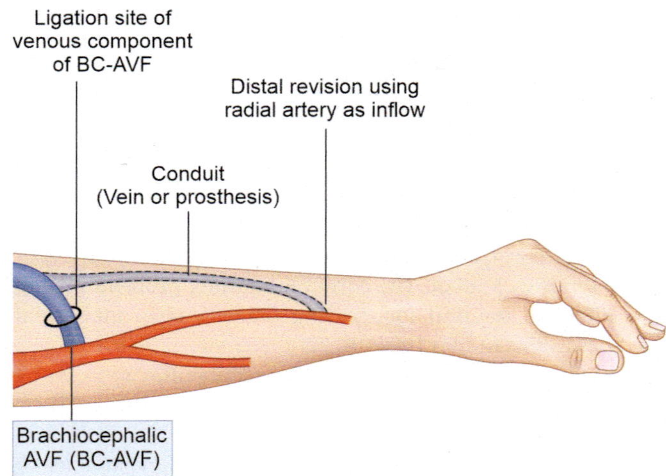

Fig. 5: Revision Using Distal Inflow.

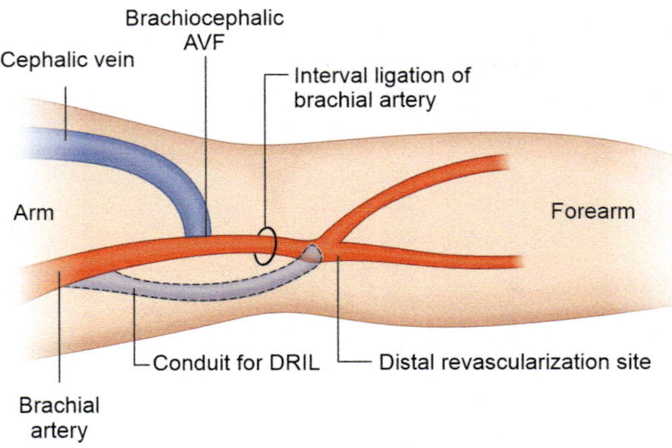

Fig. 6: DRIL (Distal Revascularization with Interval Ligation) procedure.

even broken using a bigger balloon using an angioplasty technique. If a band is too loose, the procedure is easily repeated because it is minimally invasive. The MILLER procedure can be safely performed in an outpatient setting.[8] Studies show up to 94% immediate success with the MILLER technique of banding in patients with high-flow AVFs.[13]

The *Revision Using Distal Inflow (RUDI) technique* **(Fig. 5)** is based on the theory that access flow will decrease once inflow is provided by a smaller caliber forearm artery. Tortuous AVFs may allow this intervention without the need for an additional conduit, but often harvesting of the saphenous vein or the use of a prosthetic graft is required.[14] This technique is an open salvage procedure in which the AVF is ligated at its origin from the venous limb. The distal radial/ulnar artery is then used as the inflow, which is anastomosed to the venous end of the ligated AVF using a saphenous or basilic vein graft or a prosthesis as a conduit to reach the venous end of the original AVF.[15] Studies show an 82% successful outcome in patients treated with the RUDI technique for correction of high-flow AVF, over a 12-month follow-up period.[15]

Distal Revascularization with Interval Ligation (DRIL) **(Fig. 6)** is a procedure to treat symptomatic ischemic steal but has been noted to decrease the Qa in high-flow AVFs. In this procedure, a bypass graft is inserted with its origin from the AVF artery above the AVF and it ends with an end-to-side anastomosis again to the same artery, but distal to the AVF, thus achieving distal revascularization. Interval ligation is the simple cutting and tying of the AVF artery distal to the AVF but proximal to the bypass graft anastomosis.[16] Thus, DRIL involves revision using distal inflow, which involves ligating the fistula and then reattaching it more distally with jump grafts.[12] Most studies done on the DRIL method have used improvement in distal hypoperfusion as the study outcome. Further studies or secondary analyses need to be done in order to analyze the efficacy of the DRIL procedure in reducing the flow in high-flow AVFs.

CONCLUSION

High-flow AVFs are often an under-recognized yet significant cause for heart failure among patients on HD. They can also cause other complications such as central vein stenosis, aneurysmal dilatations of AVF, and distal steal. The management of high-flow AVFs usually involves the medical management of HOHF. The decision regarding surgical correction needs to be taken on an individualized basis weighing both patient factors and the expertise of the vascular team.

REFERENCES

1. Basile C, Lomonte C. The complex relationship among arteriovenous access, heart, and circulation. Semin Dial. 2018;31(1):15-20.
2. House AA, Wanner C, Sarnak MJ, Piña IL, McIntyre CW, Komenda P, et al. Heart failure in chronic kidney disease: conclusions from a Kidney Disease: Improving Global Outcomes (KDIGO) Controversies Conference. Kidney Int. 2019;95(6):1304-17.
3. Beathard GA, Lok CE, Glickman MH, Al-Jaishi AA, Bednarski D, Cull DL, et al. Definitions and End Points for Interventional Studies for Arteriovenous Dialysis Access. Clin J Am Soc Nephrol CJASN. 2018;13(3):501-12.

4. Basile C, Lomonte C, Vernaglione L, Casucci F, Antonelli M, Losurdo N. The relationship between the flow of arteriovenous fistula and cardiac output in haemodialysis patients. Nephrol Dial Transplant Off Publ Eur Dial Transpl Assoc - Eur Ren Assoc. 2008;23(1):282-7.
5. Aitken E, Kerr D, Geddes C, Berry C, Kingsmore D. Cardiovascular changes occurring with occlusion of a mature arteriovenous fistula. J Vasc Access. 2015;16(6): 459-66.
6. Sequeira A, Tan TW. Complications of a high-flow access and its management. Semin Dial. 2015;28(5):533-43.
7. Saleh MA, El Kilany WM, Keddis VW, El Said TW. Effect of high flow arteriovenous fistula on cardiac function in hemodialysis patients. Egypt Heart J. 2018;70(4):337-41.
8. Miller GA, Hwang WW. Challenges and management of high-flow arteriovenous fistulae. Semin Nephrol. 2012;32(6):545-50.
9. Schuman E, Ronfeld A, Barclay C, Heinl P. Comparison of clinical assessment with ultrasound flow for hemodialysis access surveillance. Arch Surg. 2007;142(12):1129-33.
10. Jayroe H, Foley K. Arteriovenous Fistula. In: StatPearls [Internet]. Treasure Island (FL): StatPearls Publishing; 2024 [cited 2024 Dec 14]. Available from: http://www.ncbi.nlm.nih.gov/books/NBK559213/ [Last accessed June, 2025].
11. Davison BD, Polak JF. Arterial injuries: a sonographic approach. Radiol Clin North Am. 2004;42(2):383-96.
12. Chang RS, Hu JR, Beckman JA, Forbes RC, Shawar SH, Concepcion BP. High output heart failure associated with arteriovenous fistula in the setting of kidney transplantation. Kidney Int Rep. 2020;6(2):544-51.
13. Miller GA, Goel N, Friedman A, Khariton A, Jotwani MC, Savransky Y, et al. The MILLER banding procedure is an effective method for treating dialysis-associated steal syndrome. Kidney Int. 2010;77(4):359-66.
14. Mallios A, Jennings WC. Endovascular Revision Using Distal Inflow: EndoRUDI. Eur J Vasc Endovasc Surg. 2020;60(1):144.
15. Kordzadeh A, Garzon LAN, Parsa AD. Revision using distal inflow for the treatment of dialysis access steal syndrome: A Systematic Review. Ann Vasc Dis. 2018;11(4): 473-8.
16. Field M, Blackwell J, Jaipersad A, Wall M, Silva M, Morgan R, et al. Distal revascularisation with interval ligation (DRIL): an experience. Ann R Coll Surg Engl. 2009;91(5):394-8.

CHAPTER

26 Stenosis or Thrombosis of Vascular Access

26.1 CENTRAL VEINS

Gireesh Reddy G, Sahil Arora, Cherin Josi C, Sumiran Mahajan, Dwarak S, Dileep Kumar P

DEFINITION AND CLINICAL SIGNIFICANCE OF CENTRAL VEIN STENOSIS AND THROMBOSIS[1-5]

- Central vein stenosis (CVS) refers to the pathological narrowing or occlusion of the large veins within the thoracic cavity, including the superior vena cava (SVC), brachiocephalic veins, subclavian veins, and jugular veins.
- Thrombosis describes the formation of a blood clot within these vessels, which can partially or completely obstruct blood flow.
- Clinically, CVS and thrombosis represent critical complications, particularly in patients with chronic kidney disease (CKD) requiring long-term hemodialysis.
- The clinical significance of CVS and thrombosis is profound, given their potential to severely compromise vascular access sites, vital for dialysis procedures.
- Patients with CVS often present with significant morbidity including debilitating symptoms such as upper limb swelling, venous hypertension, dyspnea, chest wall collateral vein enlargement, and recurrent vascular access dysfunction.
- CVS directly impacts a patient's quality of life (QoL) and survival by limiting dialysis efficacy and increasing procedural complexity and healthcare utilization.
- Recognizing and managing CVS and thrombosis early and effectively are paramount to sustaining adequate dialysis therapy, reducing hospitalization rates, and ultimately improving patient outcomes and QoL.

EPIDEMIOLOGY: PREVALENCE AND INCIDENCE IN DIALYSIS AND NONDIALYSIS POPULATIONS[6-8]

Global Overview

Central vein stenosis and thrombosis are significant complications in patients requiring central venous access, particularly those undergoing hemodialysis. Globally, the prevalence of CVS among hemodialysis patients ranges from *16% to more than 40%*, with higher rates observed in individuals with prolonged catheter use and multiple catheter insertions. The incidence of new-onset CVS in this population is approximately *7–10% per year*, with thrombosis complicating CVS occurring at a rate of *5–10% per year*.

Indian Context

In India, the epidemiology of CVS and thrombosis among hemodialysis patients reflects both global trends and region-specific factors:

- *Prevalence:* A prospective observational study conducted at a tertiary care center in South India reported a *13.1% prevalence* of CVS among 152 patients on maintenance hemodialysis. The brachiocephalic vein was the most commonly affected site, accounting for *65%* of cases.
- *Risk factors:* The high prevalence of CVS in Indian hemodialysis patients is attributed to factors such as emergency presentations necessitating temporary catheter insertions.

Implications for Practice

The Indian data underscore the need for:

- *Early planning:* Timely creation of arteriovenous fistulas to minimize catheter dependence
- *Surveillance:* Regular monitoring for signs of CVS in high-risk patients, including those with a history of central venous catheterization
- *Preventive strategies:* Adoption of best practices for catheter insertion and maintenance to reduce the incidence of CVS and thrombosis.

Risk Factors Influencing Epidemiology

- *Duration and site of catheter placement:* Subclavian veins are most commonly involved due to anatomical constraints and catheter-induced endothelial trauma.
- *Type and frequency of interventions:* Recurrent interventions and prolonged use of temporary catheters significantly increase the risk.
- *Demographic factors:* Age, diabetes, obesity, smoking status, hypercoagulability states, malignancy, and inflammatory conditions may elevate risk.

Geographic and Demographic Variability

- Slight geographical variations are noted, possibly linked to regional differences in vascular access practices and clinical guidelines.
- No significant gender predisposition; however, elderly patients and those with higher body mass index (BMI) appear to have modestly increased risks.

RISK FACTORS FOR CENTRAL VEIN STENOSIS AND THROMBOSIS

Understanding risk factors for CVS and thrombosis is critical for prevention, early identification, and effective management. Several key risk factors significantly contribute to the development and progression of CVS, as given in the following text.

Central Venous Catheters

Central venous catheters (CVCs) represent the single most important modifiable risk factor for CVS and thrombosis, especially in dialysis patients.

- *Duration of catheterization:*
  - Prolonged dwell times significantly increase endothelial trauma, inflammation, and fibrosis.
  - Catheter use exceeding 90 days markedly escalates the risk, with stenosis prevalence approaching 50% after prolonged catheterization, particularly via subclavian veins.
- *Site of catheter placement:*
  - Subclavian vein catheterization has the highest risk due to anatomical constraints (clavicle and first rib compression).[9]
  - Internal jugular vein (IJV) catheterization, though relatively safer, still poses a considerable risk, especially with repeated insertions.
- *Multiple and emergency insertions:*
  - Frequent catheter insertions and emergency placements increase endothelial damage, resulting in inflammation, hyperplasia, and eventual stenosis formation.
  - Each catheter insertion significantly compounds risk.
- *Catheter size and material:*
  - Larger bore and stiffer catheters cause more endothelial injury, enhancing stenosis likelihood.
  - Catheter materials with higher stiffness or lack of biocompatibility amplify endothelial injury.

Pacemaker and Implantable Cardioverter-defibrillator Leads[10,11]

Pacemaker and implantable cardioverter-defibrillator (ICD) leads positioned within central veins represent an important risk factor due to sustained mechanical trauma.

- *Mechanical trauma:*
  - Constant contact of device leads with vein walls induces endothelial injury, fibrosis, and stenosis.
  - Long-term presence (years to decades) exponentially increases the risk of stenosis and thrombosis.
- *Inflammatory response:* Foreign body reaction around leads further exacerbates vessel wall damage and fibrosis, predisposing to thrombosis and stenosis.
- *Lead number and configuration:* Multiple-lead configurations (such as dual-chamber or biventricular pacing) increase vessel wall irritation, heightening the stenosis risk.

Previous Interventions and Procedures

- *Repeated angioplasty or stenting:*
  - Repeated endovascular interventions create cumulative endothelial injury and intimal hyperplasia.
  - Recurrent procedures strongly correlate with accelerated stenosis and restenosis rates, emphasizing the need for careful intervention planning.

- *Surgical procedures:*
    - Prior thoracic surgeries, especially those involving venous reconstruction or manipulation, significantly increase the risk of CVS.
    - Scarring, altered vessel anatomy, and postoperative inflammation are key contributors.
- *Radiation therapy:* Thoracic radiation for malignancies leads to vascular endothelial injury, inflammation, and accelerated fibrosis, significantly elevating stenosis risk.

Patient-specific Risk Factors[12,13]

Several intrinsic patient-related factors can independently predispose to CVS and thrombosis:

- *Age:* Older patients exhibit greater endothelial vulnerability and decreased reparative capacity, elevating risk.
- *Hypercoagulability:* Conditions such as inherited thrombophilia, malignancies, nephrotic syndrome, or inflammatory diseases enhance thrombotic risk.
- *Diabetes mellitus and obesity:* These conditions promote chronic inflammation and endothelial dysfunction, substantially increasing CVS risk.
- *Smoking:* Tobacco use induces systemic inflammation and endothelial injury, potentiating stenosis and thrombosis development.
- *Hemodialysis-specific factors:* In dialysis patients, additional unique factors play critical roles:
    - *High-flow arteriovenous access:* Arteriovenous fistulas or grafts with very high blood flow cause turbulent flow and endothelial trauma within the central veins, increasing stenosis formation.
    - *Hyperdynamic circulation:* Dialysis patients often exhibit hyperdynamic circulation, leading to persistent endothelial shear stress and vessel remodeling.
    - *Uremia and calcium-phosphate disorders:* Uremic toxins, altered calcium-phosphate metabolism, and chronic inflammation foster accelerated vascular calcification and stenosis.

CLINICAL MANAGEMENT IMPLICATIONS[14,15]

Understanding these hemodynamic alterations guides clinical management toward:

- Early recognition and intervention in CVS to maintain optimal dialysis efficacy[15]
- Careful hemodynamic monitoring (e.g., access pressures, recirculation tests) to detect and manage complications proactively
- Judicious selection of access placement sites to minimize hemodynamic sequelae
- Aggressive management of stenosis through timely balloon angioplasty or stenting, reducing the likelihood of downstream hemodynamic consequences.

CLINICAL PRESENTATION

Central vein stenosis and thrombosis have distinct clinical manifestations resulting primarily from impaired venous drainage, venous hypertension, and secondary hemodynamic alterations. Recognizing these presentations promptly is crucial to initiating appropriate diagnostic and therapeutic measures.

Symptoms

Patients typically present with symptoms reflective of increased venous pressure and impaired venous drainage, commonly including the following:

- *Extremity edema:*
    - Often unilateral, involving the arm on the side of vascular access or catheter placement
    - In advanced cases, bilateral edema may develop due to central venous occlusion at the confluence points of brachiocephalic veins or SVC
    - Edema may progressively worsen during dialysis sessions due to increased venous return through dialysis access.[16]
- *Venous hypertension:*
    - Clinically evident as prominent, tortuous superficial veins on the upper extremity, chest wall, and shoulders due to collateral circulation attempting to bypass central obstruction
    - Elevated venous pressure measurements in dialysis circuits (>200 mm Hg) strongly suggest CVS.[17,18]
- *Dilated chest-wall veins:*
    - Visible dilatation of collateral veins on the chest and upper abdomen (often termed "caput medusae")
    - Indicates chronicity and severity of stenosis or occlusion.[19]
- *Facial swelling and plethora:*[20]
    - Noticeable puffiness of the face, neck, and periorbital region
    - Often aggravated by recumbent positions, due to gravity-dependent venous return obstruction

  - Severe forms may present as cyanosis or facial plethora (reddening due to venous engorgement).
- *Respiratory distress:*[21]
  - Dyspnea or shortness of breath, primarily due to elevated central venous pressure causing pulmonary congestion and pleural effusions
  - Patients may report exacerbation of respiratory symptoms when lying down (orthopnea), reflecting increased thoracic venous pressure.

Differential Diagnoses[22-25]

Clinical manifestations of CVS may overlap significantly with other conditions, requiring careful differentiation.

- *Superior vena cava syndrome (SVCS):*
  - Presents with upper-body edema, facial swelling, cyanosis, and respiratory distress
  - Commonly secondary to extrinsic compression by tumors or mediastinal masses rather than intrinsic venous stenosis
  - Radiological imaging and patient history (malignancy) help differentiate from dialysis-associated CVS.
- *Thoracic outlet syndrome (TOS):*
  - Occurs due to compression of the neurovascular structures passing through the thoracic outlet (first rib, clavicle, and scalene muscles)
  - Patients present predominantly with positional symptoms, arm paresthesia, weakness, or intermittent edema worsened by overhead activity.
  - Typically diagnosed via provocative maneuvers and imaging studies demonstrating extrinsic compression.
- *Congestive heart failure (CHF):*
  - May present similarly with facial and peripheral edema, pleural effusions, and shortness of breath
  - Differentiation is primarily clinical, based on a detailed cardiovascular history (cardiac disease, reduced ejection fraction), echocardiography findings, and elevated cardiac biomarkers [e.g., brain natriuretic peptide (BNP)].
- *Deep vein thrombosis (DVT) of upper extremities:*
  - Presents with sudden onset of painful swelling of the affected extremity
  - Typically identified using duplex ultrasound imaging
  - Clinical history and imaging help distinguish isolated extremity DVT from central venous obstruction.

Clinical Evaluation and Importance

Early recognition and appropriate differentiation from similar clinical entities are crucial for optimal therapeutic intervention. Clinicians must maintain high suspicion, especially in dialysis patients or individuals with CVCs/devices, to reduce complications and ensure effective dialysis.

DIAGNOSTIC APPROACH

- Clinical evaluation and physical examination
- *Noninvasive modalities:*
  - Duplex ultrasonography: Diagnostic role and limitations
  - Magnetic resonance venography (MRV)
  - Computed tomography venography (CTV)
- *Invasive modalities:*
  - Digital subtraction venography (DSV): Gold standard
  - Pressure gradient measurements

Clinical Evaluation and Physical Examination

The diagnostic journey begins with a meticulous clinical evaluation:

- *Detailed history:*
  - Assessment of previous catheter placements, dialysis history, pacemaker implantation, and prior vascular interventions
  - Documentation of symptom onset, progression, severity, and positional variations
- *Physical examination:*
  - Inspection for visible edema of the extremities, face, and neck
  - Evaluation for collateral venous circulation: Dilated chest-wall veins (indicative of chronic obstruction)
  - Palpation and auscultation of dialysis access sites to assess for pulsation, thrill, and bruit changes (loss of thrill or bruit suggests dysfunction)
  - Assessment for signs of venous hypertension: Persistent swelling, cyanosis, or facial plethora
  - Measurement of arm circumference to quantify edema severity objectively

Invasive Modalities[26,27]

Invasive diagnostic methods offer definitive evaluation and precise characterization of CVS:

Digital Subtraction Venography—Gold Standard

- *Diagnostic role:*
  - Remains the definitive gold standard for diagnosing central venous stenosis
  - Real-time, high-resolution visualization of central venous anatomy, precise determination of stenosis severity, and identification of collateral circulation
  - Essential for interventional planning, offering immediate opportunity for simultaneous therapeutic interventions
- *Procedure:*
  - Typically performed via femoral or peripheral vein puncture
  - Contrast administration under fluoroscopy allows detailed visualization of central veins and associated stenosis or occlusion
- *Advantages:*
  - Immediate confirmation of stenosis or thrombosis.
  - Allows concurrent intervention (angioplasty, stenting)
- *Limitations:*
  - Invasive, involving risk of bleeding, infection, contrast-induced reactions, and radiation exposure
  - Operator expertise critical for accurate interpretation and safe intervention.

Pressure Gradient Measurements

- *Diagnostic role:*
  - Provides objective hemodynamic confirmation of clinically significant stenosis
  - Measures trans-stenotic pressure gradients to quantitatively assess stenosis severity.
- *Clinical criteria:*
  - A significant pressure gradient typically defined as ≥5–10 mm Hg across a lesion, confirming hemodynamic importance
  - Correlates well with symptomatic venous hypertension and clinical severity.
- *Advantages:*
  - Objective and quantifiable evidence of lesion severity
  - Aids clinical decision-making regarding intervention.
- *Limitations:*
  - Requires invasive catheter placement
  - Affected by systemic hemodynamic variations during the measurement.

Practical Diagnostic Algorithm (Recommended Clinical Approach)

A logical, stepwise approach to diagnosis is as follows:

- *Clinical suspicion (history, symptoms, physical exam):* Identify high-risk patients (dialysis access dysfunction, prior catheters, pacemaker devices).
- *Initial noninvasive assessment (duplex ultrasound):* Quick preliminary assessment to exclude thrombosis or localized peripheral stenosis.
- *Confirmatory imaging (MRV or CTV):* Clarifies stenosis severity, extent, anatomy, and collateral circulation prior to invasive planning.
- *Definitive diagnostic evaluation (DSV with pressure measurements):* Gold standard for final confirmation, intervention planning, and execution.

MANAGEMENT STRATEGIES

- Indications for watchful waiting
- *Medical therapy:* Anticoagulants, antiplatelet agents
- *Preventive measures:* Minimizing central catheter use, catheter care protocols.

Conservative Management

Conservative management forms the foundational approach to CVS, especially in patients with mild or asymptomatic lesions. It involves careful monitoring, medical therapy, and targeted preventive strategies aimed at delaying disease progression, reducing symptoms, and minimizing the need for invasive interventions.

Indications for Watchful Waiting (Observation)

Watchful waiting or conservative monitoring is recommended under specific clinical scenarios:

Clinical criteria:

- *Asymptomatic stenosis:* Incidentally detected stenosis without associated clinical symptoms or hemodynamic complications
- *Mild symptoms:* Mild, transient swelling or minimal venous hypertension symptoms without significant interference with dialysis function
- *Stable hemodynamics:* Stenosis does not significantly impair dialysis flow rates or cause substantial access dysfunction (venous pressure <200 mm Hg).

Rationale:

- Intervening prematurely in asymptomatic or minimally symptomatic stenosis may accelerate recurrent restenosis due to procedural injury, potentially exacerbating vascular complications.

- Regular monitoring ensures timely identification of symptom progression or hemodynamic deterioration, prompting intervention at the appropriate time.

Recommended surveillance protocols:

- Regular clinical follow-ups (every 3–6 months)
- Periodic duplex ultrasonography to monitor venous flow and lesion progression
- Monitoring dialysis parameters (venous pressures, blood flow rates, recirculation studies).

Medical Therapy: Anticoagulants and Antiplatelet Agents

Medical therapy complements conservative management by reducing thrombotic risk, especially important in high-risk patients or those with recurrent thrombotic complications.

Anticoagulants [heparin, low molecular weight heparins, warfarin, direct oral anticoagulants (DOACs)]:

- *Indications:*
    - Known hypercoagulable states (inherited/acquired thrombophilias)
    - History of recurrent thrombosis associated with CVCs or devices
- *Mechanism of action:* Prevent thrombin formation, fibrin stabilization, and propagation of thrombus.
- *Clinical evidence:* Routine anticoagulation reduces catheter-related thrombosis risk but is balanced against bleeding risks, particularly in dialysis populations.
- *Cautions and monitoring:*
    - Requires careful monitoring [prothrombin time/international normalized ratio (PT/INR) for warfarin, renal function for DOACs]
    - Consider bleeding risk, especially important postdialysis due to prolonged hemostasis.

Antiplatelet agents (aspirin, clopidogrel):

- *Indications:*
    - High-risk patients for stenosis progression or thrombosis with minimal bleeding risk
    - After angioplasty or stenting to prevent early restenosis/thrombosis
- *Mechanism of action:* Inhibit platelet aggregation, activation, and thrombus formation
- *Clinical evidence:* Evidence is mixed; aspirin or clopidogrel may reduce thrombosis and restenosis risk postintervention.
- *Cautions and monitoring:* Monitor for bleeding complications, particularly gastrointestinal bleeding or prolonged access-site bleeding post dialysis.

Guideline recommendations:

- Individualize anticoagulant/antiplatelet therapy based on risk–benefit analysis considering thrombosis versus bleeding risk.
- Consider routine aspirin/clopidogrel following stent placement, typically for 1–6 months, guided by clinical judgment.

Preventive Measures[14,28]

Preventing central venous stenosis and thrombosis is paramount, particularly in dialysis patients, who are inherently at higher risk.

Minimizing central venous catheter use:

- *Early fistula creation:*
    - Early referral for native AV fistula placement, reducing catheter dependency.
    - National Kidney Foundation's KDOQI guidelines advocate early AV fistula creation (Stage IV CKD) to reduce CVS risk.
- *Avoid subclavian vein catheterization:*
    - Subclavian sites demonstrate the highest risk of stenosis due to anatomical and mechanical constraints.
    - Preferred sites are IJV, associated with lower stenosis risks.

Optimal catheter management protocols:[29-32]

- *Catheter insertion techniques:*
    - Real-time ultrasound guidance for accurate placement, reducing multiple punctures and endothelial trauma
    - Strict aseptic technique using sterile ultrasound gel and advanced biodefense formulations like SQ53 to minimize infection risk, indirectly reducing thrombosis risk.
- *Routine catheter care:*
    - Proper catheter securement to prevent mechanical injury
    - Regular flushing protocols to maintain catheter patency and minimize thrombotic complications
    - Use of citrate-based lock solutions or low-dose heparin lock protocols to prevent catheter-related thrombosis.

Patient and staff education:

- Training dialysis nurses and medical staff regarding optimal catheter management and care

- Patient education about signs of catheter-related complications and proper catheter care practices.

Endovascular Interventions

Endovascular interventions constitute the primary treatment for clinically significant CVS, aiming to restore venous patency, alleviate symptoms, optimize dialysis efficacy, and improve QoL **(Table 1)**.

Balloon Angioplasty[33,34]

Percutaneous transluminal balloon angioplasty (PTBA) is the cornerstone and initial therapeutic choice for symptomatic central venous stenosis.

Technique:

Access and imaging:
- Typically performed through femoral or peripheral veins
- Diagnostic venography to clearly define lesion anatomy and severity

Procedure:
- Guidewire placement across the stenotic lesion under fluoroscopic guidance
- A balloon catheter is advanced over the wire, inflated at high pressure (typically 8–20 atm) to mechanically disrupt intimal hyperplasia and dilate the lesion.

Postdilatation assessment: Venography and pressure gradients postdilatation confirm technical success, ideally achieving minimal residual stenosis (<30%) and pressure gradients ≤3 mm Hg.

TABLE 1: Types of refractory stenosis and their first-line and second-line techniques.

Indication	First-line technique	Second-line technique
Short-segment refractory stenosis	Direct reconstruction (anastomosis)	Venous bypass
Long-segment refractory stenosis	Venous bypass	Segmental reconstruction (patch angioplasty)
Total occlusion refractory to CTO	Venous bypass or segmental reconstruction	Hybrid surgical–endovascular approach

(CTO: chronic total occlusion)

Indications:
- Symptomatic CVS (upper limb edema, venous hypertension, dialysis dysfunction)
- First-line therapy due to minimally invasive nature and immediate symptom relief potential.

Outcomes:
- Technical success rates are high (85–95%).
- Immediate clinical relief from symptoms and significant hemodynamic improvement are often achieved.

Limitations:
- *Elastic recoil:* Immediate postprocedure recoil (elastic recoil) can limit durable vessel dilation.
- *Restenosis rates:*
  - High recurrence rates (40–70%) within 6–12 months due to ongoing endothelial injury and neointimal hyperplasia
  - Frequent repeat interventions often necessary, influencing patient morbidity and healthcare resources.

Stenting[35,36]

Stenting provides scaffold support to maintain patency following suboptimal balloon angioplasty results or recurrent stenosis.

Indications:
- Failure of balloon angioplasty (residual stenosis >30% or rapid recurrence)
- Long-segment stenoses or lesions refractory to angioplasty alone
- Recurrent stenosis causing repeated symptomatic presentations.

Choice of stents:
- *Self-expanding stents:*
  - Preferred for central venous use due to superior flexibility and adaptability to vessel diameter changes
  - Wallstent (braided stainless steel) is commonly used.
- *Balloon-expandable stents:*
  - Less flexible, mainly reserved for rigid, short segments or cases requiring precise deployment
  - Increased risk of fracture or deformation due to venous anatomical movements.

Outcomes and patency rates:

- Technical success rates exceed 95%.
- Improved primary patency compared to angioplasty alone (50–70% at 6–12 months)
- Secondary patency (following repeat interventions) typically exceeds 80% at 12 months.

Risks of restenosis:

- Neointimal hyperplasia through stent interstices
- Stent fractures and deformation due to mechanical stress
- Potential thrombosis, necessitating long-term antiplatelet or anticoagulant therapy.

Advanced Techniques for Chronic Total Occlusion[36-42]

Chronic total occlusion (CTO) presents unique challenges, requiring specialized advanced interventional techniques to successfully recanalize totally occluded central veins.

- *Sharp recanalization:*
  - *Technique:* Dedicated sharp-tipped devices or needles (e.g., Colapinto, Rösch-Uchida needle) to traverse tough, fibrotic occlusions
  - *Application:* Effective when standard wire techniques fail
  - *Limitation:* Higher risk of vessel perforation, requiring expert hands
- *Radiofrequency (RF) wire perforation (PowerWire®, Baylis RF system):*
  - *Technique:* RF energy delivered through specialized wires allowing controlled passage through dense fibrotic lesions
  - *Advantage:* Precise, controlled perforation minimizing vessel injury
  - *Limitations:* Requires specialized equipment, cost implications, expert use
- *Laser recanalization (excimer laser):*
  - *Technique:* Uses high-energy laser pulses to vaporize and fragment fibrotic and thrombotic occlusions
  - *Advantages:* Effective in calcified, fibrotic, and thrombus-rich occlusions.
  - *Limitations:* Risk of vessel perforation or dissection, high cost, specialized operator training required
- *Retrograde approaches:*
  - *Technique:* Approach occlusions from the opposite direction (e.g., from dialysis access sites retrogradely)
  - *Advantage:* High technical success for challenging CTO lesions refractory to antegrade recanalization
  - *Clinical applications:* Complex SVC or brachiocephalic vein occlusions with significant collateral circulation
- *Intravascular ultrasound (IVUS)-guided procedures:*
  - *Technique:* Real-time IVUS imaging guides wire advancement, ensuring luminal positioning and avoiding perforation.
  - *Advantages:* Enhanced visualization of vessel structure, precise lesion characterization, and improved procedural safety.
  - *Clinical applications:* Complex CTO cases where fluoroscopic visualization alone is inadequate.
  - *CrossBoss/Stingray System:* Facilitates precise controlled re-entry into true lumen, particularly useful in complex lesions
  - *Outback® catheter:* Needle-based device allowing controlled vessel re-entry, highly effective in tough occlusions
- *Hybrid techniques:*
  - Combining multiple advanced techniques (e.g., antegrade/retrograde approach, sharp recanalization plus IVUS, re-entry devices).
  - Maximizes procedural success, minimizes risk.

CLINICAL RECOMMENDATIONS AND ALGORITHMIC APPROACH

- *Initial approach:* Balloon angioplasty for uncomplicated, short-segment stenosis
- *Recurrent or refractory stenosis:* Consider stenting
- *Complex or total occlusions (CTO):* Advanced techniques (sharp recanalization, retrograde approaches, IVUS guidance, hybrid methods) in specialized centers by experienced interventionalists
- Long-term patient outcomes hinge upon meticulous technique selection, appropriate patient selection, and vigilant postprocedural management strategies (antiplatelet or anticoagulation protocols, close surveillance for restenosis).

SURGICAL OPTIONS FOR CENTRAL VEIN STENOSIS AND THROMBOSIS

Endovascular interventions have dramatically advanced the management of CVS; however, surgery remains essential for patients in whom these minimally invasive approaches are unsuccessful, contraindicated, or unsuitable. Surgical management, while more invasive, offers definitive and durable solutions in selected complex cases, thereby playing a vital role in comprehensive care.

Indications for Surgical Intervention[43]

Surgical treatment is reserved for specific clinical scenarios wherein endovascular interventions have been exhausted or cannot be safely pursued:

- *Endovascular intervention failure:*
  - Repeated failure of balloon angioplasty or stenting
  - Severe restenosis refractory to multiple endovascular attempts
  - Technical impossibility to cross CTOs despite advanced interventional techniques
- *Contraindications to endovascular procedures:*
  - Severe contrast allergy or severe anaphylactic reactions
  - Critical renal insufficiency with contraindication to contrast administration
  - Patients with prohibitive bleeding risks or complex anatomical considerations
- *Long-segment occlusion:*
  - Extensive lesions or complex anatomical deformities involving large segments of central veins
  - Occlusion involving significant segments of the SVC or bilateral brachiocephalic veins

Surgical Techniques

Meticulous surgical expertise and careful preoperative planning form the cornerstone of successful venous reconstruction surgery. Two primary surgical approaches dominate clinical practice: (1) Venous bypass surgery and (2) venous reconstruction (direct surgical repair).

Venous Bypass Surgery

Venous bypass creates an alternative conduit around severely stenotic or occluded venous segments, restoring efficient venous drainage and relieving venous hypertension:

Technique:

- *Patient preparation and imaging:* Preoperative venography, CTV, or MRV to delineate lesion extent
- *Choice of graft:*
  - Autologous veins (e.g., greater saphenous vein) preferred due to reduced infection risk and superior long-term patency
  - Synthetic grafts [e.g., expanded polytetrafluoroethylene (ePTFE)] may be necessary when autologous veins are insufficient or unsuitable.
- *Procedure:*
  - Creation of precise proximal and distal anastomoses around the stenotic segment, meticulously preserving the surrounding anatomical structures
  - Ensuring proper orientation and tension-free graft placement to minimize complications and enhance patency

Preferred graft conduits:

- *Autologous vein grafts:* Superior patency, lower infection risk
- *ePTFE or Dacron synthetic grafts:* Considered when autologous veins not viable, albeit associated with slightly higher thrombosis and infection risks

Venous Reconstruction (Direct Surgical Repair)[44,45]

Venous reconstruction encompasses direct surgical repair techniques, including resection and end-to-end anastomosis, vein patch angioplasty, or segmental reconstruction with vein or prosthetic patches.

Technique:

- *Direct venous repair:* Resection of stenotic segments followed by meticulous end-to-end vein anastomosis with precision suture technique (monofilament polypropylene sutures)
- *Patch angioplasty:* Enlargement of narrowed segment via longitudinal incision and placement of autologous vein or synthetic patch to widen the stenosed lumen significantly
- *Segmental reconstruction:* Replacement of extensive fibrotic segments with graft segments to restore venous patency in complex chronic occlusions.

Key surgical considerations:

- Precise dissection and mobilization of venous segments to ensure tension-free reconstruction
- Minimized handling of vein segments to reduce endothelial damage and promote better healing and reduced thrombosis risk.

Outcomes and Patency Rates[46]

Surgical venous reconstructions offer definitive solutions in well-selected cases, with substantial improvements in clinical symptoms and dialysis function:

- *Primary patency rates:*
  - Venous bypass: *60–80% at 1 year*, with meticulous technique and patient selection

- Direct surgical reconstruction: *50–70% at 1 year*, depending on the complexity of the lesion and the quality of venous segments involved
- *Secondary patency (postreintervention) rates:* Approaching 80–90% at 1–2 years with rigorous follow-up, anticoagulation therapy, and appropriate secondary interventions (angioplasty/stenting) when needed.

COMPLICATIONS OF INTERVENTION

- *Immediate complications:* Vessel rupture, hemorrhage, tamponade
- *Delayed complications:* Thrombosis, restenosis, infection
- *Management of complications:* Covered stents, surgical backup, pericardial drainage.

Delayed Complications

Delayed complications typically manifest days to months following the procedure and can significantly compromise long-term outcomes.

Thrombosis

Etiology:
- Endothelial injury during angioplasty or stenting
- Suboptimal blood flow dynamics postintervention
- Hypercoagulability or inadequate anticoagulation/antiplatelet therapy.

Clinical presentation:
- Recurrent swelling, pain, or complete loss of dialysis access functionality
- Decreased dialysis efficacy, increased venous pressures.

Management strategies:
- Prompt diagnosis via duplex ultrasound or venography
- Anticoagulation adjustments (heparinization or systemic anticoagulants)
- Endovascular thrombolysis [catheter-directed thrombolysis using agents like tissue plasminogen activator (tPA) or urokinase]
- Mechanical thrombectomy or repeat angioplasty/stenting.

Restenosis

Etiology:
- Intimal hyperplasia and fibrosis post balloon angioplasty or stenting
- Elastic recoil not adequately controlled.

Clinical presentation:
- Recurrent clinical symptoms (edema, venous hypertension)
- Dialysis dysfunction or access site high venous pressures.

Management strategies:
- Regular follow-up surveillance via clinical examination and ultrasound
- Repeat angioplasty (possibly with drug-coated balloons)
- Stenting (self-expanding stents for longer-term patency)
- Surgical revision or reconstruction in recurrent refractory cases.

Infection[47]

Etiology:
- Procedural contamination, compromised sterile technique
- Implantation of prosthetic materials (stents, grafts).

Clinical presentation:
- Fever, chills, bacteremia, local site redness, swelling, purulent drainage
- Systemic infection signs in severe cases (endocarditis, sepsis).

Management strategies:
- Blood cultures, imaging studies for abscesses or infection localization
- Empirical broad-spectrum antibiotics adjusted by cultures
- Surgical drainage of infected hematomas or abscesses
- Potential removal of infected stents or grafts in refractory infections.

Advanced Management Strategies for Complications

Covered Stents (Stent-Grafts)[48,49]

Covered stents are essential for managing vessel perforation, rupture, and bleeding:
- Immediate sealing of perforations or disruptions
- Devices include Viabahn, Fluency, and Gore stent-grafts
- High technical success, effective in acute emergencies.

Surgical Backup[50,51]

It is vital in any advanced interventional setting:
- Immediate surgical consultation availability mandatory

TABLE 2: Clinical algorithm for complication management.

Complication	*Immediate action*	*Definitive management*	*Follow-up care*
Vessel rupture/ perforation	Balloon tamponade, fluid resuscitation	Covered stent, surgical repair if needed	ICU monitoring, repeat imaging
Hemorrhage	Compression, transfusion as needed	Surgical exploration, vessel repair	Hematoma monitoring
Tamponade	Echocardiogram-guided pericardiocentesis	Surgical pericardial window if necessary	ICU care, serial echo
Thrombosis	Immediate anticoagulation	Catheter-directed thrombolysis, thrombectomy	Anticoagulants/antiplatelets
Restenosis	Surveillance imaging	Repeat angioplasty/stent, drug-coated balloon	Close surveillance, secondary prevention
Infection	Cultures, antibiotics initiation	Surgical drainage, removal of infected implants	Prolonged antibiotic therapy, close follow-up

- Prepared for thoracotomy or sternotomy for uncontrolled bleeding or vessel rupture
- Emergency vascular surgical expertise significantly improves survival and reduces morbidity.

Pericardial Drainage[52]

Immediate access to echocardiographic and percutaneous drainage skills:

- Rapid percutaneous drainage crucial in cardiac tamponade
- Surgical pericardial window creation may be required in persistent or complicated cases.

PREVENTIVE MEASURES AND RECOMMENDATIONS

- *Rigorous adherence to optimal technique:*
  - Appropriate balloon sizing and careful inflation pressures
  - Gentle manipulation of wires and catheters, meticulous procedural planning
- *Real-time imaging guidance:* Fluoroscopy and IVUS significantly reduce procedural complications.
- *Anticoagulation and antiplatelet protocols:* Individualized according to thrombotic and bleeding risk factors
- *Skilled operator and multidisciplinary team:*
  - Critical to identify and manage complications promptly
  - Dedicated interventional and surgical backup essential
- *Regular follow-up surveillance:* Early detection and timely management of delayed complications significantly improve outcomes.

Clinical Algorithm for Complication Management (Table 2)

Clinical algorithm for complication management is given in **Table 2**.

Conclusion

Complication management in central vein interventions demands preparedness, vigilance, meticulous procedural technique, and swift, decisive action. Recognizing potential complications and possessing the skills and tools to manage them promptly ensure patient safety, enhance long-term outcomes, and elevate clinical standards globally.

Future Directions and Research Priorities

- Development of improved biomaterials, drug-eluting stents/balloons, and biodegradable scaffolds to enhance long-term patency
- Prospective, randomized clinical trials evaluating innovative interventions, preventive strategies, and QoL outcomes.
- Enhanced patient-specific predictive modeling to identify individuals most likely to benefit from specific interventions, tailoring therapy accordingly.

VISIONARY FUTURE RESEARCH ROADMAP IN CENTRAL VEIN STENOSIS AND THROMBOSIS

These pioneering topics represent strategic avenues for advanced translational and clinical research, aimed at significantly improving clinical outcomes, procedural success, and patient QoL.

Future Directions and Research Priorities in Central Vein Stenosis and Thrombosis

Advancements in managing CVS and thrombosis depend significantly on innovative research, novel technologies, and personalized clinical approaches. The next era of CVS management must focus on groundbreaking developments in biomaterials, rigorous clinical trials, personalized medicine, and predictive modeling to optimize patient outcomes, enhance vessel patency, and improve quality of life.

Development of Advanced Biomaterials and Innovative Device Technologies

The future of CVS management lies significantly in sophisticated biomaterials and cutting-edge device technologies. These innovations will directly impact restenosis rates, intervention durability, and patient morbidity.

Next-generation drug-eluting stents and balloons

- *Innovative pharmacological agents:* Exploration of novel antiproliferative and anti-inflammatory agents superior to existing paclitaxel and sirolimus derivatives, offering more durable inhibition of neointimal hyperplasia and fibrosis.
- *Enhanced drug delivery mechanisms:* Novel coatings ensuring sustained, uniform, and targeted drug delivery directly to affected vessel segments, significantly reducing restenosis risks.

Biodegradable stents and scaffolds

- *Temporary scaffold solutions:* Fully bioresorbable scaffolds designed to provide initial support, followed by controlled biodegradation once the vessel integrity stabilizes
- *Benefits:*
  - Eliminates risks associated with permanent stents (late thrombosis, fracture)
  - Enables vessel remodeling, growth in pediatric populations, and reduces long-term foreign body-related complications.

Improved vascular grafts and prosthetics

- *Advanced biological and synthetic materials:* Development of grafts incorporating tissue-engineered materials, bioactive surfaces, or biomimetic coatings enhancing endothelialization, biocompatibility, and reducing infection and thrombosis risks.
- *Integration of nanotechnology and smart biomaterials:* Biomaterials with self-healing properties, responsive drug release capabilities, and real-time monitoring of graft function.

Clinical and Translational Research Infrastructure Development

Strengthening the research ecosystem by developing robust infrastructure supports innovation, accelerates translation from bench to bedside, and fosters sustainable clinical improvements:

- *Advanced imaging and intervention centers:* Specialized global centers equipped with cutting-edge imaging technologies (IVUS, MRV, advanced fluoroscopy) dedicated to high-quality research and complex interventions
- *Global research networks and partnerships:* International collaborations fostering knowledge exchange, technology transfer, and standardized protocols ensuring global best practices
- *Dedicated vascular research fellowships and training programs:* Specialized training fostering next-generation clinical leaders adept in innovative research methodologies, device development, and patient-centered outcome measurement.

Hydrophilic-coated PICC lines and catheters

- *Research significance:* Investigating the effectiveness of hydrophilic coatings on peripherally inserted central catheters (PICCs) and dialysis catheters in reducing thrombosis, infection, endothelial damage, and subsequent stenosis.
- *Potential advantages:*
  - Reduced catheter-related thrombotic complications
  - Improved patient comfort and catheter longevity
  - Decreased rates of intimal hyperplasia and stenosis due to minimized endothelial irritation
- *Future research directions:*
  - Prospective randomized trials comparing hydrophilic-coated catheters vs. standard catheters.
  - Long-term outcomes analysis assessing stenosis incidence, patency, infection rates, and patient comfort.

  Research priority is given in **Table 3**.

Strategic Vision and Recommendations

- Foster interdisciplinary collaboration between clinicians, pharmacologists, bioengineers, and regulatory authorities globally.

TABLE 3: Research priority.

Research domain	*Clinical objective*	*Recommended study designs*	*Anticipated impact*
Hydrophilic-coated PICC lines/ catheters	Reduce thrombosis, infection, stenosis risk	Randomized clinical trials, cohort studies	Reduced complications, improved outcomes
Sirolimus/paclitaxel-coated balloons	Durable restenosis prevention	Multicenter randomized trials	Enhanced long-term patency, fewer interventions
Ramatroban	Prevent vascular calcification, inflammation	Preclinical, phase II-III clinical trials	Reduced stenosis and calcification, improved vascular health
HIF pathway-inhibiting DuStats	Prevent neointimal hyperplasia postintervention	Preclinical, translational, Clinical trials	Enhanced patency postangioplasty/stenting
FORS Cath Lab Technology	Optimize procedural accuracy, reduce radiation	Comparative clinical trials, cost analysis	Safer, more precise, radiation-free interventions

- Establish dedicated research funding streams and investigator-initiated studies focusing on these cutting-edge innovations.
- Facilitate rapid translation of promising pre-clinical findings to clinical application through accelerated regulatory pathways and global clinical collaboration.

Conclusion and Legacy Impact

- Exploring these visionary research domains promises to revolutionize the management of CVS and thrombosis profoundly. These innovations can significantly enhance clinical outcomes, reduce patient morbidity, improve healthcare resource utilization, and redefine standards of patient-centered care.
- By investing collective clinical and research energies into these pioneering pathways, the future of CVS management will reach unprecedented heights—transforming patient experiences, clinical outcomes, and healthcare delivery worldwide for decades to come.

Summary and Clinical Impact

Understanding prognostic factors, patency rates, and quality-of-life outcomes postintervention in CVS guides clinicians in personalized patient management. Meticulous preventive strategies, optimal procedural techniques, diligent follow-up, and patient-centered care ensure significantly improved patient outcomes, durable vessel patency, and sustained quality-of-life enhancements.

Prevention and Future Directions

- Preventative strategies in dialysis populations
- Emerging technologies and stent materials
- Advances in drug-eluting balloons and stents
- Ongoing clinical trials and future research directions.

Expert Recommendations and Guidelines

- Summary of guidelines from major vascular societies [Kidney Disease Outcomes Quality Initiative (KDOQI), Society for Vascular Surgery (SVS), Cardiovascular and Interventional Radiological Society of Europe (CIRSE)]
- Algorithmic approach to management decisions based on latest evidence.

EXPERT RECOMMENDATIONS AND GUIDELINES FOR CENTRAL VEIN STENOSIS AND THROMBOSIS

Management of CVS and thrombosis benefits substantially from adherence to expert consensus recommendations provided by leading vascular and nephrology societies globally. This summary synthesizes current evidence-based guidance from the Kidney Disease Outcomes Quality Initiative (KDOQI), Society for Vascular Surgery (SVS), and Cardiovascular and Interventional Radiological Society of Europe (CIRSE).

Summary of Guidelines from Major Vascular Societies

Kidney Disease Outcomes Quality Initiative

KDOQI provides comprehensive guidelines, particularly addressing CVS in dialysis patients:

- *Prevention:*
  - Minimize central catheter usage and prioritize AV fistulas and grafts.
  - Strict adherence to aseptic insertion practices, employing sterile antiseptic solutions and sterile ultrasound gel universally
- *Diagnosis:*
  - Early duplex ultrasound or venography upon clinical suspicion of CVS
  - Regular monitoring of dialysis-access blood flow and venous pressure
- *Interventions:*
  - Balloon angioplasty as first-line intervention
  - Stent placement reserved for angioplasty failures or rapid recurrence
  - Surgical options considered in refractory cases after multiple failed endovascular attempts.

Society for Vascular Surgery

The SVS offers detailed procedural guidance emphasizing vascular surgical principles:

- *Preventive recommendations:*
  - Careful catheter selection and placement techniques to reduce vessel trauma
  - Rigorous skin antisepsis and sterile barrier techniques
- *Interventional recommendations:*
  - Balloon angioplasty remains first-line therapy; stenting recommended for lesions resistant to angioplasty alone
  - Preference for self-expanding stents due to superior flexibility and reduced risk of fracture
  - Routine imaging and clinical surveillance postintervention to facilitate early re-intervention, improving long-term patency
- *Surgical management recommendations:*
  - Surgical bypass or reconstruction reserved for endovascular failures, complex or extensive lesions
  - Autologous vein grafts preferred; synthetic grafts when necessary.

Cardiovascular and Interventional Radiological Society of Europe

The CIRSE emphasizes minimally invasive, image-guided approaches and advanced procedural techniques:

- *Diagnostic guidance:*
  - DSV as gold standard; IVUS recommended for complex lesions
  - Pressure gradient measurements (>3 mm Hg gradient indicating significant stenosis)
- *Interventional techniques:*
  - Preference for balloon angioplasty first; drug-coated balloons/stents for restenosis management
  - CTO interventions employing advanced techniques (sharp recanalization, RF wires, laser, hybrid approaches)
  - Consideration of covered stents for complex stenoses or vessel rupture scenarios
- *Follow-up protocols:*
  - Intensive ultrasound and MRV/CTV-based surveillance protocols
  - Timely reinterventions for preserving secondary patency.

Algorithmic Approach to Management Decisions (Based on Latest Evidence)

Step-by-Step Master Clinical Algorithm

Step 1: Clinical assessment and initial diagnosis

- Clinical symptoms (swelling, venous hypertension, dialysis dysfunction)
- Duplex ultrasound screening; confirmatory venography or advanced imaging (MRV/CTV)

Step 2: Primary management decision

Scenario	***Recommended action***
Mild stenosis, asymptomatic	Conservative management (watchful waiting, surveillance imaging)
Symptomatic moderate–severe stenosis	*First-line:* Balloon angioplasty
Immediate post-angioplasty failure/elastic recoil	Immediate re-angioplasty ± stent placement

Step 3: Advanced intervention for recurrent/complex cases

Scenario	***Recommended action***
Angioplasty failure, rapid recurrence	Self-expanding stent placement
CTO or complex stenosis	Advanced CTO techniques (sharp recanalization, RF wire, laser, hybrid approaches)
Vessel rupture or perforation	Immediate covered stent placement; surgical backup

Step 4: Refractory or recurrent complex stenosis

Scenario	Recommended action
Multiple endovascular failures	Surgical reconstruction (venous bypass, vein patch angioplasty)

Step 5: Preventive and follow-up protocols

- *Immediate postprocedure:*
  - SQ53 antiseptic platform application; sterile ultrasound gel for imaging guidance.
  - Initiate tailored anticoagulation or antiplatelet therapy.
- *Long-term surveillance:*
  - Regular ultrasound/MRV/CTV imaging every 3–6 months post-intervention
  - Prompt re-intervention at early signs of restenosis
- *Long-term preventive measures:*
  - Minimize catheter use; transition early to AVFs or AVGs.
  - Optimize management of hypercoagulability and inflammatory states.

Summary of Clinical Recommendations (Integrated Guidelines)

Clinical aspect	Unified master recommendations
Prevention	Minimize catheter use; rigorous antisepsis (SQ53), sterile ultrasound gel
Diagnostic strategy	Duplex ultrasound first-line; DSV and IVUS for detailed lesion characterization
Primary intervention	Balloon angioplasty first-line, selective stenting if required
Advanced intervention	CTO methods (sharp, RF, laser); covered stents for complex lesions
Surgical management	Reserved for multiple endovascular failures
Follow-up	Rigorous imaging surveillance and tailored re-intervention

Future Directions Based on Society Recommendations

- Global harmonization of clinical protocols and recommendations.
- Continued updating of guidelines based on evolving evidence from rigorous clinical trials.
- Integration of innovative technologies (drug-coated balloons/stents, biodegradable scaffolds, advanced antiseptics) into official guidelines upon robust clinical validation.

CONCLUSION

Central vein stenosis and thrombosis remain significant clinical challenges, particularly in dialysis-dependent, oncology, pediatric, and cardiac device patients. This comprehensive chapter has synthesized current global evidence, practical recommendations, advanced techniques, and innovative research horizons—establishing a definitive resource to guide optimal patient care worldwide.

Essential Takeaways

- *Definition and clinical significance:* CVS critically impacts patient morbidity, dialysis efficacy, and quality of life. Early recognition and proactive management are imperative.
  - *Epidemiology and risk factors:* High prevalence in dialysis populations; central catheter usage, pacemaker leads, and previous interventions constitute major risks.
  - *Pathophysiology:* Intimal hyperplasia, fibrosis, thrombosis, and endothelial injury are central mechanisms contributing to CVS development. Understanding Virchow's triad (endothelial injury, stasis, hypercoagulability) underpins clinical strategies.
  - *Clinical presentation:* Symptoms including extremity edema, venous hypertension, dilated chest-wall veins, facial swelling, and dialysis dysfunction warrant immediate investigation.
  - *Diagnostic approach:* Duplex ultrasound as initial diagnostic modality; MRV and CTV provide detailed imaging. DSV remains gold standard; IVUS adds critical intraprocedural insights.
- *Management strategies:*
  - *Conservative:* Appropriate for asymptomatic or mild stenosis; proactive preventive measures essential.
  - *Endovascular:* Balloon angioplasty primary method; stenting for restenosis or angioplasty failure. Advanced CTO techniques are critical in refractory cases.
  - *Surgical:* Reserved for complex lesions and multiple endovascular failures; venous bypass or reconstruction provide durable solutions.

- *Complication management:*
  - Immediate identification and decisive management of complications (vessel rupture, tamponade) with covered stents, surgical backup, and pericardial drainage essential
  - Vigilant surveillance for delayed complications (restenosis, thrombosis, infection) is critical for maintaining long-term patency.
- *Special populations:*
  - Pediatric patients require meticulous vessel preservation strategies.
  - Oncology patients present unique management challenges related to hypercoagulability and extrinsic compression.
  - Heart failure and pacemaker patients necessitate an integrated multidisciplinary approach focusing on device-related stenosis prevention and management.
- *Prognosis and outcomes:*
  - Primary and secondary patency rates vary by intervention; rigorous follow-up protocols and tailored anticoagulation therapy significantly enhance outcomes.
  - Effective management translates into profound quality of life improvements and significant healthcare cost reductions.
- *Innovations and preventive strategies:* Incorporation of advanced antiseptic biodefense platforms (SQ53) and universal use of sterile ultrasound gel significantly reduce catheter-related complications and enhance outcomes.
- *Expert guidelines:*
  - Adherence to evidence-based guidelines from KDOQI, SVS, and CIRSE ensures consistent, high-quality care.
  - Structured, algorithmic approaches guide precise, timely clinical decisions.

Reinforcement of Key Concepts and Practical Clinical Pearls

Clinical pearls for prevention and early management:

- Minimize central catheter use; prioritize AV fistulas and grafts.
- Universal implementation of advanced antiseptic strategies (SQ53) and sterile ultrasound gel use for catheter insertion, maintenance, and imaging procedures significantly reduces infection and stenosis risk.

Clinical pearls for diagnostics:

- Always initiate diagnostic workup promptly upon symptom recognition.
- Combine duplex ultrasound for screening with definitive venography and IVUS for complex lesion assessment and intervention planning.

Clinical pearls for endovascular interventions:

- Balloon angioplasty as first-line therapy; reserve stents (preferably self-expanding or covered) for refractory or recurrent cases.
- Master advanced CTO intervention techniques, enhancing procedural success in complex cases.

Clinical pearls for surgical management:

- Surgical approaches (venous bypass, reconstruction) crucial after multiple endovascular failures; meticulous surgical technique essential for long-term success.

Clinical pearls for complication management:

- Maintain readiness for immediate covered stent placement or surgical backup to rapidly address vessel rupture or complications.
- Proactively manage thrombosis, restenosis, and infection through regular surveillance, prompt reinterventions, and tailored medical therapies.

Clinical pearls for special populations:

- Pediatric management must focus on long-term vessel preservation and minimally invasive strategies.
- Oncology-related CVS mandates close coordination with oncology teams for integrated therapeutic decisions.
- Cardiac device-related stenosis requires coordinated electrophysiological and vascular management.

Clinical pearls for enhancing prognosis:

- Continuous patient surveillance, personalized anticoagulant protocols, and timely interventions significantly improve vessel patency.
- Employ validated quality-of-life instruments to objectively assess and enhance patient-centered outcomes.

Clinical pearls for future innovations:

- Advance global clinical trials evaluating innovative biomaterials, biodegradable scaffolds, drug-coated balloons/stents, and pharmacological interventions (e.g., Ramatroban, DuStats) targeting CVS pathophysiology.

- Integrate cutting-edge imaging technologies (FORS Cath Labs) into standard clinical practice, enhancing procedural precision and patient safety.

Visionary Outlook

By implementing rigorous evidence-based strategies, fostering innovative research, and embracing technological advances, the global clinical community will significantly elevate standards of care for patients suffering from CVS and thrombosis. The recommendations and insights detailed herein will guide clinicians worldwide, ensuring enduring improvements in patient outcomes and healthcare quality, setting a legacy standard for decades to come.

Master Clinical Recommendation Summary Table

Domain	*Recommended actions*
Prevention and antisepsis	Prioritize AV access; universal SQ53 and sterile ultrasound gel use
Diagnosis	Duplex ultrasound, confirmatory DSV/IVUS
Endovascular intervention	Balloon angioplasty; stent if required; advanced CTO methods
Surgical intervention	Reserved for refractory cases
Complication management	Immediate covered stenting; surgical backup readiness
Special populations	Tailored approaches for pediatric, oncology, and cardiac patients
Prognosis optimization	Rigorous surveillance, early reintervention, personalized anticoagulation
Innovations and future research	Advanced biomaterials, pharmacological interventions, enhanced imaging

- *Clinical presentation:* In the same study, *47%* of patients presented with arm edema, *29%* with facial swelling, and *11%* experienced prolonged bleeding from the arteriovenous fistula postdialysis.
- *Outcomes:* Angioplasty was performed in nine patients, achieving a primary success rate of *66%* and a 6-month patency rate of *44.4%*. Notably, *55%* of patients required termination of their vascular access due to complications.

REFERENCES

1. Echefu G, Stowe I, Lukan A, Sharma G, Basu-Ray I, Guidry L, et al. Central vein stenosis in hemodialysis vascular access: clinical manifestations and contemporary management strategies. Front Nephrol. 2023;3:1280666.
2. Proksch DM, Rodriguez LE, Rathore A, Steerman SN, Panneton JM. A comparison of stenting versus hemodialysis reliable outflow graft for hemodialysis patients with recurrent central venous obstructions. J Vasc Surg Venous Lymphat Disord. 2021;9(5):1136-44.
3. Krishna VN, Eason JB, Allon M. Central Venous Occlusion in the Hemodialysis Patient. Am J Kidney Dis. 2016;68(5):803-7.
4. https://evtoday.com/articles/2010-june/treating-cvd-in-the-dialysis-patient.
5. Adwaney A, Lim C, Blakey S, Duncan N, Ashby DR. Central venous stenosis, access outcome and survival in patients undergoing maintenance hemodialysis. Clin J Am Soc Nephrol. 2019;14(3):378-84.
6. Agarwal AK. Central vein stenosis. Am J Kidney Dis. 2013;61(6):1001-15.
7. Al-Balas A, Almehmi A, Varma R, Al-Balas H, Allon M. De Novo Central Vein Stenosis in Hemodialysis Patients following initial tunneled central vein vatheter placement. Kidney360. 2021;3(1):99-102.
8. Sohail MA, Vachharajani TJ, Anvari E. Central venous catheters for hemodialysis-the myth and the evidence. Kidney Int Rep. 2021;6(12):2958-68.
9. Borgquist O, Naddi L, Božović G, Hellberg M, Annborn M, Sjövall F, et al. Central venous stenosis after subclavian versus internal jugular dialysis catheter insertion (CITES) in adults in need of a temporary central dialysis catheter: study protocol for a two-arm, parallel-group, non-inferiority randomised controlled trial. Trials. 2023;24(1)327.
10. Timal RJ, Karalis I, Cabezas JMM, Rotmans JI, Hensen LCR, Buiten MS, et al. Development of central venous stenosis upon ICD implantation in dialysis patients: a non-negligible issue. Cardiol Cardiovasc Med. 2022;6(2):171-88.
11. Roşu CD, Bolintineanu SL, Căpăstraru BF, Iacob R, Stoicescu ER, Petrea CE. Risk factor analysis in vascular access complications for hemodialysis patients. Diagnostics (Basel). 2025;15(1):88.
12. Haridas S, Abraham S, Padmanabhan A, Kumar S. WCN25-4569 Central Venous Stenosis, Risk Factors, and Outcome in Patients Undergoing Maintenance Hemodialysis: A Single-Center Experience from South India. Kidney International Reports. 2025;10(2):S454-5.
13. Shiri P, Rezaeian S, Abdi A, Jalilian M, Khatony A. Risk factors for thrombosis in dialysis patients: a comprehensive systematic review and meta-analysis. J Vasc Nurs. 2024;42(3):165-76.
14. Lok CE, Huber TS, Lee T, Shenoy S, Yevzlin AS, Abreo K, et al. KDOQI clinical practice guideline for vascular access: 2019 Update. Am J Kidney Dis. 2020;75(4 Suppl 2):S1-S164.
15. Kitrou P, Katsanos K, Karnabatidis D. Management of central venous stenoses and occlusions. Cardiovasc Intervent Radiol. 2023;46(9):1182-91.

16. Agarwal AK, Patel BM, Haddad NJ. Central vein stenosis in hemodialysis vascular access: clinical manifestations and contemporary management strategies. Kidney360. 2022;3(1):75-86.
17. Quaretti P, Galli F, Moramarco LP, Formica M, Maestri M, Corti R, et al. Management of central vein stenosis and occlusion in hemodialysis patients: results of a prospective study. J Vasc Access. 2016;17(2):124-30.
18. Kian K, Shapiro M, Salman L, Beathard G, Agarwal A, Misra S, et al. Management of central vein stenosis in hemodialysis patients. Semin Dial. 2018;31(5):441-6.
19. Levit RD, Cohen RM, Kwak A, Kim HS, Prombo J, Vesely TM, et al. Central venous stenosis in hemodialysis patients: prevalence and efficacy of endovascular treatment. Kidney Int. 2006;69(4):701-7.
20. Doty DB, Baker WH, Weir EK. Superior vena cava syndrome: clinical diagnosis and management. Am J Med Sci. 1981;282(1) 40-51.
21. Vachharajani TJ, Asif A, Tee A, Misra S, Beathard G, Jennings WC, et al. Central vein stenosis: a nephrologist's perspective. Semin Dial. 2020;33(4):291-300.
22. Povlsen B, Hansson T, Povlsen SD. Treatment for thoracic outlet syndrome. Cochrane Database Syst Rev. 2014;(11):CD007218.
23. Illig KA, Donahue D, Duncan A, Freischlag J, Gelabert H, Johansen K, et al. Reporting standards of the Society for Vascular Surgery for thoracic outlet syndrome. J Vasc Surg. 2016;64(3):e23-e35.
24. Yancy CW, Jessup M, Bozkurt B, Butler J, Casey DE Jr, Colvin MM, et al. 2022 AHA/ACC/HFSA guideline for the management of heart failure. J Am Coll Cardiol. 2022;79(17):e263-421.
25. Mustafa S, Stein PD, Patel KC, Otten TR, Holmes R, Silbergleit A. Upper extremity deep venous thrombosis. Chest. 2003;123(6):1953-6.
26. Forauer AR, Theoharis CG, Dasika NL. Percutaneous transluminal angioplasty for treatment of central venous stenosis in hemodialysis patients: correlation between clinical outcome and central venous pressure measurements. J Vasc Interv Radiol. 2000;11(10):1231-7.
27. MacRae JM, Dipchand C, Oliver M, Moist L, Lok C, Clark E, et al. Arteriovenous access failure, stenosis, and thrombosis. Can J Kidney Health Dis. 2016;3:2054358116669126.
28. Trerotola SO, Ponce P, Stavropoulos SW, Mondschein JI, Shlansky-Goldberg RD, Soulen MC, et al. Central venous stenosis: clinical features and endovascular management. Semin Intervent Radiol. 2011;28(4):401-10.
29. O'Grady NP, Alexander M, Burns LA, Dellinger EP, Garland J, Heard SO, et al. Guidelines for the prevention of intravascular catheter-related infections. Clin Infect Dis. 2011;52(9):e162-93.
30. Loveday HP, Wilson JA, Pratt RJ, Golsorkhi M, Tingle A, Bak A, et al. epic3: National evidence-based guidelines for preventing healthcare-associated infections in NHS hospitals in England. J Hosp Infect. 2014;86(Suppl 1):S1-70.
31. Agarwal AK, Roy-Chaudhury P, Mounts P, Hurlburt E, Pfaffle A, Poggio EC. Taurolidine/Heparin Lock Solution and Catheter-Related Bloodstream Infection in Hemodialysis: a randomized, double-blind, active-control, phase 3 study. Clin J Am Soc Nephrol. 2023;18(11):1446-55.
32. El-Sharkawy MM, Abdelgawad MA, Gad OE, Emara AA. Effect of taurolidine-citrate-heparin lock solution on inflammatory response and hemodialysis adequacy in hemodialysis patients with tunneled catheters. J Egyptian Soc Nephrol Transplant. 2023;23(2):1-7.
33. Trerotola SO, Stavropoulos SW, Mondschein JI, Soulen MC, Shlansky-Goldberg RD, Tuite CM, et al Treatment of central venous stenosis in hemodialysis patients: results of angioplasty and stent placement. Radiology. 2000;217(2):738-42.
34. Bakken AM, Hagen SM, Mokrzycki MH, Kirsch CM, Allon M. Long-term outcomes of percutaneous angioplasty for central venous stenosis in hemodialysis patients. J Vasc Surg. 2007;45(4):776-83.
35. Kundu S, Haskal ZJ, Vesely TM, Trerotola SO, Soulen MC, O'Malley ME, et al. Use of stents in treating central venous stenoses and occlusions in hemodialysis patients: indications, techniques, and outcomes. Am J Roentgenol. 2010;195(3):693-9.
36. Quinn SF, Keller FS, Velez M, Mikkelsen R. Percutaneous transluminal angioplasty versus stent placement for the treatment of central venous stenoses in hemodialysis patients: prospective randomized trial. J Vasc Interv Radiol. 1995;6(6):851-5.
37. Gray RJ, Levitin A, Buck D, Brown DB, Horton KM, Nikolic B, et al. Sharp recanalization of chronic central venous occlusions in hemodialysis patients. J Vasc Interv Radiol. 2005;16(5):653-61.
38. Bream PR, Friedman KD, Day JD, Rilling WS, Darcy MD, Hicks ME. Use of radiofrequency wire for recanalization of central venous occlusions in hemodialysis patients. J Vasc Interv Radiol. 2003;14(7):915-22.
39. Kuo MD, Cummings KW, Kothary N, Sze DY. Excimer laser-assisted recanalization of chronic total occlusions of the central veins. J Vasc Interv Radiol. 2003;14(8):939-45.
40. Funaki B, Lorenz JM, Hoffer EK, Rosenblum JD, Stavropoulos SW, Madden JF, et al. Retrograde recanalization of central venous occlusions via hemodialysis access. Am J Roentgenol. 2005;185(6):1640-4.
41. Witte M, Kiefhaber TR, Jonsson P, Venbrux AC, Simons ME. Intravascular ultrasound in the diagnosis and treatment of central venous stenosis and occlusion in hemodialysis patients. J Vasc Interv Radiol. 2007;18(9): 1101-7.
42. Rajan DK, Patel NH, Valji K, Patel NH, Valji K, Valji K, et al. Combined antegrade and retrograde approach for recanalization of chronic central venous occlusions. J Vasc Interv Radiol. 2008;19(2 Pt 1):195-200.
43. Agarwal AK, Al-Ali F, Bajwa TA, Beathard GA, Asif A. Central vein stenosis in hemodialysis vascular access:

clinical manifestations and management. Semin Dial. 2020;33(4):291-300.

44. Gupta A, Kaufman J, Chandra S, Hulbert J. Surgical reconstruction of central veins for dialysis access. Ann Vasc Surg. 2011;25(2):252-60.
45. Schanzer H, Veith FJ, Lipman JM, Sasahara AA, Ascer E. Surgical management of central venous obstruction in hemodialysis patients. J Vasc Surg. 1986;3(6):924-31.
46. Kian K, Agarwal AK, Beathard GA, Hanson S, Lorenzen M, Mannick J. Surgical bypass for central venous stenosis or occlusion in hemodialysis patients. J Vasc Access. 2009; 10(3):178-83.
47. van Roeden S, van Oevelen M, Abrahams AC, Dekker FW, Rotmans JI, Meijvis SCA. The best solution down the line: an observational study on taurolidine-versus citrate-based lock solutions for central venous catheters in hemodialysis patients. BMC Nephrol. 2021;22(1):308.
48. Vesely TM, Guimaraes AS, Harmsen WS, Valji K, Trerotola SO. Use of stent-grafts to repair hemodialysis graft-related pseudoaneurysms and to salvage thrombosed stent-grafts. J Vasc Interv Radiol. 2005;16(6):739-49.
49. Nassar GM, Sorial EE, Kallail KJ. Stent graft salvage of ruptured dialysis access. Semin Dial. 2015;28(5):540-5.
50. Gupta A, Kaufman J, Chandra S, Hulbert J. Surgical management of central venous obstruction in hemodialysis patients. Ann Vasc Surg. 2011;25(2):252-60.
51. Mickley V. Central venous stenosis in hemodialysis patients: incidence, endovascular management, and prevention. Curr Opin Nephrol Hypertens. 2008;17(6): 629-32.
52. Tsang TS, Freeman WK, Barnes ME, Reeder GS, Packer DL, Hagler DJ, et al. Percutaneous echocardiographically guided pericardiocentesis in cardiac tamponade. N Engl J Med. 2002;347(21):1695-702.

26.2 ARTERIOVENOUS FISTULA AND GRAFTS

Venkatesh Rajkumar S, Nikhil Sharma, Varinder Singh Bedi

INTRODUCTION

Arteriovenous fistulas (AVFs) and arteriovenous grafts (AVGs) are the cornerstone of vascular access for hemodialysis, offering durable conduits for patients with end-stage renal disease (ESRD). As the preferred modality recommended by the National Kidney Foundation's Kidney Disease Outcomes Quality Initiative (NKF KDOQI), AVFs provide superior longevity and lower infection rates compared to catheters, while AVGs serve as a vital alternative when native vessels are inadequate.[1] However, their efficacy is frequently compromised by thrombosis and stenosis, which account for the majority of access failures and pose significant challenges in interventional nephrology. Understanding and managing these complications is paramount to improving patient outcomes and reducing the burden of repeated interventions.

The clinical significance of these issues is underscored by their prevalence. Data from the United States Renal Data System (USRDS) indicate that approximately 40% of AVFs fail to mature or thrombose within 2 years of creation, while AVGs experience primary patency loss in 50–60% of cases within the first year.[2] Stenosis, often a precursor to thrombosis, develops in up to 70% of AVFs and AVGs due to neointimal hyperplasia and hemodynamic stress, necessitating frequent surveillance and intervention.[3] These failures not only disrupt dialysis schedules but also increase morbidity, healthcare costs, and reliance on temporary catheters—options associated with higher mortality risks.

This chapter explores the pathophysiology, epidemiology, diagnosis, management, and prevention of AVF and AVG thrombosis and stenosis, with a focus on the interventionalist's role. By integrating current evidence and clinical strategies, it aims to equip practitioners with the tools to preserve vascular access longevity. From endovascular techniques to emerging preventive therapies, the discussion highlights advances that shape the future of hemodialysis care.

PATHOPHYSIOLOGY OF THROMBOSIS AND STENOSIS

Thrombosis and stenosis represent the leading causes of AVF and AVG failure in hemodialysis patients, undermining the lifeline of renal replacement therapy. Understanding their pathophysiology is critical for interventionalists tasked with preserving vascular access. Both conditions stem from a complex interplay of endothelial injury, hemodynamic forces, and inflammatory responses, though their manifestations differ between AVFs and AVGs due to anatomical and material distinctions.

In AVFs, stenosis typically arises from neointimal hyperplasia, a proliferative response to shear stress and turbulent flow at the venous anastomosis.[4] High-pressure arterial blood entering a low-pressure vein triggers endothelial damage, recruiting fibroblasts and smooth muscle cells that deposit extracellular matrix, narrowing the lumen.[5] Thrombosis often follows as stagnant flow activates the coagulation cascade, with fibrin and platelet aggregation occluding the vessel.[1] Studies estimate that 80% of AVF thromboses are preceded by significant stenosis, highlighting their mechanistic link.[6]

Arteriovenous grafts, constructed from synthetic materials such as polytetrafluoroethylene (PTFE), exhibit distinct pathology. Stenosis predominantly occurs at the venous outflow due to intimal hyperplasia, exacerbated by foreign body reactions to the graft. The lack of native endothelium in AVGs promotes platelet adhesion and thrombus formation, with rates of thrombosis reported at 0.5–2 events per patient-year—higher than AVFs.[7] Compliance mismatch between the rigid graft and flexible vein further amplifies shear stress, accelerating stenosis.[8]

Inflammation plays a pivotal role in both access types. Cytokines like interleukin-6 and tumor necrosis factor-alpha, elevated in uremic states, amplify neointimal growth and prothrombotic tendencies.[9] Additionally, oxidative stress from dialysis itself damages endothelium, compounding injury. In AVFs, smaller vein diameter (<2.5 mm) correlates with early stenosis, while in AVGs, repeated cannulation disrupts graft integrity, seeding thrombi.[10]

These processes underscore the need for targeted interventions. For instance, addressing upstream stenosis via angioplasty can restore flow and avert thrombosis, while anti-inflammatory strategies remain underexplored. The distinct etiologies—venous remodeling in AVFs versus graft-related reactions in AVGs—demand tailored approaches in interventional nephrology, balancing immediate patency with long-term access survival.

EPIDEMIOLOGY AND RISK FACTORS OF ARTERIOVENOUS FISTULA AND ARTERIOVENOUS GRAFT THROMBOSIS AND STENOSIS

Thrombosis and stenosis remain critical barriers to maintaining vascular access for hemodialysis patients, with distinct epidemiological patterns in India and Asia. In India, where hemodialysis serves over 150,000 ESRD patients annually, AVFs are the predominant access type, yet failure rates are notable.[11] Studies from the Indian population indicate that 35–45% of AVFs fail within 2 years, often due to thrombosis preceded by stenosis, while AVGs, though less common, show primary patency loss in 55–65% of cases within 1 year.[12] Across Asia, the Dialysis Outcomes and Practice Patterns Study (DOPPS) reports AVG thrombosis rates of 0.5–1.8 events per patient-year, higher than AVFs (0.1–0.6), reflecting regional reliance on synthetic grafts in some settings.[13] These figures highlight a significant burden, particularly in resource-constrained environments where timely intervention is challenging.

Risk factors driving these complications are diverse and pronounced in the Indian/Asian context. Patient-specific factors dominate, with diabetes mellitus—affecting 50–60% of Indian dialysis patients—accelerating neointimal hyperplasia and thrombosis via microvascular damage and inflammation. Hypertension, nearly ubiquitous in 85–95% of Asian ESRD cohorts, amplifies shear stress, increasing stenosis risk by 1.8-fold in AVFs.[14] Older age (>65 years), prevalent in India's aging dialysis population, and female sex, linked to smaller vein diameters (<2.5 mm), further heighten vulnerability, with women showing 30% higher early failure rates. Smoking, a rising concern in urban Asia, compounds endothelial injury, elevating thrombosis odds by 1.4 times.[15]

Access-related risks are equally significant. In AVFs, preoperative vein diameters below 2.5 mm, common in Indian patients with suboptimal vasculature, correlate with a 45% increased stenosis risk, while arterial insufficiency from atherosclerosis—often undiagnosed—precipitates thrombosis. AVGs face heightened risks from their PTFE composition, triggering foreign body reactions that double venous outflow stenosis rates compared to AVFs. Repeated cannulation, exacerbated by inconsistent technique in overburdened dialysis units, damages graft walls, raising failure risk by 25–35%.

Procedural factors in India amplify these challenges. Suboptimal anastomosis angles (>90°), frequent in less-specialized centers, disrupt flow and foster stenosis, while delayed surveillance—due to limited imaging access—misses early lesions. For AVGs, cannulation within 2 weeks of placement, sometimes unavoidable in urgent cases, triples thrombosis risk. Mitigating these risks through improved patient screening, surgical expertise, and access care protocols is essential for interventionalists in this region.

DIAGNOSIS OF ARTERIOVENOUS FISTULA AND ARTERIOVENOUS GRAFT THROMBOSIS AND STENOSIS

Diagnosing thrombosis and stenosis in AVFs and AVGs is pivotal in interventional nephrology, ensuring timely interventions to maintain hemodialysis access. A comprehensive approach integrating physical examination, Doppler ultrasound, CT venography, and a modality combining diagnosis and intervention delivers precise detection of complications, from peripheral to central venous lesions, optimizing patient management.

Physical examination provides the initial, cost-efficient assessment of access health. A functional AVF displays a palpable thrill and a soft, continuous bruit on auscultation; stenosis is suggested by a weakened thrill, high-pitched or discontinuous bruit, or prolonged postdialysis bleeding (>10 minutes), while thrombosis shows as an absent thrill and bruit. In AVGs, these signs persist, though thrombus may cause firmness or increased pulsatility beyond a stenosis due to synthetic material. Precision in technique is key, as a 50% reduction in thrill strength can indicate stenosis exceeding 50% luminal narrowing, triggering further diagnostics.

Doppler ultrasound, a noninvasive mainstay, offers detailed hemodynamic insights. It identifies stenosis with peak systolic velocity (PSV) >400 cm/s or a ratio >2:1 (stenotic vs. upstream segment), signaling >50% narrowing in AVFs and AVGs, while thrombosis appears as absent flow with echogenic clot.[16] Flow rates below 600 mL/min highlight dysfunction, aiding early intervention. Its contrast-free application enhances utility, though operator skill influences accuracy.

Computed tomography venography plays a crucial role in detecting central venous lesions, particularly when peripheral diagnostics suggest upstream obstruction. Using contrast-enhanced imaging, it visualizes stenosis or thrombosis in the subclavian or brachiocephalic veins—common in patients with prior catheter use—offering high sensitivity (>90%) for lesions missed by Doppler due to depth or bony interference.[17] While less routine due to radiation and contrast risks, it is invaluable for planning central interventions.

A modality combining diagnosis and intervention, such as contrast injection under fluoroscopy, provides definitive assessment and immediate therapeutic options. It maps stenosis—often juxta-anastomotic in AVFs, venous outflow in AVGs—and thrombus extent, confirming >50% luminal reduction per intervention criteria. Its dual role facilitates procedures such as angioplasty, though cost and radiation limit its use to complex cases.[18] Together, these tools form a diagnostic continuum, addressing both peripheral and central pathology.

MANAGEMENT

Introduction to Managing Arteriovenous Access Complications

Thrombosis and stenosis in AVFs and AVGs are significant challenges in hemodialysis, compromising vascular access patency and patient outcomes. Effective management requires a spectrum of techniques tailored to the lesion's characteristics, location, and patient factors. Endovascular approaches dominate due to their minimally invasive nature and high success rates, while hybrid open methods address more complex cases.

Endovascular Techniques

Balloon angioplasty

Plain old balloon angioplasty: Plain old balloon angioplasty (POBA) is a key initial treatment for stenotic lesions in AVFs and AVGs. Using a balloon catheter inflated at the stenosis site, POBA mechanically dilates the vessel to improve blood flow, particularly for focal, short-segment stenoses. Restenosis is common, often requiring reintervention.

High-pressure balloons are designed to treat resistant stenoses in AVFs and AVGs, particularly in fibrotic or calcified segments. Capable of inflating to 20–30 atm, these noncompliant balloons deliver consistent radial force to expand narrowed vessels. Technical success, defined as residual stenosis <30%, exceeds 90%.[3] However, 6-month primary patency rates range from 40 to 60%, reflecting the need for adjunctive therapies to sustain outcomes.[4] Risks, though uncommon (1–2%), include vessel rupture or dissection, underscoring the importance of skilled execution. **Figures 1A to C** shows POBA of an immature right radiocephalic AVF with good results.

Drug-coated balloons (DCBs): Drug-coated balloons deliver antiproliferative agents (e.g., paclitaxel) to inhibit neointimal hyperplasia, a primary cause of restenosis.

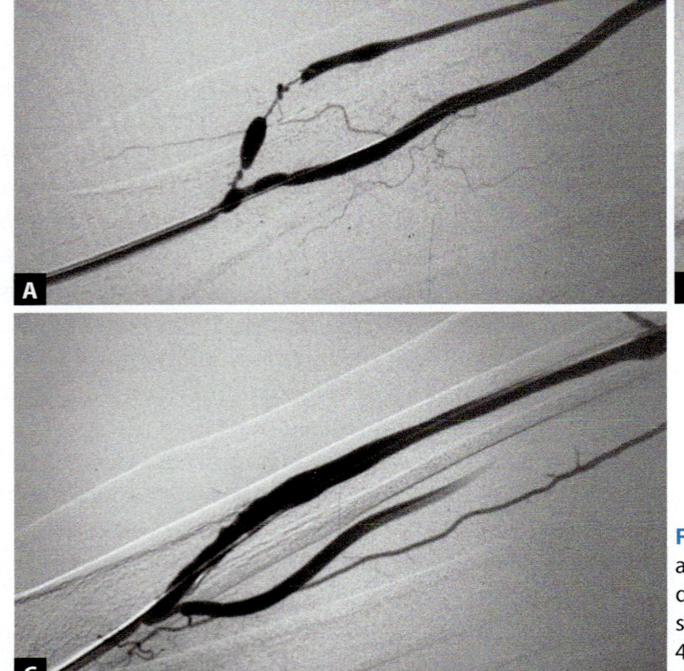

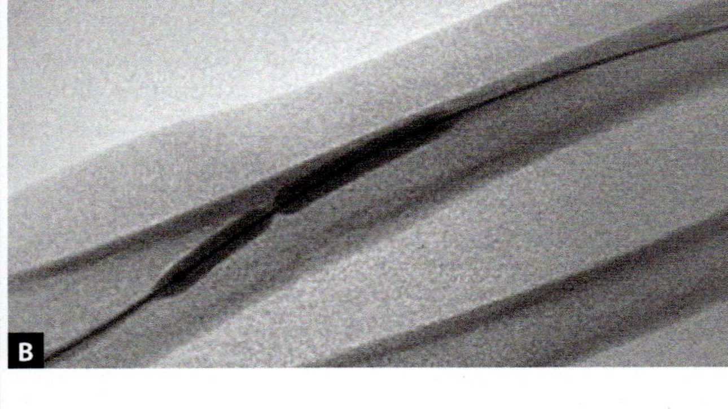

Figs. 1A to C: (A) Markedly narrowed anastomotic and juxta-anastomotic segments: Radial angiogram through the right distal radial artery shows a markedly narrowed juxta-anastomotic segment of a right radiocephalic fistula; (B) PTA with a 4 mm × 40 mm mustang balloon catheter; (C) Radial angiogram post-PTA shows a good final result.

Deployed after standard angioplasty, DCBs enhance vessel patency by reducing smooth muscle proliferation. In the IN.PACT AV randomized trial, 12-month target-lesion primary patency was 63.8% with DCB versus 43.6% with plain balloon angioplasty; the DCB arm also required fewer reinterventions through 12 months.[20] DCBs excel in recurrent or complex stenoses, though cost and limited long-term data constrain their routine use. They represent a valuable tool in the endovascular arsenal.

Stents in arteriovenous fistula and arteriovenous graft salvage: Stents play a critical role in maintaining patency across the AV access circuit, addressing stenoses unresponsive to angioplasty alone. Their applications vary by location and lesion type, offering mechanical support to ensure adequate dialysis flow.

- *Supera stent in the cephalic arch:* The cephalic arch, prone to stenosis in brachiocephalic fistulas, poses challenges due to its curvature and mechanical stress. The Supera stent, with its interwoven nitinol structure, provides flexibility and durability, adapting to the vessel's dynamic motion. Studies show a 1-year primary patency rate of ~75% and a low fracture rate of 5%, outperforming traditional stents in this region.[21] Its unique design minimizes kinking, making it ideal for the cephalic arch, though cost considerations may limit its use.
- *Stents for central venous lesions:* Central venous stenoses (e.g., subclavian or brachiocephalic veins) impair outflow and elevate venous pressures, often requiring stents when angioplasty fails. Self-expanding nitinol stents are preferred for their adaptability to large, variable-diameter veins. Technical success exceeds 90%, with 6-month patency rates of 60–70%.[22] In-stent restenosis, however, affects up to 40% of cases within a year, often necessitating reintervention.[19] Antiplatelet therapy post-stenting is commonly employed, though its efficacy remains under evaluation.
- *Other stent applications:* Stents are also deployed in venous outflow, graft–vein anastomosis, and intragraft regions. Balloon-expandable covered stents effectively manage vessel ruptures or pseudoaneurysms, while self-expanding bare-metal stents suit tapering peripheral veins. Guidelines recommend stenting for residual stenosis >30% postangioplasty or rapid restenosis.[18] In venous outflow of AVGs, 6-month primary patency reaches 50–60%, with secondary patency up to 80% after reinterventions.[23]

Stent considerations and limitations: Use of stent carries risks, including in-stent restenosis from neointimal hyperplasia, the "stent jail" effect limiting future surgery, and rare migration (1–2%). Precise sizing and deployment, along with follow-up imaging, mitigate these issues. Drug-eluting stents, an emerging option, may reduce restenosis but require further validation in AV access.

Mechanical Thrombectomy Devices

Cleaner XT: The Cleaner XT, a rotating sinusoidal-wire device, fragments wall-adherent thrombus and is particularly useful in tortuous or aneurysmal segments. In a single-centre series, technical and clinical success rates were 88%, meeting KDOQI targets for early outcomes.[24] It is effective for soft, gelatinous clots, minimizing thrombolytic use and reducing procedure duration.

Penumbra indigo system: The Penumbra system employs aspiration and separation to extract firm, organized clots, with a 90% success rate and low embolization risk.[25] It excels in dense thrombus cases, complementing the Cleaner XT based on clot composition.

In addition to the Cleaner XT and Penumbra Indigo System, other devices include Solitaire and Trevo, stent retrievers that capture clots in their mesh for removal, and AngioJet, which uses high-pressure saline jets to break up and aspirate clots.

Pharmacologic thrombolysis with actilyse (rt-PA): Actilyse (rt-PA) dissolves fibrin-rich clots through catheter-directed infusion (2–10 mg), administered as a pulse spray or continuous drip. Combined with mechanical thrombectomy, it restores patency in 80% of cases, excelling in acute or extensive thrombosis.[26] Bleeding risks (5–10%), such as access-site hematomas, limit its use to scenarios where mechanical methods alone fail. Contraindications include recent surgery or active bleeding.

Hybrid Open Thrombectomy

Fogarty balloon: In hybrid thrombectomy, a Fogarty balloon catheter is inserted surgically, advanced to the thrombus, and inflated to extract it. Success rates exceed 90%, particularly for adherent clots resistant to endovascular techniques.[27] Vessel trauma (2–5%) may occur, often requiring adjunctive angioplasty. Its reliability makes it a key hybrid tool.

Adherent clot catheter: This advanced catheter features a specialized tip to engage organized clots, achieving 95%

removal with reduced trauma (10% vs. 25% with Fogarty) and shorter procedure times.[27] It minimizes embolization, enhancing outcomes in complex cases.

PREVENTION

Strategies to Prevent Thrombosis and Stenosis in Arteriovenous Fistulas and Grafts

Preventing thrombosis and stenosis in AVFs and AVGs is critical to maintaining vascular access patency and minimizing interventions.

Pharmacologic Interventions

Pharmacologic agents like antiplatelets and anticoagulants aim to reduce thrombotic risk, with efficacy varying by access type and patient factors.

- *Antiplatelet therapy:* Low-dose aspirin (75–100 mg daily) reduces thrombosis in AVGs by 20–30%, though its benefit in AVFs is less clear.[4] Clopidogrel (75 mg daily) is an alternative for aspirin-intolerant patients, but bleeding risks (5–10%) and costs limit its use.[28] Dual antiplatelet therapy shows mixed results and increased bleeding, making it less routine.
- *Anticoagulation:* Warfarin lowers thrombosis rates in AVGs by 25–35% in hypercoagulable patients but requires monitoring due to a 15–20% bleeding risk.[25] Newer oral anticoagulants (e.g., apixaban) show early promise with fewer bleeding events, though further research is needed.[29]

Access Care Protocols

Effective access care and surveillance reduce mechanical damage and enable early intervention.

- *Cannulation techniques:* The buttonhole method for AVFs minimizes vessel trauma and aneurysm risk but demands strict infection control. In AVGs, rotating cannulation sites cuts stenosis risk by 15–20%.
- *Surveillance programs:* Routine flow monitoring (e.g., Doppler ultrasound) detects stenoses early. KDOQI guidelines suggest intervention at flow rates below 600 mL/min (AVFs) or 400–500 mL/min (AVGs), or stenosis >50%, reducing thrombosis by 30–40%.[30]

These practices enhance access durability and reduce urgent procedures.

Emerging Preventive Therapies

Innovative approaches target underlying causes of stenosis and thrombosis.

- *DCBs:* Prophylactic DCB use in high-risk areas may reduce restenosis by 25% at 12 months, pending cost-effectiveness data.
- *Bioengineered grafts:* Heparin-bonded grafts improve 1-year patency by 20% over standard PTFE, as per the RCT data.[31]
- *Wearable devices:* Continuous flow sensors could cut access failures by 40%, though adoption hurdles remain.[32]

These advances hold potential but require further validation.

Ultrasound-guided Arteriovenous Fistuloplasty

Ultrasound-guided balloon angioplasty of AVFs offers a safe, effective, and radiation-free alternative to fluoroscopy-guided procedures. For interventional nephrologists working in resource-constrained environments, mastering this easy technique can dramatically expand access to AVF salvage procedures. Unlike central venous interventions, the superficial course of peripheral AVFs allows excellent real-time USG visualization for both diagnostic and therapeutic procedures. Studies have shown that, when performed by trained operators, USG-guided angioplasty yields comparable outcomes to fluoroscopic approaches, with the added benefits of reduced cost and no radiation exposure.[33]

Step-by-Step Technique

The procedure begins with a detailed Doppler ultrasound assessment to identify the stenosis, its severity, and extent. After sterile preparation and local anesthesia, venous access is obtained using a 20G IV cannula under ultrasound guidance. A 0.035-inch mini-guidewire is introduced, followed by insertion of a 5 Fr or 6 Fr vascular sheath, with the choice guided by vessel size and anticipated balloon dimensions. The sheath is typically placed near the outflow tract and directed retrogradely for juxta-anastomotic and mid-venous stenoses and anterogradely for outflow lesions. Through the sheath, a 0.014-inch floppy-tipped wire is used to traverse the stenosis. Navigation challenges, such as the guidewire entering tributaries, are resolved by real-time ultrasound-guided redirection. Once across the lesion, a noncompliant balloon—size based on adjacent vein diameter and severity of stenosis—is advanced over the wire and inflated usually to 8–10 atm under USG visualization. Multiple inflations may be required to achieve luminal gain.[34] **Figures 2 and 3** illustrate the

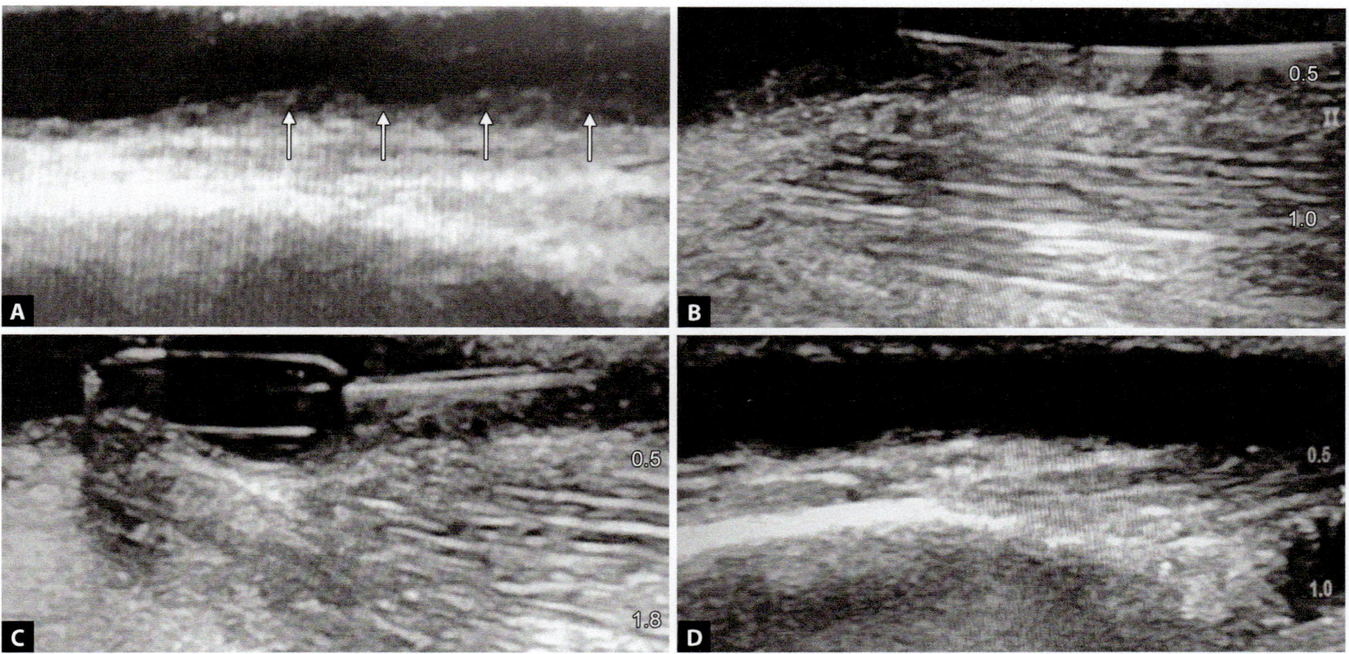

Figs. 2A to D: AV fistula balloon angioplasty under USG guidance for a case of long segment stenosis. (A) 2.5 cm long stenotic segment in mid venous segment of a radiocephalic AV fistula; (B) 4.5 × 1.5 mm angioplasty balloon passed over an 0.014-inch wire and placed at the stenotic segment; (C) The balloon was inflated to 10 atm pressure; (D) Resolution of stenosis after balloon dilatation.

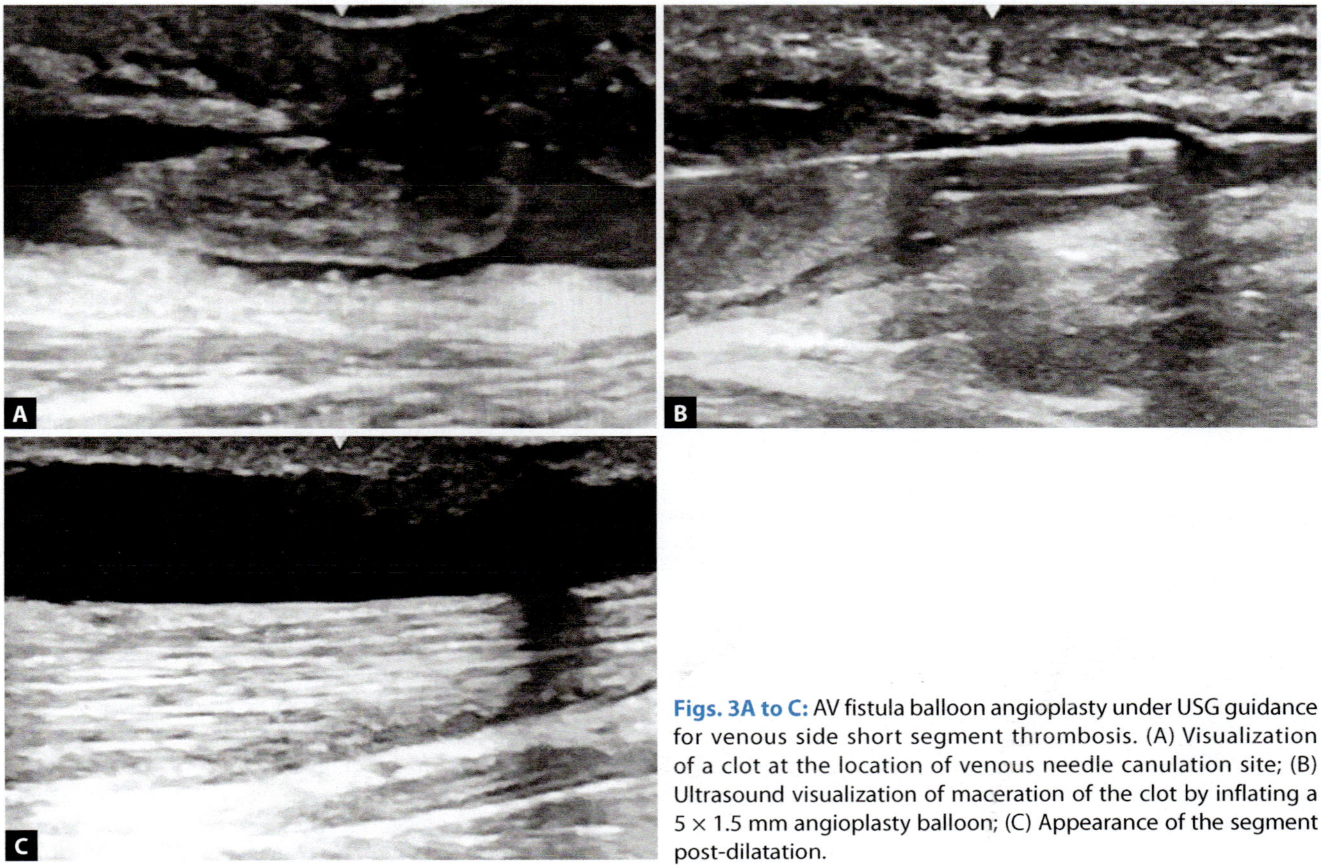

Figs. 3A to C: AV fistula balloon angioplasty under USG guidance for venous side short segment thrombosis. (A) Visualization of a clot at the location of venous needle canulation site; (B) Ultrasound visualization of maceration of the clot by inflating a 5 × 1.5 mm angioplasty balloon; (C) Appearance of the segment post-dilatation.

ultrasound visualization of balloon dilatation during the procedure.

POINTS TO CONSIDER AND COMPLICATION MANAGEMENT

Ultrasound guidance allows dynamic visualization of the balloon inflation and the vein wall, enabling prompt identification of dissection flaps or incomplete dilation. Minor bleeding at the access site is common and typically resolves with manual compression. However, bleeding risk increases with the use of larger (6 Fr) sheaths and should be anticipated in patients with fragile vessels. In cases of partial dissection, balloon tamponade can effectively seal the flap. Immediate postprocedure dialysis should demonstrate improved flow and normalized venous pressures. Restenosis remains a limitation and may occur within 6–12 months; however, reintervention is usually successful. Data suggest that with appropriate technique and follow-up, reintervention-free patency rates of over 85% at 6 months can be achieved.[35]

CONCLUSION

The realm of interventional nephrology stands at a pivotal juncture, where the challenges posed by thrombosis and stenosis in AVFs and AVGs demand both ingenuity and teamwork. These vascular access issues are more than technical hurdles—they are vital to the well-being of hemodialysis patients, shaping their treatment experience and longevity. Rather than merely reacting to complications, the field is shifting toward a forward-thinking stance, fueled by cutting-edge developments like advanced imaging, minimally invasive procedures, and novel materials that promise to redefine how we safeguard these lifelines.

The landscape of interventional nephrology is poised for significant evolution, driven by innovations that aim to enhance the longevity and functionality of AVFs and AVGs. Advances in artificial intelligence (AI) and machine learning are paving the way for predictive models that analyze Doppler ultrasound data and flow metrics to forecast complications such as stenosis and thrombosis, enabling preemptive interventions. Concurrently, the advent of bioengineered grafts—featuring endothelial cell linings or nanotechnology-enhanced surfaces—offers promise in reducing thrombogenicity and intimal hyperplasia, key contributors to access failure. These developments, herald a future where vascular access complications are not only treated with greater precision but potentially averted, positioning interventionalists at the forefront of improving hemodialysis outcomes.

REFERENCES

1. Lok CE, Huber TS, Lee T, Shenoy S, Yevzlin AS, Abreo K, et al. KDOQI Clinical Practice Guideline for Vascular Access: 2019 Update. Am J Kidney Dis. 2020;75(4 Suppl 2):S1–S164.
2. United States Renal Data System (USRDS). 2023 USRDS Annual Data Report: Epidemiology of kidney disease in the United States. Bethesda (MD): National Institutes of Health, National Institute of Diabetes and Digestive and Kidney Diseases; 2023.
3. Tessitore N, Lipari G, Bedogna V, Poli A, Baggio E, Loschiavo C, et al. Can blood flow surveillance and pre-emptive repair of subclinical stenosis prolong the useful life of arteriovenous fistulae? Nephrol Dial Transplant. 2004;19(9):2325-33.
4. Roy-Chaudhury P, Sukhatme VP, Cheung AK. Hemodialysis vascular access dysfunction: a cellular and molecular viewpoint. J Am Soc Nephrol. 2006;17(4):1112-27.
5. Lee T, Roy-Chaudhury P. Advances and new frontiers in the pathophysiology of venous neointimal hyperplasia and dialysis access stenosis. Adv Chronic Kidney Dis. 2009;16(5):329-38.
6. National Kidney Foundation. KDOQI Clinical Practice Guidelines for Vascular Access: 2006 Update. Am J Kidney Dis. 2006;48(Suppl 1):S176-S247.
7. Maya ID, Oser R, Saddekni S, Barker J, Allon M. Vascular access stenosis: comparison of arteriovenous grafts and fistulas. Am J Kidney Dis. 2004;44(5):859-65.
8. Jeong Y, Yao Y, Yim EKF. Current understanding of intimal hyperplasia and effect of compliance in synthetic small-diameter vascular grafts. Biomater Sci. 2020;8(16):4383-95.
9. Hu K, Guo Y, Li Y, Lu C, Cai C, Zhou S, et al. Oxidative stress: An essential factor in the process of arteriovenous fistula failure. Front Cardiovasc Med. 2022;9:984472.
10. Smith GE, Gohil R, Chetter IC. Factors affecting the patency of arteriovenous fistulas for dialysis access. J Vasc Surg. 2012;55(3):849-55.
11. Sahasrabudhe P, Bindu A. Nuances of arteriovenous fistula creation for vascular access in hemodialysis. Indian J Plast Surg. 2021;54:257-63.
12. Sahasrabudhe P, Dighe T, Panse N, Deshpande S, Jadhav A, Londhe S. Prospective long-term study of patency and outcomes of 505 arteriovenous fistulas in patients with chronic renal failure: authors' experience and review of literature. Indian J Plast Surg. 2014;47(3):362-9.
13. Pisoni RL, Zepel L, Fluck R, Lok CE, Kawanishi H, Süleymanlar G, et al. International differences in the location and use of arteriovenous accesses created for hemodialysis:

results from the Dialysis Outcomes and Practice Patterns Study. Am J Kidney Dis. 2018;71(4):469-78.

14. Kim IS, Kim S, Yoo T-H, Kim J-K. Diagnosis and treatment of hypertension in dialysis patients: a systematic review. Clin Hypertens. 2023;29:24.
15. Hoffstaetter T, Silpe J, Delijani D, Landis GS, Etkin Y. Sex disparities in arteriovenous fistula maturation outcomes. Ann Vasc Surg. 2023;95:197-202.
16. Bandyk DF, Hodgkiss-Harlow KD. Color duplex ultrasound in dialysis access surveillance. In: AbuRahma AF, Perler BA, editors. Noninvasive Vascular Diagnosis. Cham: Springer; 2021. pp. 1-21.
17. Collin G, Jones RG, Willis AP. Central venous obstruction in the thorax. Clin Radiol. 2015;70(6):654-60.
18. Dariushnia SR, Walker TG, Silberzweig JE, Annamalai G, Krishnamurthy V, Mitchell JW, et al. Society of Interventional Radiology Standards of Practice Committee. Quality Improvement Guidelines for Percutaneous Image-Guided Management of the Thrombosed or Dysfunctional Dialysis Circuit. J Vasc Interv Radiol. 2016;27(10):1518-30.
19. Aktas A, Bozkurt A, Aktas B, Kirbas I. Percutaneous transluminal balloon angioplasty in stenosis of native hemodialysis arteriovenous fistulas: technical success and factors affecting postprocedural patency. Diagn Interv Radiol. 2015;21(2):160-6.
20. Holden A, Haruguchi H, Suemitsu K, Isogai N, Ross J, Hull J, et al. IN.PACT AV Access randomized trial: 12-month clinical results demonstrating the sustained treatment effect of drug-coated balloons. J Vasc Interv Radiol. 2022;33(8):884-94.e7.
21. D'Cruz RT, Leong SW, Syn N, Tiwari A, Sannasi VV, Singh Sidhu HR, et al. Endovascular treatment of cephalic arch stenosis in brachiocephalic arteriovenous fistulas: a systematic review and meta-analysis. J Vasc Access. 2019;20(4):345-55.
22. Çildağ MB, Öztürk VS, Özgür R, Köseoğlu ÖFK. Primary patency rates of endovascular interventions in hemodialysis patients with central venous stenosis and occlusions. Acta Angiol. 2021;27(1):17-21.
23. Huber TS, Carter JW, Carter RL, Seeger JM. Patency of autogenous and polytetrafluoroethylene upper extremity arteriovenous hemodialysis accesses: a systematic review. J Vasc Surg. 2003;38(5):1005-11.
24. Huan KWSJ, Tan CS, Chua D, Yap CJQ, Tan RY, Chong TT. The Cleaner XT™ device as an endovascular adjunct for pharmacomechanical thrombolysis of thrombosed arteriovenous fistulas and grafts. Ann Vasc Dis. 2020;13(4):1-7.
25. Marcelin C, D'Souza S, Le Bras Y, Petitpierre F, Grenier N, van den Berg JC, et al. Mechanical thrombectomy in acute thrombosis of dialysis arteriovenous fistulae and grafts using a vacuum-assisted thrombectomy catheter: a multicenter study. J Vasc Interv Radiol. 2018;29(7):993-7.
26. Sofocleous CT, Hinrichs CR, Weiss SH, Contractor D, Barone A, Bahramipour P, et al. Alteplase for hemodialysis access graft thrombolysis. J Vasc Interv Radiol. 2002;13(8):775-83.
27. Yang YS, Han KD, Choi EH, Park YS, Seo YH, Kim CS. Clinical experience with a hybrid procedure using the adherent clot catheter for salvage of thrombosed hemodialysis access: a comparison with the standard Fogarty balloon catheter. Vasc Specialist Int. 2015;31(1):25-31.
28. Dember LM, Beck GJ, Allon M, Delmez JA, Dixon BS, Greenberg A, et al. Dialysis Access Consortium Study Group. Effect of clopidogrel on early failure of arteriovenous fistulas for hemodialysis: a randomized controlled trial. JAMA. 2008;299(18):2164-71.
29. Crowther MA, Clase CM, Margetts PJ, Julian J, Lambert K, Sneath D, et al. Low-intensity warfarin is ineffective for the prevention of PTFE graft failure in patients on hemodialysis: a randomized controlled trial. J Am Soc Nephrol. 2002;13(9):2331-7.
30. Schmidli J, Widmer MK, Basile C, de Donato G, Gallieni M, Gibbons CP, et al. Editor's Choice – Vascular Access: 2018 Clinical Practice Guidelines of the European Society for Vascular Surgery (ESVS). Eur J Vasc Endovasc Surg. 2018;55(6):757-818.
31. Shemesh D, Goldin I, Hijazi J, Zaghal I, Berelowitz D, Verstandig A, et al. A prospective randomized study of heparin-bonded graft (Propaten) versus standard graft in prosthetic arteriovenous access. J Vasc Surg. 2015;62(1):115-22.
32. Pullano S, Oliva G, Laganá F, Fiorillo A, Pratticò D, Presta P, et al. Development of a Wearable Device for Arteriovenous Fistula Monitoring. 2024. pp.1-4.
33. Malik J, Tuka V, Kasalova Z, Bezdekova V, Svobodova J, Malikova H, et al. Real-time ultrasound-guided percutaneous transluminal angioplasty of hemodialysis arteriovenous fistulas: a feasibility study. J Vasc Access. 2015;16(6):446-51.
34. Arun Thomas ET, Pookunju S, Joseph R. USG guided AV fistula balloon angioplasty for optimizing cost-efficiency and accessibility: a comprehensive analysis of technical aspects and outcome. Kidney Int Rep. 2025;10(2):S418-9. Abstract WCN25-2645.
35. Tessitore N, Bedogna V, Poli A, Lipari G, Bassi P, Bedogna V, et al. Dialysis outcomes of stenosis angioplasty under ultrasound versus fluoroscopic guidance in native arteriovenous fistulae: a prospective study. J Vasc Access. 2021;22(1):42-8.

CHAPTER 27

Pseudoaneurysm and Hemorrhage

Krishnaswamy Sampathkumar, Prabhu Kumarappan Chidambaram

CASE SCENARIO

A 54-year-old female presented with complaints of pain in the left arm for the past 3 weeks associated with swelling of the whole limb for 2 months. The patient underwent left brachial artery-axillary vein arteriovenous graft (AVG) 2 years back which is being used for hemodialysis since then.

On examination, diffuse pitting edema of the left arm was noted. A 4 × 4 cm pulsatile tender swelling in the upper arm over the left brachioaxillary AVG was seen. Blanching was present in the palm of hand. Sensation was intact, and there were no neurological deficits. Doppler and CT venogram showed a pseudoaneurysm of AVG with stenosis of axillary vein just distal to its venous end **(Fig. 1)**.

Central veins were patent. A diagnosis of a pseudoaneurysm of AVG with severe venous hypertension due to outflow vein stenosis was made. She was managed surgically by excision of the pseudoaneurysm segment of AVG and interposition graft bypass with proximalization of venous anastomosis to normal portion of the axillary vein. There was immediate reduction in the pain followed by resolution of arm edema. She could be reinitiated onto hemodialysis using the same AVG **(Fig. 2)**.

INTRODUCTION

The term *aneurysm* describes dilatation of any blood vessel. Aneurysms can be true or false (pseudoaneurysm). The distinction of true or false aneurysms is dependent on whether it is a dilatation of the entire vascular wall (i.e., true aneurysm) or there is a defect in the vascular wall with locally contained hematoma (i.e., pseudoaneurysm), the wall of the pseudoaneurysm being formed by connective tissue formed in reaction to the contained hematoma. A neck which connects the affected artery and the main body of the aneurysm can be imaged by a Doppler ultrasonography which picks up active blood flow.[1]

INCIDENCE

Aneurysm formation is a known complication of hemodialysis arteriovenous grafts (AVG) and fistulas, as the arteriovenous access is subjected to repeated trauma during puncture for dialysis. The incidence is estimated at 2–10% during the functional life of a graft.[2] Pseudoaneurysm of an arteriovenous fistula (AVF) is less frequent compared to AVG. True aneurysms are reported in up to 17% of AVF.[3]

ETIOLOGY AND PATHOPHYSIOLOGY

- Puncture related
- Infection
- Surgical complication—anastomotic suture disruption

Arteriovenous graft, in particular, is at an increased risk than AVF because of degradation of the graft material caused by repeated needle punctures. Different puncture techniques may exert different effects on vascular access dilatation. Three options for puncture have been routinely used: (1) Rope ladder, (2) area puncture, and (3) buttonhole technique. It has been suggested that aneurysm formation was usually a result of the area puncture technique.[4]

Pseudoaneurysms also develop at the anastomosis site secondary to suture line dehiscence due to a faulty surgical technique in the postoperative period or can occur later as a complication of infection. In this scenario, anastomosed arteries are often involved leading to life-threatening secondary hemorrhage.[5]

Pseudoaneurysms are frequently caused or accompanied by pre- or postaneurysm stenosis or central vein stenosis. A hemodynamically significant proximal stenosis leads to aneurysmal dilatation due to raised intraluminal pressure.[6] In contrast to autogenous access, grafts do not dilate but false aneurysms develop at puncture sites.[7]

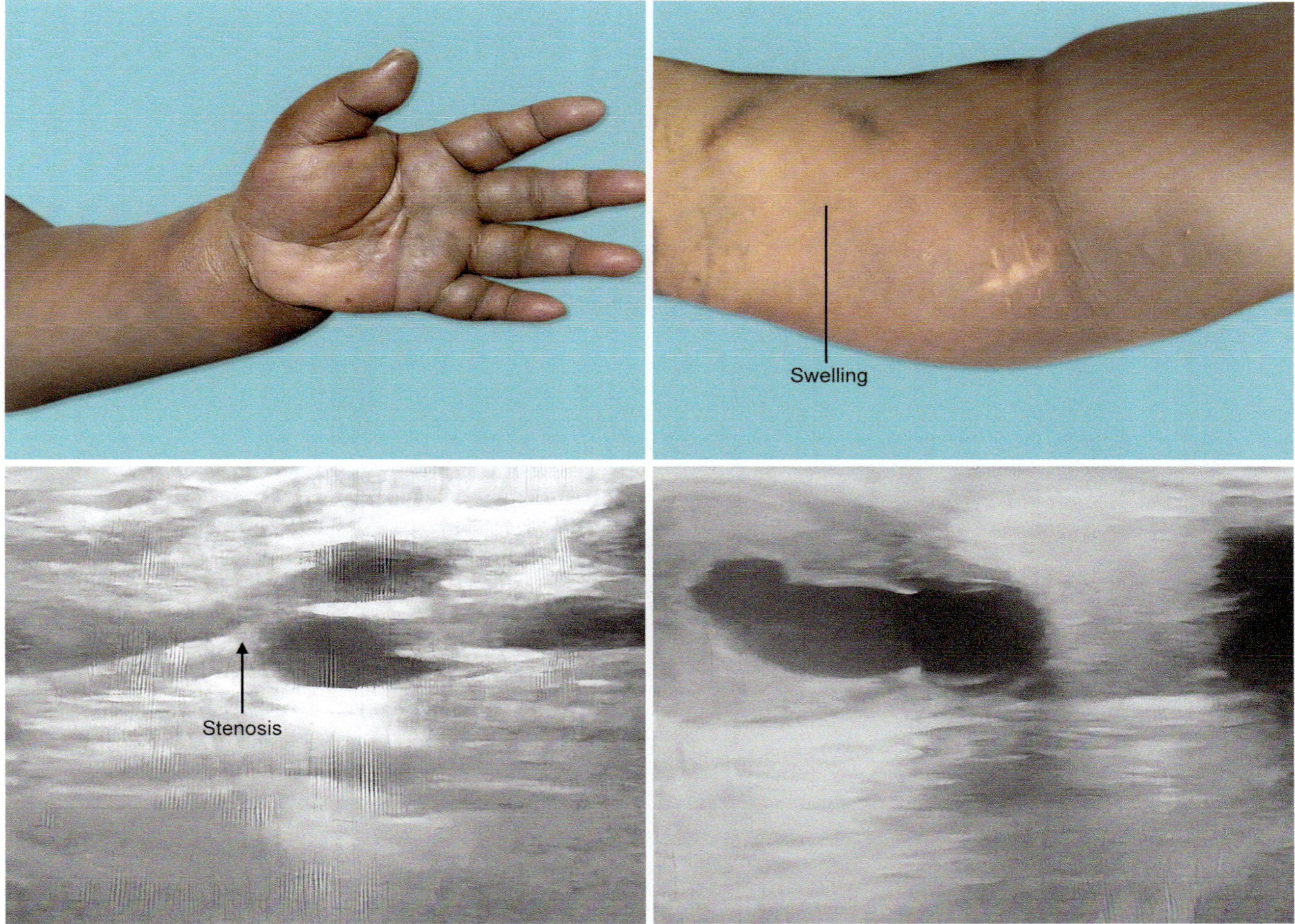

Fig. 1: Severe edema of hand and forearm. Tender swelling in the upper arm in the arteriovenous graft site. Ultrasound showing a tight stenosis in the axillary vein just distal to the anastomosis and a large pseudoaneurysm with disrupted graft surface.

Diagnosis

Arteriovenous access pseudoaneurysm is usually diagnosed clinically and confirmed by ultrasound examination.

Clinical features of pseudoaneurysm:

- Pulsatile swelling
- Pain during dialysis
- Progressive shiny skin over the swelling
- Purulent discharge
- Skin ulceration
- Bleeding

Investigations

Doppler Ultrasound

Doppler ultrasound diagnoses a pseudoaneurysm accurately. The typical ultrasound appearance of a pseudoaneurysm is an echolucent sac that is pulsatile. On color Doppler, a swirling flow pattern is noted within this sac. On spectral waveform analysis, the characteristic "to-and-fro" flow pattern can be noted which is pathognomonic for a pseudoaneurysm.[8]

CT angiogram or MR angiogram is required only when the sac is extending across the tissue planes which could not be discerned by ultrasound and to find out additional access or graft tears. CT venogram also identifies associated central venous or outflow venous stenosis/occlusions.

Complications

Bleeding, thrombosis, and infection are the three major complications. Of this, life-threatening hemorrhage is the most dreaded one.

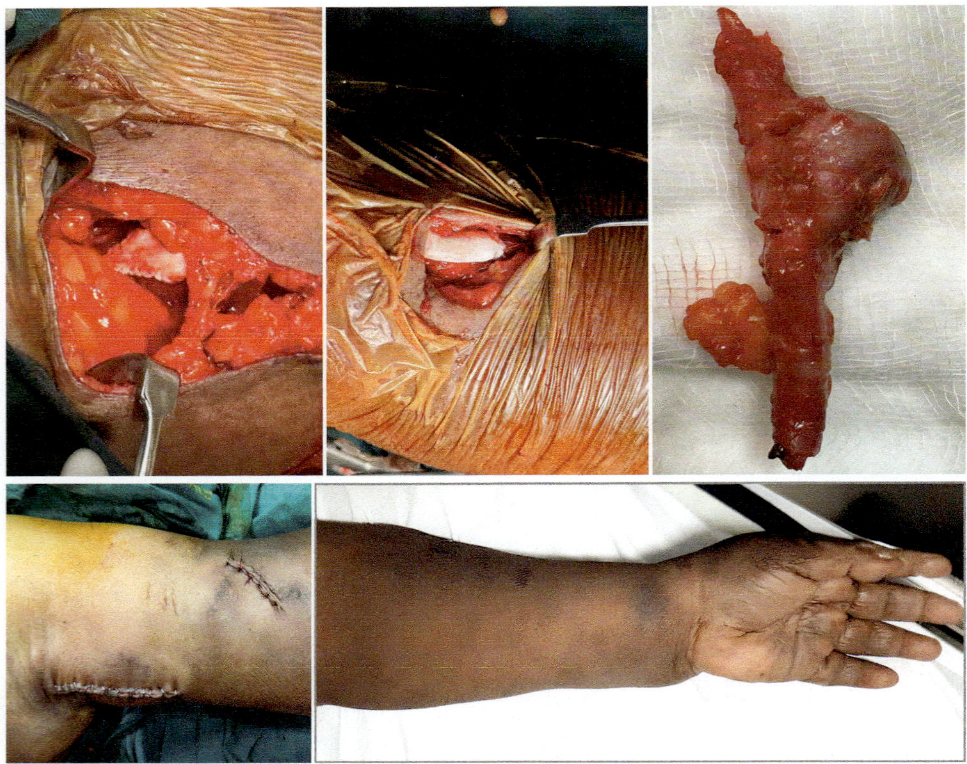

Fig. 2: Proximalized graft to venous anastomosis and graft-to-graft anastomosis. Separate sterile tunnel used for the jump graft. Complete resolution of edema in postoperative day 1.

HEMORRHAGE

Inherently, patients on hemodialysis have an increased bleeding tendency which is multifactorial. Defective aggregation of platelets, reduced thromboxane A2 and nitric oxide generation, defective fibrinogen, von Willebrand factor (vWF), and GPIIb–IIIa complex interplay are implicated in abnormal platelet-to-platelet and platelet-to-vessel wall interactions leading to bleeding.

Hemorrhage is encountered in two situations. The first one is during the perioperative period with intra- and postoperative bleeding or hematoma formation. The second situation occurs after dialysis characterized by a failure of hemostasis at the puncture sites. This may manifest as external bleeding, hematoma, or pseudoaneurysm.[3]

Preventive measures to avoid hemorrhage and pseudoaneurysm are:

- Adequate preparation of patient:
  - Maintenance of a hematocrit >30%
  - Adequate dialysis before any intervention
  - Monitoring bleeding time and coagulation parameters
- Proper cannulation technique
- Arteriovenous access and graft surveillance
- Medical management to correct coagulopathy and control bleeding
  - 1-deamino-8-d-arginine vasopressin (DDAVP)
  - Cryoprecipitate
  - Estrogen

Dialysis nurses quality education and audit programs: Use of proper cannulation technique, rotation of cannulation site, and avoiding one-site cannulation are some of the ways recommended for prevention of aneurysm and pseudoaneurysm in dialysis access. Cannulation should be avoided in the affected area, especially when the overlying skin is thin and shiny making it vulnerable for bleeding and infection. Regular discussions, audit, and root cause analysis should be included in the training programs of dialysis nurses and technicians. When a pseudoaneurysm is diagnosed, monthly AVG surveillance and 3-monthly AVF surveillance using ultrasound are of paramount importance.[7]

Pain during dialysis is a symptom that an aneurysmal fistula is progressing to complications. Abnormal bleeding not controlled by regular compression techniques raises caution for an imminent rupture.

Nonsurgical Interventions to Control Bleeding

Digital Compression

Direct digital compression is an effective and the most commonly used method for needle hole bleeding in dialysis rooms. However, only digital compression is not enough in many circumstances, especially in the aneurysmal fistula vein/graft. Recent studies have shown effective use of specialized dressings and compression techniques in such situations.

- *Special dressings*:
    - Chitosan-based dressings
    - Cellulose-based gauze
    - Thrombin-soaked gauze
    - Poly-N-acetyl glucosamine–based patch

  Postcannulation bleeding time was compared between standard and specialized dressings in four studies and found that use of specialized dressings decreased bleeding time by 35–74%. No adverse effects of using specialized dressings were reported. However, there are no specific recommendations about which dressing types to use and when to use them. A disadvantage of chitosan and cellulose-based dressing is the cost. Moreover, there are no comparative studies which have shown better efficacy.[9]
- *Mechanical compression devices:*
    - Tourniquet application
    - Adjustable clamps
    - Bottle cap compression

A study by Abidian et al. has shown successful use of torniquet placed on AVF/AVG postcannulation and found to have good bleed control and prevents formation of pseudoaneurysm. But the study has no control group.[10] Greenstein et al. reported successful use of bottle cap in controlling bleed outside the dialysis unit until it was removed in the operation theater. These methods do act as temporizing measures prior to operative management and control bleeding that could not be achieved by conventional compression methods. No adverse effects are reported with the usage of compression devices.[11]

The use of adjustable clamps on vascular access sites was associated in one study with more consistent pressure measurement across the fistula, compared with the two-finger compression technique.[12] Similarly, chronic use of a sleeve compression device on the aneurysmal parts of AVF has not been found to be associated with aneurysmal expansion, increased bleeding, or thrombosis. It is thus possible that clamp use to manage postcannulation bleeding could lead to lower AVF thrombosis rates.[13]

PSEUDOANEURYSM MANAGEMENT

Surgical repair is the standard treatment for AVG pseudoaneurysms, especially when the pseudoaneurysm diameter is more than twice the diameter of the graft. However, in recent times, other minimally invasive treatment alternatives are successfully used such as endovascular stent graft repair with comparable results in selected patients.

Other bedside procedures used in pseudoaneurysm management are ultrasound-guided manual compression and thrombin injection with good outcomes in selected cases.

Indications for management of autogenous access and AVG pseudoaneurysm are:

- *Urgent:*
    - Ulcerated or necrotic skin
    - Bleeding
- *Nonurgent:*
    - Cannulation difficulty due to aneurysm
    - High output congestive heart failure due to aneurysm
    - Disfigurement impacting a patient's body image
    - Infection

Management of an AV access pseudoaneurysm depends on the size, site (puncture site vs. anastomotic), and etiology (sterile vs. infectious).

Small Saccular Pseudoaneurysms

Small pseudoaneurysms with narrow necks and no signs of infection may be amenable to thrombin injection or ultrasound compression. This noninvasive technique may be attempted before resorting to surgical or endovascular alternatives in selective cases, whereas large pseudoaneurysm requires surgical or endovascular management.

Various Modalities of Treatment

Ultrasound-guided Compression

The digital compression given directly over the connection between the cavity and the outflow vein is localized by the ultrasonography. The time needed to occlude the pseudoaneurysm usually ranges from 20 to 45 minutes. Several sittings may be required once or twice a day.

Witz et al. reported three cases of AVF pseudoaneurysms treated successfully by ultrasound-guided compression (UGC) using manual compression directly over the pseudoaneurysm cavity identifiable by the ultrasonography.[14]

In the largest series published to date, success rates ranged from 74 to 93%. Multiple factors impede successful ultrasound-guided compression including:

- Anticoagulation
- Size of pseudoaneurysm
- Patient compliance

Complications include rupture of pseudoaneurysm and thrombosis of AV access.[15]

Balloon-assisted/Percutaneous Thrombin Injection

It is a routinely used procedure for femoral artery pseudoaneurysms with small neck. It can be administered in percutaneous fashion under ultrasound guidance with or without balloon occlusion of the pseudoaneurysm.

In the balloon occlusion method, the balloon is inflated across the neck of pseudoaneurysm under fluoroguidance and thrombin is injected into the sac under USG guidance. A 5-minute inflation of balloon is ideal. This technique can be used in small to moderately wide-neck pseudoaneurysms. Apart from few case reports and series, no trials are available for this modality.

The most significant complications of this procedure include thrombosis of the native artery or vein if thrombin is inadvertently injected into these vessels. Anaphylaxis has been reported with bovine preparations but is rare.[16]

Large Puncture Site Pseudoaneurysm

In the acute setting, large nonresolving puncture-related pseudoaneurysms generally require surgical repair. However, recent studies show comparable results with endovascular stent graft repair with acceptable outcomes.

Endovascular Management

Endovascular management of arteriovenous access or AVG pseudoaneurysm involves deployment of covered stents, also known as stent grafts across the aneurysmal segment of the access or graft, thereby excluding the aneurysmal portion devoid of high-pressure blood flow and causing decompression of pseudoaneurysm preventing rupture of the aneurysm.

Stent grafts are constructed with expanded polytetrafluoroethylene (ePTFE) or woven polyester material (Dacron) lining a metal stent. It has been hypothesized that the synthetic material in the stent graft external to metal stent allows for better incorporation into the surrounding tissue and thereby reduces the chance of development of pseudoaneurysms after repeated needle puncture.

Various stent grafts are available in the Indian market like Fluency Plus (BD), Covera Plus (BD), and Wallgraft (Boston Scientific) which were successfully used in the management of fistula pseudoaneurysms.

Initial attempts at endovascular management of pseudoaneurysms deployed detachable balloons to promote thrombosis. Subsequently, other investigators described the successful stent graft repair of AV access pseudoaneurysms.

It can be considered as an alternative to open repair in patients who are anatomically suitable candidates.

Suitable candidates for endovascular stent graft placement are:

- Puncture site pseudoaneurysm:
  - Short segment and small size
  - Not involving arterial anastomosis
- No signs of infection
- Arteriovenous access characteristics:
  - Appropriate diameter of the access vein
  - Appropriate landing zones (>10 mm proximal and distal to aneurysm)

Contraindications

- Any signs of local or systemic infection
- *Larger diameter of access vein landing zones (>10–12 mm):* As the available stent grafts are available in maximum diameter of 14–15 mm

Nonavailability of graft during emergency situations also plays a role in decision-making.

Procedure

A standard antegrade or retrograde angiogram is performed to evaluate the access vein or graft including the arterial anastomosis and outflow veins, as well as the central venous system. Measurements of the proximal and distal landing zone diameters as well as the diameter and neck diameter of the pseudoaneurysm were then obtained. Appropriate stent graft is selected with 10–15% oversizing, i.e., 1–1.5 mm greater than the diameter of the access vein or graft. The stent graft length was determined by allowing for coverage of at least a 10 mm segment of landing zone, both proximal and distal to the pseudoaneurysm. A stent graft is then deployed over a hydrophilic wire and ballooned using the same size balloon as the stent for complete opposition of stent graft to the vein or graft wall. Completion angiogram is taken to check for exclusion of pseudoaneurysm and for any endoleaks. Associated stenosis in the outflow vein or central vein is further corrected.[17]

Advantages

- Endovascular repair permits immediate use of the access site.
- Identification and angioplasty of stenosis in adjacent sites at the same setting is possible.

Outcome

Criado et al. found that exclusion of pseudoaneurysms can be achieved with a high degree of technical success, low morbidity rate, and short hospital stay.[18]

Wong et al. showed that 1-, 6-, and 12-month primary patency rates were 89.2%, 55.5%, and 22.0%, respectively. The 1-, 6-, and 12-month secondary patency rates were 100%, 88.6%, and 78.6% respectively. These stent grafts can be immediately used for dialysis with no need for bridging catheters placement.[19]

Complications

Infection and thrombosis are the main complications. Wong et al. showed late complications of infections at 17.1% and thrombosis at 37.1%, which is comparable with the 11–41% infection rate of AVGs without a stent/stent graft. Other complications include protrusion of stent grafts through the skin ulcer and stent fractures but are rare.[19]

Stent graft pseudoaneurysm repair and stent graft cannulation for hemodialysis are not approved by the US Food and Drug Administration owing to the absence of well-conducted prospective studies and high-quality evidence, but present studies are showing good comparable outcomes to open surgical repair.

Infected Pseudoaneurysm

Pseudoaneurysms related to infection, particularly with grafts, require surgery. Endovascular repair is contraindicated in the presence of infection.

Surgical Management

Surgical repair is the standard treatment for arteriovenous access/grafts and pseudoaneurysms and remains the gold standard treatment. With the advent of endovascular interventions for pseudoaneurysm, the situations considered for surgical revision include **(Fig. 3)**:

- Exposed graft with overlying skin erosion
- Erythematic, purulent discharge or a draining sinus tract, which are signs of local infection
- Rapidly expanding aneurysm
- Ulceration and bleeding

Surgical intervention is usually required in the presence of pseudoaneurysm with local or systemic infections.

The recommended surgical treatment for infected pseudoaneurysm depends on:

- Extent of infection
- Type of AV access conduit (autogenous vs. prosthetic)
- Bacterial etiology
- Functional status of the AV access (patent or occluded)

Surgical options:

- Access-preserving procedures
- Total excision with ligation of access

Access-preserving procedures:

- Excision and repair with primary suturing
- Segmental access excision with interposition grafting

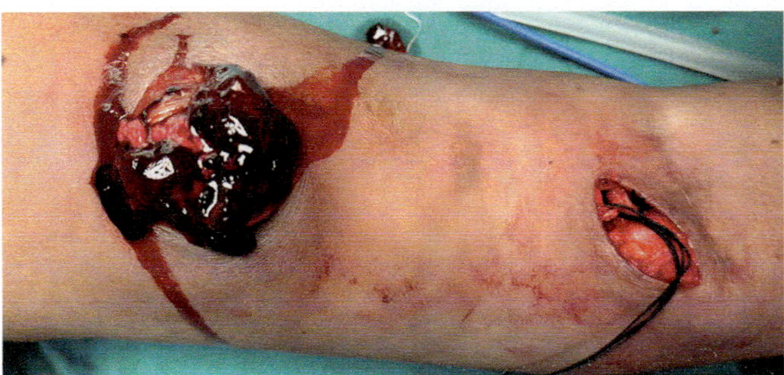
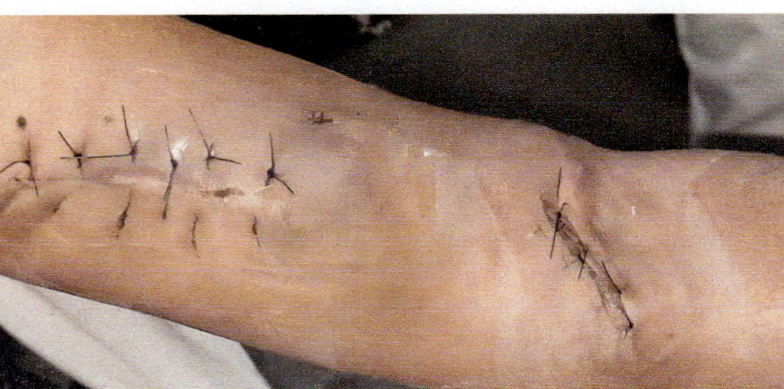

Fig. 3: Ruptured pseudoaneurysm in a post-transplant patient with hematoma and severe pain managed by excision of pseudoaneurysm and thrombophlebitic fistula vein.

Excision and repair with primary suturing: Puncture site pseudoaneurysm with intact wall of the access and without any infection can be excised and the neck of the aneurysm closed primarily using prolene sutures.

Segmental access excision and interposition graft reconstruction: This procedure is recommended when:

- Loss of integrity in the anterior wall of graft or access vein
- Signs of infection confined to a segment of access

In more than half of infected AV accesses, infection is confined to a focal segment of the graft. Segmental access excision with placement of a new jump graft through a sterile field should be considered in these situations.

Total or subtotal AV access excision: This should be performed for infected conduits when:

- Access is causing septicemia
- Access is occluded
- Infection is due to *Pseudomonas* spp. or other aggressive bacteria
- The entire AV access is involved with infection as manifested by pus or fluid surrounding the entire conduit
- Conduit is completely unincorporated

The combined presence of bleeding, proximity to an anastomosis, and local site infection is more likely to result in sacrifice of the access.

Anastomotic pseudoaneurysms with infection may require ligation of the brachial artery with a jump graft to distal clean artery in a sterile field. In these dire situations, ligation of the brachial artery is well tolerated due to collateral flow **(Fig. 4)**.[9]

Georgiadis et al. reported that the mean primary patency after salvage is 93%, 82%, 57%, and 32% at 3, 6, 12, and 24 months, respectively.[20]

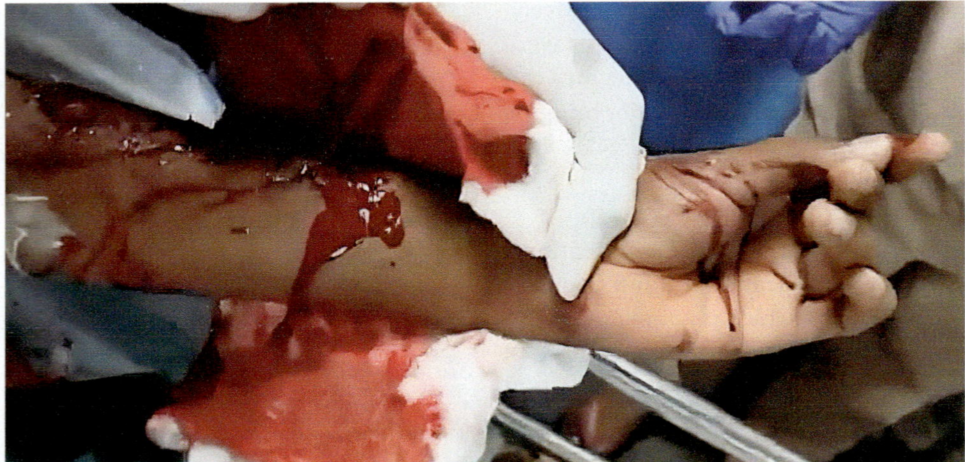

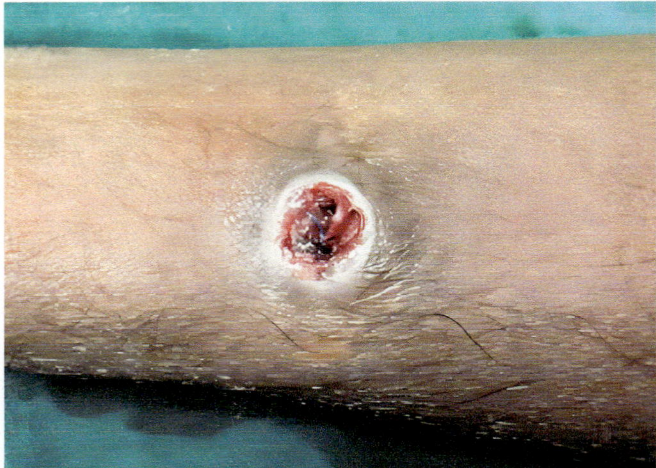

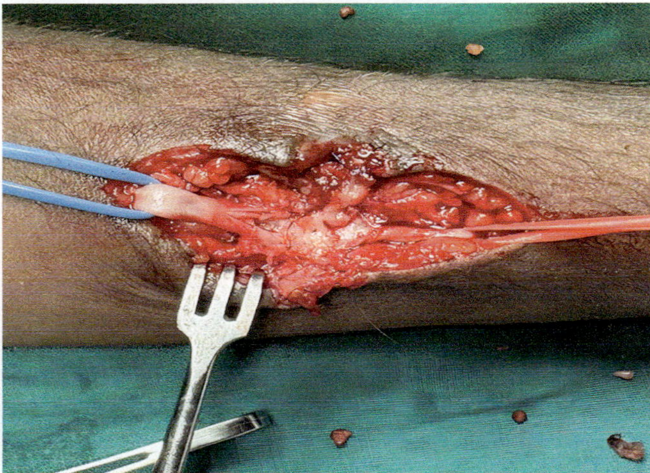

Fig. 4: Active bleeding from an infected fistula anastomosis site. Anastomotic pseudoaneurysm with disrupted anastomosis managed by ligation of radial artery and excision of aneurysm.

CONCLUSION

Arteriovenous access or graft pseudoaneurysms is a treatable complication. Preventive steps taken in dialysis units in the form of regular training sessions on a correct access cannulation technique for dialysis nurses and technicians will go a long way to reduce its incidence. Early recognition and endovascular/surgical management will prolong the patency of the access. Hemorrhage due to pseudoaneurysm is an emergency and early intervention is pivotal in reducing morbidity and mortality.

REFERENCES

1. Sidawy A, Perler B. Rutherford's Vascular Surgery and Endovascular Therapy, 9th edition. Philadelphia: Elsevier; 2019. pp. 877-8.
2. Palder SB, Kirkman RL, Whittemore AD, Hakim RM, Lazarus JM, Tilney NL. Vascular access for hemodialysis. Patency rates and results of revision. Ann Surg. 1985;202:235-9.
3. Padberg FT, Calligaro KD, Sidawy AN. Complications of arteriovenous hemodialysis access: Recognition and management. J Vasc Surg. 2008;48(5):55-80.
4. Hsiao JF, Chou HH, Hsu LA, Wu LS, Yang CW, Hsu TS, et al. Vascular changes at the puncture segments of arteriovenous fistula for hemodialysis access. J Vasc Surg. 2010;52(3):669-73.
5. Lazarides MK, Georgiadis GS, Argyriou C. Aneurysm formation and infection in AV prosthesis. J Vasc Access. 2014;15(7):120-4.
6. Barshes NR, Annambhotla S, Bechara C, Kougias P, Huynh TT, Dardik A, et al. Endovascular repair of hemodialysis graft-related pseudoaneurysm: an alternative treatment strategy in salvaging failing dialysis access. Vasc Endovascular Surg. 2008;42(3):228-34.
7. Schmidli J, Widmer MK, Basile C, de Donato G, Gallieni M, Gibbons CP, et al. Editor's Choice - Vascular Access: 2018 Clinical Practice Guidelines of the European Society for Vascular Surgery (ESVS). Eur J Vasc Endovasc Surg. 2018;55(6):757-818.
8. Abu-Yousef MM, Wiese JA, Shamma AR. The "to-and-fro" sign: duplex Doppler evidence of femoral artery pseudoaneurysm. AJR Am J Roentgenol. 1988;150(3):632-4.
9. Milosevic E, Forster A, Moist L, Rehman F, Thomson B. Non-surgical interventions to control bleeding from arteriovenous fistulas and grafts inside and outside the hemodialysis unit: A scoping review. Clin Kidney J. 2024;17(5):sfae089.
10. Abidian M, Broxton-Key R, Rawls F. Safety and efficacy of a novel compression hemostatic device for vascular access: a quality improvement study. J Am Soc Nephrol. 2023;34:541.
11. Greenstein R, Nawrocki P, Nesbit C. Bottle it up: Prehospital management of an AV fistula bleed using a bottle cap. Am J Emerg Med. 2023;67:197.
12. Álvaro Cristóbal A, París Boal C, Blanco Velasco N, Sanchidrián SM, Mayoral-Peñas A, José Arévalo Manso J, et al. Hemostasis of arteriovenous fistula: Comparison of direct two-finger pressure to an adjustable device. Nefrologia. 2021;41(5):566-72.
13. Joseph T, Sulzbach C, Bhattarai P, Nguyen T, Khan F, Verma N, et al. Benefits of compression therapy in dialysis patients with aneurysmal AV fistulas. Vascular. 2017;25:46.
14. Witz M, Werner M, Bernheim J, Shnaker A, Lehmann J, Korzets Z. Ultrasound-guided compression repair of pseudoaneurysms complicating a forearm dialysis arteriovenous fistula. Nephrol Dial Transplant. 2000;15(9):1453–4.
15. Eisenberg L, Paulson EK, Kliewer MA, Hudson MP, DeLong DM, Carroll BA. Sonographically guided compression repair of pseudoaneurysms: further experience from a single institution. Am J Roentgenol. 1999;173(6):1567-73.
16. Giordano G, Sollami OR, Meo D, Piana S, Lentini V, Magnano San Lio V. Balloon-assisted, ultrasound-guided percutaneous real-time thrombin injection, for the arteriovenous fistula pseudoaneurysm treatment. Radiol Case Rep. 2023;18(2):524-6.
17. Shah AS, Valdes J, Charlton-Ouw KM, Chen Z, Coogan SM, Amer HH, et al. Endovascular treatment of hemodialysis access pseudoaneurysms. J Vasc Surg. 2012;55(4):1058-62.
18. Criado E, Marston WA, Ligush J, Mauro MA, Keagy BA. Endovascular repair of peripheral aneurysms, pseudoaneurysms, and arteriovenous fistulas. Ann Vasc Surg. 1997;11(3):256-63.
19. Wong WK, Su TW, Cheng WL, Yang HT, Wei WC, Ko PJ. Endovascular Stent Graft Repair is an Effective and Safe Alternative Therapy for Arteriovenous Graft Pseudoaneurysms. Eur J Vasc Endovasc Surg. 2016; 52(5):682-8.
20. Georgiadis GS, Lazarides MK, Panagoutsos SA, Kantartzi KM, Lambidis CD, Staramos DN, et al. Surgical revision of complicated false and true vascular access-related aneurysms. J Vasc Surg. 2008;47(6):1284-91.

CHAPTER 28

Accessory Veins: Identification and Management

Arushi Nautiyal, J Balasubramaniam

CASE SCENARIO

A 60-year-old male underwent a left-sided radiocephalic arteriovenous fistula (AVF) formation 2 months back; however, cannulation is difficult with poor inflows 7–10 cm beyond anastomosis. Infiltration injuries are common, making its use unreliable. The patient was advised for AVF assessment.

INTRODUCTION

The success of the arteriovenous access circuit for hemodialysis is dependent upon the integrity of both the inflow and the outflow segments. A good arterial inflow limb would require an adequate caliber vessel capable of dilatation post arteriovenous fistula (AVF) creation. Similarly, the venous outflow segment requires various attributes to allow for successful realization as an access for hemodialysis. Such requirements include a long, superficial, straight cannulation segment of vein, central and peripheral venous patency, distensible vein capable of supporting increased blood flow, and absence of stenotic venous areas in the outflow segment that fail to dilate. The presence of significant accessory veins in the outflow segment can divert blood flow from the main fistula vein interfering in its remodeling and contributing to fistula failure.

Accessory veins are superficial veins draining into the larger, named superficial veins which are utilized for AVF formation.[1] They are normal anatomical structures and can be single or multiple and should be actively sought during fistula formation[2] **(Fig. 1)**. Also known as venous tributaries or side branches, accessory veins contribute to an inconsistent venous anatomy as opposed to the arterial vasculature utilized in AVF creation.[1] Collateral veins may develop in the presence of downstream stenosis and divert flow in a similar fashion to accessory veins; they are, however, not a part of normal venous anatomy

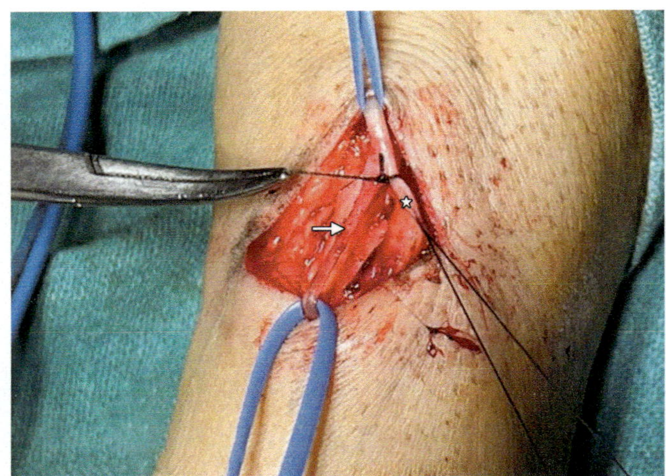

Fig. 1: Radiocephalic arteriovenous fistula (AVF). Arrow represents cephalic vein and star represents accessory vein.

unlike accessory veins. Distinguishing between the two may be difficult; an accessory vein with low flow may develop significant increase in flow in the presence of venous stenosis and despite correction of the stenosis, flow may continue in the accessory vein, impeding fistula development.[3]

Valves are often present within accessory veins near their drainage into the main fistula vein; if competent, they will not allow backflow of blood. However, blood stasis would eventually lead to thrombosis and scarring and the accessory venous segments may act as a tethering point for the main fistula vein, altering its anatomy. If the valves are incompetent or become so due to increased flow, there would be diversion of blood into these venous tributaries which could lead to poor fistula maturation and dysfunction.[1] Presence of accessory veins may be helpful in some scenarios. In a situation with adequate inflow, they may develop to form alternative cannulation segments; however, they can be tortuous and may be anatomically placed in a manner not amenable to comfortable cannulation or long-term use. Accessory veins may also be useful in case of thrombosis of the main fistula vein, where they could provide patent options for cannulation. It has also been observed that the presence of accessory veins is associated with a lower thrombotic burden in case of thrombosis of the main fistula vein, making thrombectomy procedures easier.[4] Accessory veins mostly pose a difficulty in forearm fistulas; upper arm and especially the basilic vein rarely have any significant side branches.[5] Younger patients are also likely to have a greater number of accessory veins, possibly owing to increased physical activity.[3]

An early fistula failure is defined as the inability to use a fistula at any point or one which fails within 3 months of use.[2] Many causes may contribute to such a development, such as inflow problems arising from the use of small caliber artery or atherosclerotic disease which can be avoided to some extent by appropriate selection of vessels or be due to the more common cause of juxta-anastomotic stenosis, a phenomenon which may be amenable to intervention. Outflow issues contributing to fistula failure include small caliber or fibrotic vein, which fails to dilate or due to accessory veins which could siphon blood flow from the main venous segment, thus preventing its adequate dilatation and arterialization.[6,7]

DETECTION OF ACCESSORY VEINS

Accessory veins can occasionally be seen on physical examination preoperatively, especially with application of tourniquet in mid forearm or arm, more likely to be picked up so in thin individuals. They are also usually not well picked up on conventional color Dopplers used for preoperative fistula assessment. Wong et al. followed up patients undergoing radiocephalic AVF formation to assess maturation. They used color Doppler ultrasound along with a pulse-generated runoff system preoperatively, and by using this combination they were able to identify accessory veins in 20 out of 60 patients. The majority had a single major branch with two patients having two branches and two more having three branches within 5 cm of the wrist. They also identified on postoperative follow-up that major branches within 5 cm of anastomosis were associated with fistula failure.[8] Planken et al., in a small prospective study, using contrast-enhanced MR angiography preoperatively, identified accessory veins with vessel diameter >70% of the main cephalic vein to be a significant cause of nonmaturation of radiocephalic AVF, though the use of this modality in advanced kidney failure patients may be problematic due to the need for gadolinium-based contrast agents.[9]

Intraoperative ultrasound may also be useful in evaluating venous anatomy and accessory veins, especially under the effect of anesthesia, as regional block causes a venodilation effect due to sympathetic blockade improving the evaluation of venous anatomy.[10,11]

Any accessory veins encountered during fistula creation should be ligated and thus made nonfunctional by the surgeon. Accessory veins which were missed or remained unencumbered operatively would also receive an increased blood flow following anastomosis, and even small veins are likely to augment and undergo remodeling alongside main venous outflow segment.[5] They may thus become an alternative cannulation site beside main venous segment or may hinder fistula development by diverting blood flow, which tends to be the more usual outcome, necessitating dealing with accessory veins preferably in the operative stage itself. If not ligated during AVF creation, an intervention, which could be surgical or endovascular, could be warranted to manage accessory veins in the setting of nonmaturation, delaying use of AVF and becoming a financial burden.[4]

Postoperatively, when evaluating for fistula failure, it is necessary to rule out accessory veins. They may be visible or be palpable on physical examination.[12] A thrill is present in a fistula and the same can be traced proximally; however, when a significant accessory vein is present, the thrill may disappear beyond it, signifying the poorly formed venous outflow. The thrill felt at the arterial anastomosis also normally disappears upon proximal manual occlusion of the fistula; however, if an accessory vein present below the point of occlusion is diverting flow, the thrill does not disappear and upon palpation of the fistula downward a thrill would be felt at the site of the accessory vein. The whole venous segment may thus be examined by moving point of occlusion progressively downstream of the fistula (proximally) and observing for the point of recurrence of thrill which would mark a significant accessory vein.[6]

When evaluating an immature fistula, duplex scan can help identify possible culprit accessory veins as well as perforators which branch deep to anastomosis. Fistulograms are imperative prior to planned secondary ligation of accessory veins as they best showcase flow diversion.[12,13] Caputo et al., in a retrospective analysis, found that routine color duplex scans done 4–6 weeks' post-AVF formation were more sensitive in picking up abnormal findings needing reintervention including accessory veins as compared to physical examination alone, which helped in achieving functional patency.[14] Etkin et al. also observed the utility of color Doppler scans done routinely for access evaluation at 8 weeks, even comparing with fistulography results for detecting accessory veins.[15] Thus, the policy of routine Doppler scans to assess a maturing fistula should be advocated in vascular access centers wherever possible, to pick up early remediable lesions and reduce catheter dependency.

In the presence of a downstream stenosis in the fistula outflow, an accessory vein would become more prominent. It is thus imperative in such situations to first resolve the stenosis and then assess the significance of the accessory vein, as the blood flow diversion may become inconsequential upon removing downstream stenosis.[2] In a retrospective analysis by Engstrom, the presence of accessory veins with coexisting venous stenosis was the most common pattern seen in nonmaturing AVF.[5] The presence of multiple factors responsible for fistula nonmaturation should always be considered, as an inadequate evaluation can lead to unsuccessful interventions.

Multiple studies have provided evidence of successful salvage of immature fistulas, associated with good primary and secondary patency rates. Thus, a full evaluation of contributing lesions and possible interventions with Doppler and angiographic studies should be attempted prior to abandoning access. Accessory vein obliteration has been found to be often necessitated in such situations when dealing with outflow problems.[5,16,17]

DETERMINING THE SIGNIFICANCE OF ACCESSORY VEINS

There is no consensus for determining the significance of accessory veins identified when evaluating an immature fistula, especially when other factors such as upstream or downstream stenosis may be in play. However, certain characteristics have been described to be of importance; some studies have shown a proximity with the anastomosis (usually within 5 cm) to be of more significance,[8] whereas some operators determine the significance of accessory veins by their size (>3 mm), advocating for ligating all such accessory veins as visualized or palpated along the main vein.[13] Engstrom et al., in a retrospective study, were able to identify a fall in fistula caliber postaccessory vein to have an important association with fistula nonmaturation. This fall corroborates with a difference in the diameters of the main fistula vein before and beyond an impeding accessory vein. Coil embolization of accessory veins which caused a diameter difference (fistula caliber) of >5% was more likely to be associated with successful maturation than in those without, though this did not reach statistical significance. The authors also noted that nonmaturing fistulas with accessory veins would usually be accompanied by stenosis.[5] Haq et al. used various computational fluid dynamics simulations to assess blood flows in fistulas; they identified accessory veins with diameters >60% of the fistula vein to be associated with >20% of blood flow from fistula. They also found that presence of multiple accessory veins compounded flow diversion and branching of accessory veins with diameters around 50% of fistula vein with branches of similar diameters produced more steal, though the distance from anastomosis or angle of accessory vein did not make any difference.[4]

ACCESSORY VEIN OBLITERATION

In the absence of randomized controlled data, evidence on the benefit of accessory vein obliteration is debatable. It is available from large single-center studies done in a retrospective or prospective manner. In a retrospective analysis including 145 fistulas, 20 cases (14%) had accessory veins as the sole cause for fistula immaturity with 76 (52%) having coexisting stenosis and accessory veins.[5] Another prospective study found accessory veins as the primary cause in only 4 out of 119 fistulas (3.4%) and with co-existing stenosis in 35 patients (29.4%), though close to 75% of fistulas under study had multiple contributing lesions.[16] The data is also disputed on the basis of differences in vascular cannulation when assessing immature fistulas, which have been proposed to present different findings.[18] Turmel-Rodrigues et al. in a prospective study of forearm fistulas including 69 patients found stenosis to be the main causative factor in immature fistulas and did not identify any significant accessory vein needing intervention. They undertook feeding artery cannulation for angiographic studies which they considered superior to assess the significance of detected lesions which were all stenotic in nature.[18] Whereas Beathard et al., in a multicenter case series including 100 fistulas, found accessory veins alone as primary lesion in 12% of cases, they utilized a venous cannulation for fistula assessment and inflow was evaluated via reflux angiogram, which could lead to high pressures and impression of increased flow through accessory veins; however, the authors described a 100% success rate in fistulas where accessory vein obliteration was performed when considered significant.[17] Thus, accessory veins do seem to contribute to fistula failure; however, defining their significance in a particular case is difficult and often subjective despite imaging studies such as Doppler and fistulograms, which provide information on diameters and flow through accessory veins.[4]

To enable fistula maturation, accessory veins' obliteration can be achieved via open surgical method, percutaneously or endovascularly. These measures would redirect inflow toward the main fistula vein, allowing for greater likelihood of fistula success.

In the surgical technique, an accessory vein is identified via fluoroscopy or ultrasound and marked on skin. An incision is placed above, and the tissue is dissected till the vein is localized and then ligated using a 4-0 silk tie. Fluoroscopy can be done postprocedure to confirm its closure.[12,19] In the endovascular technique, once an accessory vein is identified via angiogram, coils are utilized to cause embolization and closure of the vein. More than one coil may be required to complete the procedure. Coils can lead to development of pain and local irritation from thrombophlebitis.[4,12] Coils may also migrate and even enter pulmonary circulation with possibility of complications; thus, after determining the size of the target accessory veins on angiography, coils around 1–2 mm larger are inserted for vein obliteration, which is confirmed angiographically.[3] As many cases of accessory vein intervention also require management of stenosis, doing vein obliteration endovascularly allows for multiple procedures to be done in the same sitting.

Endovascular is also the preferred technique in case of deep accessory veins not amenable for open surgical or percutaneous management. Faiyaz et al., described a percutaneous technique in managing accessory veins, with successful maturation in 15 out of 17 fistulas. After marking the accessory vein by angiography close to its entry point into the fistula, the vein was ligated using 2-0 prolene curved needle suture inserted adjacent to the vein, directed underneath the vein and then exited onto the opposite side without any tissue cut down, sutures were removed after 2 weeks. Only one case had recanalization of accessory vein requiring repeat procedure and also suffered from stitch abscess requiring incision and

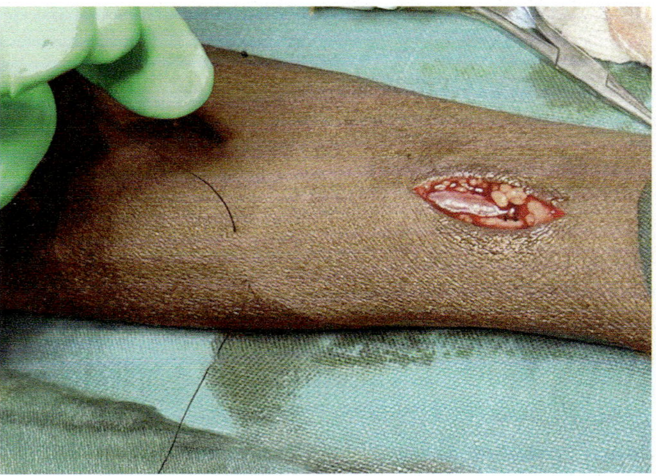

Fig. 2: Accessory vein as seen on physical examination.

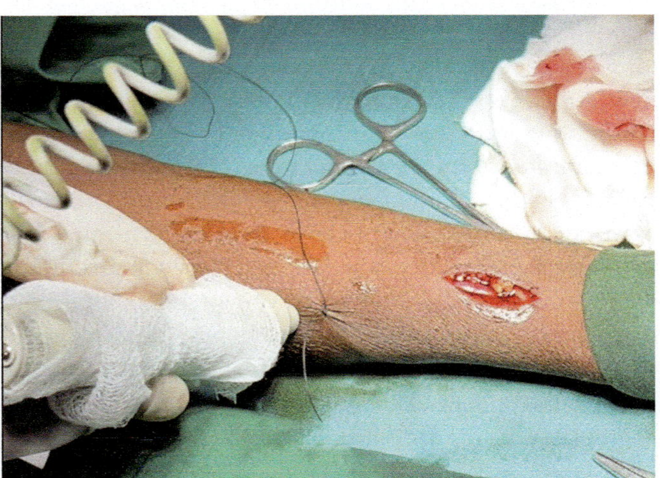

Fig. 3: Percutaneous closure of accessory vein confirmed on Doppler.

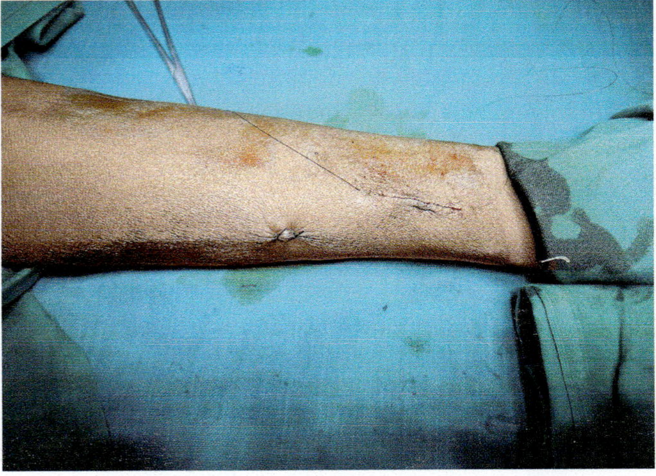

Fig. 4: Final step of percutaneous technique.

drainage.[20] **Figures 2 to 4** illustrating the percutaneous technique.

Nikam et al. reported on accessory vein endovascular coiling studied retrospectively in 42 patients at a single center; they also included patients with late failure of AVF (more than 3 months of use), with the median time of needing intervention being 11.9 months in late failure. Majority of the procedures included angioplasty and coil embolization; only 2 cases of accessory vein obliteration needed further interventions (in other accessory veins) as opposed to a larger number for angioplasty, signifying a low recurrence rate.[3] Yan et al., in a retrospective review, analyzed surgical versus endovascular management of accessory veins. They reported a greater technical success with surgical management and lesser need for reintervention as compared to those managed endovascularly; however, no difference was seen in long-term outcomes.[21] Nauwelaers et al. described a new surgical technique performed in three patients with failure to mature due to accessory veins, which involved the rejoining of the arm veins to create a single outflow vessel.[22] Bae et al. reported on this technique of forced maturation in 23 patients in a retrospective analysis. Rejoining was considered in patients where a main outflow vessel could not be identified. Veins whose combined diameters exceeded 6 mm and were within the range of each other underwent rejoining. They reported a primary patency rate of 82% at 1 year; 34.8% needed an additional angioplasty during the follow-up period (mean 965 days).[23]

Continuing case discussion: Physical examination of the fistula showed poor thrill in the proximal aspect of AVF. Color Doppler picked up a significant accessory vein 5 cm from anastomosis, with diameter similar to outflow venous vein segment with no other possible culprit lesions. Significant divergent flow is demonstrated on angiography and following selective catheterization of the accessory vein, coils are advanced for its obliteration, confirmed angiographically.

CONCLUSION

Presence of accessory veins and their augmentation post-AVF formation can often interfere with vascular access usage. Thus, any accessory veins identified during surgical AVF creation should be ligated. Accessory veins as a prominent cause of fistula failure should especially be considered in forearm fistulas and should be evaluated for in routine physical and Doppler surveillance examinations post-AVF creation. Accessory veins can be managed by various techniques to allow for better fistula maturation and usage; however, concomitant proximal stenosis should always be sought and managed as well.

REFERENCES

1. Shenoy S. Surgical anatomy of upper arm: what is needed for AVF planning. J Vasc Access. 2009;10(4):223-32.
2. Beathard GA. An algorithm for the physical examination of early fistula failure. Semin Dial. 2005;18(4):331-5.
3. Nikam M, Popuri RK, Inaba A, Taylor U, Farquharson F, Mitra S, et al. Arteriovenous fistula failure: is there a role for accessory draining vein embolization? J Vasc Access. 2012;13(4):498-503.
4. Haq NU, Albaqumi M. Accessory vein obliteration criteria for immature fistulae: a modest proposal for an old paradigm. Semin Dial. 2014;27(5):E51-4.
5. Engstrom BI, Grimm LJ, Ronald J, Smith TP, Kim CY. Accessory veins in nonmaturing autogenous arteriovenous fistulae: analysis of anatomic features and impact on fistula maturation. Semin Dial. 2015;28(3):E30-4.
6. Beathard GA. Physical Examination of the Dialysis Vascular Access. Semin Dial. 1998;11:231-6.
7. Dixon BS. Why don't fistulas mature? Kidney Int. 2006;70(8):1413-22.
8. Wong V, Ward R, Taylor J, Selvakumar S, How TV, Bakran A. Factors associated with early failure of arteriovenous fistulae for haemodialysis access. Eur J Vasc Endovasc Surg. 1996;12(2):207-13.
9. Planken RN, Tordoir JH, Duijm LE, de Haan MW, Leiner T. Current techniques for assessment of upper extremity vasculature prior to hemodialysis vascular access creation. Eur Radiol. 2007;17(11):3001-11.
10. Mousa AY, Dearing DD, Aburahma AF. Radiocephalic fistula: review and update. Ann Vasc Surg. 2013;27(3):370-8.
11. Renaud CJ, Leong CR, Bin HW, Wonh JCL. Effect of brachial plexus block-driven vascular access planning on primary distal arteriovenous fistula recruitment and outcomes. J Vasc Surg. 2015;62(5):1266-72.
12. Haq NU, Althaf MM, Lee T. Accessory Vein Obliteration for Early Fistula Failure: A Myth or Reality? Adv Chronic Kidney Dis. 2015;22(6):438-45.
13. McLafferty RB. Techniques to enhance arteriovenous fistula maturation. Perspect Vasc Surg Endovasc Ther. 2009;21(1):41-5.
14. Caputo BC, Leong B, Sibona A, Jhajj S, Kohne C, Gabel J, et al. Arteriovenous fistula maturation: Physical exam versus flow study. Ann Vasc Surg. 2021;77:16-24.
15. Etkin Y, Talathi S, Rao A. The role of duplex ultrasound in assessing AVF maturation. Ann Vasc Surg. 2021;72:315-20.
16. Nassar GM, Nguyen B, Rhee E, Achkar K. Endovascular treatment of the "failing to mature" arteriovenous fistula. Clin J Am Soc Nephrol. 2006;1(2):275-80.

17. Beathard GA, Arnold P, Jackson J, Litchfield T; Physician Operators Forum of RMS Lifeline. Aggressive treatment of early fistula failure. Kidney Int. 2003;64(4):1487-94.
18. Turmel-Rodrigues L, Mouton A, Birmelé B, Billaux L, Ammar N, Grézard O, et al. Salvage of immature forearm fistulas for haemodialysis by interventional radiology. Nephrol Dial Transplant. 2001;16(12):2365-71.
19. Beathard GA, Settle SM, Shields MW. Salvage of the nonfunctioning arteriovenous fistula. Am J Kidney Dis. 1999;33(5):910-6.
20. Faiyaz R, Abreo K, Zaman F, Pervez A, Zibari G, Work J. Salvage of poorly developed arteriovenous fistulae with percutaneous ligation of accessory veins. Am J Kidney Dis. 2022;39:824-27.
21. Yan Q, Miserlis D, Jayakumar L, Brahmbhatt R, Mitromaras C, Sideman MJ, et al. Management of arterio-venous side branches during maturation: ligation or coil embolization. Ann Vasc Surg. 2022;82:52-61.
22. Nauwelaers S, Lansink W, Schroë H, Lauwers G. Surgical rejoining of small arm veins to enhance dialysis fistula maturation. J Vasc Access. 2020;21(1):105-9.
23. Bae M, Lee CW, Chung SW, Huh U, Kim J, Jeong H, et al. Rejoining Veins for Forced Maturation of Small-Caliber Arteriovenous Fistula. Ann Vasc Surg. 2024;104:268-75.

CHAPTER 29

Steal Syndrome and Ischemia

Vipul Prakash Sanghavi, Aadil Beigh

CASE SCENARIO

Mr X is a 69-year-old male with end-stage renal disease (ESRD) secondary to diabetes, who has been undergoing maintenance hemodialysis (HD) three times a week for the past 2 years. Initially, he used a left radiocephalic arteriovenous fistula (RC AVF), which failed due to downstream stenosis which resulted in thrombosis following an episode of intradialytic hypotension. His current dialysis access is a left brachiocephalic (BC) AVF constructed 2 weeks ago, with good thrill, bruit, and distal pulsation. Additionally, he has a right internal jugular vein (IJV) uncuffed HD catheter.

Mr X has a history of poorly controlled type 2 diabetes mellitus (DM), diagnosed with diabetic kidney disease 15 years ago, along with hypertension, coronary artery disease, and chronic smoking.

One week after the BC AVF construction, Mr X presented with symptoms of paresthesia, coldness, and severe pain in his left hand. On examination, a weak radial pulse was noted, but the AVF exhibited a good thrill and bruit. His left hand appeared colder than the right, with a capillary refill time exceeding 5 seconds and visible pallor.

A Doppler ultrasound revealed a patent fistula with a flow rate of 1,800 mL/min, accompanied by flow reversal in the distal radial artery, which suggested a high-flow AVF with arterial steal. These clinical findings, along with the duplex ultrasound, confirmed a diagnosis of dialysis access-associated steal syndrome (DASS).

Summary: Mr X, with ESRD secondary to diabetes, presents with symptoms of DASS following recent BC AVF construction, including paresthesia, coldness, and pallor of the left hand.

Intervention: A left upper limb angiogram was performed, which did not reveal any central venous or cephalic arch stenosis and had absent blood flow to the hand distal to the AVF. Manual compression of the AVF improved hand circulation, confirming the diagnosis of steal syndrome. The MILLER (Minimally Invasive Limited Ligation Endoluminal-assisted Revision) banding technique was applied, using a 4-mm intraluminal balloon as a sizing dowel and 2-0 prolene sutures to band the vessel. This procedure successfully restored hand circulation while maintaining AVF flow. Following the intervention, Mr X experienced significant symptomatic relief and remained asymptomatic, with no further issues related to his dialysis access.

INTRODUCTION

Ischemia caused by the creation of an arteriovenous graft (AVG) or arteriovenous fistula (AVF) as dialysis access is a rare but dreadful complication. Ischemia can occur due to various factors, most commonly reduced blood flow to the distal extremity caused by blood diversion through the AVF or AVG[1] **(Fig. 1)**.

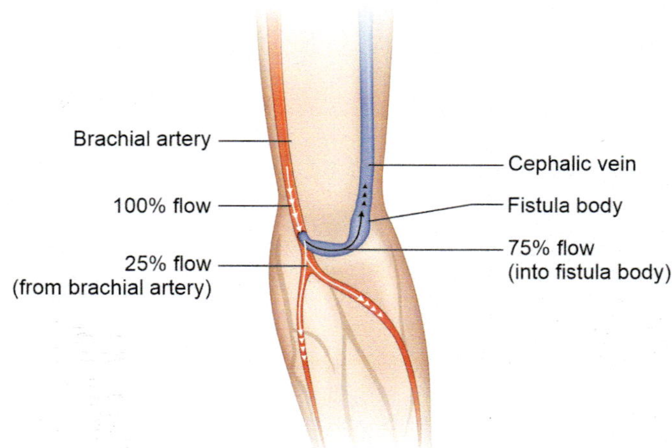

Fig. 1: Dialysis access-associated steal syndrome.
Source: Miller et al.[5]

Dialysis access-associated steal syndrome (DASS) is a more comprehensive term that encompasses the various causes of access-induced ischemia. It can present with either high or low AV access flows necessitating individualized treatment approaches.

Ischemic monomelic neuropathy (IMN), a variant of DASS, may lead to irreversible neurological deficits and demands an aggressive and immediate management strategy.

A clinician and patients need to understand DASS since its consequences can lead to limb dysfunction or even the loss of a limb.

PREVALENCE

Dialysis access-associated steal syndrome is the clinical manifestation of this ischemia, and its prevalence ranges from 4 to 10%, depending on the type and location of the AV access.[2]

The severity of DASS[3] can vary, with symptoms ranging from mild to life-threatening requiring immediate intervention. A study by Zanow et al.[4] on 4,863 patients identified the incidence of DASS in various types of fistulas and grafts: Snuffbox AVF (0%), radiocephalic AVF (0.3%), brachiobasilic AVF (3.7%), brachiocephalic/basilic AVF (5.2%), and polytetrafluoroethylene AVG (2.2%).

PATHOPHYSIOLOGY

To understand the pathophysiology of DASS, it is essential to first grasp the hemodynamic changes that occur after the creation of an arteriovenous (AV) access.

Brachial artery normally has approximately 80 mL/min of blood flow which increased approximately 10-fold after the creation of AV access,[6] typically ranging from 600 to 800 mL/min. To accommodate this surge in volume, both the inflow artery and the outflow vein undergo dilation,[7] a process facilitated by the release of nitric oxide.

Hemodynamics of AV access involves four primary vascular components:

1. *Feeding artery to the AV access (arterial inflow):* The artery supplying blood to the AV access
2. *AV access (outflow resistance):* The access itself provides a pathway for blood flow.
3. *Arterial supply distal to the arterial anastomosis of the AV access:* Artery that supplies the distal extremity beyond the AV access connection
4. *Collaterals:* Additional arteries that help to supply blood to the distal areas in case the main arterial flow is compromised.

TABLE 1: Pathophysiology of dialysis access-associated steal syndrome.

Pathophysiology	*Etiology*
Access inflow reduction	Atherosclerotic lesion in the feeding artery upstream to the anastomosis
Excess of steal from the anastomosis	Larger anastomosis or multiple arteriovenous access
Compromised flow in distal arteries (radial, ulnar, interosseous)	Atherosclerotic lesion in the arteries distal to AV access
Lack of dilatation in distal arteries and arterioles	Uremic milieu, medial arterial calcinosis, diabetic microangiopathy
Venous hypertension ("stagnant HAIDI" variant)	Side-to-side anastomosis on the vein, outflow stenosis

These four vascular beds interact in a delicate balance, and any disruption in this system can lead to the development of DASS **(Table 1)**.

Causes for the above pathophysiology:

- *Access inflow reduction:* Stenosis in the subclavian, axillary, brachial, or proximal radial arteries
- *Higher distal arterial resistance:* Peripheral vascular disease, Raynaud's phenomenon, systemic sclerosis, diabetes mellitus, prior history of instrumentation
- *Lower venous outflow resistance:* Creation of a larger anastomosis (artery to vein/artery to graft) resulting in retrograde flow from the "high-resistance" arterial bed (distal arteries) into the "low-resistance" venous system (AV access)
- *Impaired adaptation of inflow, outflow, and collaterals:* DM is a risk factor leading to a complex hemodynamic imbalance that causes DASS.

RISK FACTORS

Risk factors are:

- DM
- Female gender
- Smoking
- Coronary artery disease
- Peripheral vascular disease
- Previous history of DASS with AV access

CLINICAL PRESENTATION

The onset of DASS symptoms tends to be more acute following the creation of an AVG as compared to an AVF, where symptoms usually develop in a subacute to chronic manner.

This onset of symptoms can be classified into acute and chronic forms:

- The acute form often presents immediately after access surgery, with symptoms such as a cold, pale, or bluish painful hand with sensorimotor neurodeficit, which requires prompt intervention. This acute ischemia typically develops within hours to days and may either worsen or resolve over time.
- The chronic form of DASS develops more gradually, often weeks to months after access placement, and tends to be progressive. Symptom-wise, it includes nail changes, digital ulcerations, gangrene, and muscle atrophy.

Both acute and chronic forms of DASS can range in severity, from mild to severe symptoms.

Clinical symptoms in increasing severity:[8]

- Mild pain during dialysis at the AV access site or distally
- Nail changes
- Occasional tingling
- Extremity coolness
- Tingling and numbness in hand and fingers
- Muscle weakness
- Pale to whitish or cyanotic fingernail beds
- Rest-pain
- Sensory and motor function deficit
- Fingertip ulcerations
- Tissue loss

Dialysis access-associated steal syndrome is also known as hemodialysis access-induced distal ischemia (HAIDI) which is staged as per the severity of symptoms.

Staging of DASS as per severity[9] is given in **Table 2**.

TABLE 2: Clinical staging of dialysis access-associated steal syndrome as per the severity of symptoms.

Stage	*Clinical signs/symptoms*
Grade 1	No clear symptoms, but few signs of mild ischemia may be observed
Grade 2a	Complaints during an hemodialysis (HD) session or hand exercise: *Tolerable pain*, cramps, paraesthesia, numbness, or disturbing coldness in the finger or hand
Grade 2b	Complaints during an HD session or by use of the hand: *Intolerable pain*, cramps, paraesthesia, numbness, or disturbing coldness in the finger or hand
Grade 3	Rest pain or motor dysfunction of fingers or hand, upper limb
Grade 4a	Limited tissue loss (ulceration/necrosis), potential for preservation of hand function if ischemia is reversed
Grade 4b	Irreversible tissue loss and significant hand functioning; requires amputation and impossible to preserve or reverse hand functioning

DIAGNOSIS

A detailed clinical history and examination can often lead to the diagnosis of steal syndrome in most cases.[10] Manual compression of the AVF, with subsequent improvement in symptoms, may help confirm the presence of the steal phenomenon.

In many instances, physical examination alone is not conclusive and requires noninvasive testing. Physiologic tests can provide additional insight, such as digital waveforms and pressures, both with and without AVF compression. Ultrasound with spectral Doppler can help identify arterial stenosis and flow reversal and quantify AV access flows. Finally, a conventional angiogram can assist in diagnosing and treating the anatomical lesions responsible for steal syndrome.

Physical symptoms:[8] Physical symptoms that may be evident during examination include:

- Pale or livid hand
- Paraesthesia, coldness of the hand
- Diminished or absent radial and ulnar pulses
- Relief of acute symptoms upon compressing the AV access
- Cyanotic fingers
- Ischemic changes (e.g., nail changes, ulcerations, necrosis, and nonhealing ulcers)
- Digital brachial index (DBI) of 0.6 or less
- Digital pressures below 50 mm Hg or nonrecordable

Imaging techniques:

- Doppler ultrasound[7,11,12]
- The most commonly used probe is a standard linear probe (7.5–20 MHz) for superficial B-mode and color Doppler examination.
- The exam should be performed in a warm environment to avoid cold surrounding-induced spasms. The patient is asked to be seated or reclined, with the arm fully exposed from axilla to fingers. It is important to ensure

that the arm is kept comfortable during the Doppler examination. It is preferable to remove compressive dressings.

- Ischemia is confirmed by reduced or absent digital artery perfusion. Symptom relief and restoration of normal distal flow after manual occlusion of the access confirm the diagnosis of steal syndrome. Since small arteries may be difficult to assess with conventional ultrasound, continuous-wave Doppler can be more effective. A dynamic maneuver can also assess increased digital perfusion after occlusion.
- A straight segment with laminar flow, located at least 5 cm from aneurysms, stenotic lesions, and anastomosis sites, allows for accurate estimation of fistula flow. In cases of proximal access complicated by DASS, low blood flow is typically associated with antegrade or bidirectional flow in the artery distal to the anastomosis, while bidirectional or retrograde flow is more common in high-flow access.
- Ultrasound evaluation can confirm the diagnosis of DASS and determine the blood flow category and its etiology. This remains a crucial step since the treatment approach varies based on the flow and lesion contributing to DASS.
- Identify arterial stenosis upstream or downstream of the anastomosis, which helps guide treatment options based on anatomical and hemodynamic data.
- Additionally, ultrasound can assess any previous AVFs on the same arm that may be ligated to reduce global AV shunting and improve distal perfusion.

Access angiography: Options like CTA, MRA, or conventional angiography are in place, but conventional angiography can be diagnostic as well as therapeutic. It provides a more detailed view of vascular anatomy, identifies stenosis or steal-related anomalies, and corrects them.

Arm elevation test during physical examination helps assess AVF collapse and the degree of steal.

DIFFERENTIAL DIAGNOSIS[13]

The differential diagnosis of DASS is given in **Table 3**.

MANAGEMENT

The management of DASS should be tailored to the clinical stage, ischemia severity, AV access type, location, and volume flow. Overall, an individual approach is needed to decide the treatment strategy.

Management Outline as per Clinical Staging

- *Grade I/IIa:* Conservative management with close observation. No intervention is necessary unless symptoms progress.
- *Grade IIb/III/IVa:* Intervention is required, depending on AV access volume flow.
- *Grade IVb:* Expectant management, often necessitating amputation.

General Management for Nonintervention Patients

For patients with mild symptoms, treatment should focus on symptom stabilization. This includes optimizing hemodynamics (particularly during HD), preventing intradialytic hypotension, and using warming gloves.

TABLE 3: Differential diagnosis (D/D) of dialysis access-associated steal syndrome.

D/D	*Clinical feature*	*Diagnostic approach*
Carpal tunnel syndrome	Tingling numbness, burning, and pain (primarily in the thumb and index, middle, and part of ring finger)	Electrophysiological tests, local part ultrasonography
Central venous occlusion	Edema of the upper extremities, face, and neck, dilated veins, tenderness, pain, and associated erythema	CT angiography or conventional angiogram
Ischemic monomelic neuropathy	Symptoms immediately after access creation, unilateral severe pain and paresthesia, and sensorimotor loss. Patent pulsations	Electrophysiological tests (acute symptoms involving multiple nerves of the upper extremity after the creation of an AVF)
Ungual onychomycosis	Subungual hyperkeratosis and onycholysis, yellow-whitish discoloration; as the disease progresses, paresthesia, pain, discomfort, and loss of dexterity	Histopathology studies, dermoscopy
Peripheral neuropathy	Throbbing sharp or burning pain, hyperesthesia	Electrophysiological tests, blood tests, nerve biopsy

Some centers practice adjustments in dialysis settings (e.g., reducing flow rates, adjusting cannulation techniques, or using different access sites) to help alleviate symptoms. Regular follow-up is essential to monitor for worsening symptoms, and patient education is crucial to prevent hand injuries.

Arteriovenous Access Preservation

Arteriovenous access for many HD patients remains a lifeline. While AV access ligation typically reverses ischemic symptoms, preserving the access should be prioritized where feasible or in cases of access crunch. The flow volume of the AV access is critical in determining treatment, as different approaches are required for high-flow and low-flow accesses.

Flow-dependent Treatment

- *High-flow AV access (>1,500 mL/min):* Flow reduction may suffice for, e.g., "precision banding".
- *Low- or normal-flow AV access (≤1,500 mL/min):* Revascularization procedures are required to alter flow hemodynamics and improve distal perfusion while maintaining AV access function.

Interventional Treatment

- Grade 2b and above invariably require intervention to prevent permanent damage.
- Various treatment options include the following:
  - *Inflow arterial stenosis:* In stenotic lesions proximal to the AV anastomosis jeopardizing flow to AVF and distal arm, an endovascular catheter-guided balloon angioplasty intervention may offer therapeutic benefits. Atherosclerotic vascular disease responsible for DASS, especially in a case of upper arm fistula, has shown favorable outcomes after endovascular intervention.[14]
  - *Distal artery occlusion:* For distal radiocephalic AVFs, occlusion of the distal artery can eliminate reversal of flow, provided the ulnar artery is patent. Prior to performing this procedure, duplex ultrasound should confirm flow reversal in the distal radial artery, and ulnar artery patency must be verified. Furthermore, an improvement in digital waveforms should be observed when the AV access or the radial artery distal to the AVF is compressed.
  - *Precision banding:* For high-flow AVFs, flow reduction using *precision banding* or partial banding of AVF can effectively treat DASS and reduce cardiopulmonary complications. The MILLER procedure or open surgical banding is used for flow reduction. Nonabsorbable sutures, small interposition grafts, or tight Dacron or polytetrafluoroethylene (PTFE) cuffs can be used for this procedure. While banding low-flow AV access can address steal, it may increase the chances of dialysis inadequacy and increase the potential risk of access thrombosis. When banding is performed with intraoperative flow monitoring, targeting approximately 400 mL/min for native fistulas and 600 mL/min for grafts, the outcomes for both access patency and dialysis adequacy are enhanced.

    The effectiveness of banding can be evaluated through measurements such as digital pressures, DBI, photoplethysmography, pulse volume recording (PVR) waveforms, or volume flow data obtained via duplex ultrasound. A small study[15] involving five patients with DASS demonstrated complete resolution of ischemic symptoms with AV access banding, showing a 5 mm intraoperative increase in the PVR waveforms. Another study by Vaes et al.[16] showed the immediate short-term success of the intervention in proximal high-flow AVF but at 1 year, nearly 50% relapsed into the high flow again **(Figs. 2 to 5)**.
  - *Revascularization procedures:* For patients where access preservation is a priority, procedures such as *distal revascularization interval ligation (DRIL), proximalization of arterial inflow (PAI),* and *revision using distal inflow (RUDI)* can be performed to improve distal perfusion but have its pros and cons **(Figs. 6A to C)**.
    - *DRIL:* In 1988, Schanzer et al. introduced this procedure to treat DASS. It involves ligating the artery distal to the access anastomosis, halting retrograde diastolic inflow into the fistula, the primary cause of steal. In distal radiocephalic fistulas, ligating the distal radial artery (DRAL) is sufficient if the ulnar artery and palmar arch are patent. In brachial AVFs and AVGs, a vein bypass is added to reroute blood flow, ensuring long-term patency.[18]

      While DRIL is pathophysiologically ideal for steal syndrome, it is complex, time-consuming, and can reduce access flow by up to 25%. It is

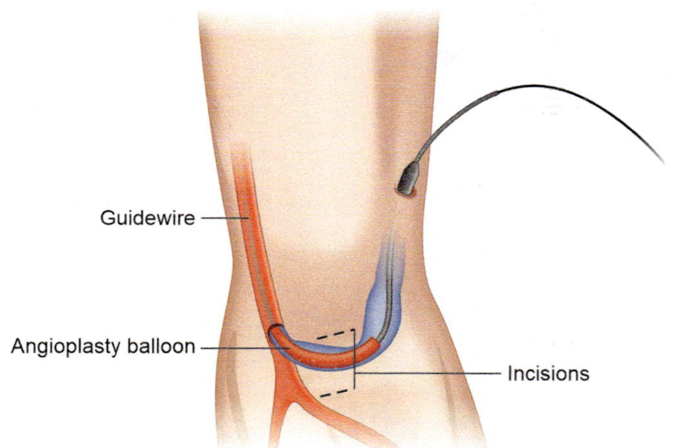

Fig. 2: An inflated angioplasty balloon is used as a sizing dowel inside the access. Two parallel, lateral 0.5 cm incisions are made approximately 1–3 cm from the arteriovenous anastomosis.
Source: Miller GA, Goel N, Friedman A, Khariton A, Jotwani MC, Savransky Y, et al. The MILLER banding procedure is an effective method for treating dialysis associated steal syndrome. Kidney Int. 2010;77(4):359-66.

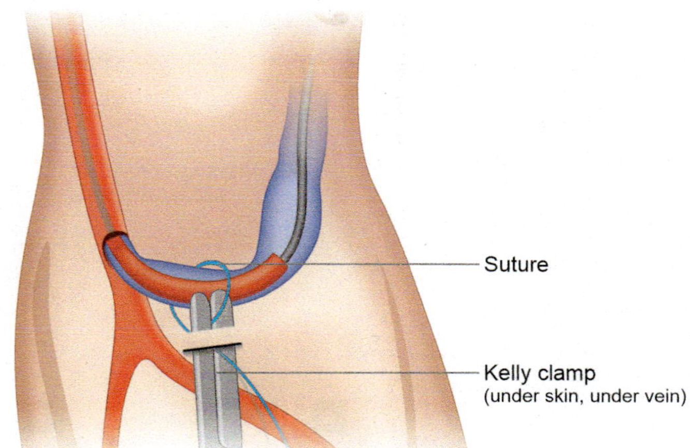

Fig. 4: The suture is looped over the access (under the skin) using a Kelly clamp.
Source: Miller GA, Goel N, Friedman A, Khariton A, Jotwani MC, Savransky Y, et al. The MILLER banding procedure is an effective method for treating dialysis associated steal syndrome. Kidney Int. 2010;77(4):359-66.

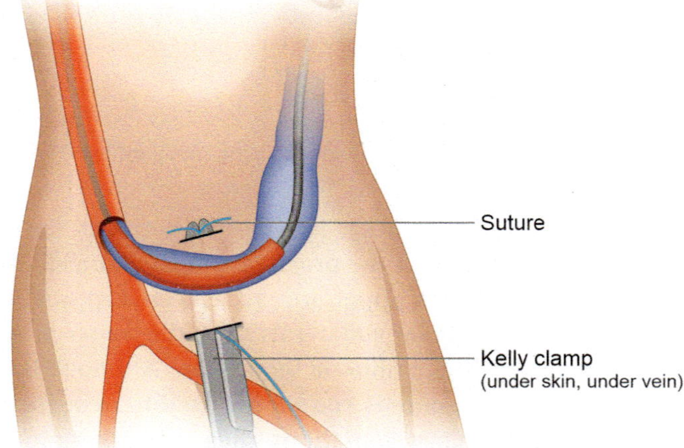

Fig. 3: A peri-access tunnel is dissected subcutaneously using Kelly clamp blunt dissection, and a 2-0 monofilament ligature of Prolene is pulled under the access.
Source: Miller GA, Goel N, Friedman A, Khariton A, Jotwani MC, Savransky Y, et al. The MILLER banding procedure is an effective method for treating dialysis associated steal syndrome. Kidney Int. 2010;77(4):359-66.

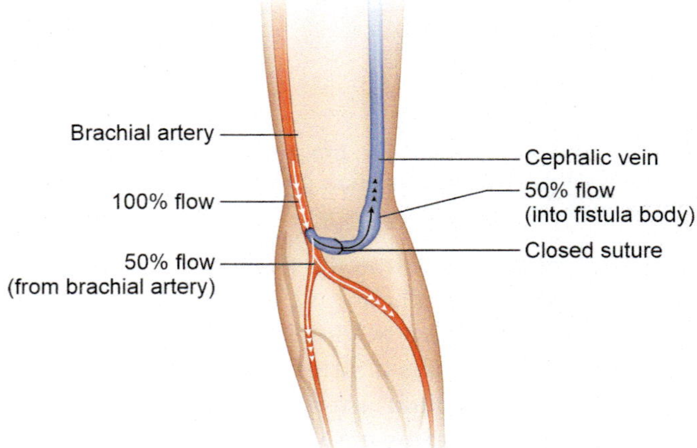

Fig. 5: Following the minimally invasive limited ligation endoluminal-assisted revision (MILLER) banding procedure, the resistance band redirects flow, improving distal perfusion, and alleviating symptoms.
Source: Miller GA, Goel N, Friedman A, Khariton A, Jotwani MC, Savransky Y, et al. The MILLER banding procedure is an effective method for treating dialysis associated steal syndrome. Kidney Int. 2010;77(4):359-66.

most effective for high-flow steal syndrome. In cases of low-flow steal syndrome, bypass without interval ligation is suggested, though clinical results are variable. The procedure generally provides immediate relief for most patients with steal symptoms.

A systematic review[19] of 22 studies concluded that in 52% of cases, the presenting grade of severity was grade 3 or 4. The overall success rate was 81% over a mean follow-up period of 22.2 months. The great saphenous vein was the most preferred conduit. Bypass thrombosis was

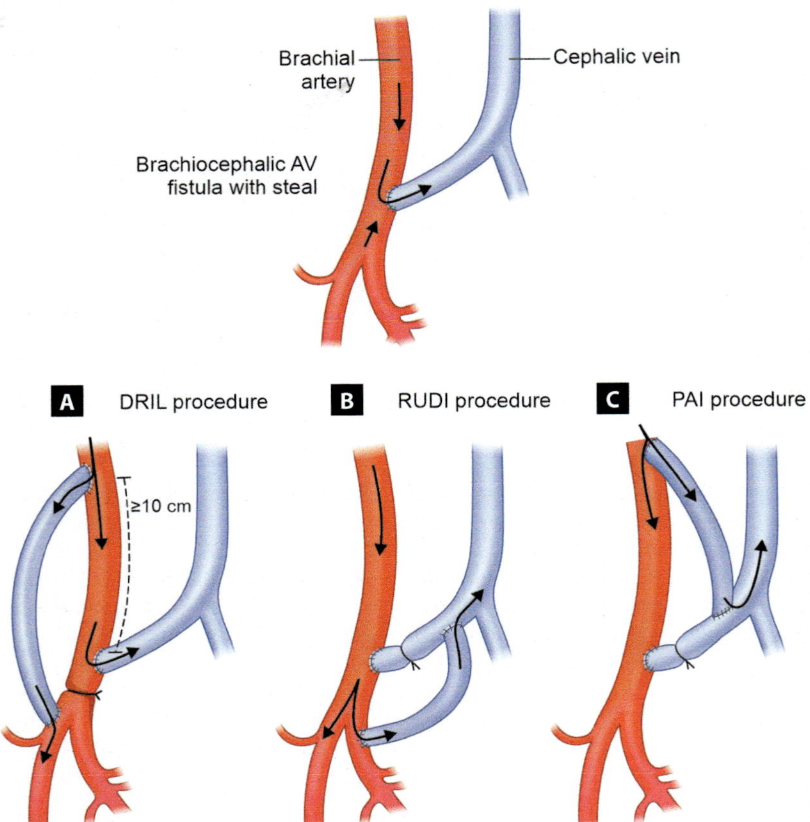

Figs. 6A to C: Revascularization procedure: (A) Distal revascularization interval ligation (DRIL); (B) Revision using distal inflow (RUDI); (C) Proximalization of arterial inflow (PAI).
Source: Al Shakarchi et al.[17]

most prevalent in the PTFE group, with a 43% overall thrombotic rate.

- *RUDI:* In this procedure, the vein is anastomosed to a more distal arterial source, such as the radial or ulnar artery, or uses a graft, while the original fistula vein is ligated just above the anastomosis. This procedure is considered effective in reducing the flow and also increases the needling area, but the prerequisite is the patent distal artery. Unlike the DRIL procedure, which focuses on preserving the extremity's circulation, the RUDI procedure prioritizes the fistula itself by maintaining the native arterial flow.
- *PAI:* Fundamentally, this procedure includes the creation of new AV anastomosis but far more centrally. The original AV anastomosis is ligated, and an interposition graft is used to connect the access vein or graft to a more central feeding artery, such as the distal brachial artery for a wrist fistula or the proximal brachial or axillary artery for an upper arm access. This approach recruits larger collaterals from the upper arm, improving peripheral blood flow. Although the PAI procedure is commonly used to treat steal syndrome, systematic studies are limited. In a notable prospective series of 30 patients, Zanow et al.[20] reported complete relief of ischemic symptoms in 84% of cases, with excellent access patency rates.
- *Arteriovenous access ligation:* In severe cases or when revascularization is not possible, and in cases of IMN, AV access ligation may be required.

ISCHEMIC MONOMELIC NEUROPATHY

Definition

Introduce IMN, a severe variant of DASS, where the ischemia leads to nerve damage and potentially permanent neurological deficits.

Clinical Features

Symptom onset typically occurs immediately after AV access placement, with neurologic symptoms being the primary concern, often without signs of hand tissue ischemia. Symptoms typically include pain, paresthesias, and numbness in the hand, along with significant motor dysfunction such as poor wrist extension, reduced function of the intrinsic hand muscles, and difficulty with thumb opposition. These deficits may progress to a claw hand deformity. The hand remains warm, with a preserved capillary refill, and a palpable radial or ulnar pulse. This lack of tissue ischemia contrasts with the clinical presentation of typical DASS.

Management

As per Kidney Disease Outcomes Quality Initiative (KDOQI) 2019, once the clinical diagnosis of IMN is made, it has been recommended to close AV access immediately. In some cases, surgical decompression of the nerve has been attempted. Despite aggressive intervention and AV access ligation, the results of treatment have been variable, with the majority of patients demonstrating only partial clinical recovery.[21,22] The duration of ischemia may decide the level of improvement after treatment, and hence an aggressive approach is needed.

PREVENTION

- *Access planning:* Careful selection of a patient and AV access sites is extremely crucial. Consider the patient's vascular anatomy, comorbidities, and risk stratify each individual for DASS.
- *Preoperative vascular mapping:* Assess the arterial and venous anatomy in depth by Doppler ultrasound. This ensures an optimal site for access creation, considering factors such as arterial size and patency.
- *Perform modified Allen's test* to evaluate the patency of both the ulnar and radial arteries, as well as the palmar arch, and to ensure that there is enough collateral circulation in the hand.
- *Careful surgical technique:* Avoid larger arteriotomy. The anastomosis should be made in a way that minimizes the risk of retrograde flow or significant disruption to the normal arterial circulation of the hand. Ideally, avoid using small arteries or those with poor collateral supply.
- *Blood flow monitoring:* Intraoperative blood flow monitoring and adjusting the anastomosis to achieve adequate flow are required. Advocate for regular monitoring of dialysis access, especially in high-risk patients, using Doppler ultrasound or clinical evaluations to detect early signs of steal syndrome.
- *Postoperative management: Hand and arm exercises:* Encourage patients to perform hand exercises that can enhance collateral circulation and promote good blood flow in the hand.
- *Careful monitoring for neurologic symptoms:* Educate your patient and as a clinician be vigilant for early signs of neurologic deficits, such as pain, paresthesia, or motor dysfunction, which could indicate developing steal syndrome. Early detection is key to effective management.

CONCLUSION

Due to the rise in the median ages of incident and prevalent hemodialysis patients and due to the growing percentages of diabetics among them, access-related ischemia has become a growing problem.

In general, the *prognosis of DASS is good with timely intervention and newer advances in treatment modality.* Early detection; appropriate treatment such as surgical revision or ligation, banding, or revascularization; and careful postoperative monitoring are critical to ensuring favorable outcomes and minimizing the risk of irreversible ischemic damage.

Delay in diagnosis or inadequate management can lead to persistent symptoms, functional impairment, and potential failure of dialysis access, which can significantly impact the patient's long-term health and quality of life.

REFERENCES

1. Davidson D, Louridas G, Guzman R, Tanner J, Weighell W, Spelay J, et al. Steal syndrome complicating upper extremity hemoaccess procedures: incidence and risk factors. Can J Surg. 2003;46(6):408.
2. van Hoek F, Scheltinga MR, Kouwenberg I, Moret KEM, Beerenhout CH, Tordoir JHM. Steal in hemodialysis patients depends on the type of vascular access. Eur J Vasc Endovasc Surg. 2006;32(6):710-7.
3. Adams A, Osman A. Dialysis access steal syndrome. J Emerg Nurs. 2020;46(4):524-6.
4. Zanow J, Petzold M, Petzold K, Kruger U, Scholz H. Diagnosis and differentiated treatment of ischemia in patients with arteriovenous vascular access. Vascular Access for Hemodialysis-VII Conference, Gore, Chicago, IL; 2001. pp. 201-9.
5. Miller GA, Goel N, Friedman A, Khariton A, Jotwani MC, Savransky Y. The MILLER banding procedure is an effective

method for treating dialysis—associated steal syndrome. Kidney Int. 2010;77(4):359-66.

6. Wedgewood KR, Wiggins PA, Guillou PJ. A prospective study of end-to-side vs. side-to-side arteriovenous fistulas for hemodialysis. Brit J Surg. 1984;71:640-2.
7. Davidson IJ, Chan D, Dolmatch B, Hasan M, Nichols D, Saxena R, et al. Duplex ultrasound evaluation for dialysis access selection and maintenance: a practical guide. J Vasc Access. 2008;9:1-9.
8. Malik J, Tuka V, Kasalova Z, Chytilova E, Slavikova M, Clagett P, et al. Understanding the dialysis access steal syndrome. A review of the etiologies, diagnosis, prevention and treatment strategies. J Vasc Access. 2008;9(3):155-66.
9. Scheltinga MR, van Hoek F, Bruijninckx CM. The time of onset in haemodialysis access-induced ischaemia (HAIDI) is related to the access type. Nephrol Dial Transpl. 2009;24(10):3198-204.
10. Mickley V. Steal syndrome—strategies to preserve vascular access and extremity. Nephrol Dial Transpl. 2008;23(1): 19-24.
11. Franco G. [Technique and results of duplex-Doppler for non-stenosing complications of vascular access for chronic hemodialysis: ischemia, steal, high flow rate, aneurysm]. J Mal Vasc. 2003;28(4):200-5.
12. Malik J, Slavikova M, Maskova J. Dialysis access-associated steal syndrome: the role of ultrasonography. J Nephrol. 2003;16(6):903-7.
13. Pirozzi N, De Alexandris L, Scrivano J, Fazzari L, Malik J. Ultrasound evaluation of dialysis access-related distal ischaemia. J Vasc Access. 2021;22(1_suppl):84-90.
14. Cheun TJ, Jayakumar L, Sideman MJ, Pounds LL, Davies MG. Upper extremity arterial endovascular interventions for symptomatic vascular access-induced steal syndrome. J Vasc Surg. 2019;70:1896.
15. Rivers SP, Scher LA, Veith FJ. Correction of steal syndrome secondary to hemodialysis access fistulas: a simplified quantitative technique. Surgery. 1992;112(3):593-7.
16. Vaes RH, Wouda R, van Loon M, van Hoek F, Tordoir JH, Scheltinga MR. Effectiveness of surgical banding for high flow in brachial artery-based hemodialysis vascular access. J Vasc Surg. 2015;61(3):762-6.
17. Al Shakarchi J, Stolba J, Houston JG, Inston N. Surgical techniques for haemodialysis access-induced distal ischaemia. J Vasc Access. 2016;17(1):40-6.
18. Schanzer H, Skladany M, Haimov M. Treatment of angio access induced ischemia by revascularization. J Vasc Surg. 1992;16:861-6.
19. Kordzadeh A, Parsa AD. A systematic review of distal revascularization and interval ligation for the treatment of vascular access-induced ischemia. J Vasc Surg. 2019;70(4):1364-73.
20. Zanow J, Kruger U, Scholz H. Proximalization of the arterial inflow: a new technique to treat access-related ischemia. J Vasc Surg. 2006;43:1216-21.
21. Scher LA, Shah AR. Vascular access neuropathic syndrome: Ischemic monomelic neuropathy. In: Wilson SE (Ed). Vascular Access: Principles and Practice, 5th edition. Philadelphia: Lippincott Williams & Wilkins; 2009. p. 182.
22. Ramdon A, Breyre A, Kalapatapu V. A Case of Acute Ischemic Monomelic Neuropathy and Review of the Literature. Ann Vasc Surg. 2017;42:301.e1-301.e5.

SECTION 7

Special Considerations in Vascular Access Procedures

CHAPTER 30

Pediatric Vascular Access

Sukanya Govindan, Srinivasavaradan Govindarajan

CASE SCENARIO

A 10-year-old boy, a known case of neurogenic bladder with chronic kidney disease stage V (estimated glomerular filtration rate 10 mL/1.73 m^2/min), has a poor appetite and protein energy wasting (PEW). He has lost 3 kg in the past 6 months and stunted on examination. Investigations showed blood urea 180 mg/dL and serum creatinine 5.1 mg/dL with metabolic acidosis. He has a residual urine output of 800–1,000 mL and is on regular clean intermittent catheterization. In view of end-stage kidney disease with chronic malnutrition, he has been planned to initiate hemodialysis after discussing it with his parents. How to proceed?

INTRODUCTION

Reliable vascular access is the Achilles heel for hemodialysis (HD). Ideal HD access should help deliver a continuous and desired blood flow to achieve the targeted clearance. Pediatric HD poses unique challenges due to smaller vessel size and the limited availability of vascular access options. Securing vascular access in children should consider functional access, which ensures effective dialysis and minimal associated complications in the long run. We aim to discuss the available options for pediatric HD access, their challenges, complications, and management with emphasis on the available evidence.[1]

OPTIONS FOR HEMODIALYSIS ACCESS

Hemodialysis access in children is limited due to their smaller-sized vessels and lesser expertise to secure the same. Available options include:

- Central venous catheters (CVC)
- Arteriovenous fistula (AVF)
- Arteriovenous graft (AVG)

Age and size of the child, vessel size and condition, anticipated time to transplantation, and patient perspective are the major factors to be considered while deciding vascular access.

Central Venous Catheters

Central venous catheters are double-lumen catheters made of polyurethane. CVCs are still the preferred access for HD as there is limited expertise for AVF due to various factors. CVCs serve as an immediate access, most suitable for acute dialysis sessions. Tunneled CVC provides longer access with a lesser infection rate. The available CVCs are discussed in the following text.

Noncuffed HD Catheter

Non-cuffed HD catheter is usually the preferred access in (1) children with acute kidney injury, (2) chronic kidney disease presenting with complications who need an urgent start of HD, (3) transplant recipients requiring temporary HD during rejection episodes, (4) bridging access for children awaiting the maturation of AVF or during periods of abdominal rest before initiation of peritoneal dialysis, and (5) plasmapheresis.

Sites of insertion preferred (in descending order):

1. Right internal jugular vein
2. Left internal jugular vein
3. Left femoral vein
4. Subclavian vein

The right internal jugular vein is preferred because it is short and straight to the heart. Subclavian veins are least preferred because they carry a high risk of developing pneumothorax and hemothorax and a higher risk of central venous stenosis in the long term. Femoral veins are preferred in acute conditions for critically ill patients with coagulopathy and acute respiratory distress syndrome. The right femoral vein is not preferred because thrombosis can affect the anastomosis for kidney transplantation. Ultrasound-guided catheter insertion has also reduced the rates of complications and failure **(Table 1)**.

Uncuffed CVCs are not tunneled; hence, there is a higher risk of infection. Kidney Disease Outcomes Quality Initiative (KDOQI) 2019 Vascular Update suggests a maximum use of 2 weeks for a temporary CVC **(Fig. 1)**.

Tunneled and Cuffed CVC

Tunneled catheters are preferred in children planning for kidney transplantation in the next 6 months or AVF failure. Tunneled catheters have cuff and the entry site is far away from the vascular access, thereby reducing the risk of infections. Vascular sites similar to the temporary catheters are accessible for tunneled catheters; however, size and length vary according to the site preferred **(Table 2)**.

Tunneled catheter placement requires fluoroscopy-guided insertion as there is a high risk of profuse bleeding if misplaced or the vessel is punctured. As per the KDOQI 2019 guidelines, tunneled catheters can be used for as long as 6 months.

Pediatric-specific challenges: The length of the catheter is longer as no specific pediatric catheters are available.

Long-term care: Exit-site care includes cleaning the exit site with chlorhexidine solution/iodine-based solution at every contact and inspecting the exit site for evidence of infection or purulent discharge. Local application of antibiotics like mupirocin and povidone-iodine has not shown proven benefits in reducing the incidence of exit-site infection. Antibiotic-based heparin locks are commonly used to prevent thrombosis. Practice varies according to the institute's policy; European Society for Clinical Nutrition and Metabolism (ESPEN) guidelines suggest the use of tissue plasminogen activator (tPA) as a locking solution. Dialysis access should be handled only by trained personnel and should not be used as intravenous access for intravenous fluids, drugs, or sampling unless in emergent conditions **(Fig. 2)**.

TABLE 1: Preferred size of central venous catheter (CVC) based on weight and age.

CVC size (Fr)	*Length (cm)*	*Weight band (kg)*
6.5	10	<7
8	11.5	7–15
10	12	15–30
11.5	13.5	>30

Complications:[2]

- Catheter-related bloodstream infection (CRBSI)
- Exit-site infection
- Thrombosis and central venous stenosis
- Bleeding/hemorrhage
- Mechanical damage
- Accidental removal

Arteriovenous Fistula

An AVF is the preferred vascular access for HD in adults. Though it is considered an ideal HD access, there is still hesitance to use it in children due to difficulties in establishing successful access, a lack of expertise among dialysis personnel in handling AVFs, and patients' denial of the procedure due to fear of repeated puncturing and pain. According to the International Pediatric HD Registry (IPHN), only 26% of children have used AVFs as HD access.

An AVF poses various advantages like higher effective access flow, longevity, and fewer infections. Hence, patients should be counseled about their benefits. Fistula First Initiative increased the usage of AVF in adults; however, it did not include children.

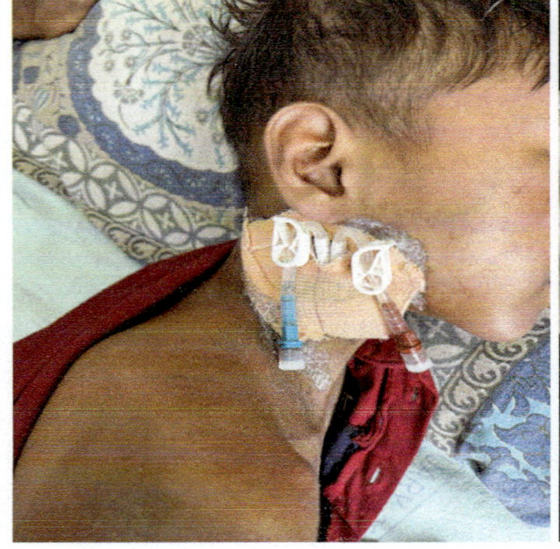
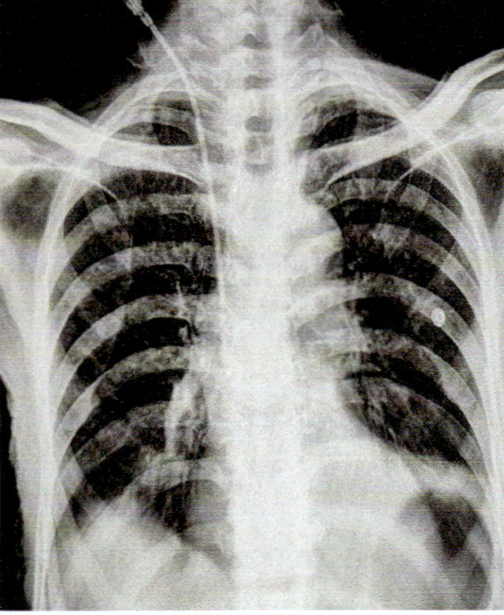

Fig. 1: Uncuffed HD catheter (11 Fr) placed in right IJV and X-ray showing placement of tip.

Sites for AVF

Preparation of AVF in children is challenging; however, the principle follows the same as in adults. AVF preparation should be planned as early as estimated glomerular filtration rate (eGFR) <30 mL/1.73 m^2 as it takes time to mature as an ideal access. In children who present with emergent indications for dialysis, a temporary catheter can be used (as discussed earlier) and can also be planned for AVF creation with the CVC as a bridging access till AVF matures. The major step in AVF preparation is vein preservation preferably in the nondominant hand (avoiding venipuncture, BB measurement). A "distal before proximal" approach is preferred in the nondominant hand followed by the dominant hand, radiocephalic AVF in the wrist being the preferred site. Other options include brachiocephalic at the elbow and brachiobasilic AVF at the upper arm which requires transpositioning due to its deeper location.

TABLE 2: Central venous catheter (CVC) size and length vary according to the site preferred.

CVC size (Fr)	*Cuff-to-tip length (cm)*	*Weight band (kg)*
12	13	<15
14	19	>15 [right internal jugular vein (IJV)]
14	23	>15 (left IJV)

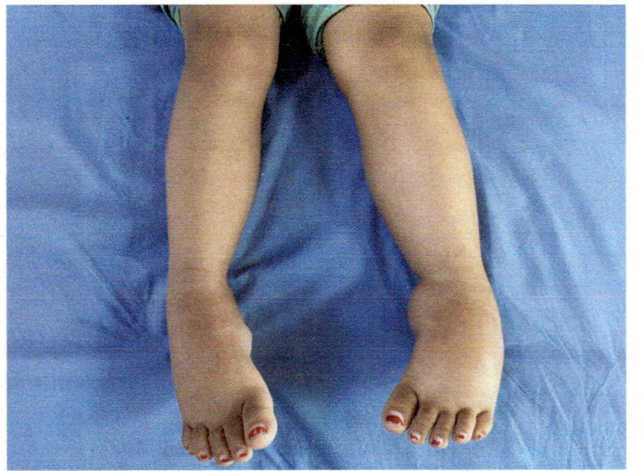

Fig. 2: Edema of left lower limb (Deep vein thrombosis of left femoral vein post-femoral vein dialysis catheter placement).

Physical examination should be performed in all children planned for AVF, to look for scars, pulse pattern of the arteries using Allen's test, and length and patency of veins. A Doppler scan shall be performed if there is any suspicion in physical examination, to assess the vessel diameter and flow. A minimum of 2.5 and 1.5 mm are suggested for venous and arterial diameter, respectively, for a successful mature AVF. In case of a previous history of HD catheter placement in the neck, venography studies are required to rule out central valve stenosis **(Fig. 3)**.[3]

Needles for Access (Table 3)

The dimensions of needles required for access are given in **Table 3 and Figure 4**.

Post-AVF Care

Children with AVF should be encouraged to perform hand exercises regularly to help in the maturation of AVF. Maturation time varies in children from 4 to 8 weeks and can be prolonged in smaller children. The appearance of a

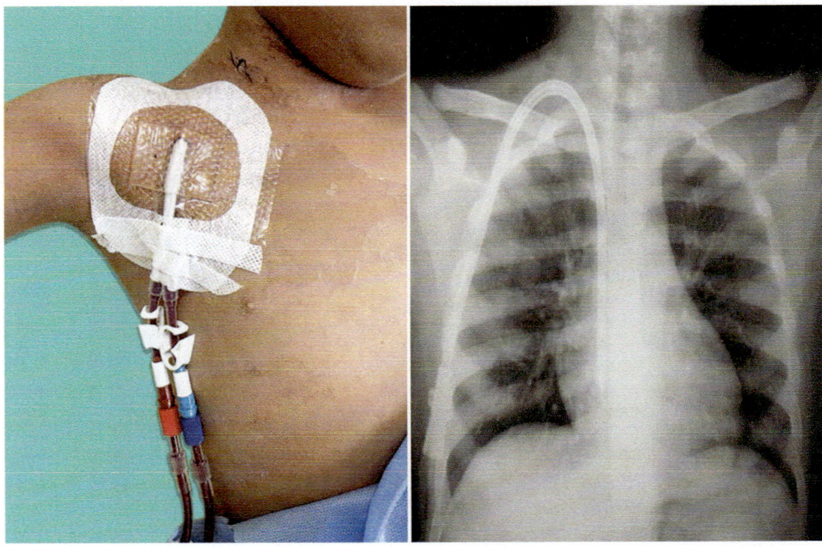

Fig. 3: Tunneled HD catheter placed in Right IJV (12 Fr pediatric, asymmetric tip).

strong thrill is a sign of maturation in the arterialized vein. KDOQI 2019 Vascular Update suggests the following criteria for the maturity of AVF in adults: (1) Flow should be >600 mL/min, (2) skin-to-vein distance is <6 mm, and (3) the internal diameter of the vein measured by USG is >6 mm. The same is considered appropriate for children as well.

Once maturation is confirmed, AVF cannulation should always be performed by trained personnel. Initially, narrow-bored cannulas are preferred to avoid bleeding or cannulation pain. Topical local anesthetics are available that can reduce pain due to pricks, thereby reducing anxiety. Cannulation techniques like the buttonhole method and the step-ladder pattern are commonly used in children.[4]

Complications

The most common complication associated with AVF in children is primary failure, majorly related to smaller vessel diameter and vasospasm. Injury, rupture, and bleeding can also happen. Other complications include stenosis or thrombosis to the inflow and can result in secondary failure. Pseudoaneurysms and steal phenomenon are other rare complications.[5]

Long-term Surveillance

Regular examination of the fistula for a palpable thrill to assess patency, augmentation test to assess the arterial inflow, and the arm-raise test to look for outflow obstruction like central venous stenosis are recommended.

TABLE 3: Needles color code, size, and target blood flow rate.

Color code	*Size (G)*	*Blood flow rate target (mL/min)*
Yellow	15	350–450 mL/min
Green	16	300–350 mL/min
Red	17	<300 mL/min

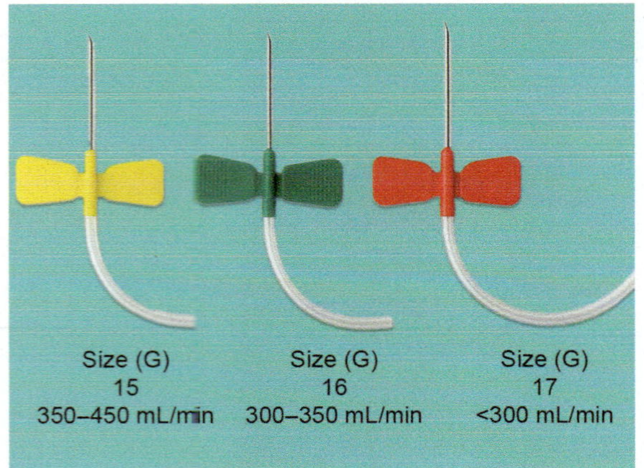

Fig. 4: AV fistula needles (Color coded).

Arteriovenous Grafts

Arteriovenous grafts are very rarely used in children due to a lack of expertise. They are made of nonimmunogenic and nonthrombotic synthetic materials that are easily accessible for cannulation. Commonly used materials include Dacron, polytetrafluorethylene (PTFE), and polyurethane. It can still be considered in children with failed AVF, need for early cannulation, or small caliber vessels. PTFE grafts are associated with postoperative edema hindering its early use. Newer composite grafts have been introduced to overcome this. Though AVGs are similar to AVFs, they are prone to a higher risk of thrombosis and stenosis.

CONCLUSION

Various vascular access for HD are available for children. Selection should be based on urgency, expertise, and patient preferences. "The fistula first" policy should be followed in nephrology centers with focused care. Vein preservation and early preparation for HD access are the key. Long-term surveillance for complications helps in early detection and prolongs access survival.

REFERENCES

1. Shroff R, Calder F, Bakkaloğlu S, Nagler EV, Stuart S, Stronach L, et al. Vascular access in children requiring maintenance haemodialysis: a consensus document by the European Society for Paediatric Nephrology Dialysis Working Group. Nephrol Dial Transplant. 2019;34(10):1746-65.
2. Borzych-Duzalka D, Shroff R, Ariceta G, Yap YC, Paglialonga F, Xu H, et al. Vascular access choice, complications, and outcomes in children on maintenance hemodialysis: Findings from the International Pediatric Hemodialysis Network (IPHN) Registry. Am J Kidney Dis. 2019;74(2):193-202.
3. Lok CE, Huber TS, Lee T, Shenoy S, Yevzlin AS, Abreo K, et al. KDOQI Clinical Practice Guideline for Vascular Access: 2019 Update. Am J Kidney Dis. 2020;75(4):S1-164.
4. Chand DH, Valentini RP, Kamil ES. Hemodialysis vascular access options in pediatrics: considerations for patients and practitioners. Pediatr Nephrol. 2009;24(6):1121-8.
5. Raina R, Mittal A, Sethi SK, Chakraborty R. Challenges of vascular access in the pediatric population. Advances in Chronic Kidney Disease. 2020;27(3):268-75.

CHAPTER 31

Vascular Access in Patients with Coagulopathy

Abhijit Madhav Konnur, Sishir Dashrathmal Gang

CLINICAL SCENARIO

Mr ABC, a 65-year-old male with a history of end-stage renal disease (ESRD) secondary to diabetic nephropathy, presents to the emergency department with worsening uremic symptoms, including nausea, volume overload, and hyperkalemia. He has been receiving hemodialysis via an arteriovenous (AV) fistula, but it recently thrombosed. Attempts at declotting have failed, and he requires urgent dialysis.

His past medical history includes atrial fibrillation on warfarin, cirrhosis with mild thrombocytopenia (platelet count 75,000/μL), and a recent gastrointestinal bleed. Laboratory findings reveal an elevated international normalized ratio (INR) of 2.1 and an activated partial thromboplastin time (aPTT) of 45 seconds. Given his coagulopathy and the urgency of dialysis, a tunneled dialysis catheter is planned for central venous access.

Clinical decision-making:

- *Site selection:* The right internal jugular (IJ) vein is preferred due to its lower risk of complications compared to the subclavian or femoral veins. A lower platelet count of <50,000/μL should make femoral vein access preferable as external compression is possible in case of bleeding. Ultrasound guidance is utilized to minimize vascular injury.
- *Coagulation management:* Warfarin is withheld, and fresh frozen plasma (FFP) is preferred over injectable vitamin K as a vascular access is required urgently on a background of disordered clotting time. Given mild thrombocytopenia, platelet transfusion is necessary only if persistent bleeding occurs and is contraindicated as a prophylactic strategy.
- *Procedure:* Under strict aseptic technique and ultrasound guidance, a 14.5 Fr tunneled catheter is inserted into the right IJ vein. Meticulous hemostasis is ensured, and postprocedural monitoring by both close physical examination and radiological imaging, if required, is undertaken.
- *Postprocedure care:* The patient is closely monitored for hematoma, bleeding, and catheter function. Dialysis is initiated successfully, and anticoagulation is carefully resumed after risk stratification.

This case highlights the challenges of vascular access in ESRD patients with coagulopathy, emphasizing individualized anticoagulation management and ultrasound-guided techniques to reduce complications.

INTRODUCTION

Patients who have had a history of stroke, venous thromboembolic events, malignancy, or significant cardiovascular disease require assessment for thromboembolic risk and thrombolytic therapy. This is necessitated by high fatality rates of 17.5% for mechanical heart valves, 5–10% for venous thromboembolism (VTE), and 37% for embolic strokes. The management plan varies depending on patient-specific factors, including the underlying condition requiring anticoagulation, the type of procedure, and the pharmacokinetics of the anticoagulant. Coagulopathy with derangement of coagulation balance to either side can result in serious and unfortunately fatal complications for patients undergoing procedures.

End-stage renal disease (ESRD) associated coagulopathy leads to both bleeding and thrombotic events with uremic toxins and platelet dysfunction playing important roles. Hemodialysis (HD) procedure also contributes to these coagulation abnormalities.

Coagulation Disorders in End-stage Renal Disease

Bleeding Risk

Increased accumulation of uremic toxins leads to platelet dysfunction and impaired hemostasis, increasing the risk of bleeding. Platelet dysfunction is both intrinsic and related to impaired platelet–vessel wall interaction, precipitating hemorrhagic tendencies. Patients with ESRD have impaired platelet function, including reduced platelet activation, recruitment, adhesion, and aggregation. Spontaneous bleeding can occur at cutaneous, mucosal, and serosal sites, as well as retroperitoneal or intracranial hemorrhages.

Thrombotic Risk

Patients with ESRD are at an increased risk for both arterial and VTE.

Hemodialysis itself can trigger thrombotic events due to chronic platelet activation from contact with artificial surfaces. Endothelial dysfunction, inflammation, and comorbidities further contribute to the thrombotic risk. Thrombotic complications can occur in vascular access sites, as well as in coronary, cerebral, and retinal arteries.

Hemodialysis and Coagulation

Hemodialysis, while essential for eliminating uremic toxins, can also contribute to coagulation abnormalities. Repeated heparin administration during HD may further influence the coagulation system. The HD process itself can contribute to bleeding due to contact with artificial surfaces and the potential for blood pressure fluctuations.

KEY TOPICS

Indications for Anticoagulation

- Atrial fibrillation, deep vein thrombosis (DVT), pulmonary embolism, mechanical heart valves, and history of stroke or coronary artery bypass grafting
- An estimated 250,000 patients in the United States require anticoagulation cessation for surgery annually.

Types of Anticoagulants and Their Mechanisms

- *Antiplatelet agents:* Aspirin, nonsteroidal anti-inflammatory drugs (NSAIDs), clopidogrel, prasugrel, ticagrelor, cangrelor **(Table 1)**.
- *Vitamin K antagonists (VKA):* Warfarin (long-acting, requires careful monitoring).
- *Direct oral anticoagulants (DOACs):* Rivaroxaban, apixaban, edoxaban, dabigatran (shorter half-life, predictable effects) **(Table 2)**.
- *Parenteral anticoagulants:* Heparin [unfractionated heparin (UFH) and low molecular weight heparin (LMWH)], fondaparinux **(Table 3)**.

Assessment of Perioperative Risk

- *Thromboembolic risk:*
  - *Stroke risk:* Evaluated using CHA_2DS_2-VASc score for atrial fibrillation and consideration of recent thromboembolism. The CHA_2DS_2-VASc score is a point-based predictive tool used to determine annual stroke risk assessment in patients with nonvalvular atrial fibrillation (NVAF) with risk factors like age, heart conditions, and vascular diseases designated with points.
    - C: ongestive heart failure
    - H: ypertension
    - A: ge >75 years (2 points)
    - D: iabetes mellitus
    - S: troke/TIA (2 points)
    - V: ascular disease
    - A: ge 65–74 years
    - S: ex category (female)

Each risk factor contributes a certain number of points (1 or 2), and the total score determines the patient's risk level.

TABLE 1: Types of antiplatelet agents and their mechanisms.

Agent	*Time to maximum antiplatelet effect*	*Half-life*	*Comments*
Aspirin	30 minutes	15–30 minutes	Antiplatelet effect appears within 1 hour and persists for at least 4 days after the last dose
Clopidogrel	3–7 days	8 hours	More rapid inhibition of platelet function can be achieved with loading dose; antiplatelet effect lasts up to 10 days after the last dose
Ticagrelor	1.5 hours	7 hours	Residual antiplatelet effect decreased to 30% after 2.5 days
Prasugrel	30 minutes	7 hours	Antiplatelet effect lasts 5–7 days after the last dose
Ticlopidine	1–3 hours	24–36 hours	Antiplatelet effect lasts for 5–7 days after the last dose

TABLE 2: Types of direct oral anticoagulants (DOACs) and their mechanisms.

	Apixaban	*Rivaroxaban*	*Edoxaban*	*Dabigatran*
Classification	Selective direct Xa inhibitor	Selective direct Xa inhibitor	Selective direct Xa inhibitor	Selective thrombin inhibitor
Metabolism	25% renal, 75% biliary	66% renal, 33% biliary	50% renal, 50% biliary	80% renal, 20% biliary
Half-life	8–15 h	5–9 h 9–12 h (elderly)	10–14 h	12–17 h 14–17 h (elderly)
Rescue/antidote	• KCENTRA 5,000 units • Non-ICH bleeding or need for urgent/ emergent invasive procedure: KCENTRA 50 unit/kg (maximum 5,000 units)	• KCENTRA 5,000 units • Non-ICH bleeding or need for urgent/ emergent invasive procedure: KCENTRA 50 unit/kg (maximum 5,000 units)	KCENTRA 5,000 units	• Only DOAC with antidote: Idarucizumab (Praxbind) • Only DOAC that can be moderately reversed by dialysis

(ICH: intracranial hemorrhage)

TABLE 3: Types of parenteral anticoagulants.

Heparin	*Protamine dose*	*Withhold time*	*Comments*
Unfractionated heparin	1 mg per 100 units of heparin		Full-dose (50 mg) protamine indicated in patients needing reversal <60 minutes after heparin bolus administration
Enoxaparin	8 hours: 1 mg for every 1 mg of enoxaparin; >8 hours: 0.5 mg for every 1 mg of enoxaparin	Withhold 1 dose if prophylactic dose used; withhold 2 doses if therapeutic dose used	Reversal may not be necessary for >12–24 hours since the last enoxaparin dose in normal renal function
Dalteparin	8 hours: 1 mg of protamine for every 100 units of dalteparin; >8 hours: 0.5 mg for every 100 units of dalteparin	Withhold 1 dose before high-risk procedure	Reversal may not be necessary for >12–24 hours since the last dalteparin dose in normal renal function

Risk stratification

Low risk: Score of 0

Moderate risk: Score of 1

High risk: Score of 2 or higher

Why it is important?

The CHA_2DS_2-VASc score helps clinicians determine the need for anticoagulation (blood-thinning medication) to reduce the risk of stroke in patients with atrial fibrillation.

Anticoagulation guidelines: Patients with a score of 2 or higher are generally recommended to receive anticoagulation.

Patients with a score of 1 may be considered for either aspirin alone or full anticoagulation, depending on individual circumstances.

CHA_2DS_2-VASc score versus CHADS2 score: The CHA_2DS_2-VASc score is more inclusive of common stroke risk factors than the older $CHADS_2$ score.

- *Venous thrombosis risk:*
  - *Acuity of clot:* Most recurrences and embolization occur within 30 days and decrease significantly after 3 months.
  - *Clot type and location:* DVT is more complicated than superficial vein thrombosis, and proximal DVT (e.g., popliteal) causes more recurrences than distal DVT (calf veins).
  - Cancers, obesity, hormone replacement therapy, long-term immobilization, and certain thrombophilia (APLA syndromes) have strong associations with risk.
- *Mechanical heart valves:* Stopping anticoagulations for even a short period of time is associated with high thrombosis risk (1–7%) for any mechanical valvular prosthesis. It is higher for mitral and aortic valves and is uncomfortably high for bioprosthetic and endovascularly deployed valves.
- *Coronary artery disease:* Coronary artery disease is highly prevalent among patients with ESRD/HD and

coronary percutaneous interventions (PCI) have been increased by nearly 50% over the past decade. After PCI with stent placement, guidelines recommend dual antiplatelet therapy (DAPT). Unfortunately, there is no specific tailored pharmacotherapy approach defined for this frail population who are mostly excluded from large randomized clinical trials (RCTs). In patients treated with stents who are to undergo subsequent procedures that mandate discontinuation of $P2Y_{12}$ receptor inhibitors, guidelines recommend that aspirin be continued if at all possible and thienopyridine restarted as soon as possible after the procedure. Aspirin should only be discontinued if the known bleeding risks are similar to or more severe than the observed cardiovascular risks of aspirin withdrawal. In patients who require early (<6 months) noncardiac surgery within placement of a drug-eluting stent (DES), the American College of Chest Physicians guidelines suggest continuing DAPT around the time of surgery instead of stopping, depending on the bleeding risk intrinsic to each kind of intervention. Clinical judgment is key to identifying patients at high risk of perioperative thrombotic events as those who have received a bare-metal stent (BMS) within 1 month or a DES within 6 months, those who have received a DES >12 months but remain at risk of stent thrombosis or life-threatening complications for unfavorable anatomic or procedural characteristics (i.e., long stented segments, multiple stenting, overlapping stents, small vessels, bifurcation lesions, left main, last remaining vessel), or those with unfavorable clinical characteristics [i.e., recent acute coronary syndrome (ACS), history of stent thrombosis, left ventricular ejection fraction, chronic kidney disease, diabetes mellitus]. The need for keeping such high-risk patients on aspirin alone, clopidogrel alone, or both during the procedure period should be individualized.

- *Bridging therapy:* Oral $P2Y_{12}$ receptor inhibitors (clopidogrel, prasugrel, or ticagrelor) increase the risk of bleeding complications in those requiring any invasive procedure within the preceding 5–7 days before discontinuation. If bridging is necessary, antiplatelet agents should be preferred over anticoagulants, because platelet accumulation at sites of vascular injury is well known as the primary event in arterial thrombosis. Importantly, UFH makes platelets more reactive to activation by other agonists such as adenosine diphosphate and binds to the glycoprotein IIb/IIIa receptor on the platelet, resulting in a prothrombotic effect. Therefore, bridging with heparin can actually be potentially harmful. Although low-molecular-weight heparin does not stimulate platelets like UFH, this does not have platelet inhibitory effects, which remain key for bridging.

  On this background, the only approved agents with fast-acting and potent platelet inhibitory effects with relatively short duration of action are the small-molecule intravenous glycoprotein IIb/IIIa antagonists (e.g., tirofiban, eptifibatide). Cangrelor is a nonthienopyridine adenosine triphosphate analog that reversibly binds to the $P2Y_{12}$ receptor, and, unlike clopidogrel, prasugrel, and ticagrelor, it is administered intravenously with a rapid onset and offset of effect. In comparison with glycoprotein IIb/IIIa inhibitors, cangrelor features more desirable characteristics because of its faster offset and specificity to the $P2Y_{12}$ receptor. In addition, different from glycoprotein IIb/IIIa inhibitors, dose-finding studies designed to achieve a "thienopyridine-like" platelet inhibitory effect were specifically conducted for cangrelor to reduce the risk of bleeding with prolonged infusion. These pharmacological properties make cangrelor the ideal drug to be considered for bridging patients to surgery (BRIDGE) trial. In brief, after discontinuation of the $P2Y_{12}$ inhibitor as per guideline recommendations (7 days before surgery for prasugrel, 5 days before surgery for clopidogrel or ticagrelor), bridging with tirofiban or eptifibatide should be initiated ≈72 hours before surgery and continued up to 4–6 hours from surgery. In patients with renal impairment (creatinine clearance <50 mL/min), a dose reduction is warranted (0.05 µg/kg/min for tirofiban, 1.0 µg/kg/min for eptifibatide) and earlier suspension (8–12 hours) should be considered. After noncardiac surgery, irrespective of bridging strategy, clopidogrel should be resumed with a loading dose as soon as oral administration is possible. If oral administration of clopidogrel is not possible, postsurgery bridging with an intravenous agent should be considered.
- *Bleeding risk assessment:* Patients with congenital bleeding diathesis, disseminated intravascular coagulation, sepsis, or renal dysfunction have acquired coagulopathy with elevated bleeding. A bleeding episode within 3 months of a procedure has an increased risk.

Patients are assessed with the help of HAS-BLED score as this score is validated to predict bleeding rates in patients with NVAF who are on long-term VKA anticoagulation. It is purely patient characteristic specific and not procedure risk specific and has moderate performance for prediction. Predictors of bleeding were history of mechanical heart valve and HAS-BLED score >3 **(Tables 4 and 5)**.

The BleedMAP score assigns 1 point each for the following race factors: History of *Bleed*ing, mitral *M*echanical heart valve, Active cancer, and low *Pl*atelet count. A score of >3 reflects >10% major bleeding rates for all patients and >12% bleeding associated with bridging therapy with LMWH.

- *Procedure-associated bleeding risk:* A two-tier procedure-related bleeding risk categorization has low-risk procedures (<1.5% rate of major bleeding) which rarely have hemorrhagic complications or occur in areas where bleeding is easy to diagnose and control. High bleeding risk procedures (>1.5% rate of major bleeding) have high hemorrhagic complications or in surgical sites where bleeding will be difficult to diagnose and control (e.g., intra-abdominal cavity, lung tissues, and retroperitoneal area) procedures.

Preprocedure laboratory testing: For a high-risk procedure, it is recommended to do hemoglobin, platelet count, prothrombin time (PT), activated partial thromboplastin time (aPTT), or anti-Xa testing for patients receiving UFH. Fibrinogen levels are recommended for patients with cirrhosis. DOAC-specific assays or similar assays should be done. An international normalized ratio (INR) <1.8 may be safe for a renal biopsy, but INR <1.5 is recommended for arterial interventions.

TABLE 4: Conditions and their points.

Condition	*Points*
H—Hypertension	1
A—Ab(N) liver/renal	1 point each
S—Stroke	1
B—Bleeding	1
L—Labile international normalized ratios (INRs)	1
E—Elderly (>65 years)	1
D—Drugs or alcohol	1 point each

TABLE 5: Score and bleeds.

Score	*Bleeds (per 100 patient-years)*
0	1.13
1	1.02
2	1.88
3	3.74
4	8.770
5	12.5

- *Laboratory parameters for low bleeding risk procedures* can be safely performed at INR >1.5 or platelet count >20,000/cmm that include central venous catheter (CVC) insertions or removal, paracentesis, thoracentesis, and angiography.

Abnormalities in PT and INR are not associated with increased bleeding during CVC insertions. There is absence of clinically significant bleeding in patients with elevated INR who did not receive FFP and underwent CVC interventions.

Central venous catheter placement is the most common intervention that requires prophylactic platelet transfusion in the world. Platelet count threshold recommendations for platelet transfusions prior to interventions vary significantly between countries (<50,000/cmm in the United Kingdom, 30,000/cmm in Belgium, 20,000/cmm in the United States, and 10,000/cmm in Germany) unless there are other risk factors for bleeding. A 2015 review by American Association of Blood Banks (AABB) recommends prophylactic platelet transfusion for platelet counts <20,000/cmm for patients undergoing elective CVC placement. There is a higher incidence of hematoma with platelet count <10,000/cmm.

In the absence of an overt of bleeding and an expected PT of <18 seconds, periprocedural testing of PT and aPTT measurement is not warranted. The 2012 American College of Cardiology/Society for Cardiovascular Angiography and Interventions (ACC/SCAI) consensus document recommends deferring elective coronary angiography for patients on long-term warfarin till INR <1.8 for femoral artery access and <2.2 for radial artery access.

For patients with minimal risk factors for bleeding, screening coagulation laboratory testing is not routinely recommended. It is recommended for patients on VKA or UFH or who have a history of bleeding diathesis. Target and correct INR <2–3 or less and consider platelet transfusion if platelet count <20,000/cmm.

For arterial access with low bleeding risk, INR threshold <1.8 for femoral access and <2.2 for radial access is recommended.

- *Laboratory parameters for high bleeding risk procedures:* Platelet count of >50,000/cmm and an INR <1.5 have been the standard threshold at which a major surgery can be performed successfully.
  - *Image-guided liver biopsy:* Platelet counts >50,000/cmm are strongly recommended to avoid significant bleeding. Coagulation parameter thresholds are not well defined in the medical literature to provide a recommendation.
  - *Lumbar puncture:* The AABB has chosen to recommend a very liberal platelet count of 50,000/cmm as a threshold for lumbar puncture. Single-agent antiplatelet agents may be safe for certain high bleeding risk procedures such as solid organ biopsy, percutaneous endoscopic gastrostomy (PEG), and percutaneous nephrolithotomy. Bleeding complications were <0.6% for patients who have taken aspirin within 10 days of biopsy. Patients who use clopidogrel within 5 days of undergoing core biopsy of solid organs (liver, lung, kidneys, or retroperitoneal areas) revealed very less major complication rates (1 in 63). Of these, 76% had taken aspirin within 5 days of the procedure.
  - *Coagulation parameters:* Correct INR to within a range of <1.5–1.8 and consider platelet transfusion if platelet count <50,000/cmm.
- *Laboratory parameters for patients with chronic liver disease:* The American Association for Study of Liver Disease (AASLD) has clearly stated that PT and INR in patients with cirrhosis do not correlate with bleeding, and any attempt to correct with plasma is ineffective and likely to be detrimental in most patients with cirrhosis. Splenomegaly plays a central role in thrombocytopenia due to rapid splenic sequestration of platelets. These patients will exhibit a poor incremental response to repeated platelet transfusions increasing the risk of transfusion-related circulatory overload, elevated portal presses, and bleeding. PT/INR and platelet counts have been shown to be poor predictors of bleeding risk in patients with chronic liver disease. Hyperfibrinolysis is an emerging concept and major cause of bleeding, and the assessment of fibrinogen level in patients with chronic liver disease is of value. The AASLD has recommended that presence of hyperfibrinolysis or clinical evidence of disseminated intravascular coagulation should preclude an invasive procedure. Cryoprecipitate replacement is to be considered in patients with low fibrinogen levels.

- *Bridging therapy considerations:* Bridging requirements differ before and after a planned procedure. Before a procedure, bridging is necessary if there is very high thrombosis risk to minimize the time of anticoagulation. A parenteral agent, typically heparin, is given after the effect of an oral agent, usually warfarin, has waned. Bridging after a procedure involves giving a parenteral agent till the oral anticoagulant effect of warfarin is takes effect or before a DOAC is given.

Bridging can be associated with excessive bleeding. The Bridge or continue Coumadin for device surgery randomized controlled trial showed that patients in whom therapeutic anticoagulation with a VKA was maintained with an INR goal of <3 on the day of the procedure experienced significantly less bleeding than those who were randomized to undergo temporary interruption of the VKA agent and bridging with heparin. The role of Coumadin in preventing thromboembolism in atrial fibrillation patients undergoing catheter ablation trial study demonstrated that patients who continue vitamin K anticoagulation with the INR goal of 2–3 experience lower rates of minor bleeding and thromboembolic events than patients who undergo anticoagulation interruption and bridging with LMWH before catheter ablation for atrial fibrillation. In another study comparing various bridging strategies (none, prophylactic-dose heparin, full-dose heparin) after stopping warfarin in mostly minor procedures (60%), the rate of thrombosis was 0.8% and the rate of bleeding was 3.2%. Patients on full-dose heparin or LMWH experienced increased bleeding risk. Similarly, in another study comparing bridging versus no bridging patients on warfarin for secondary prevention of VTE undergoing surgical procedures, there was a 17-fold higher risk of bleeding for patients receiving bridging. Hence, bridging strategies should be utilized judiciously, mainly for high-risk thromboembolic patients (e.g., mechanical heart valves, recent stroke, or VTE).

MANAGEMENT STRATEGIES

Management strategies for new vascular access are shown in **Flowchart 1**.

- *For VKA (warfarin):* Stop 5 days before surgery, bridge with LMWH if high risk, and resume 12–24 hours postoperatively.
- *For DOACs:* Stop 24–48 hours before surgery (longer if high bleeding risk or poor renal function) and resume within 24–48 hours postoperatively. Treatment can be resumed with prophylactic or therapeutic dose of anticoagulation or antiplatelet agent. Following a procedure is based on the risk of postprocedural bleeding versus the patient's risk of thromboembolic events. Resumption of treatment with prophylactic or therapeutic dose of anticoagulation or antiplatelet agent following a procedure is based on risk of post procedure of bleeding versus the patient's risk of thromboembolic events. As a common recommendation among guidelines, DOACs should be held 3 half-life times before low-risk procedures and 5 half-life times before high-risk procedures. For low-bleeding-risk procedures, rivaroxaban, apixaban, and dabigatran are interrupted 24 hours before surgery in patients with CrCl >50 mL/min. If the renal function are compromised (CrCl <50 mL/min), drugs are suspended 2 days before the procedure. Regardless of renal function, all drugs were reinitiated at 48 hours for high-bleeding-risk surgical procedures and 24 hours for low-bleeding-risk procedures.
- *For antiplatelet therapy:* Generally continued, but dual therapy (aspirin + clopidogrel) should be assessed case by case.

The timing of restitution of anticoagulation and antiplatelet agents after a procedure is shown in **Flowchart 2**.

The option available is to restart at a low dose, maintenance dose, or loading dose. Clopidogrel may require loading dosing, but it is best to involve the cardiovascular specialist for risk assessment to decide dosing.

DOACs: In low bleeding risk procedures, dabigatran was restarted at a low dose of 75 mg on the night of the procedure (4 hours after neuraxial anesthesia) with full dose from the next morning. In high bleeding risk procedures, dabigatran was restarted at a full dose 48 hours after the procedure or later.

Flowchart 1: New vascular access management strategies.

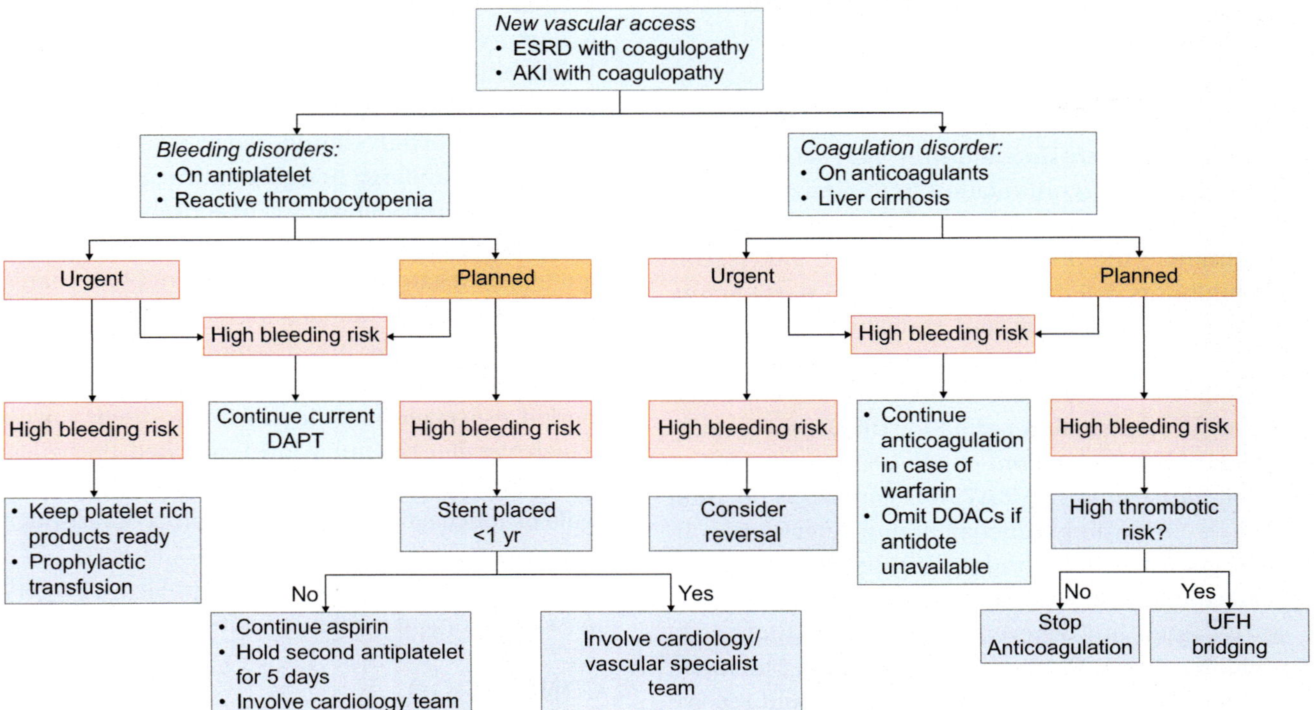

(AKI: acute kidney injury; DAPT: dual antiplatelet therapy; DOACs: direct oral anticoagulants; ESRD: end-stage renal disease; UFH: unfractionated heparin)

Flowchart 2: Timing of restitution of anticoagulation and antiplatelet agents after a procedure.

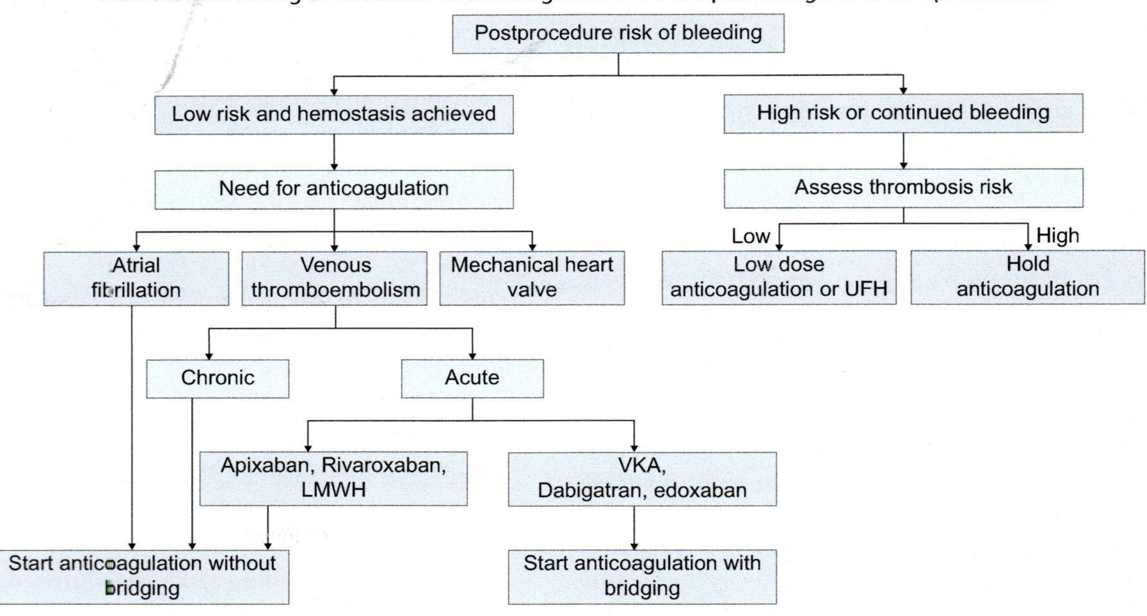

(LMWH: low molecular weight heparin; UFH: unfractionated heparin; VKA: vitamin K antagonist)

Emergency reversal of anticoagulation:

- *Warfarin:* Vitamin K, FFP, prothrombin complex concentrate (PCC)
- *DOACs:* Andexanet alfa (for factor Xa inhibitors), Idarucizumab (for dabigatran).
- *Heparin:* Protamine sulfate

Special considerations:

- *Neuraxial anesthesia:* Requires precise timing of anticoagulant discontinuation to minimize bleeding risks. Recent multisociety consensus guidelines recommend the discontinuation of a DOAC (factor Xa inhibitors 3–5 days; dabigatran 4–5 days) before a neuraxial procedure and restarting of DOAC 24 hours after the procedure. For patients with a high thrombotic risk, bridging strategy may be warranted as the discontinuation period for DOAC is unusually extended in this situation.
- *Atrial fibrillation:* The 2017 ACC consensus decision pathway regarding anticoagulation interruption in patients with NVAF undergoing procedures states that patients with low risk should not receive bridging anticoagulation whereas those with high risk, including those with a recent stroke (within 3 months), should. Patients at intermediate risk should receive individualized strategies based on a multidisciplinary team recommendation after assessment of their bleeding and thrombotic risk profile. The CHA_2DS_2-VASc score helps in decisions regarding bridging strategies in patients with NVAF.
- *Venous thromboembolism:* Decisions are based on acuity (<3 months), location (proximal/distal DVT), and clinical context (provoked/unprovoked). Postprocedural patients with an acute episode of thrombotic event should receive rivaroxaban or apixaban or undergo bridging anticoagulation if they were on warfarin, dabigatran, or edoxaban.
- *Mechanical heart valves:* The AHA/ACC has issued guidelines regarding the management of mechanical heart valves. The management of antithrombotic therapy should take into account the valve type and location and number of valves in the periprocedural period, especially for patients with prosthetic valves. If a high bleeding risk procedure is required, the patient's cardiology team should guide strategies regarding brief hold of anticoagulation versus periprocedural bridging strategy.
- *Patients with coronary stents:* Delay elective surgery if possible; if urgent, continue aspirin.

CONCLUSION

The perioperative management of anticoagulation requires balancing thromboembolic and bleeding risks.

Current guidelines emphasize individualized decision-making based on patient-specific factors, surgical risk, and the type of anticoagulant used. Bridging therapy should be reserved for high-risk cases, while most patients can be managed through strategic anticoagulation interruption.

ACKNOWLEDGMENT

The authors thank Mr Nitiraj Shete for graphics support.

SUGGESTED READING

1. Bashir S, Mukund A, Syed RF, Nayak SL, Rastogi A, Sarin SK. Combined Fluoroscopy and Ultrasound-Guided Transjugular Kidney Biopsy in Cirrhotic Patients. J Vasc Interv Radiol. 2018;29(5):696-703.
2. Capodanno D, Angiolillo DJ. Management of antiplatelet therapy in patients with coronary artery disease requiring cardiac and noncardiac surgery. Circulation. 2013;128(25):2785-98.
3. Novelli PM, Tublin JM, Orons PD. Correcting Coagulopathy for Image-Guided Procedures. Semin Intervent Radiol. 2022;39(4):428-34.
4. Patel IJ, Rahim S, Davidson JC, Hanks SE, Tam AL, Walker TG, et al. Society of Interventional Radiology Consensus Guidelines for the Periprocedural Management of Thrombotic and Bleeding Risk in Patients Undergoing Percutaneous Image-Guided Interventions-Part II: Recommendations: Endorsed by the Canadian Association for Interventional Radiology and the Cardiovascular and Interventional Radiological Society of Europe. J Vasc Interv Radiol. 2019;30(8):1168-84.e1.
5. Summaria F, Giannico MB, Talarico GP, Patrizi R. Antiplatelet Therapy in Hemodialysis Patients Undergoing Percutaneous Coronary Interventions. Nephrourol Mon. 2015;7(4):e28099.
6. Wiltrout C, Kondo KL. Correction of coagulopathy for percutaneous interventions. Semin Intervent Radiol. 2010;27(4):338-47.

CHAPTER 32

Vascular Access in Patients with Complex Anatomy

Sachin S Soni, Sanjay Srinivas, Umapati N Hegde

INTRODUCTION

Hemodialysis (HD) is a life-sustaining treatment for individuals with end-stage renal disease (ESRD). Vascular access is the lifeline and the Achilles heel for ESRD patients on HD. Providing an adequate dialysis access continues to challenge nephrologists as dialysis patients live longer and exhaust their access options. The ideal vascular access for HD is the arteriovenous fistula (AVF), which offers numerous advantages, including better long-term patency, fewer complications, and lower infection rates than other access. A distal-most possible location is chosen to create AVF to preserve proximal venous capital for future use if needed. When an AVF is not viable or cannot be used immediately, a tunneled dialysis catheter can serve as a temporary or long-term access solution. These catheters are inserted into central veins such as the internal jugular, subclavian, or femoral vein, providing an alternative route for dialysis.

VASCULAR ACCESS IN PATIENTS WITH COMPLEX ANATOMY

The radiocephalic AVF (RC-AVF) at the wrist, initially described by Brescia-Cimino in 1966, remains the preferred vascular access (VA). When vessels at the wrist area are unsuitable for creating RC AVF, brachiocephalic AVF (BC-AVF) at the elbow area is the next option. These conventional VAs are created in patients with normal vascular anatomy. Other options must be explored in patients with complex vascular anatomy due to the poor quality of the cephalic vein or radial artery. We shall discuss possible options in this chapter.

ARTERIOVENOUS FISTULA

Ulnar Basilic Fistula

In those patients where the RC-AVF either is not possible or has failed, the ulnar-basilic fistula is a viable alternative. It has an adequate 1-year patency rate. This type of AVF needs more extensive dissection; the basilic vein is thin and is more prone to spasms than the cephalic vein.[1,2] A recent study suggested that the prone position of a patient may be more comfortable for both the operator and the patient when creating ulnar-basilic AVF.[3]

Radiobasilic Transposition

Radiobasilic transposition is possible for patients when the cephalic vein in the forearm is inadequate. The basilic vein from the medial aspect of the forearm is mobilized and transposed in a subcutaneous tunnel toward the radial artery to create an anastomosis.[4]

Forearm Loop Transposition

When the radial artery is unsuitable for RC AVF at the wrist level, the cephalic or basilic vein can be transposed and placed in a loop to be anastomosed with the proximal radial artery in the antecubital fossa.[5]

Gracz Arteriovenous Fistula

The perforating vein in the antecubital fossa can be anastomosed with a proximal radial or brachial artery. This method helps achieve arterialization of both the cephalic and the basilic veins. Gracz described this technique,[6] and was subsequently modified by Konner et al.[7]

Brachiobasilic Arteriovenous Fistula with Transposition

In patients unsuitable for RC-AVF or BC-AVF, brachiobasilic AVF is an option. As the basilic vein lies in the deeper plane of the arm in proximity to the neurovascular bundle, its superficialization and transposition are needed.[8] Transposition can be a single-step or two-step procedure. As the name suggests, in a single-step surgery, both anastomosis and transposition are performed simultaneously. The basilic vein is dissected and transposed, establishing a new trajectory, followed by the end-to-side anastomosis with the brachial artery. This approach reduces the time needed for the first cannulation. It eliminates the need for a second surgery; still, it is associated with more mechanical complications such as kink and swing-site stenosis as the transposition is done using an unarterialized vein.[9]

In a two-stage procedure, the first step involves anastomosis between the basilic vein and the brachial artery. Following a maturation assessment by Doppler ultrasound, usually after 4 weeks, the second procedure is executed to superficialize and/or transpose the vein.[10]

Brachiobrachial Arteriovenous Fistula

An AVF between the brachial vein and the brachial artery is a possible VA in desperate situations. Brachial veins are generally in pairs lying on either side of the brachial artery. As a first step, anastomosis between the brachial artery and vein is created in the antecubital fossa. After 4–6 weeks, maturation assessment is done, and superficialization of the arterialized brachial vein is executed **(Figs. 1A to C)**. However, this technique's major drawbacks include a high initial failure rate of up to 53% and low primary patency after a year (35–40%), limb edema, and difficulty in cannulation of the superficialized vein.[11]

Arteriovenous Fistula in the Lower Limb

When the upper limb cannot be a site for AVFs or grafts, as in cases of bilateral central venous stenosis or with exhausted sites in the upper limb, lower limb AVF can be considered. *Femoral vein transposition (FVT)* AVF can be one of the described options.[12] According to reports, the 1-year primary patency rates for FVT range from 73 to 91%.[13] Extensive surgical dissection, the risk of distal ischemia, and wound complications have been major deterrents to its widespread use. The *laterolateral femorofemoral AVF* with anastomosis between the distal femoral artery and the superficial femoral vein is an alternative VA. This approach avoids ligation of the distal popliteal vein.[14] Tibiosaphanous AVF created around the ankle region is also described through case reports.[15]

ARTERIOVENOUS GRAFTS

Using arteriovenous graft (AVG) as a VA is a viable and suitable option. It has lesser failure rate and shorter maturation time, is easier for needling, and is technically less complex than native AVF.[16,17] AVG facilitates secondary native VA in that it helps dilate previously unsuitable veins in the arms to create an AVF. However, AVGs are more expensive and are associated with more morbidity. Expanded polytetrafluoroethylene (PTFE) is the recommended material for creating AVGs. This material has been shown to have better integration rates and less infection risk. A bilayer PTFE prosthesis reinforced with a third elastomer layer can create an immediate puncture AVG to allow cannulation after 24 hours. A bioengineered prosthesis manufactured from a polyester matrix and sheep collagen has also demonstrated promising results.[18]

The AVG can be implanted in a straight line or a loop shape. The prosthesis length should be 20–40 cm with a diameter of 6–8 mm.[16,19] Arteries or veins identified for the anastomosis should not be <4 mm, and the anastomosis is end-to-side type.[16] Arterial anastomosis should be performed as distal as possible, and the order of preference is the brachial artery in the antecubital fossa, brachial artery in the arm, and brachial artery close to the axilla and axillary artery. The venous anastomosis can be performed on the veins in the antecubital fossa or above the elbow, as well as in the cephalic, basilic, axillary, subclavian, and jugular veins.

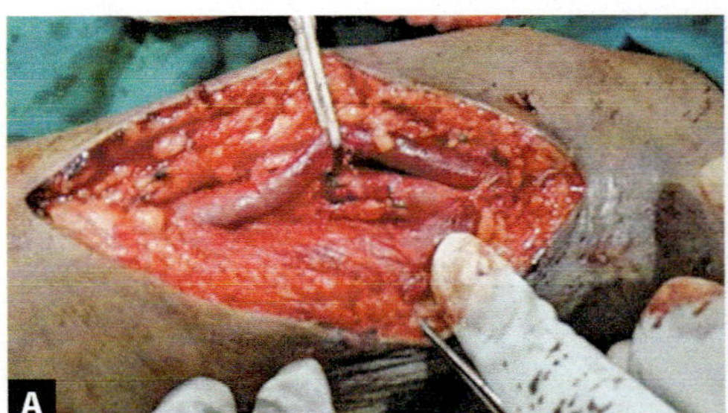

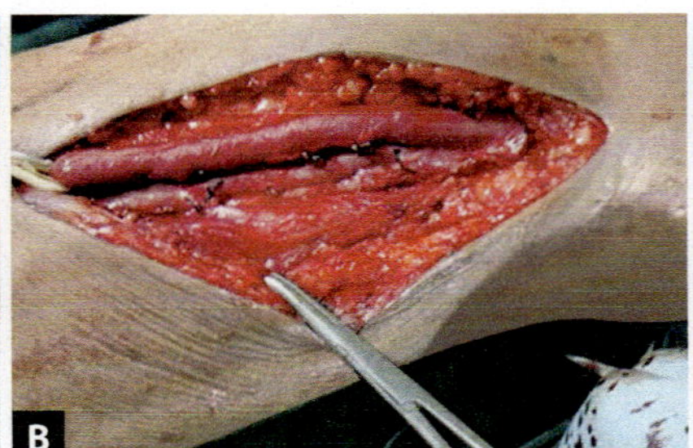

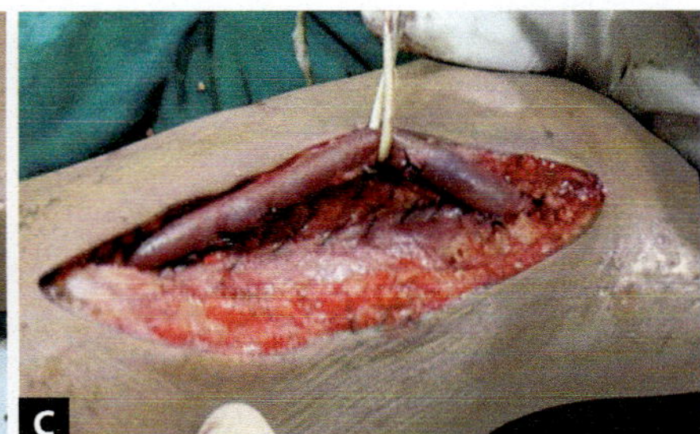

Figs. 1A to C: Steps in brachial vein transposition: (A) Arterialized brachial vein which runs parallel to brachial artery being separated very carefully; (B) Artery and vein after complete separation; (C) Muscle and fascia layer between the artery and vein is sutured. Now, the artery lies in its anatomical location and the arterialized brachial vein is completely superficialized.

An AVG can also be placed in the lower limb. A PTFE graft between the common femoral or superficial femoral artery and the common femoral, superficial femoral or long saphenous vein, placed in a loop configuration in the subcutaneous plane of the anterior aspect of the thigh, is one option.[20] Another option is a mid-thigh (proximal to patella) graft arterial anastomosis with superficial femoral artery and venous with popliteal vein. Suprapubic femoral-femoral graft from the femoral artery to the contralateral femoral vein is also described in the literature.

TABLE 1: Vascular access options (arteriovenous fistula or arteriovenous graft) in patients with complex anatomy.

Arteriovenous fistula	*Arteriovenous graft*
Upper limb: • Ulnarbasilic • Radiobasilic • Brachiobasilic (Transposition) • Brachiobrachial (Transposition)	*Upper limb:* • Radio-antecubital straight graft • Brachio-antecubital loop graft • Radio-antecubital loop graft • Brachioaxillary straight graft • Brachiobrachial straight graft • Brachioaxillary loop graft • Brachiobrachial loop graft
Lower limb: • Femorofemoral • Tibiosaphenous	*Lower limb:* • Femorofemoral (upper thigh) • Femoropopliteal (mid-thigh) • Suprapubic femorofemoral crossover
	Chest wall: • Axilloaxial graft • Necklace graft • Subclavian-subclavian graft • Internal jugular vein (IJV) to subclavian graft
Arterioarterial prosthetic graft and right atrial appendage graft	
Arterio-arterial prosthetic graft: • Brachial arterioarterial graft • Axillary arterioarterial graft • Femoral arterioarterial graft	*Right atrial (RA) appendage graft:* • Axillary artery to atrial appendage • Brachial artery to atrial appendage • Subclavian artery to atrial appendage • Axillary vein to atrial appendage

When there are extensive occlusions of venous trunks, both in upper and lower limbs, some exotic AVGs are described, like axillary artery to axillary vein over anterior chest wall or necklace graft from axillary artery to contralateral axillary vein. A summary of possible VAs in patients with complex vascular anatomy is shown in **Table 1**.

Arterial–arterial Prosthetic Loop Graft

Arterial–arterial prosthetic loop (AAPL) grafts are indicated if sufficient venous drainage is not possible due to occlusions of prominent deep veins or if the increased cardiac output exerts too much strain on the heart. This essentially creates an interposition graft in continuity with the artery placed in an accessible position to cannulate **(Figs. 2A to C)**. The graft may be straight (parallel to the artery), a loop graft or an omega loop graft. A study by Khafagy et al.[21] analyzed 35 brachial arterioarterial prosthetic loops **(Figs. 6A to D)**. The primary patency rates were 87.9%, 70.4%, and 38.8% at 12, 24, and 36 months, respectively. The secondary patency rates were 90.7%, 80.3%, and 67.6% at 12, 24, and 36 months, respectively.[21] Zanow et al. reported 36 AAPLs as vascular access (axillary

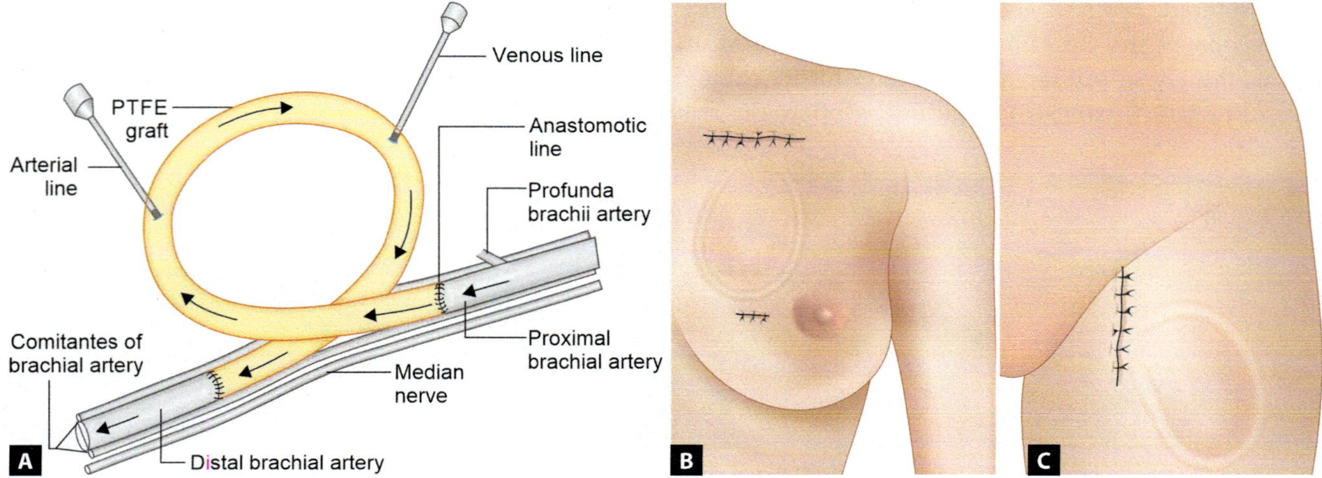

Figs. 2A to C: Arterial–arterial prosthetic loop (AAPL) graft. (A) Brachial arterio-arterial prosthetic loops; (B) Axillary chest loops; (C) Femoral arterial prosthetic loops. (PTFE: polytetrafluoroethylene)

chest loop—31 and femoral loop—5). The primary patency rate was 73% and the secondary patency rate was 96% at 1 year, whereas at 3 years the patency rates were 54% and 87%, respectively.[22] AAPL showed promising results with low complication rates, but there is a potential chance for limb ischemia. Thrombosis occurred in 20–42% of grafts.[21,22]

Right Atrial Appendage Graft

A large-diameter externally reinforced PTFE (GoreTex), autologous veins or bovine carotid artery graft can bypass the obstructed vein and be anastomosed to the right atrial appendage. This technique bypassed lesions in the subclavian vein,[23] the innominate vein/superior vena cava junction, and the distal axillary vein. RA graft may be used to bypass between upper limb arteries to the right atrial appendage to create new access for dialysis, i.e., axillary artery to atrial appendage[24] **(Figs. 3A and B)**, brachial artery to atrial appendage, or subclavian artery to atrial appendage. The right atrium can be used as a direct outflow for an AVG. This requires cardiac exposure via a thoracotomy or sternotomy and anastomosis of a graft to the right atrial (RA) appendage. El-Sabrout[25] described the mean patency of 15.4 months ranging from 1.5 to 52 months, with 78% patency at 3 months and 44% 1-year patency.

TUNNELED DIALYSIS CATHETERS

If the dialysis initiation is urgent or emergent, the patient may not have had a choice of vascular access and initiated with a CVC. Tunneled dialysis catheters (TDCs) are used as temporary access points before permanent access can be created. They are inserted into large veins such as the internal jugular, subclavian, or femoral vein and tunneled under the skin to minimize the risk of infection. Tunneled catheters are helpful for short-term dialysis but carry a higher risk of complications, especially infections, thrombosis, and catheter-related bloodstream infections (CRBSIs), compared to AVF. Postinsertion imaging should be considered to avoid mispositioning of CVCs.[26]

Tunneled Dialysis Catheter Placement in Difficult Situations

When right internal jugular vein (IJV) is not available for placement of tunneled dialysis catheters, the sites preferred in order of catheter placement are left IJV, external jugular vein (EJV), femoral veins, subclavian veins, translumbar inferior vena cava (IVC),[27] and transhepatic inferior vena cava.

For several reasons, the right IJV is preferred over the left[28] **(Fig. 4)**. Left IJV requires the hemodialysis central venous catheter (HD-CVC) to make two right angle bends and an anteroposterior bend over the pulmonary arch before reaching the superior vena cava (SVC), thereby potentially leading to more chances of encountering resistance while advancing the wire, dilators, sheath, and subsequently, the catheter[29] **(Table 2)**.

Important considerations for the left IJV tunneled catheter: To minimize complications, fluoroscopy or ultrasound is crucial for real-time needle visualization, guidewire, and catheter placement. Malposition is more likely to occur when inserting a split-tipped catheter through the left

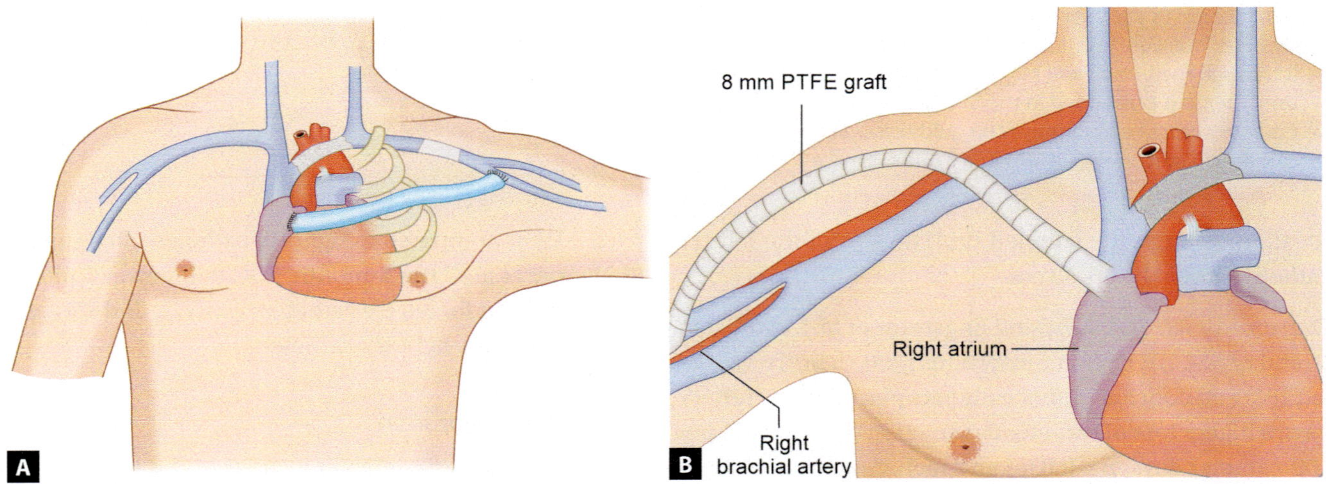

Figs. 3A and B: Right atrial (RA) appendage graft. (A) Bypass graft from axillary vein to atrium; (B) Brachial artery to right atrium. (PTFE: polytetrafluoroethylene)

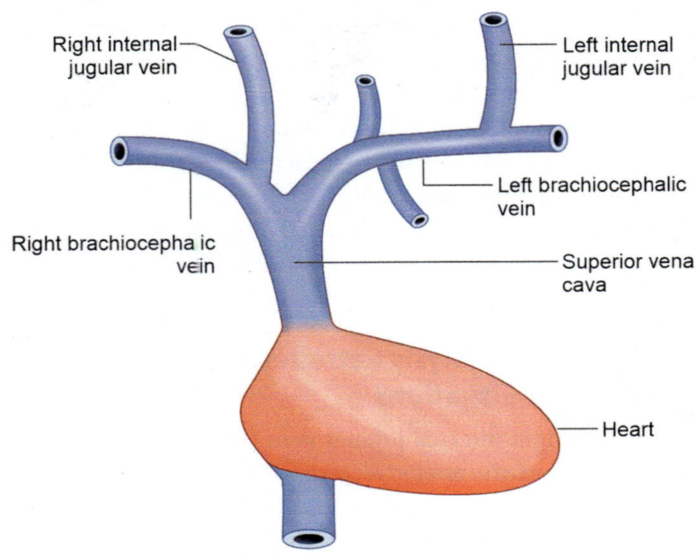

- (I) *Size:* The right IJ vein is dominant and wider in diameter in most people.
- Right IJ vein diameter (median diameter 17 mm, range 13–20 mm) and left IJ vein diameter (median diameter 13 mm, range 10–16 mm)
- The cross-sectional area of the right IJ vein (median 160 mm^2, range 108–235 mm^2) was larger than the left IJ vein (median 102 mm^2, range 63–168 mm^2)
- (II) *Anatomy:* The right IJ vein follows a straight course into the right brachiocephalic and superior vena cava and hence allows for easier passage and less trauma as compared to the left IJ vein, which has two 90° turns and more tributaries

Fig. 4: Right and left internal jugular vein (IJV) anatomy and why right IJV is preferred as the first option for vascular access.

TABLE 2: Key steps of a left internal jugular vein (IJV) tunneled cuffed catheter (TCC) insertion.

Steps for left IJV placement	***Challenges during left IJV placement***
• *Patient preparation:* The patient is supine, with the head slightly turned away from the insertion site. A sterile field was established, including draping and antiseptic skin preparation • *Landmark identification:* Locate the left IJV by identifying the clavicle's sternocleidomastoid muscle and the medial border • *Venous access:* Using an ultrasound probe, guide a needle to puncture the left IJV at a 30–45° angle. Aspirate to confirm blood return • *Guidewire insertion:* Introduce a guidewire via the needle into the vein and advance it into the superior vena cava • *Subcutaneous tunnel creation:* Make a small incision at a selected site on the chest, typically below the clavicle. Using a tunneling device, make a subcutaneous passageway from the skin incision to the vein puncture site • *Catheter insertion:* Insert the TCC over the guidewire, guiding it through the tunnel and into the vein. Advance the catheter until the tip is positioned in the SVC RA junction • *Catheter securement:* Remove the guidewire. Secure the catheter in place with sutures or a fixation device	• *Complex venous anatomy:* The left brachiocephalic vein is typically longer and has more tributaries compared to the right, making it easier to accidentally enter a smaller branch instead of the main vein • *Sheath kinking:* When advancing the catheter through the sheath, the tip can kink at the junction where the left brachiocephalic vein meets the left IJV, especially if the insertion angle is not optimal • *Catheter mispositioning:* The catheter tip might be directed into smaller tributaries, leading to improper placement and potential complications • *Increased risk of complications:* Compared to the right side, a left IJV insertion may have a slightly higher chance of complications like pneumothorax, arterial puncture, or damage to nearby structures due to the anatomical variations

IJV than through the stepped tip. The size of the left IJV catheter should be 26–33 cm.

Outcome of left IJV catheters: Engstrom et al.[30] evaluated a total of 532 IJV catheter insertions (398 right IJV vs. 194 left IJV) and concluded that catheters placed in the left IJV have a higher rate of catheter dysfunction (0.25 vs. 0.11 per 100-catheter days; $p = 0.036$) and higher rates of catheter-related infection (0.50 vs. 0.27 per 100 catheter days; $p = 0.005$) as compared to right IJV catheters. In a study by Shingarev et al.,[31] the 6-month TDC patency at 6 months and 12 months for left IJV catheters was 37% and 6% versus 54% and 35% for right IJV catheters.

External Jugular Vein

The EJV is a superficial vein located in the neck, formed by joining the posterior division of the retromandibular vein with the posterior auricular vein. EJV is preferred for venous access, as it is superficial, easily approachable, and dilated due to its attachment with the investing layer of deep cervical fascia, which prevents it from collapsing. EJV TDC insertion should be done under ultrasound and fluoroscopic guidance to minimize complications, define the venous anatomy, and ensure the correct position. If the EJV is found to be collapsed, it may be made more prominent by performing the Valsalva maneuver or creating a humming sound.

Steps of EJV TDC insertion: The steps of insertion of the right EJV are shown in **Figure 5**. A retrospective study comparing right EJV versus left IJV tunneled catheter by Wang et al.[32] concluded that right EJV might be superior to left IJV as an alternative insertion route for TDC placement in hemodialysis patients whose right IJVs are unavailable. The mean cumulative catheter patency was significantly higher in the right EJV group (382.04 ± 33.55 vs. 261.36 ± 20.81 days) compared with that in the left IJV group and 61.9% right EJV catheter survival at 240 days compared to 46.4% in left IJV. Vats et al.[33] concluded that EJ blood flow outcomes at 30th day and 90th day were comparable to LIJ and RIJ. In a study by Behera et al.,[34] it was found that EJV TDC insertion has a reasonable technical success rate when performed under fluoroscopy. It is associated with an acceptable rate of catheter dysfunction, especially thrombosis, which is more common in EJV opening into subclavian veins.

Subclavian Catheterization

Infraclavicular subclavian vein catheterization has become a well-established technique. Supraclavicular approach is less practiced even though it has advantages, including a well-defined insertion landmark (the clavis sternomastoid angle), a shorter distance from skin to the vein, a larger target area, a straighter path to the superior vena cava, less proximity to the lung, and fewer complications of pleural or arterial puncture.

A subclavian vein tunneled catheter is generally considered to have a higher risk of complications such as pneumothorax and arterial puncture with potential outcomes including increased risk of thrombosis, hematoma formation, and pneumothorax; however, it has a lower risk of catheter-related bloodstream infection than other sites. The subclavian vein often forms a right angle with the SVC, and an advancing stiff dilator and peel-away sheath can cause a vascular injury.[35] However, raising the patient's arm can alter the position of the

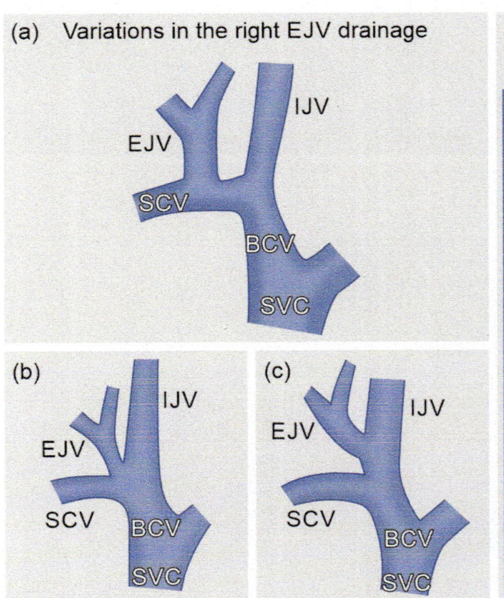

Steps of EJV TDC insertion

- Choose the appropriate size TCC (19 cm, 23 cm, or 28 cm). The procedure should be done under fluoroscopy and preferably USG guidance to minimize complications.
- Trendelenburg position with the head turned to the contralateral side to make the EJV prominent. The puncture site is about 1 cm cranial to the clavicle.
- After local anesthesia, EJV is punctured using an 18 g introducer needle, and a 5 mL diluted contrast can define the course of EJV.
- J-tip of the 150 cm hydrophilic guidewire is passed and positioned in IVC.
- After placing the catheter on the chest wall appropriate exit sites and tunnel lengths are planned, and a 5 mm incision is made. 3–4 mm incision is given lateral to the insertion site, and blunt dissection is done at the venotomy site.
- The tunneller creates a subcutaneous tunnel of the required length. A catheter is tunneled through it to keep the Dacron cuff 2 cm deep to the exit site.
- After using sequential dilators to dilate the venotomy site, the final trocar with a peel-away sheath is inserted into the vein. The catheter is inserted through the sheath, with the tip in the mid-right atrium. Blood flow is checked and tip position is confirmed using fluoroscopy. Catheter ports are locked with heparin
- The venotomy site is sutured, and hemostasis is achieved with firm pressure over the tunnel.

Variations in the right EJV regarding its opening into proximal veins. It opens into (a) SVC, (b) the confluence of SVC and IJV, or (c) directly into the IJV.
(IJV: internal jugular vein; EJV; external jugular vein; SCV: subclavian vein; BCV: brachiocephalic vein; SVC: superior vena cava)

Fig. 5: Variation in the external jugular vein and steps of insertion of tunneled cuffed catheter (TCC) in right external jugular vein.

guidewire and, therefore, change the favorable angle of the vein (right angle to obtuse angle) relative to the SVC for this placement as shown in **Figures 6A to D**.[35] The risk of developing CVS has been reported to be as high as 30–50% with subclavian vein catheters as compared to around 10% with an internal jugular vein THDC,[36,37] limiting its use due to compromising future AVF creation. Randomized catheter placement in an internal jugular vein or subclavian by Zafarghandi et al., followed for 6 months, showed no difference in infection or thrombosis resulting in extraction; however, the failure rate was significantly higher in cases with internal jugular vein catheter.[38]

Femoral Vein Tunneled Catheter

A femoral vein tunneled catheter, sometimes used for long-term vascular access, is often considered a less ideal choice due to a higher risk of complications than other sites such as the IJV. The steps of insertion of femoral TDC are shown in **Figures 7A to C**.

Specific Challenges with Femoral Vein Tunneled Catheter Placement and Outcome

The femoral vein can be relatively superficial and prone to movement, making accurate placement challenging, especially in patients with obesity or poor vascular access.

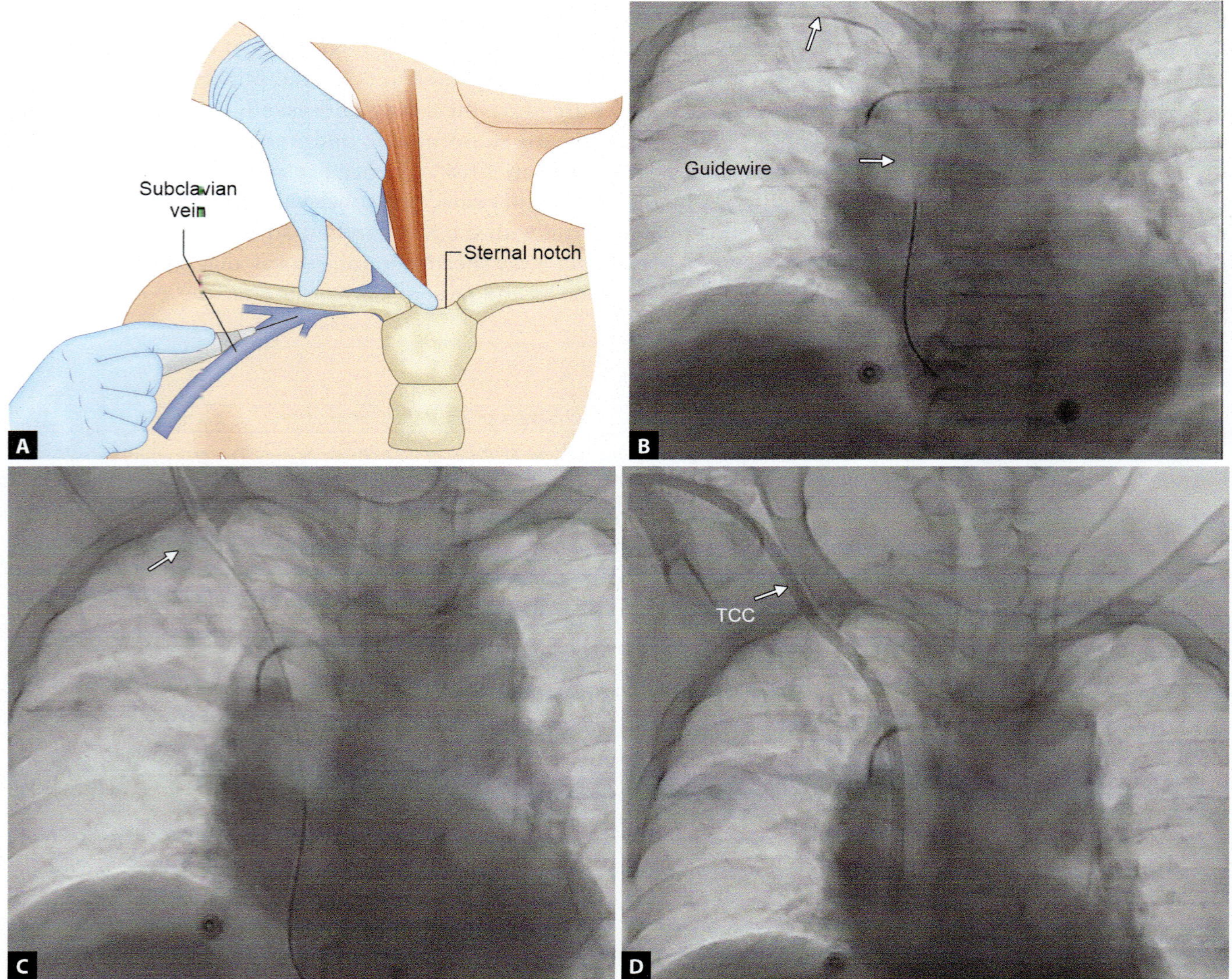

Figs. 6A to D: Right subclavian vein tunneled cuffed catheter (TCC). (A) Anatomical landmark—subclavian vein puncture; (B) Right angle of the subclavian vein to SVC; (C) Raising arm, changed from acute to obtuse; (D) TCC in the right subclavian vein.

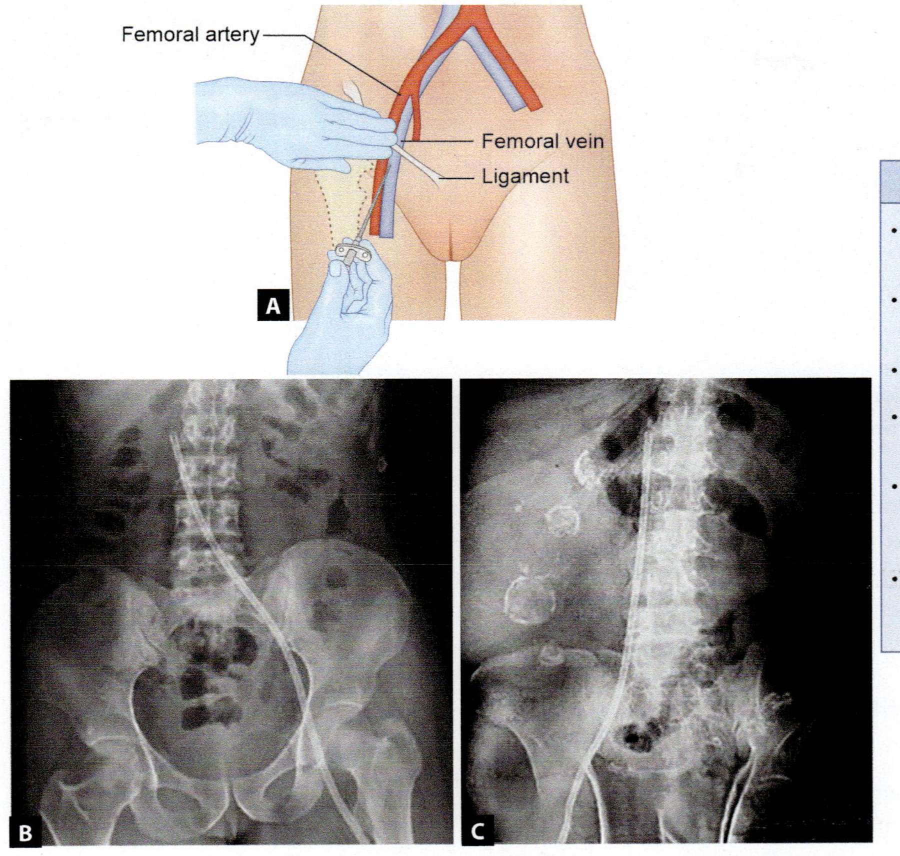

Steps of femoral vein TCC placement

- An 18-gauge needle is used to puncture the femoral vein, and a guidewire is inserted through the needle.
- A subcutaneous tunnel is created using a tunneling device, and the exit site is placed on the lateral thigh, away from the groin.
- The catheter is attached to the tunneler and pulled through the tunnel.
- After using sequential dilators to dilate the venotomy site, the trocar with a peel-away sheath is inserted into the vein.
- The catheter is pushed into the sheath, the tip is positioned in the IVC using fluoroscopic guidance and the sheath is peeled away. The catheter is secured with sutures.
- Fluoroscopic images are taken to assess the catheter tip position and to check for kinking, and flow is confirmed.

Figs. 7A to C: Steps of insertion of femoral tunneled cuffed catheter (TCC) and tip placement. (A) Anatomical landmark—femoral vein puncture; (B) Tip low in inferior vena cava (IVC); (C) Tip high in IVC.

Due to the proximity to the groin, femoral catheters are more prone to infection than other sites. The femoral vein is relatively large, with slower blood flow, which can increase the risk of blood clots forming around the catheter tip. It is also susceptible to kinking or occlusion due to leg movement, increasing the chance of clotting. The study by Sethi et al.[39] concluded that tunneled femoral catheters revealed low catheter survival (30, 60, 90, and 180 days were 81%, 29%, 18%, and 12.5%, respectively) and significant complications (deep venous thrombosis—15.7% and malfunction/occlusion). Burton et al.[40] showed that factors such as advanced age, diabetes, and left-side femoral vein catheter insertion were associated with a higher catheter failure rate. In a retrospective review, Herrington et al.[41] showed no benefit in routinely adding prophylactic anticoagulation in patients with TFC to reduce the rates of catheter-related deep venous thrombosis. In a study by Zaleski et al., the technical success of placement and initial function was 100%.[42] The 30-, 60-, and 180-day primary patency rates were 78%, 71%, and 55%, respectively, and secondary patency rates were 95%, 83%, and 61%, respectively. The femoral catheter flow rate is better, and so is the URR with high tip placement compared to low tip placement.[43]

SOLUTIONS AND APPROACHES TO CATHETER PLACEMENT

To optimize catheter placement and minimize complications, ultrasound guidance helps identify the optimal access point, ensures proper positioning of the catheter, and reduces the risk of complications such as arterial puncture or inadvertent catheter malposition. Preprocedural venography can be used to evaluate the patency of veins and guide catheter placement in patients with complicated central venous anatomy.

Unconventional Exit Site for Tunneled Catheters

Cognitively impaired patients often manipulate their catheters, risking infection, bleeding, or complete removal of their TDCs when the catheters are tunneled over the

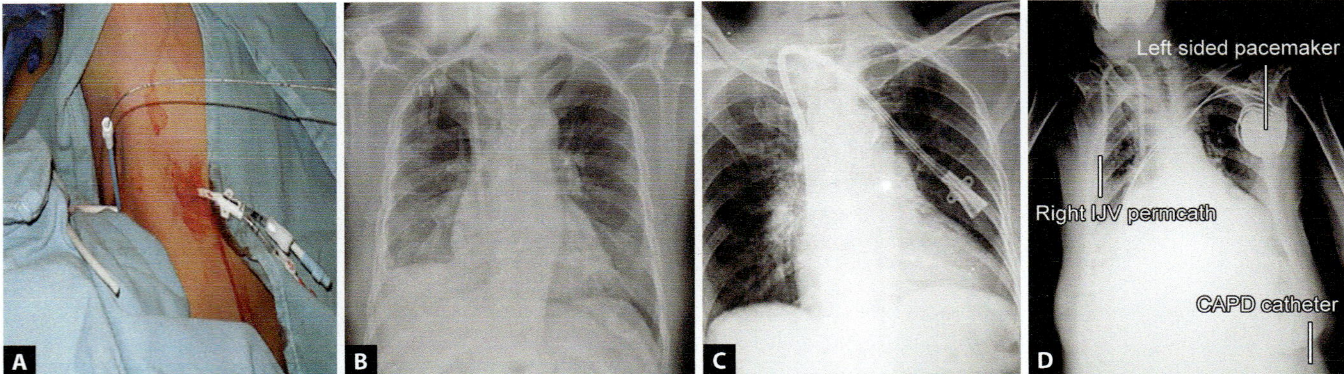

Figs. 8A to D: The catheter with an unusual exit site position and tunneled cuffed catheter (TCC) with pacemaker. (A) A subcutaneous tunnel in the back; (B) Chest X-ray: TCC exit site in the back; (C) TCC with exit site left chest; (D) TCC in right-sided pacemaker on left.

anterior chest. To potentially circumvent this, a technique was developed that tunnels the catheter posteriorly over the patient's shoulder[44] **(Figs. 8A to C)**. Although self-manipulation of hemodialysis catheters and the associated complications.

Tunneled Catheter in a Patient with a Permanent Pacemaker

Pacemaker wires have been implicated as a cause of central vein stenosis and as an occult cause of ipsilateral arteriovenous access failure in HD patients. During catheter insertion or catheter replacement, pacemaker wire dislocation is possible. Teruya et al.[45] reported subclavian stenosis (venous hypertension, arm swelling) after 1 year in 71% of patients with ipsilateral hemodialysis transvenous pacemakers and AV access; hence, the placement of AV access ipsilateral to a transvenous pacemaker is not suggested as shown in **Figure 8D**. A recent study by Asif et al.[46] has, thus, proposed using an epicardial approach to place pacemakers/automatic implantable cardioverter defibrillators (AICDs) to prevent the associated complication of CVS and infection with the transvenous approach.

Unconventional Sites for Temporary Cuffed Catheter

The unconventional sites for TCC placement are chosen as a last resort to maintain hemodialysis. According to Sakarachi et al.,[47] end-stage vascular access (ESVA) is anatomically classified into three classes: (1) No upper limb vascular access option, (2) no lower limb vascular access option, and (3) no vascular access options at any site, which means all sites are exhausted. In an Indian scenario, ESVA is considered when there is no option for any conventional access.

Unconventional access should be considered in patients with failed conventional access or as a transit to renal transplantation for preservation of femoral veins or for sustenance of hemodialysis among patients with ESVA. Placement of TCC in the IVC can be by translumbar approach or transhepatic approach.

Case Scenario

A 57-year-old male patient on maintenance hemodialysis for 8 years presented to the emergency department with complaints of anasarca, breathlessness at rest, palpitation with pulmonary edema needing oxygen, uremic fetor, and acidotic breathing. He underwent his last dialysis a week back due to failure of all dialysis access. He had failed AVFs over both upper limbs, bilateral thrombosed IJVs with venous congestion involving the face and both upper limbs, and engorged veins over the chest, suggestive of associated central venous stenosis.

This case is a classic example of a patient classified as ESVA. With the ongoing diabetic pandemic, improved finances of the population, good government support, and easy accessibility to hemodialysis, more and more aged population are opting for dialysis. Improved dialysis techniques have improved long-term survival on hemodialysis, which significantly increases the patient pool with access problems.

The only emergency option for dialysis access in such a patient would be the placement of TCC in IVC using the translumbar or transhepatic vein approach.

Translumbar IVC TCC (Video 1)

The translumbar approach to IVC was first described by Kenney et al. in 1985 as providing total parenteral nutrition. Many authors have described this approach as a safe, reliable, and suitable option for hemodialysis among patients with ESVA.[48-51]

The translumbar catheter set differs from the conventional one with a longer (20 cm) introducer needle, 80-cm guidewire, serial dilators, peel-away sheath, and a 55-cm cuffed double-lumen catheter.

Imaging: Imaging of IVC can be done using ultrasound, C-arm, or fluoroscopy. Imaging the spine helps prevent the introducer needle from crossing the midline, avoiding the risk of aortic puncture. Flushing the marginally patent femoral vein in few selected patients with contrast helps to highlight the IVC for better guidance.

Most of these patients come for an emergency procedure, in pulmonary edema with severe tachypnea. It may be challenging to image in such a situation and hence, the IVC puncture turns out to be a blind procedure even by the experienced and skilled person. The steps of placement and advantages are shown in **Table 3** and **Figures 9A to E.**

A retrospective study by Mori et al.[51] placed 40 catheters in 22 HD patients (26 TLCs and 14 THCs). It showed that translumbar catheters have better catheter survival compared to transhepatic [591 (283–2,372) vs. 261 (35–1,329) days]. The reasons for removing the catheter were dysfunction or thrombosis (60%), followed by infection (20%) and exposure to a cuff (15%). An Indian single-center, unpublished data by Shrinivas[52] with 30 translumbar IVC permcath procedures showed good long-term outcomes with average catheter survival of 22 months, 55% catheters lasting more than a year and the longest functioning catheter recorded at 55 months. 37% of these patients were recorded to have definitive successful outcomes. 26% underwent a successful AVF recreation and 11% underwent a successful renal transplant.

Transhepatic IVC TCC

This technique involves the placement of a tunneled dialysis catheter through the right or middle hepatic veins across the IVC into the right atrium. Ultrasound guides the introducer needle into the right or middle hepatic veins at the anterior or mid-axillary line level as shown in **Figures 10A to C**. The right hepatic vein is preferred over the middle hepatic vein due to its lateral position. The left hepatic vein should be avoided due to its vital structures and proximity to the hepatic hilum. Portal veins, which lie more medially, have echogenic margins on ultrasound, differentiating them from the hepatic veins. Hepatic vein cannulation requires an introducer needle and dilators to pass through the hepatic parenchyma, which carries the risk of bleeding. Bleeding diathesis and shrunken liver are relative contraindications for the procedure. After placing the guidewire and serial dilation, the permcath insertion technique is like conventional TCC. It is desirable to place the Catheter tip in the right atrium.

Without meaningful data, the available literature suggests transhepatic IVC as a viable proposition for patients with ESVA,[47] and with good long-term catheter

TABLE 3: Technique and advantages of translumbar tunneled catheter.

Technique of placement of translumbar catheter	***Advantages of translumbar tunneled catheter***
• Procedure is performed with patient in prone position or left lateral position (obese and tachypneic patients) • A point is marked 2 cm above the highest point of right iliac crest. Introducer needle is passed through the point at an angle 45° medially and 45° cranially, directing it anterior to the body of vertebra simultaneously avoiding crossing midline of spine using USG/fluoroscopy • A give-away feel with a free and continuous flow of blood indicates inferior vena cava (IVC) puncture • The needle position is confirmed by flushing dye to highlight the IVC • Guidewire is passed till the right atrium • Remaining steps of serial dilation and placing catheter using peelaway sheath is like the conventional tunneled cuffed catheter (TCC) placement • It is desirable to have the tip of the catheter in the left atrium	• Preserves femoral and iliac veins for future transplant • Does not interfere in squatting, sleeping, or head movements • Less risk for deep vein thrombosis (DVT), infections, catheter migration, breaking of catheter or fracture • No prophylaxis for thrombosis

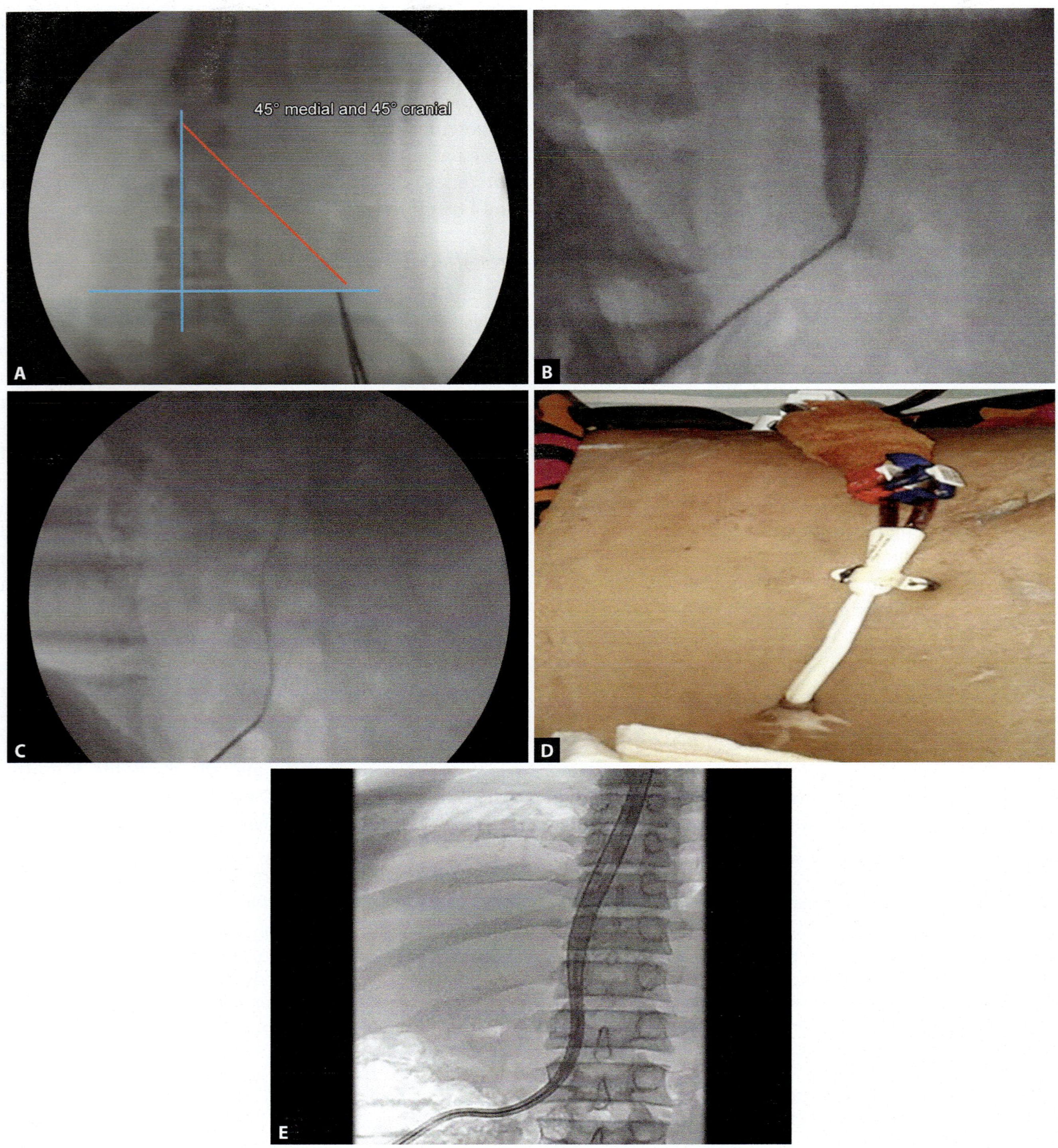

Figs. 9A to E: Steps of trans-lumbar tunneled cuffed catheter (TCC) placement. (A) Red line of the direction of needle for inferior vena cava (IVC); (B) Confirming needle position by dye study; (C) Guidewire into IVC via introducer needle; (D) Translumbar tunneled dialysis catheter (TDC) connected to dialysis; (E) Dialysis catheter in the IVC **(Video 1)**.

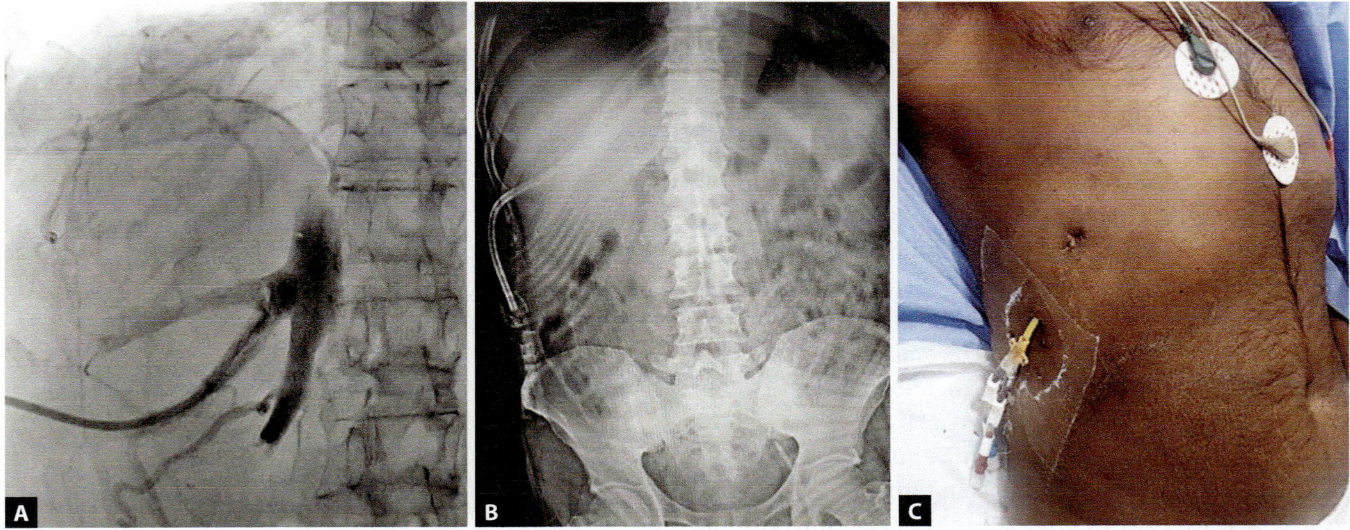

Figs. 10A to C: Transhepatic tunneled cuffed catheter (TCC) placement. (A) Inferior vena cava (IVC) highlighted transhepatic approach; (B) Transhepatic IVC permcath position; (C) Transhepatic IVC permcath.

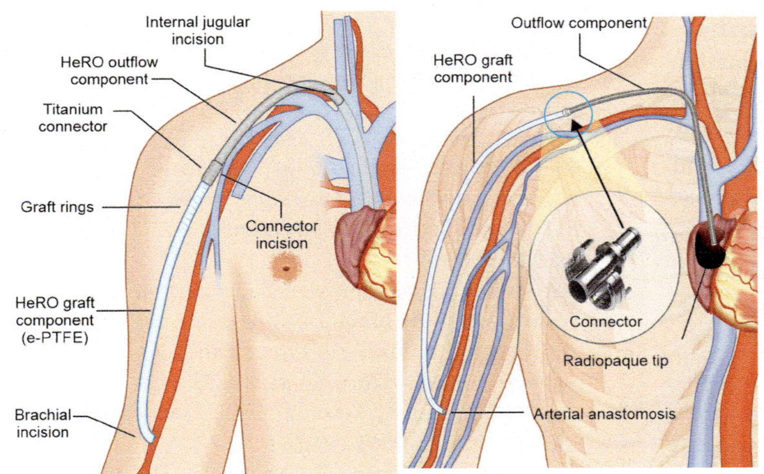

Steps of insertion of HeRO graft

- A small incision is made in the neck, and IJV is cannulated using an 18 G needle.
- If the veins are blocked or narrow, venoplasty may be performed to open the vessel.
- The graft component is attached to an artery in the arm, and the outflow component is connected to the top of the graft component.
- The graft is tunneled under the skin from the arm to the shoulder area.
- The end of the outflow component is placed into the neck, and the tip is in the right atrium. The outflow component is connected to the graft via a titanium connector. Blood flow is confirmed.
- The incisions are closed with stitches.

Fig. 11: The Hemodialysis Reliable Outflow (HeRO) graft components and steps of insertion. (e-PTEF: expanded polytetrafluoroethylene)

survival and minimal procedural complications.[53] In a retrospective review by Smith et al.,[54] 21 transhepatic hemodialysis catheters were placed in 16 patients, and 100% technical success was achieved. 21 catheters needed 30 exchanges, and device failure was the most common reason for catheter exchange. A study by El Gharib et al.[55] placed 25 transhepatic access in 23 patients' catheters, which achieved good long-term functionality within 90–300 days.

There are no absolute contraindications for both procedures as this procedure is an attempt to save the lives of the patients, who otherwise would lose their lives in the absence of access.

Hemodialysis Reliable Outflow Graft

The Hemodialysis Reliable Outflow (HeRO) device is a subcutaneous, implantable graft-catheter, surgical, and endovascularly placed access offering options for failing AVF/AVG or catheter-dependent patients. HeRo graft has the following components **(Fig. 11)**: Arterial graft component [53-cm long expanded polytetrafluoroethylene (ePTFE) HD graft], titanium connector attaches the arterial graft component to the venous outflow component, and 40-cm long venous outflow ("Nitinol") component.[55] Compared with tunneled HD catheters, HeRO grafts showed 69% lower infection rates, 16–32% improved dialysis clearance, and 50% reduced maintenance interventions.[55] HeRO graft candidates should have the following characteristics evaluated before placement:[55] (1) All AV access options in the upper extremity have been exhausted; (2) the patient has an appropriately high blood pressure; (3) the patient has suitable anatomy (a) adequate inflow artery and (b) patent or correctable central venous outflow; and (4) the life plan for a patient with ESKD includes long duration of HD, at least for more than a year. The graft component requires 2–4 weeks of tissue incorporation (similar to standard ePTFE AV grafts) and is accessed in the same manner as conventional grafts.[56]

In a study by Illig et al., 55 HeRO grafts were placed under general anesthesia with a mean operative time of 70 ± 26 (38–148) minutes. At a mean follow-up of 95 (maximum 383) days, three other graft infections have occurred in this group (7%), all involving the cannulatable portion of the graft and all requiring excision. Al Shakarchi et al. published a systematic review and meta-analysis examining 8 studies and 409 patients. The primary and secondary pooled patency rates in this complex dialysis patient cohort were 21.9% (9.6–37.2%) and 59.4% (39.4–78%). The dialysis access-associated steal syndrome rate was low at 6.3% (1–14.7%), as was the range of HeRO-related bacteremia (0.13–0.7 events per 1,000 days).[57]

CONCLUSION

The creation of an AVF and the placement of tunneled catheters are fundamental components of hemodialysis access. While AVFs are the preferred option due to their durability and lower complication rates, they can be challenging to create in patients with poor vascular anatomy, previous access failures, or comorbid conditions. In these cases, tunneled catheters can provide an alternative but have complications such as infection and thrombosis. Managing these difficult situations requires a multidisciplinary approach, careful presurgical planning, advanced imaging techniques, and skilled surgical intervention. By adopting a tailored approach, clinicians can improve outcomes for patients with challenging vascular access issues.

REFERENCES

1. Sharma S, Bera S, Goyal VD, Gupta V, Bisht N. Ulnar-basilic arteriovenous fistula for hemodialysis access: Utility as the "second procedure" after radio cephalic fistula. Ann Vasc Dis. 2021;14(2):132-8.
2. Liu W, Lagaac R, Pettigrew GJ, Callaghan CJ. Outcomes after ulnar-basilic arteriovenous fistula formation. Ann Vasc Surg. 2013;27(2):232-7.
3. Gołębiowski T, Jerzak P, Letachowicz K, Konieczny A, Kusztal M, Gołębiowski M, et al. Prone Position Facilitates Creation of Ulnar-Basilic Arteriovenous Fistula. J Clin Med. 2022;11(9):2610.
4. Silva MB, Hobson RW, Pappas PJ, Haser PB, Araki CT, Goldberg MC, et al. Vein transposition in the forearm for autogenous hemodialysis access. J Vasc Surg. 1997;26(6):981-6; discussion 987-8.
5. Hossny A. Brachiobasilic arteriovenous fistula: Different surgical techniques and their effects on fistula patency and dialysis-related complications. J Vasc Surg. 2003;37(4):821-6.
6. Gracz KC, Ing TS, Soung LS, Armbruster KF, Seim SK, Merkel FK. Proximal forearm fistula for maintenance hemodialysis. Kidney Int. 1977;11(1):71-5.
7. Konner K, Hulbert-Shearon TE, Roys EC, Port FK. Tailoring the initial vascular access for dialysis patients. Kidney Int. 2002;62(1):329-38.
8. Ozhan A, Memetoglu ME, Kehlibar T, Bastopcu M, Yilmaz M, Karakaya C, et al. Transposition of brachiobasilic arteriovenous fistulas: One-stage or two-stage technique and factors affecting the early maturation. Ther Apher Dial. 2021;25(5):636-41.
9. van Dellen D, Junejo M, Khambalia H, Campbell B. Transposition of brachiobasilic arteriovenous fistulae: improving the cosmetic effect without compromising patency. Ann R Coll Surg Engl. 2016;98(1):24-8.
10. Tan TW, Farber A. Brachialbasilic autogenous access. Semin Vasc Surg. 2011;24(2):63-71.
11. Torina PJ, Westheimer EF, Schanzer HR. Brachial vein transposition arteriovenous fistula: is it an acceptable option for chronic dialysis vascular access? J Vasc Access. 2008;9(1):39-44.
12. Parekh VB, Niyyar VD, Vachharajani TJ. Lower Extremity Permanent Dialysis Vascular Access. Clin J Am Soc Nephrol. 2016;11(9):1693-702.
13. Antoniou GA, Lazarides MK, Georgiadis GS, Sfyroeras GS, Nikolopoulos ES, Giannoukas AD. Lower-extremity arteriovenous access for haemodialysis: A systematic review. Eur J Vasc Endovasc Surg. 2009;38(3):365-72.
14. Cerri J, Ramacciotti E, Gomes M, Tedeschi Filho W, Piccinato CE. Latero-lateral femoro-femoral arteriovenous fistula: a new surgical approach for hemodialysis patients with no vascular access. Acta Cir Bras. 2011;26(1):72-6.

15. Mandwar M, Seth A, Sharma A, Kenwar DB, Patil SS, Singh S. Outcome of tibio-saphanous arteriovenous fistula in patients with failed upper extremity dialysis access: A report of two cases. J Vasc Access. 2022;23(3):481-4.
16. Akoh JA. Prosthetic arteriovenous grafts for hemodialysis. J Vasc Access. 2009;10(3):137-47.
17. Urbanes AQ. Interventional nephrology: When should you consider a graft? Clin J Am Soc Nephrol CJASN. 2013;8(7):1228-33.
18. Palumbo R, Niscola P, Calabria S, Fierimonte S, Bevilacqua M, Scaramucci L, et al. Long-term favorable results by arteriovenous graft with Omniflow II prosthesis for hemodialysis. Nephron Clin Pract. 2009;113(2):c76-80.
19. Polo JR, Ligero JM, Diaz-Cartelle J, Garcia-Pajares R, Cervera T, Reparaz L. Randomized comparison of 6-mm straight grafts versus 6- to 8-mm tapered grafts for brachial-axillary dialysis access. J Vasc Surg. 2004;40(2):319-24.
20. Khadra MH, Dwyer AJ, Thompson JF. Advantages of polytetrafluoroethylene arteriovenous loops in the thigh for hemodialysis access. Am J Surg. 1997;173(4):280-3.
21. Khafagy T, Regal S, ElKassaby M, Saad E. Early results of brachial arterio-arterial prosthetic loop (AAPL) for hemodialysis. Eur J Vasc Endovasc Surg. 2016;51(6):867–71.
22. Zanow J, Kruger U, Petzold M, Petzold K, Miller H, Scholz H. Arterioarterial prosthetic loop: a new approach for hemodialysis access. J Vasc Surg. 2005;41(6):1007-12.
23. Glass C, Maevsky V, Massey T, Illig K. Subclavian vein to right atrial appendage bypass without sternotomy to maintain arteriovenous access in patients with complete central vein occlusion, a new approach. Ann Vasc Surg. 2009;23(4):465-8.
24. Chauhan Y, Zubair MM, Inkollu S, Peden EK. Axillary artery to right atrial graft for dialysis access using an autologous femoropopliteal vein. Ann Vasc Surg. 2017;45:262.e7-262.e10.
25. El-Sabrout RA, Duncan JM. Right atrial bypass grafting for central venous obstruction associated with dialysis access: another treatment option. J Vasc Surg. 1999;29(3):472–8.
26. Nazarian GK, Bjarnason H, Dietz CA, Bernadas CA, Hunter DW. Changes in Tunneled catheter tip position when a patient is upright. J Vasc Interv Radiol. 1997;8(3):437-41.
27. Lok CE, Huber TS, Lee T, Shenoy S, Yevzlin AS, Abreo K, et al. KDOQI Clinical Practice Guideline for Vascular Access: 2019 Update. Am J Kidney Dis. 2020;75(4, Supplement 2):S1-64.
28. Tartière D, Seguin P, Juhel C, Laviolle B, Mallédant Y. Estimation of the diameter and cross-sectional area of the internal jugular veins in adult patients. Crit Care Lond Engl. 2009;13(6):R197.
29. Sharma M, Tong WL, Thompson D, Vachharajani TJ. Placing an appropriate tunneled dialysis catheter in an appropriate patient including the nonconventional sites. Cardiovasc Diagn Ther. 2023;13(1):281-90.
30. Engstrom BI, Horvath JJ, Stewart JK, Sydnor RH, Miller MJ, Smith TP, et al. Tunneled internal jugular hemodialysis catheters: Impact of laterality and tip position on catheter dysfunction and infection rates. J Vasc Interv Radiol. 2013;24(9):1295-302.
31. Shingarev R, Barker-Finkel J, Allon M. Natural history of tunneled dialysis catheters placed for hemodialysis initiation. J Vasc Interv Radiol. 2013;24(9):1289-94.
32. Wang P, Wang Y, Qiao Y, Zhou S, Liang X, Liu Z. A retrospective study of preferable alternative route to right internal jugular vein for placing tunneled dialysis catheters: Right external jugular vein versus left internal jugular vein. PLoS One. 2016;11(1):e0146411.
33. Vats HS, Bellingham J, Pinchot JW, Young HN, Chan MR, Yevzlin AS. A comparison between blood flow outcomes of tunneled external jugular and internal jugular hemodialysis catheters. J Vasc Access. 2012;13(1):51-4.
34. Behera V, Ahmad S, Sinha S, G GR, Srikanth K, Ghosh I, et al. Tunneled dialysis catheter insertion in external jugular vein by nephrologists. Indian J Nephrol. 2025;35(1):46-52.
35. Yoo J, Shim DJ, Kim D, Baek SH, Park CS, Lee JW. Placement of a subclavian tunneled hemodialysis catheter with the patient's arm raised may reduce the risk of complications: Two cases report. J Korean Soc Radiol. 2023;84(2):477.
36. Hernández D, Díaz F, Rufino M, Lorenzo V, Pérez T, Rodríguez A, et al. Subclavian vascular access stenosis in dialysis patients: natural history and risk factors. J Am Soc Nephrol. 1998;9(8):1507-10.
37. Schillinger F, Schillinger D, Montagnac R, Milcent T. Post catheterisation vein stenosis in haemodialysis: comparative angiographic study of 50 subclavian and 50 internal jugular accesses. Nephrol Dial Transplant. 1991;6(10):722-4.
38. Zafarghandi MR, Nazari I, Taghavi M, Salimi J, Moini M, Askarpour S. Comparison of results of placement of cuffed -tunneled hemodialysis catheter in internal jugular vein with subclavian vein for long -term dialysis. Pol Przegl Chir. 2013;85(3):133-6.
39. Sethi J, Gaur M, Rathi M, Kohli H. Tunneled femoral vein catheterization for long-term hemodialysis – Experience from a tertiary care center. Indian J Nephrol. 2022;32(4):371.
40. Burton KR, Guo LLQ, Tan KT, Simons ME, Sniderman KW, Kachura JR, et al. Patency of femoral tunneled hemodialysis catheters and factors predictive of patency failure. Cardiovasc Intervent Radiol. 2012;35(6):1396-402.
41. Herrington WG, Nye HJ, Haynes RJ, Winearls CG, Vaux EC. Does Prophylactic anticoagulation reduce the risk of femoral tunneled dialysis catheter-related complications? J Vasc Access. 2013;14(2):135-42.
42. Zaleski GX, Funaki B, Lorenz JM, Garofalo RS, Moscatel MA, Rosenblum JD, et al. Experience with tunneled femoral hemodialysis catheters. Am J Roentgenol. 1999;172(2):493-6.
43. El Mahdi AM, Elkerdawi SO, Aborahma AM, Gawish RIA, Korany AO. Tunneled Femoral vein catheter for long

term haemodialysis in exhausted accesses; does high tip placement differ than low tip placement? Ain Shams J Surg. 2022;32(4):371-4.
44. Stroz MJ, Nathoo B, Stroz PM. Posteriorly tunneled dialysis catheters for permanent use in cognitively impaired patients undergoing hemodialysis. J Vasc Interv Radiol. 2014;25(10):1621-5.
45. Teruya TH, Abou-Zamzam AM, Limm W, Wong L, Wong L. Symptomatic subclavian vein stenosis and occlusion in hemodialysis patients with transvenous pacemakers. Ann Vasc Surg. 2003;17(5):526-9.
46. Asif A, Carrillo R, Garisto JD, Lopera G, Ladino M, Barakat U, et al. Epicardial cardiac rhythm devices for dialysis patients: minimizing the risk of infection and preserving central veins. Semin Dial. 2012;25(1):88-94.
47. Al Shakarchi J, Nath J, McGrogan D, Khawaja A, Field M, Jones RG, et al. End-stage vascular access failure: can we define and can we classify? Clin Kidney J. 2015;8(5): 590-3.
48. Inston N, Khawaja A, Mistry H, Jones R, Valenti D. Options for end stage vascular access: Translumbar catheter, arterial-arterial access or right atrial graft? J Vasc Access. 2020;21(1):7-18.
49. Liu F, Bennett S, Arrigain S, Schold J, Heyka R, McLennan G, et al. Patency and complications of translumbar dialysis catheters. Semin Dial. 2015;28(4):E41-7.
50. Rajan DK, Croteau DL, Sturza SG, Harvill ML, Mehall CJ. Translumbar placement of inferior vena caval catheters: a solution for challenging hemodialysis access. Radiogr Rev Publ Radiol Soc N Am Inc. 1998;18(5):1155-67; discussion 1167-70.
51. Mori JR, Alguiar JR, Oviedo CP, Munares PM, Sánchez ML, Linares MC, et al. Translumbar and transhepatic haemodialysis catheters: A viable option. Nefrol Engl Ed. 2019;39(1):88-90.
52. Srinivasa S, Exotic Locations—Tunneled Cuffed Catheters (TCC). 1st AVATAR INDIA conference, Bangalore, July 2024.
53. Smith TP, Ryan JM, Reddan DN. Transhepatic catheter access for hemodialysis. Radiology. 2004;232(1):246-51.
54. El Gharib M, Niazi G, Hetta W, Makkeyah Y. Transhepatic venous catheters for hemodialysis. Egypt J Radiol Nucl Med. 2014;45(2):431-8.
55. Tabriz DM, Arslan B. HeRO Graft: Indications, Technique, Outcomes, and Secondary Intervention. Semin Interv Radiol. 2022;39(1):82-9.
56. Lawson JH, Niklason LE, Roy-Chaudhury P. Challenges and novel therapies for vascular access in haemodialysis. Nat Rev Nephrol. 2020;16(10):586-602.
57. Al Shakarchi J, Houston JG, Jones RG, Inston N. A Review on the hemodialysis reliable outflow (HeRO) graft for haemodialysis vascular access. Eur J Vasc Endovasc Surg. 2015;50(1):108-13.

CHAPTER

33

Cardiac Rhythm Devices and Vascular Access

Valentine Lobo

INTRODUCTION

Cardiovascular disease is the primary cause of mortality in patients with chronic kidney disease (CKD), irrespective of the stage of CKD. Data from the United States Renal Data System database suggests that more than one-third of cardiac deaths are attributable to arrhythmias. Causes of arrhythmias are multifactorial including myocardial ischemia, which is common in CKD, autonomic imbalance, chronic inflammation, left ventricular hypertrophy, and electrolyte imbalances, all of which occur with an increased frequency. The frequency of sick sinus syndrome with predisposition to supraventricular tachycardia or tachycardia–bradycardia is also higher and increases the need for permanent pacemaker (PM) implantation in patients on maintenance hemodialysis (MHD). Data from the CRAH-ILR (Cardio Renal Arrhythmia Study in Hemodialysis using Implantable Loop Recorders) study showed that bradycardia appeared to be a particular problem in dialysis patients with a five times higher risk than the non-CKD population. CKD patients on dialysis, thus, appear to be at a very significantly higher risk for developing tachyarrhythmias, bradyarrhythmias, cardiac failure, and sudden cardiac death and have an increased need for cardiac implantable electronic devices (CIEDs) such as permanent PMs, implantable cardioverter-defibrillators (ICDs), or cardiac resynchronization devices.[1] Studies suggest that the use of these devices reduced mortality by 42%.[2] Survival benefit related to ICD therapy in sudden cardiac death (SCD) survivors was observed in dialysis patients leading to secondary prevention; however, no role in primary prevention has been shown in randomized or nonrandomized studies.[3] Cardiac resynchronization therapy (CRT) improves outcomes in patients with systolic heart failure and CKD, with expected benefits outweighing the risks, despite a more complex implantation procedure at all levels of baseline renal insufficiency and should be offered to CKD patients, if indicated.

Most of these devices contain an electrical pulse generator placed in a subcutaneous pocket in a minor surgical procedure, with transvenous leads to the cardiac chambers, via puncture of the subclavian/axillary vein or cephalic vein.

The CKD population undergoing dialysis therefore has an increased need for implantable cardiac devices which compete for the patient's veins with dialysis catheters and AV fistulas. This incidence has been estimated to be around 10% of the dialysis population in the United States, ICD in 6.1%, and a PM in 4.4%.

CARDIAC DEVICES AND VASCULAR ACCESS—COMPETING FOR VASCULAR "REAL ESTATE"

As dialysis vascular access is also either AV (fistulas and grafts) or venovenous [central venous catheters (CVCs)], the interaction with electrical leads in competing space increases the risk of infectious and vaso-occlusive complications. Leads of PMs and ICDs can cause central venous stenosis or damage to the tricuspid valve with regurgitation or be a conduit for bacterial colonization and infective endocarditis.

In the non-CKD population, central venous obstruction may be either asymptomatic or symptomatic to life threatening in the case of superior vena cava (SVC) obstruction, but in patients on hemodialysis, an ipsilateral AV fistula is more likely to uncover an occult stenosis of a central vein. Studies suggest that both the incidence and severity of obstructive lesions in such patients may be higher as also the chances of a lesion being rendered symptomatic by the creation of an ipsilateral AV access.

The cumulative incidence of asymptomatic lead-related venous obstruction (LVRO) has been reported to be

5% at 5 years after implantation with a median recognition at 0.6 years, in the most recent large study of almost 650,000 patients.[4] The incidence was slightly higher at 6.5–6.8% in patients who underwent revision procedures. Studies in patients undergoing revision of leads or device upgrade showed a higher incidence of LRVO (25–35%), while very limited studies involving symptomatic patients found an incidence of 0.5–0.9%.[5] The true incidence of all patients with CIEDs may currently be underestimated. One study estimated the incidence of subclavian stenosis caused by PM leads in hemodialysis patients at 70%.[6] A situation may also arise with CIED presence on one side and the lack of suitable vessels for AV fistula on the contralateral arm.

Box 1 shows the risk factors for central venous stenosis following CIED from the largest study.

Frequent recurrent endothelial trauma caused by device leads, especially when endothelialized, excites a proliferative and inflammatory reaction, which results in stenosis and significant luminal narrowing. The incidence of central venous stenosis has been shown to be affected by both the frequency of cannulation and the duration of use, particularly relevant for CIED leads which are required lifelong. The prevalence was 3.4%, 29.4%, and 53.8% with a history of 0–1 versus 2–3 versus 4 or more central venous cannulations, respectively.[7]

Interventions may be required for a manifest central venous stenosis caused by a combination of device leads and ipsilateral vascular access and include:

- AV fistula ligation—avoided as far as possible
- Repeated angioplasty with or without stent placement

One retrospective study on 32 patients identified 20 patients with contralateral and 12 with ipsilateral AV access and PMs.[8] Among the group with contralateral access and device, 50% (10) underwent an intervention [50% (10) had PTA and 20% (2) had stents placed]. An average of 3.6 PTAs per patient (range 1–12) was performed, for central stenosis related to the ICD on the ipsilateral side. Among those with ipsilateral device and access, 75% (9) had PTA and 33% (3) had stents placed for an average of 2.8 PTAs per patient (range 1–6). The average time to the first PTA was 9.5 months (range 1–27 months). Although there was no difference in intervention rates between patients' ipsilateral and contralateral accesses and devices, the time to intervention was shorter in patients who had AV access on the ipsilateral side to their PM (9.5 months vs. 19.5 months; $p < 0.05$), with no difference in patency rates ($p = 0.68$).

BOX 1: Risk factors for central venous stenosis following CIED from the largest study.

- Anemia
- Non-White race
- Chronic kidney disease
- CIED with >1 lead
- Number of central venous cannulations
- Hypertension
- Ischemic heart disease
- Liver disease (cirrhosis and other)
- Peripheral vascular disease
- Pulmonary conditions
- Solid organ or hematological malignancies

(CIED: cardiac implantable electronic device)

Procedure-related complications including damage to CIED leads are rare. Prior CIED leads removal if stent placement is needed in order to avoid entrapment of CIED leads by the stent is recommended.

Dialysis patients are at a higher risk for CIED-related *infections*, including endocarditis. Bacteremias have been noted to be more common in the hemodialysis population with CIED-related infections compared with localized infections in nondialysis populations (300.3 vs. 6.1 per 100,000 persons).[2] Devices were preserved more often in the dialysis population and this may have contributed to a higher 90-day mortality (13.7 vs. 5.9%). Polyzos et al. in a systematic review listed the risk factors for device-related infections as shown in **Table 1** with the odds ratio (OR) for end-stage renal disease (ESRD) being highest.[8]

Simultaneous use of CIED and either temporary or tunneled cuffed central venous catheters posed the greatest risk of SVC stenosis, catheter-related blood stream infection (CRBSI), and infective endocarditis. A functioning AV fistula or AV graft may become unusable and/or unsalvageable with central venous stenosis caused by a CIED and the resulting venous hypertension and edema.

CARDIAC IMPLANTABLE ELECTRONIC DEVICE PROCEDURE IN A PATIENT WITH CHRONIC KIDNEY DISEASE

The above underscores the importance of considering the need for a future or existing hemodialysis vascular access when a CIED is implanted, especially since the nondominant side is preferred for both the CIED and the

TABLE 1: Risk factors for CIED-related infections.

Risk factors	*OR with 95% CI*
Patient related	
DM	2.08 (1.62–2.67)
ESRD	8.73 (3.42–22.31)
COPD	2.95 (1.78–4.90)
Steroid use	3.44 (1.62–7.32)
Prior device infection	7.84 (1.94–31.60)
CKD	3.02 (1.38–6.64)
Malignancy	2.23 (1.26–3.95)
Cardiac failure	1.65 (1.14–2.39)
Preprocedure fever	4.27 (1.13–16.12)
Postoperative hematoma	8.46 (4.01–17.86)
Reintervention for lead dislodgement	6.37 (2.93–13.82)
Device replacement/revision	1.98 (1.46–2.70)
Lack of antibiotic prophylaxis	0.32 (0.18–0.55)
Temporary pacing	2.31 (1.36–3.92)
Generator change	1.74 (1.22–2.49)
Inexperienced operator	2.85 (1.23–6.58)
Abdominal generator pocket	4.01 (2.48–6.49)
Presence of epicardial leads	8.09 (3.46–18.92)
Positioning of two or more leads	2.02 (1.11– 3.69)
Dual-chamber system	1.45 (1.02–2.05)

(CI: confidence interval; CIEDs: cardiac implantable electronic devices; CKD: chronic kidney disease; COPD: chronic obstructive pulmonary disease; DM: diabetes mellitus; ESRD: end-stage renal disease; OR: odds ratio)

AVF, and the one may not be foreseen at the time the other is implanted.

Preservation of all peripheral and central veins is paramount in patients of CKD on current or future RRT. CIED implantation must therefore include careful consideration of:

- The type and possible location of the device, vascular anatomy (previous catheters or infected devices, AVF presence)
- The patient's expectations (prognosis, quality of life)
- Consultation with a vascular access specialist in patients with CKD grade 4 or 5 to decide optimal site for future AV fistula/graft placement

Evaluation should include:

- Physical examination, obtaining the history of previous vessel cannulation and ultrasound mapping

TABLE 2: Alternatives to transvenous implantation of CIEDs in hemodialysis patients.

CIED option	*Comment*
Leadless pacemaker, subcutaneous ICD (S-ICD), endocardial LV pacing using ultrasound	Preferred although no data regarding long-term outcomes
Surgically implanted epicardial system	Needs thoracotomy concerns about higher risk of lead malfunction; minimally invasive technique available
Low lateral thoracic or axillary implantation	In patients with limited prepectoral options (previous pocket infection); involves axillary vein puncture
Femoral/iliac pacing	In bilateral subclavian vein occlusion/superior vena cava syndrome; poor hygiene (diapers) or local skin infection; risk of lead fracture in walking patients are issues—use of the iliac vein should limit the risk

(CIEDs: cardiac implantable electronic devices; ICD: implantable cardioverter-defibrillator)

- Venography, including central veins, in case of any doubts or a history of previous catheters

Because of the complications that arise in patients with limited vascular space and the need for one or more procedures, innovations and alternatives need to be considered when placing a CIED in a patient needing hemodialysis. **Table 2** summarizes the available options for patients requiring both a CIED and a hemodialysis vascular access.

Leadless devices or transcutaneous pacing may eliminate the need for venous access of CIED leads and the infective complications they are associated with. Leadless PMs may also be a useful option when subclavian or brachiocephalic vein stenosis has been caused by prior central vein use for dialysis catheters. Other options in patients requiring both dialysis and cardiac devices include consideration of peritoneal dialysis or epicardial leads, subcutaneous ICD, or leadless PMs.

The Micra IDE study, Micra CA study, and the Micra PAR study were three prospective nonrandomized trials that evaluated the safety and performance of the Micra Transcatheter Pacing System[7] in a total of 2,819 patients, 201 (7%) of whom were on dialysis at the time of Micra device implantation with an average follow-up of 6 months at analysis. The technical success of the procedure was 98%

(197 of 201) with a median procedure time of 27 minutes. 11 major complications occurred in 9 patients (4.5%), including four device pacing issue events, implantation attempt), two pericardial effusion/perforation events, both resulting in deaths and three other events, one of which was also fatal. Overall, the complication rate in dialysis patients was slightly elevated (4.9 vs. 3.2%) though not significant. No bacteremia or systemic infection was noted.

Single-chamber leadless permanent PMs have recently been compared with transvenous PMs in a cohort of 384 dialysis patients studied over 14 years and the all-cause mortality rate was significantly lower in leadless pacemaker compared to transvenous pacemaker [hazard ratio (HR) = 0.68, 95% confidence interval (95% CI 0.47–0.99)], with no significant difference in cardiac arrests or other complications over a 90-day period, but significantly fewer endocarditis or device-related infections with leadless PMs (0 case vs. 4 four cases in the transvenous group, HR 0.37, 95% CI 0.14–0.98).[8]

Hospital lengths of stay were also significantly lower. Currently, the use of leadless PMs has increased from 1% to just below 10% over the last 7–8 years.[9]

Peritoneal dialysis should be seriously considered as an option, if the patient's condition allows; however, it may be limited by treatment failure. If the indication for CIED is nonurgent and implantation can wait 4 weeks, a more appropriate order of action would be PD catheter implantation, followed by a peritoneal equilibration test (PET) after 4 weeks to assess suitability followed by CIED implantation, in an uncomplicated/efficient PD course.

If a leadless device is not possible, a careful site selection for both CIED and vascular access is mandatory. Early planning and creation of an AVF on the contralateral side to the CIED prior to initiating RRT (e.g., a right-sided device in a patient with a need for a left radiocephalic AVF) and avoiding the use of a central venous catheter would be the ideal strategy in CKD patients with preimplanted pacemakers or ICDs. Because implanting or removing a central venous catheter can result in lead dislodgement, an assessment of a patient's intrinsic rhythm prior to undertaking such a procedure is mandatory as cardiac standstill may occur during the procedure. An additional precaution is the use of a temporary backup PM through a different access. An ideal site for a new CVC is the side opposite the CIED, ensuring that the subcutaneous tunnel of the catheter and the pocket of the CIED are at a safe distance. Catheter replacement or exchange should be performed in the cardiac catheter suite using appropriate imaging for tip positioning without interfering with the CIED leads.

Epicardial leads require a surgery that is more invasive and may be associated with increased morbidity but have the advantage of preserving the dialysis vascular access. Newer minimally invasive epicardial approaches, with robotic assistance, allow the leads to traverse the subcutaneous tissue without a vascular puncture, eliminating vascular injury or pneumothorax and almost completely eliminating lead dislodgement. Results from non-CKD studies suggest that results are further enhanced by the use of steroid eluting epicardial leads with a comparable survival to transvenous leads even in pediatric patients.

Subcutaneous ICDs (S-ICDs) in MHD patients offer the advantage of minimally invasive surgery and lower risk of stenosis or infection of the ventral veins compared with endocardial devices although they are limited by lack of possibility of permanent pacing.

The indications for S-ICDs are summarized in **Box 2**.

In a study comparing 18 S-ICD implantations in HD patients with 68 matched controls, there was no statistically significant difference in procedural complications between the two groups. The hospital stay was longer in HD patients (3.6 ± 5.14 vs. 1.69 ± 2.29 days, $p = 0.021$) but there was no device or blood stream infection in the HD group, compared with five device infections in the non-HD group over a follow up of >7 months. The incidence of inappropriate shocks was similar in both groups while all appropriate shocks were successful in terminating ventricular tachyarrhythmias in both groups though patients on hemodialysis had worse long-term mortality, compared with non-HD patients.[10]

A similar study on SICD implantation due to cardiomyopathy between 27 non-HD and HD patients showed no complications requiring surgical reintervention in

BOX 2: Indications for SICD in dialysis patients.

- Central venous occlusion from prior catheterization
- Ipsilateral dialysis access—AVF or TCC
- Prior bacteremia with transvenous ICDs
- Younger age
- Hypertrophic cardiomyopathy
- Congenital cardiomyopathies, or inherited channelopathies

(AVF: arteriovenous fistula; ICDs: implantable cardioverter-defibrillators; SICD: subcutaneous implantable cardioverter-defibrillator; TCC: tunneled cuffed catheter)

HD patients versus six patients in the nondialysis cohort, eventhough dialysis patients were older and more likely to be diabetic.

Wearable cardiac defibrillator is a short-term option in patients requiring temporary RRT or initiating MHD in the setting of an acute cardiac illness like an acute coronary syndrome where cardiac function may be expected to improve over a period of time where a CIED implantation is impossible due to uncontrolled infection.

VASCULAR ACCESS IN A PATIENT WITH A CARDIAC IMPLANTABLE ELECTRONIC DEVICE

Central vein stenosis can occur in almost 70% of dialyzed patients with an ipsilateral AVF and CIED, approximately 1 year after AVF construction, although long-term patency of ipsilateral and contralateral AVF and CIED are similar. Ipsilateral CIED and central venous hemodialysis catheter, either temporary or cuffed tunneled, carries the highest risk of symptomatic central venous stenosis and endovascular infection with potentially lethal complications.

Interventions reported in studies on patients with CIEDs, undergoing vascular access creation, have included CIED extraction (74.0%) and percutaneous revascularization (26.0%). Balloon venoplasty, thrombolysis, stenting, and thrombectomy are the more frequently performed interventions with drug-coated devices and surgical bypass infrequently used in 2.2% and 1% of cases, respectively. Patients with SVC obstruction were more likely to undergo extraction compared with other LRVO patients (18% vs. 11%, respectively). Extraction and venoplasty in this study appeared to be mutually exclusive with very few patients crossing over and most significantly 90% of patients whose devices were extracted did not require reinsertion.

A summary of recommendations regarding CIED and vascular access in patients on maintenance HD is given in the following text.

CASE SCENARIO

A 74-year-old diabetic CKD patient-initiated dialysis through a previously constructed left radiocephalic AV fistula in May 2021. After 6 months, his fistula began yielding poor flows (<200 mL/min) on dialysis with frequent alarms. Clinical examination and duplex ultrasonography revealed a long stenotic segment of the radial artery with poor inflow. The patient opted to have a right internal jugular tunneled cuffed catheter (TCC) inserted for his dialysis rather than intervention on the fistula.

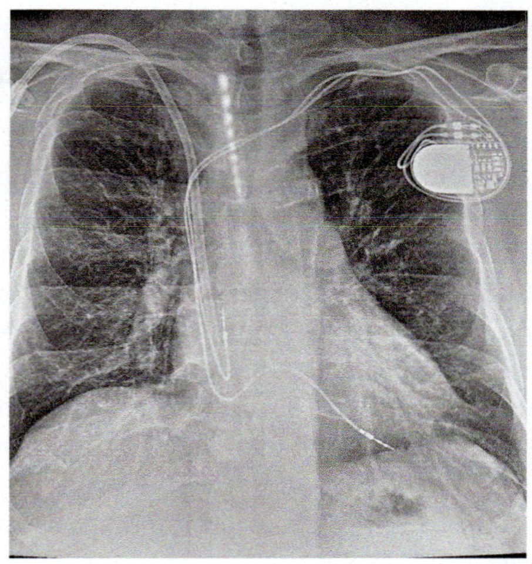

Fig. 1: Dual-chamber pacemaker inserted through left subclavian vein with right internal jugular cuffed dialysis catheter.

In July 2022, he presented with hypotension and bradycardia and his ECG revealed a complete heart block. Despite intense dialysis to correct electrolyte abnormalities, the AV dissociation persisted and he had two falls at home.

Cardiologist advised a permanent pacemaker insertion, which was placed as shown in **Figure 1**.

CONCLUSION

In the absence of randomized controlled trials, and the unlikely chance of these being performed, a pragmatic approach based on clinical experience and observations may be followed:

- Thus, AV fistula/AV graft should be created on the upper limb contralateral to the CIED, and novel devices (like leadless pacemakers, if possible) should be considered in dialysis patients.
- Avoid ipsilateral CIED and VA whenever possible.
- Avoid CVC in HD patients with a transvenous CIED or minimize duration of use if unavoidable.
- The CVC should be placed contralaterally to the transvenous CIED, with careful tunneling to avoid damage to the CIED pocket.
- ECG monitoring during CVC insertion next to the CIED lead is of paramount importance.
- CIED function must be assessed before and during the procedure with immediate access to emergency

temporary on-site pacing is necessary if maneuvers during CVC placement cause lead dislodgement.

- Percutaneous angioplasty (PTA) and proper tip location/reposition may be needed for safe catheter reimplantation or exchange while CIED leads are still in situ.
- If CIED therapy indications no longer exist in patients with limited vascular access, lead extraction can be combined with another implantation technique to reestablish and maintain central vein patency.

Miniaturization and less vascular invasive alternatives such as SICD, epicardial leads, and leadless pacemakers may be the future in patients with rapid progression of CKD, who form a special and important subset of all patients requiring CIEDs.

REFERENCES

1. Kusztal M, Nowak K. Cardiac implantable electronic device and vascular access: Strategies to overcome problems. J Vasc Access. 2018;19(6):521-7.
2. Opelami O, Sakhuja A, Liu X, Tang WH, Schold JD, Navaneethan SD. Outcomes of infected cardiovascular implantable devices in dialysis patients. Am J Nephrol. 2014;40(3):280-7.
3. Nowak K, Kusztal M. Cardiac implantable electronic devices in hemodialysis and chronic kidney disease patients: An experience-based narrative review. J Clin Med. 2021;10(8):1745.
4. El-Chami MF, Clementy N, Garweg C, Omar R, Duray GZ, Gornick CC, et al. Leadless pacemaker implantation in hemodialysis patients: Experience with the Micra transcatheter pacemaker. Clin Electrophysiol. 2019;5(2):162-70.
5. Ferro E, Kramer D, Li S, Locke AH, Misra S, Schmaier AA, et al. Incidence, treatment, and outcomes of symptomatic device lead-related venous obstruction. JACC. 2023;81(24) 2328-40.
6. Echefu G, Stowe I, Lukan A, Sharma G, Basu-Ray I, Guidry L, et al. Central vein stenosis in hemodialysis vascular access: Clinical manifestations and contemporary management strategies. Front Nephrol. 2023;3:1280666.
7. Dua A, Rothenberg KA, Mikkineni K, Sgroi MD, Sorial E, Toca MG. Secondary interventions in patients with implantable cardiac devices and ipsilateral arteriovenous access. J Vasc Surg. 2019;70(4):1242-6.
8. Polyzos KA, Konstantelias AA, Falagas ME. Risk factors for cardiac implantable electronic device infection: a systematic review and meta-analysis. Europace. 2015;17(5):767-77.
9. Panico A, Flahault A, Guillemin F, Varlet E, Couchoud C, Bauwens M, et al. Improved outcomes with leadless vs. single-chamber transvenous pacemaker in haemodialysis patients. Europace. 2024;26(11):euae257.
10. Koman E, Gupta A, Subzposh F, Saltzman H, Kutalek SP. Outcomes of subcutaneous implantable cardioverter-defibrillator implantation in patients on hemodialysis. J Interv Card Electrophysiol. 2016;45(2):219-23.

SECTION

8 Nonvascular Access Interventional Procedures

CHAPTER 34

Kidney Biopsy

Vineet Behera, Tauhidul Alam Choudhury

INTRODUCTION

Kidney biopsy is a common procedure in nephrology practice. A kidney biopsy is typically performed to diagnose or assess various kidney conditions when non-invasive tests (such as blood tests, urine tests, or imaging) are insufficient or inconclusive. Percutaneous kidney biopsy is performed under ultrasound guidance using spring-loaded automatic biopsy needles as the standard of care, mainly in nephrology and interventional radiology departments.

HISTORY

The first probable surgical kidney biopsy was probably performed as part of a renal decapsulation procedure for Bright's disease. The percutaneous kidney biopsy had been started for renal disease from the 1940s and was reported by Danish Iversen and Brun for the first time in the world in 1951. Kark and Muehrcke established the technique of percutaneous kidney biopsy in prone position using Vim Silverman needle. Thereafter, several modifications were done in the technique of kidney biopsy. Since the 1970s, ultrasound imaging has been used to localize kidneys before a kidney biopsy.

INDICATIONS[1]

Some common indications for a kidney biopsy include:

- Unexplained kidney dysfunction
- Glomerulonephritis
- Unexplained proteinuria or hematuria
- Determine etiology of chronic kidney disease
- Nephrotic syndrome
- Determine renal involvement in systemic diseases
- Unexplained renal dysfunction or proteinuria in kidney transplant

CONTRAINDICATIONS[1]

Kidney biopsy is a relatively safe procedure, but there are certain contraindications or situations where it may not be recommended. These include:

- Severe uncontrolled hypertension
- Coagulopathy or bleeding disorders
- Advanced renal dysfunction
- Small shrunken kidneys
- Active kidney or systemic infection or local skin infection
- Obvious cause of renal dysfunction such as obstruction and cystic kidney disease
- Uncooperative patients or lack of consent

Techniques

There are several types of kidney biopsy techniques used, depending on the clinical situation, patient characteristics, and the location of the kidney lesion.[1] The type of kidney biopsy chosen depends on the patient's condition (e.g., comorbidities, kidney function, and ability to tolerate procedures), the location and nature of the kidney issue, the need for a large or small tissue sample, and the skill and experience of the medical team.

The primary types of kidney biopsy[2] are as follows:

- *Percutaneous kidney biopsy:*[2] This is the most commonly used method and involves inserting a biopsy needle through the skin using anatomical landmarks or by using ultrasound/CT scan guidance. It is less invasive, with quick recovery, and minimal risk.
- *Open kidney biopsy/laparoscopic:* Open technique/laparoscopic is adopted in situations when percutaneous biopsy is not possible (e.g., due to abnormal kidney anatomy, obesity, or if percutaneous biopsy has been unsuccessful, or in situations when kidney is already exposed in an open surgery).

- *Transjugular kidney biopsy:* In this technique, a catheter is inserted into a vein in the neck (the jugular vein) and threaded to the kidney to obtain a tissue sample. This is typically done when percutaneous biopsy is not feasible (e.g., in patients with bleeding disorders).
- *Biopsy of graft kidney:* A percutaneous biopsy may be performed in a kidney transplant patient to check for signs of rejection, infection, or graft dysfunction.

PREPROCEDURE ASSESSMENT

Preprocedure assessment is essential for successful outcomes after kidney biopsy. These include clinical evaluation for blood pressure and pulse while ruling out local infections or wounds on the skin at the site of the biopsy and ascites. The patient's breath-holding ability is checked while lying in a prone position as the patient must hold breath for 20–30 seconds during the actual biopsy procedure. Though this crucial step can be a difficult task for the obese and elderly, it is usually possible in most patients with some practice.

Investigations

Investigations such as hemoglobin, platelets, and coagulation parameters should be done on the day of biopsy.[2,3] A bedside ultrasound should be done to assess kidney size, renal parenchymal echogenicity, corticomedullary differentiation, presence of cysts, and status of the pelvicalyceal system, besides ruling out ascites. Color Doppler flow imaging (CDFI) is essential to see the large-caliber intraparenchymal vessels at the lower pole **(Video 1)**.

Biopsy Needle and Tray

The biopsy tray includes sterile drapes, sterile gauze pads, surgical scalpel blade no. 11, disinfectant fluid (povidone-iodine solution), ultrasound probe sterile set (probe cover, sterile gel, rubber bands), 10-mL sterile plastic syringe, and a biopsy needle,[4] **(Fig. 1)**. An ultrasound machine with a curvilinear probe with B-mode facility, having a good resolution and color Doppler facility, should be used along with a convex array probe.

The commonly employed biopsy needle is an automatic spring-loaded disposable biopsy system (size of 16G × 10/16 cm or 18G × 16/20 cm depending on the size and age of the patient; with a tip excursion of 1.7–1.8 cm) **(Figs. 2A to C)**. A 16G needle appears to be associated with the better risk/benefit ratio in terms of glomeruli harvested and severe bleeding. A coaxial needle may also be used for doing an ultrasound-guided kidney biopsy.[3,4] The advantage of using a coaxial needle is that multiple cores of renal cortex can be taken quickly, and on completion of the procedure, glue can be injected into the biopsy tract.

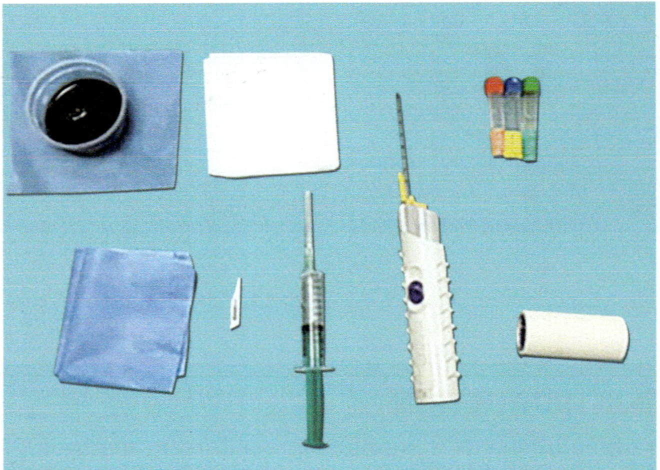

Fig. 1: The procedure tray for biopsy with cleaning gauze, povidone-iodine solution, local anesthetic solution loaded into a 10-mL syringe, spring-loaded automatic kidney biopsy needle, blade, drapes, and sample bottles.

Location and Side of Kidney

Percutaneous kidney biopsy (PKB) is usually performed on the lower pole of the left or right kidney to reduce the risk of inadvertent injury to a major vessel. The left kidney is preferred as it is visible without other organs impeding acquisition of the tissue, especially liver. However, there is a risk of splenic injury in the case of splenomegaly. The right kidney is anatomically located partially under the liver, and this position may obstruct a path to the kidney. Areas in kidney with more significant flow should be avoided to minimize the risk of bleeding. It is preferable to perform a biopsy at the level of Brodel's line, a relatively poorly vascular plane between the anterior and posterior branches of the renal artery.

PROCEDURE

Informed Consent

The patient is explained about the caudal movement of the kidney with deep inspiration and the entire procedure of the ultrasound-guided kidney biopsy along with the importance of breath holding when asked to do so.[5]

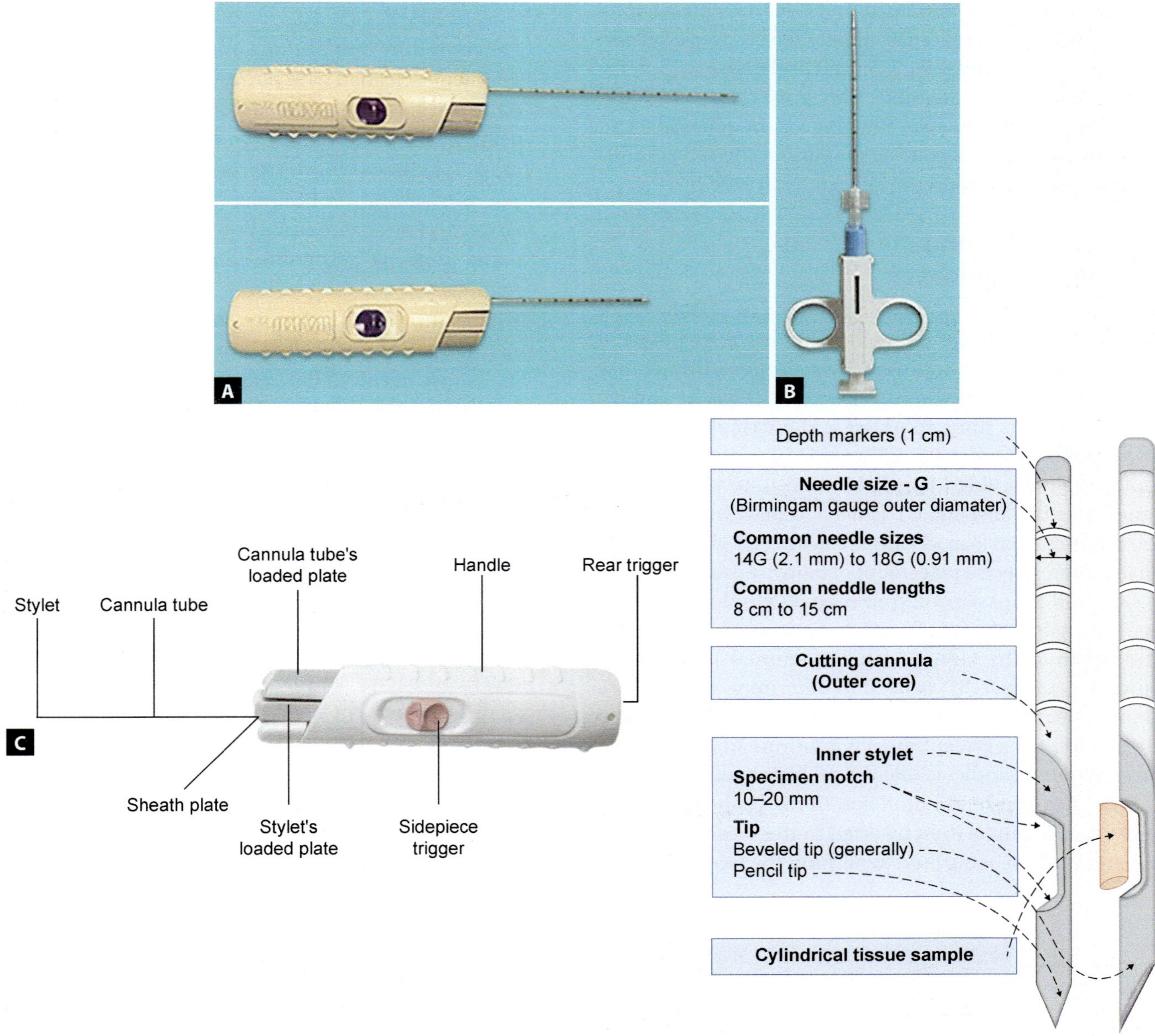

Figs. 2A to C: (A) Biopsy needle (automatic spring-loaded disposable biopsy system) of two sizes 16G × 16 cm (top) and 16G × 10 cm (below); (B) Coaxial needle biopsy gun; (C) Parts of the spring-loaded biopsy gun and parts of the biopsy needle.

Appropriate informed consent for kidney biopsy must be obtaining, after explaining the risks and possible complications.

Patient Position

The patient is placed in a prone position. Once the patient is in the prone position, they may need support, such as a pillow or sandbag placed under the abdomen, to help elevate the kidney closer to the surface of the back and reduce the physiological dorsal lordosis.[6] However, if a patient is obese, immobile, has abdominal distension, ascites, or is intubated, a lateral decubitus or sitting position may be more appropriate.

In obese patients and those who cannot lie prone, biopsy may be done in supine anterior lateral position, in which a towel is placed under the ipsilateral shoulder and gluteus to elevate the flank at an angle of 30°. The ipsilateral arm is positioned over the thorax, while the contralateral arm is abducted and used for intravenous access. The ipsilateral leg is slightly flexed over a pillow, while the contralateral leg is flexed and abducted, laying its lateral aspect on the table. This position provides full exposure of Petit's triangle, allowing for adequate space to perform ultrasound scanning and orient the ultrasound-guided puncture toward the inferior renal pole.

Ultrasound or Computed Tomography Guidance

Firstly, a preliminary ultrasound is done to visually mark the depth of the lower pole of the kidney to be biopsied in deep inspiration, followed by a proposed trajectory planning of the needle through the guide **(Figs. 3A and B)**. Then, a CDFI is done to reassess the vascularity of the lower pole of the kidney. CT-guided biopsy is similar to an ultrasound-guided biopsy but real-time visualization is not possible, Instead, CT is used to mark and measure the distance from skin to kidney capsule. CT guidance can enable more precise placement of biopsy needles.

A blind biopsy technique may be employed, which involves using ultrasound guidance to mark the surface and depth of the kidney. A probe, similar to a lumbar puncture (LP) needle, is used to determine the kidney's depth. The probe is gradually inserted towards the kidney while monitoring respiratory variations of the needle; these variations indicate that the probe is approaching the kidney. The depth and direction of the probe are noted, and a biopsy gun is then inserted to the same depth and direction before being fired to perform the biopsy.

Steps of Biopsy[6-8]

1. The procedure is to be done under sterile conditions. The skin is cleaned with povidone-iodine solution or other sterilizing solution, followed by the application of sterile drapes. A sterile window is kept within the drape for kidney biopsy access.
2. The ultrasound probe must be covered by sterile cover, and a repeat ultrasound examination is done using a sterile gel, confirming the preprocedure findings.
3. Under ultrasound guidance, an anesthetic solution (2% lignocaine) is instilled into the proposed track of the biopsy needle. If the track is long, a LP needle can be used to inject anesthesia into the deep tissues.
4. A small stab incision may be made with an 11G surgical blade to allow easy access to the spring-loaded automatic biopsy needle.
5. The biopsy needle is inserted under ultrasound guidance in the longitudinal plane of the ultrasound probe, with a cranial inclination of about 30° or 45°.
6. The biopsy needle goes through the subcutaneous tissue, the muscular planes, and the fascia till it reaches the renal capsule.
7. At this juncture, the needle tip position relative to the lower pole can be judged by changing the ultrasound probe to a horizontal plane, thereby confirming its placement at approximately 90° **(Figs. 4A and B)**.
8. A review of the proposed needle tip position should be done with the patient holding breath for a few

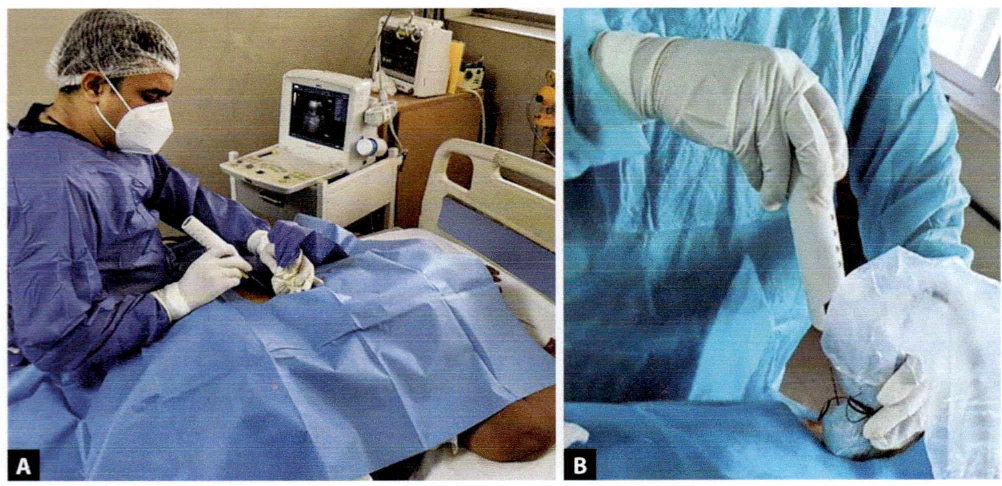

Figs. 3A and B: (A) The patient lying in a prone position, draped, and a window created for kidney biopsy under ultrasound guidance; (B) Ultrasound-guided kidney biopsy is being done by the operator.

seconds. This maneuver must be practiced prior, with the patient to allay anxiety.

9. Once the patient is holding the breath in deep inspiration, the needle tip position is confirmed at the renal capsule, and the trigger of the automatic biopsy needle is pressed.
10. The needle tip moves into the renal cortex—first, the sharp beveled tissue collector needle descends, followed by the outer needle sleeve to cover the specimen.
11. The biopsy needle is then gently withdrawn. The sample can be isolated from the tissue collector needle by retracting the outer needle sleeve and gently rolling the inner needle over the back of the operator's gloved hand.
12. The biopsy core is then transferred to a container with a solution using the plastic spatula available with the needle.
13. Two such passes are enough to collect adequate biopsy specimens. A small cortical piece (2–3 mm) can be cut out of the sample for electron microscopy.
14. The adequacy of the biopsy specimen can be checked on the bedside using a simple 10× convex hand lens.
15. The kidney biopsy specimen should be placed in a 10% neutral buffered formalin specimen vial for light microscopy, Michel's transport media, or 0.9% normal saline for immunofluorescence, and phosphate buffered 4% formaldehyde or 1% glutaraldehyde fixative for electron microscopy.
16. Post procedure, the biopsy site is compressed for a few minutes while the patient is still lying prone.
17. Thereafter, occlusive sterile dressings are applied at the site of biopsy and the patient is turned into a supine position and made to lie in bed for the next 4–6 hours.

Direction of Needle: Caudal and Cranial Techniques[8,9]

The cortex of the inferior pole of the kidney is typically targeted for native kidney biopsy. In cranial (CN) technique, the biopsy needle tip is pointed to the head at an angle of 45–60° with the participant's back. The needle is directed toward the cortex of the inferior pole of the kidney **(Fig. 5A)**. In the caudal technique, the biopsy needle tip is aimed at the legs at a 45–60° angle relative to the participant's back **(Fig. 5B)**.

Medulla Avoiding and Medulla Targeting Biopsy[9]

The kidney image is divided lengthwise into thirds, and if the site of insertion is in the middle third of the length of the kidney, then it is designated an "interpolar" biopsy. Otherwise, the biopsy is designated a "polar" biopsy. Finally, a continuation of the line of the biopsy needle is drawn. If this line crosses the medulla, the biopsy is designated as "medulla-targeting," otherwise the biopsy is designated "medulla-avoiding."

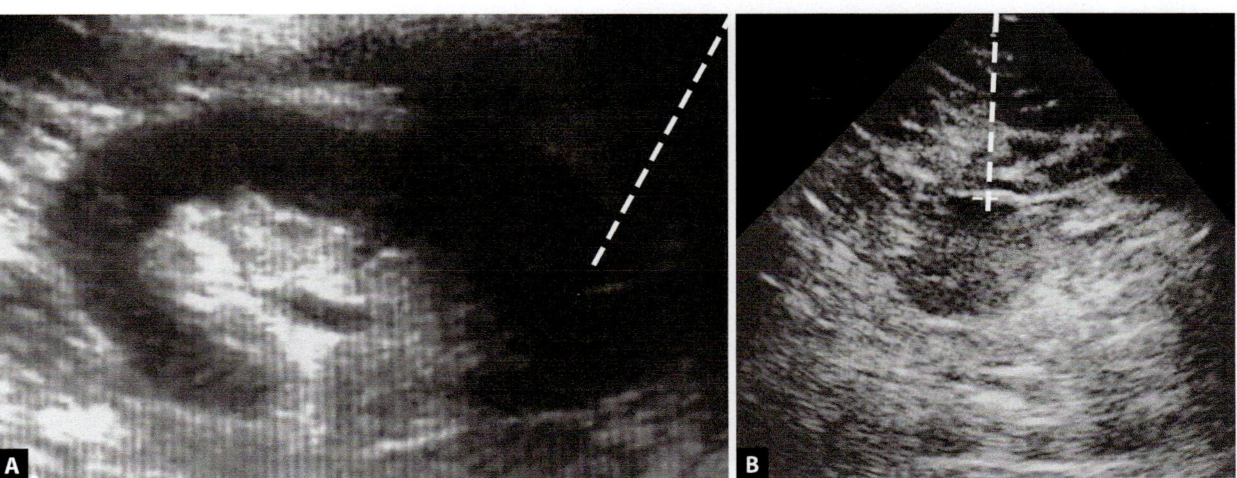

Figs. 4A and B: Ultrasound-guided biopsy of the kidney with (A) longitudinal view of kidney showing direction of needle at an angle of 45° and (B) horizontal view of kidney showing direction of needle at an angle of 90°entering the cortex.

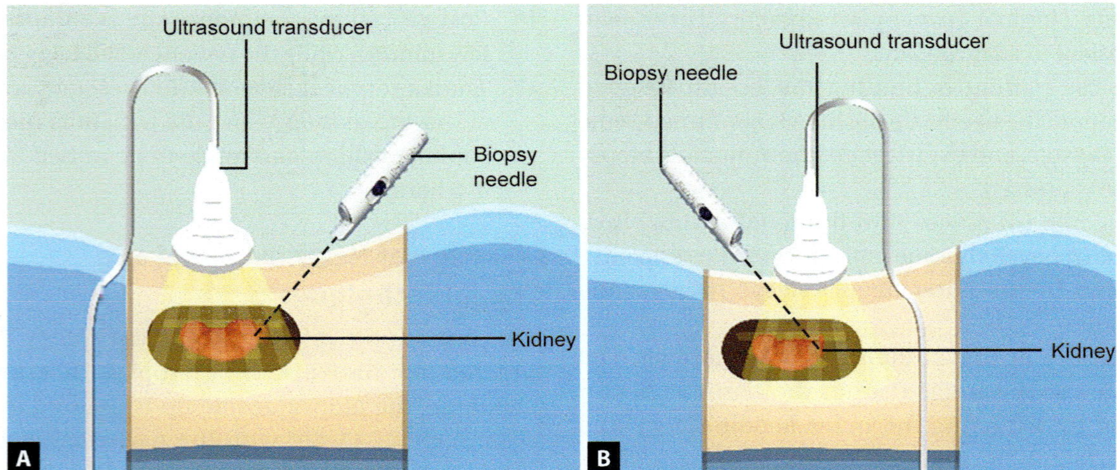

Figs. 5A and B: (A) Cranial and (B) caudal approaches of needle for kidney biopsy.

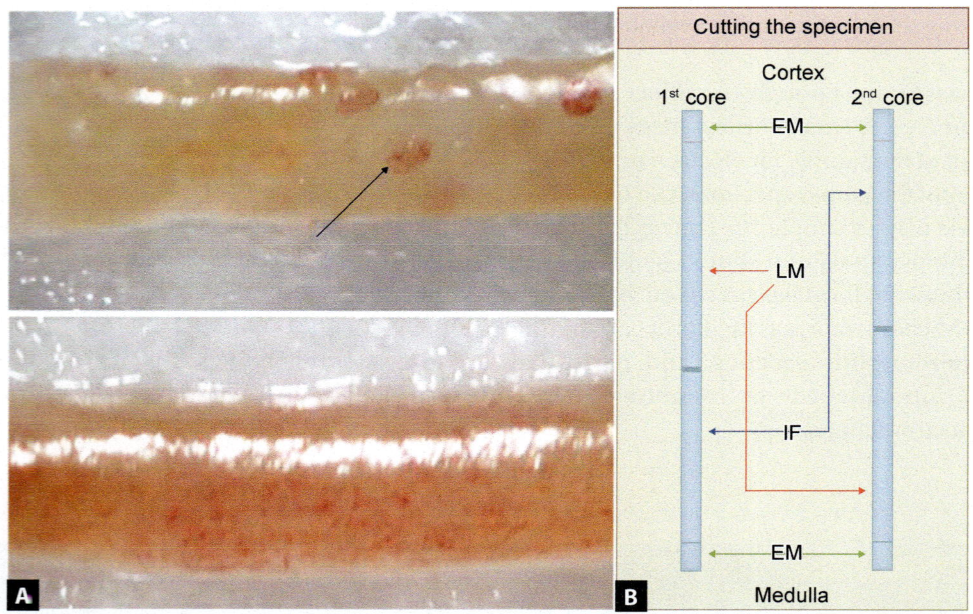

Figs. 6A and B: Magnified view of the kidney biopsy core showing the glomerulus as red dots (A) and the method of cutting for biopsy core for light microscopy (LM), immunofluorescence (IF), and electron microscopy (EM) (B).

Assessment of Biopsy Sample[10]

Biopsies are usually assessed under dissection microscope or smartphone camera in a drop of normal saline. Glomeruli appear as small red spheres in the cortex **(Figs. 6A and B)**. The tissue is placed on a glass slide with normal saline and examined with or without a cover slip on a wet mount. A trained observer can recognize fat, skeletal muscle, and other nonkidney tissue. If the specimen floats in the fixative, it is probably adipose tissue and not renal parenchyma. In this case, an additional core or divisions are required. Tissue obtained during each pass is processed according to a standard protocol to ensure adequate glomerular sampling for light microscopy (LM), immunofluorescence (IF), or electron microscopy (EM), especially when direct visualization of glomeruli is not possible.

POSTPROCEDURE MONITORING

Assessment

The patient is asked to rest for 6–12 hours after the procedure in which he is asked to avoid any undue exertion and is observed for any complications. The patient is monitored for any hematuria, pain, vital parameters, and any perinephric hematoma.[5,7] The patient's hemodynamic parameters are checked every half hour for the first hour and every 2 hours for the next 4 hours post procedure. An ultrasound and color Doppler evaluation of the kidney may be done to look for common adverse events such as hematoma, arteriovenous fistulas (AVFs), or pseudoaneurysms. The patient may be discharged after 12–24 hours depending on his condition and hospital policy.

Complications[8,10]

Kidney biopsy is generally considered a safe procedure, but, like any medical procedure, it carries some risks and potential complications **(Figs. 7A and B and Table 1)**. Most of these complications are rare and can often be managed effectively if they occur. Some common complications associated with kidney biopsy[4,8] include the following:

- *Bleeding:* It is the most common complication after kidney biopsy which may vary from minor bleeds to significant bleeding requiring further intervention or a transfusion.
- *Hematuria:* Mild or transient hematuria may occur after kidney biopsy, but most episodes are self-resolving. Severe or persistent hematuria may need further evaluation such as CT angiography or cystoscopy.
- *Pain or discomfort:* Pain at the biopsy site or in the back can occur, which is usually mild and temporary. In case of moderate-to-severe discomfort, pain relief may be used.
- *Subcapsular bleed or perinephric hematoma:* Small perinephric hematoma may occur after procedure, but most recover spontaneously without any need of intervention.
- *Retroperitoneal hematoma:* It may occur as a complication of persistent bleeding or disruption of clot over biopsy site.
- *Page kidney:* Continuous bleeding into the subcapsular space can potentially lead to compression of the kidney, a condition known as "page kidney" **(Fig. 8A)**. A large subcapsular hematoma related to page kidney can result in chronic hypertension due to persistent activation of the renin–angiotensin system.

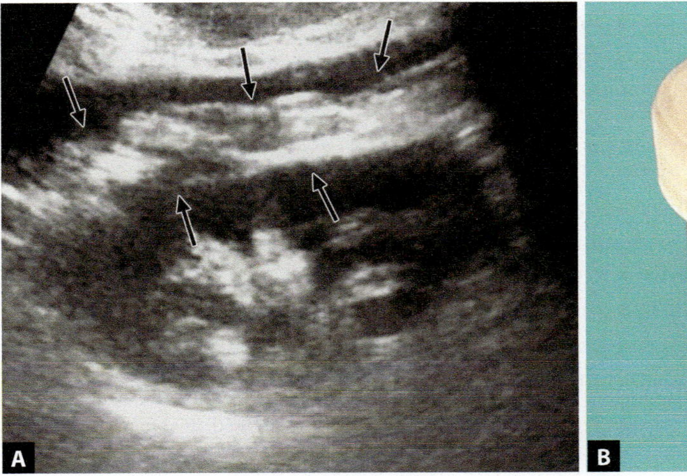

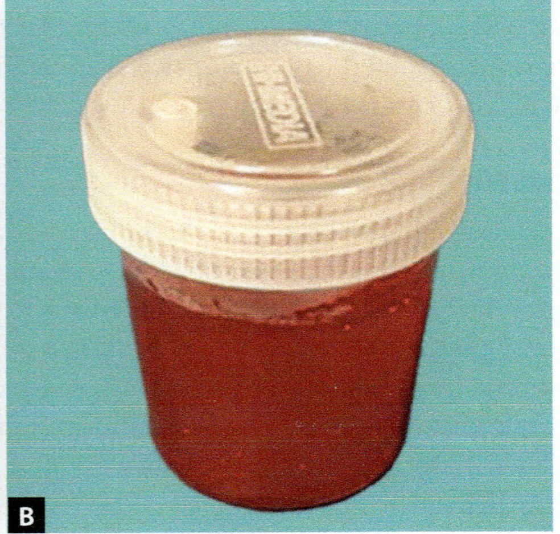

Figs. 7A and B: Common complications after kidney biopsy. (A) A subscapular hematoma on ultrasound 48 hours after the biopsy; (B) Hematuria after biopsy.

TABLE 1: Complications of kidney biopsy and their frequency.

General complications	*Bleeding-related complications*	*Serious complications*
• Pain (30–50%) • Inability to pass urine (5%) • Infection (<5%)	• Retroperitoneal bleed (5–10%) • Gross hematuria (0.4–3.5%) • Subcapsular bleed (<1%) • Perinephric hematoma (1.3–18%) • Lumbar vessel laceration (<1%)	• Arteriovenous fistula formation (<5%) • Nephrectomy 0–0.05%) • Death (0–0.06%)

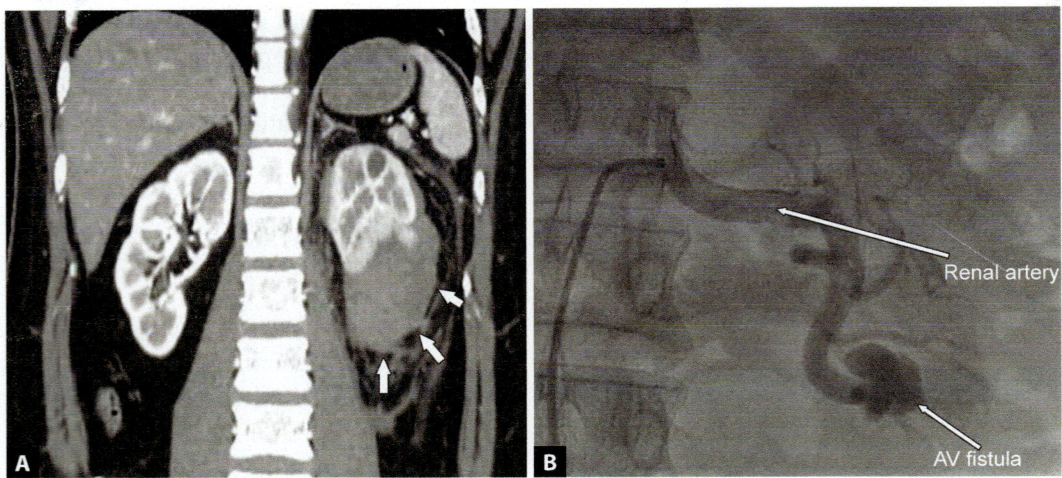

Figs. 8A and B: (A) Page kidney of left kidney after biopsy; (B) Postkidney biopsy intrarenal arteriovenous (AV) fistula undergoing coiling.

- Intrarenal pseudoaneurysm or AVF may occur after a kidney biopsy which may present as hematuria or hematoma. It may be diagnosed using a Doppler or CT angiography and may need coiling of pseudoaneurysm or AVF **(Fig. 8B)**.
- *Nephrectomy:* Nephrectomy resulting from a kidney biopsy procedure is uncommon ranging between 0.01 and 0.2%, occurring in <0.5% of cases. The mortality risk associated with a biopsy is estimated to be <0.1% in most clinical settings.

CONCLUSION

Ultrasound-guided kidney biopsy is the gold-standard technique for doing percutaneous kidney biopsy. It allows color Doppler imaging to assess preprocedure renal vascularity and postprocedure complications. Adequate experience should be gained during nephrology residency to perform a safe kidney biopsy with ultrasound guidance.

REFERENCES

1. Schnuelle P. Renal biopsy for diagnosis in kidney disease: Indication, technique, and safety. J Clin Med. 2023;12(19):6424.
2. Korbet SM. Percutaneous renal biopsy. Semin Nephrol. 2002;22(3):254-67.
3. Prasad N, Kumar S, Manjunath R, Bhadauria D, Kaul A, Sharma RK, et al. Real-time ultrasound-guided percutaneous renal biopsy with needle guide by nephrologists decreases post-biopsy complications. Clin Kidney J. 2015;8(2):151-6.
4. Schnuelle P. Renal Biopsy for Diagnosis in Kidney Disease: Indication, Technique, and Safety. J Clin Med. 2023;12(19):6424.
5. MacGinley R, Champion De Crespigny PJ, Gutman T, Lopez-Vargas P, Manera K, Menahem S, et al. KHA-CARI Guideline recommendations for renal biopsy. Nephrology (Carlton). 2019;24(12):1205-13.
6. Capretz T, Patel RM, Okhunov Z. Percutaneous renal biopsy: approach, diagnostic accuracy and risks. Curr Opin Urol. 2018;28(4):369-374.
7. Granata A, Distefano G, Pesce F, Battaglia Y, Bulzis PS, Venturini M, et al. Performing an ultrasound-guided percutaneous needle kidney biopsy: An up-to-date procedural review. Diagnostics (Basel). 2021;11(12): 2186.
8. Whittier WL. Complications of the percutaneous kidney biopsy. Adv Chronic Kidney Dis. 2012;19(3):179-87.
9. Luciano RL Moeckel GW. Update on the Native Kidney Biopsy: Core Curriculum 2019. Am J Kidney Dis. 2019;73:404-15.
10. Hogan JJ, Mocanu M, Berns JS. The native kidney biopsy: update and evidence for best practice. Clin J Am Soc Nephrol. 2016;11(2):354-62.

CHAPTER 35

Management of Complications Post-renal Biopsy

Ajit K Yadav, Anurag Gupta, Darshan Thummar, Vineeth Kurki M

CASE SCENARIO 1

A 35-year-old female patient with idiopathic nephrotic syndrome underwent percutaneous USG-guided renal parenchymal biopsy for precise diagnosis. The patient complained of mild persistent right loin pain with hematuria which failed to show clearing on successive collection of urine samples, USG screening showed sac-like structure within the renal parenchyma which on color Doppler showed aliasing suggestive of pseudoaneurysm. Due to persistent symptoms, the patient was considered for endovascular embolization **(Figs. 1A to C)**.

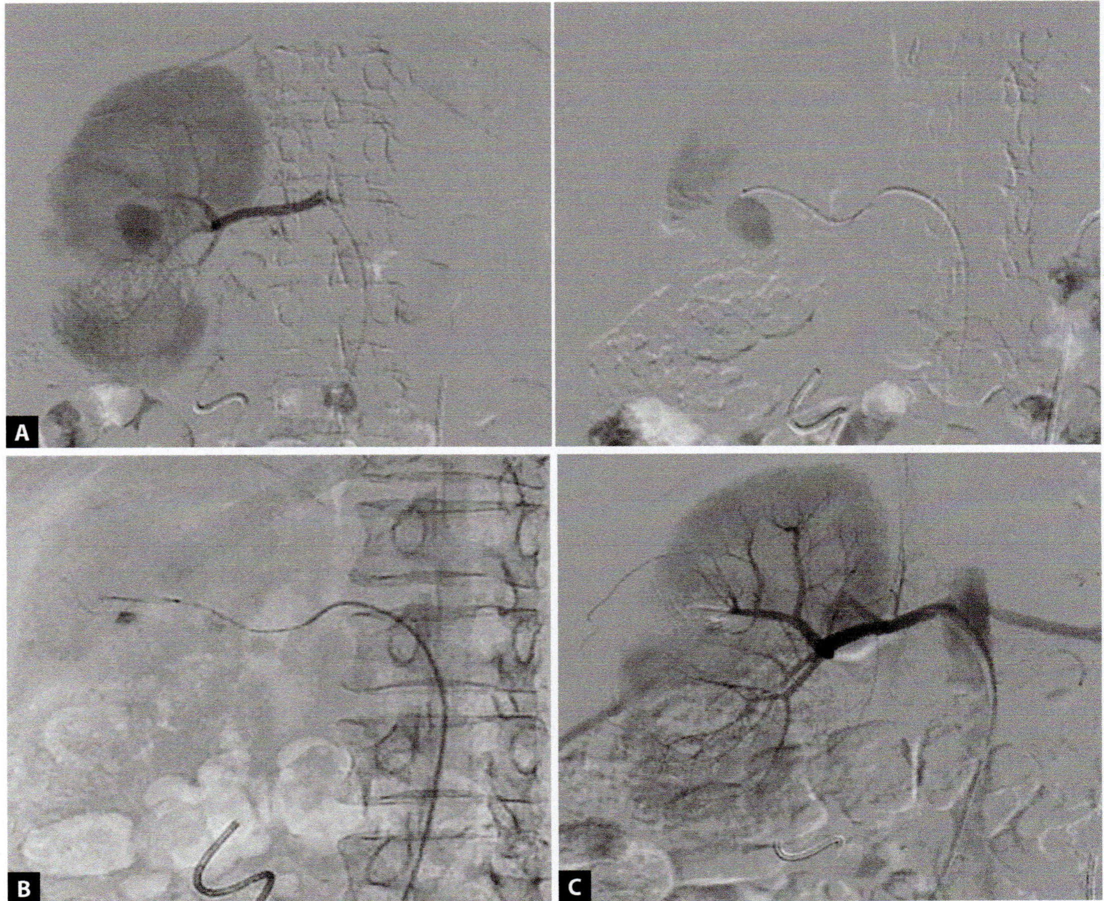

Figs. 1A to C: (A) Right image is right renal artery angiogram showing large pseudoaneurysm in mid pole and left image is selective angiogram of culprit artery of pseudoaneurysm; (B) Glue (n-Butyl cyanoacrylate) embolization of culprit artery; (C) Postembolization right renal angiogram showing complete obliteration of pseudoaneurysm and very minimal infarct (no blush area distal to embolization).

INTRODUCTION

Percutaneous renal biopsy (PRB) has been a cornerstone in diagnosing kidney disease since its inception in 1951.[1] While the procedure has undergone significant improvements, including the use of ultrasound guidance and automated biopsy systems, leading to increased safety and tissue adequacy,[2,3] it remains a high-risk procedure due to the kidney's vascularity and deep retroperitoneal location.[4]

The primary indication for native PRB is to evaluate proteinuria, microscopic hematuria, renal manifestations of systemic diseases, and unexplained renal failure. Despite its diagnostic and prognostic value, the procedure carries a risk of complications, including bleeding, which is further heightened in patients with renal disease due to uremia-associated platelet dysfunction, hypertension, and inflammatory states.[4]

COMPLICATIONS

Types of Complications

Bleeding is the most prevalent complication of PRB, with microscopic hematuria being common and not considered a complication. Other complications, though less frequent, include pain, infection, inadvertent injury to adjacent organs, perinephric hematoma, and arteriovenous fistula (AVF).[3]

A large retrospective review encompassing 2,563 percutaneous renal biopsies revealed a major bleeding rate of 2.2%, with 1.8% of patients requiring transfusions. Angiographic intervention was necessary in 0.4% of cases, and a mortality rate of 0.04% was observed.[5]

Classification of Complications

Complications following PRB can be broadly classified into minor and major categories:

- *Minor complications:* These are typically self-limiting and include hematuria, small perirenal hematomas, AVFs, and pain, all of which generally resolve spontaneously.
- *Major complications:* These require more aggressive management and include the following:
  - *Massive bleeding with hemodynamic instability:* It is characterized by significant blood loss and compromised cardiovascular function, demanding immediate intervention to stabilize the patient.
  - *Voluminous perirenal hematomas with refractory disabling pain:* Large hematomas can cause significant pain and potentially compromise renal function, necessitating pain management and potential surgical intervention.
  - *Significant hematuria with urinary tract obstruction by clots:* This can lead to urinary retention and renal dysfunction, requiring prompt intervention with clot removal and potentially stenting to maintain urinary flow.

Timing of Complications

Delayed bleeding complications are common after PRB. Studies have shown that a significant proportion of complications manifest beyond the immediate postbiopsy period. One series involving 750 adult patients demonstrated that only 67% of complications were evident at 8 hours, with 91% presenting within 24 hours. The remaining 9% of major complications were identified between 48 and 120 hours postprocedure. Another recent series demonstrated comparable results in native and transplant PRB, with 91% of major complications occurring within 12 hours and 98.4% within 24 hours. Based on these findings, many institutions routinely monitor patients for 24 hours after native renal biopsy.[6,7]

Postbiopsy renal ultrasound has been investigated as a tool for risk stratification. A study evaluating 162 patients after native PRB revealed that the presence of a hematoma 1 hour after biopsy had a 23% positive predictive value (PPV) and a 98% negative predictive value (NPV) for any major complication. Additionally, a hematoma >3 cm in size demonstrated a 44% PPV and a 97% NPV for major complications.[8]

RISK FACTORS

Hypertension

Elevated blood pressure (BP) is a significant risk factor for postbiopsy bleeding. A retrospective study demonstrated a 10-fold increase in major bleeding complications for patients with systolic BP (SBP) >140 mm Hg and diastolic BP (DBP) >90 mm Hg compared to normotensive individuals. This risk further escalated to 23 times higher for those with SBP >170 mm Hg and seven times higher for those with SBP between 141 and 170 mm Hg. DBP >90 mm Hg also exhibited a seven-fold increase in complication risk.[9] While the effect of immediate prebiopsy BP reduction on postbiopsy hemorrhage remains unstudied, some authors suggest that limited arteriolar contractility due to arteriolar hyalinosis may contribute to increased bleeding risk. Many large biopsy reviews exclude hypertensive patients or lack standardized periprocedural BP management.[4,10]

Kidney Function

Compromised kidney function is associated with an elevated risk of major complications. A meta-analysis demonstrated a higher risk for postbiopsy transfusion in patients with serum creatinine >2 mg/dL (2.1 vs. 0.4%, $p = 0.02$).[11] A large Chinese biopsy series examined 3,577 native PRBs and found that for every 1 mL/min/1.73 m^2 increase in glomerular filtration rate (GFR), there was a 4% decrease in severe bleeding risk.[12]

Thrombocytopenia and Platelet Dysfunction

The Society of Interventional Radiology (SIR) recommends holding aspirin and clopidogrel for 5 days prior to procedures with significant bleeding risk.[13] However, patients with chronic renal disease often face significant cardiovascular morbidity, and those at risk for coronary artery disease have demonstrated a 3-fold increase in major adverse cardiac events after aspirin cessation and an 89-fold increase in patients with intracoronary stents. Moreover, these patients may have stents or grafts requiring continuous antiplatelet therapy to prevent thrombosis.

Studies support periprocedural continuation of aspirin in patients with high cardiovascular risk. Thrombocytopenia has been established as an independent risk factor for postbiopsy hemorrhagic complications. The SIR recommendations for periprocedural coagulation status management include platelet transfusion for patients with counts <50,000/μL. Two studies have demonstrated an increased risk for major complications after PRB. Xu et al. observed a six-fold increased rate of major complications, and Torres Muñoz et al. demonstrated a seven-fold increased risk of major complications in patients with baseline platelet counts ≤120,000/μL.[12-15]

Platelet function is equally critical as platelet count. Uremia can cause platelet dysfunction with elevated blood urea nitrogen (BUN) levels >60 mg/dL, increasing the risk of major complications postbiopsy by up to nine times.[15] Desmopressin (DDAVP) has been shown to improve hemostasis in uremic patients.[16]

Coagulopathy

Coagulopathy is widely recognized as a risk factor for major complications. The current SIR guidelines recommend correction of intrinsic and extrinsic pathway derangements prior to PRB.[13] International normalized ratio (INR) should be <1.5, and heparin should be held or reversed for activated partial thromboplastin time (aPTT) values >1.5 times control. Novel anticoagulants should be held according to guidelines.[13]

Biopsy Needle

Biopsy needle choice has been shown to influence the major complication rate. The most commonly used automated needle sizes during PRB are 14-, 16-, and 18-gauge. Larger-gauge needles have been associated with increased major complication rates. Whittier et al. demonstrated equivalent diagnostic accuracy of 14- and 16-gauge needles, suggesting that a larger needle is not necessary.[17] Hergesell et al. showed that even with an 18-gauge needle, 99% of samples were adequate for pathological diagnosis. Employing smaller needles may decrease the risk of major complications postbiopsy. Coaxial technique was found to have significantly shorter procedural time, fewer complications (all minor), and an increased number of obtained glomerular profiles.[17-19]

MANAGEMENT: A STEP-BY-STEP APPROACH

Early Detection and Risk Assessment

Close monitoring in the immediate postprocedure period is essential to identify potential complications early. Hematoma volume assessment within the first hour postprocedure is crucial. Hematomas exceeding 40 mL are associated with a higher risk of significant complications.

Management of Minor Complications

Clear communication with patients is essential, emphasizing the expected benign course of minor complications and reassuring them about the self-limiting nature of these events. Pain relief, anti-inflammatory medications, and appropriate treatment for hematuria can be provided to alleviate symptoms and promote healing. A follow-up ultrasound at 7 days postprocedure is recommended to assess resolution of minor complications and ensure that no new abnormalities have developed.

Management of Major Complications

Immediate intensive care unit admission is necessary to stabilize the patient through fluid resuscitation, blood transfusions, and other supportive measures (**Table 1**). Angiographic imaging, either digital angiography or computed tomography angiography

TABLE 1: Complications and ideal treatment strategy.

Complications	*Management*
Major complications	
Disabling intense pain	Optimization of analgesia (use of opioids)
Hemodyamic instability with blood transfusion/gross hematuria	Endovascular treatment (Embolization)
Clot obstructing urinary tract	Irrigation with three-way probe
Minor complications	
Mild-to-moderate hematuria	Hydration
Arteriovenous fistula	Observation and conservative

(angiotomography), is crucial to precisely identify the source of bleeding and guide subsequent interventions. Conventional angiography and embolization is a minimally invasive procedure, performed by an interventional radiologist, which forms the mainstay of treatment for active bleeding. The procedure involves accessing the renal artery through either femoral or radial artery, followed by detailed anatomical angiographic study of the renal arteries and their variations, which are essential for accurate localization of the bleeding site. The renal angiogram shows main renal artery, segmental arteries and their branches followed by parenchymal blush. If complete renal parenchymal blush is not appreciated, accessory renal arteries should be searched. Renal angiogram is followed by superselective cannulation, which involves carefully guiding a microcatheter and microguidewire to the bleeding site through feeding/culprit artery, enabling precise visualization of the affected vessel. Once the bleeding vessel is identified, embolic agents are deployed to occlude the vessel and stop the hemorrhage.

Embolic agents commonly used include cyanoacrylates, polyvinyl alcohol (PVA) particles, thrombogenic coils, and gelatin sponge strips, either alone or in combination. Cyanoacrylates are usually mixed with iodized oil while PVA particles are mixed with nonionic contrast for radio-opacity. With microcatheter in the feeding or culprit artery, these embolic agents are instilled under continuous image guidance which then occlude the arteries completely. Reflux of these liquid embolic agents into other normal arteries should be avoided by controlled injection which comes with experience. Various types of coils are available; however, more commonly pushable coils are used to block the feeding/culprit arteries. Coils are placed in the microcatheter followed by injection of saline, which pushes the coil through the tip of the microcatheter placed in the required artery to occlude it. Gelatin is a temporary hemostatic agent which is biodegraded and liquefied within the body in 2–5 days. The use of gelatin has decreased due to availability of more robust agents; however, it is preferred when selective cannulation of required artery is not possible.

Embolization can lead to transient renal function impairment; however, operator experience, recent developments, and techniques, which help in more superselective cannulation of culprit arteries, minimize this risk by targeting only the bleeding vessel.[20,21] In patients with persistent gross hematuria with no angiographic abnormality, careful search should be conducted for other causes, and if unidentified, prophylactic embolization of segmental artery supplying the area of biopsy with gelatin should be considered.

Management of Pseudoaneurysms and Arteriovenous Fistulas

Most pseudoaneurysms <2.0 cm and small AVFs resolve spontaneously within 4 weeks through thrombosis. In the absence of hemodynamic instability, conservative management with close monitoring is the preferred approach. Persistent bleeding beyond 72 hours or significant postprocedure deterioration in renal function warrants interventional treatment. This involves endovascular embolization of the pseudoaneurysm or AVF, similar to the approach used for active bleeding.[20,21] In case of high-flow fistula with no intervening thin branches, venous access is necessary to avoid migration of embolic agents. Balloon catheters can be used to block the venous outflow in required cases, thus decreasing the flow in the AVF, avoiding nontarget or pulmonary embolism. A stepwise approach to management has been shown in **Flowchart 1**.

CASE SCENARIO 2

A 28-year-old female patient presented with nephrotic range proteinuria and underwent renal parenchymal biopsy from the lower pole of left kidney under USG guidance. She had persistent hematuria for which USG screening was done after 4 hours which showed features suspicious for AVF at lower pole with high PSV of 200 cm/s. She was considered for endovascular treatment **(Figs. 2A to C)**.

Flowchart 1: Clinical algorithm to manage complications following kidney biopsy.

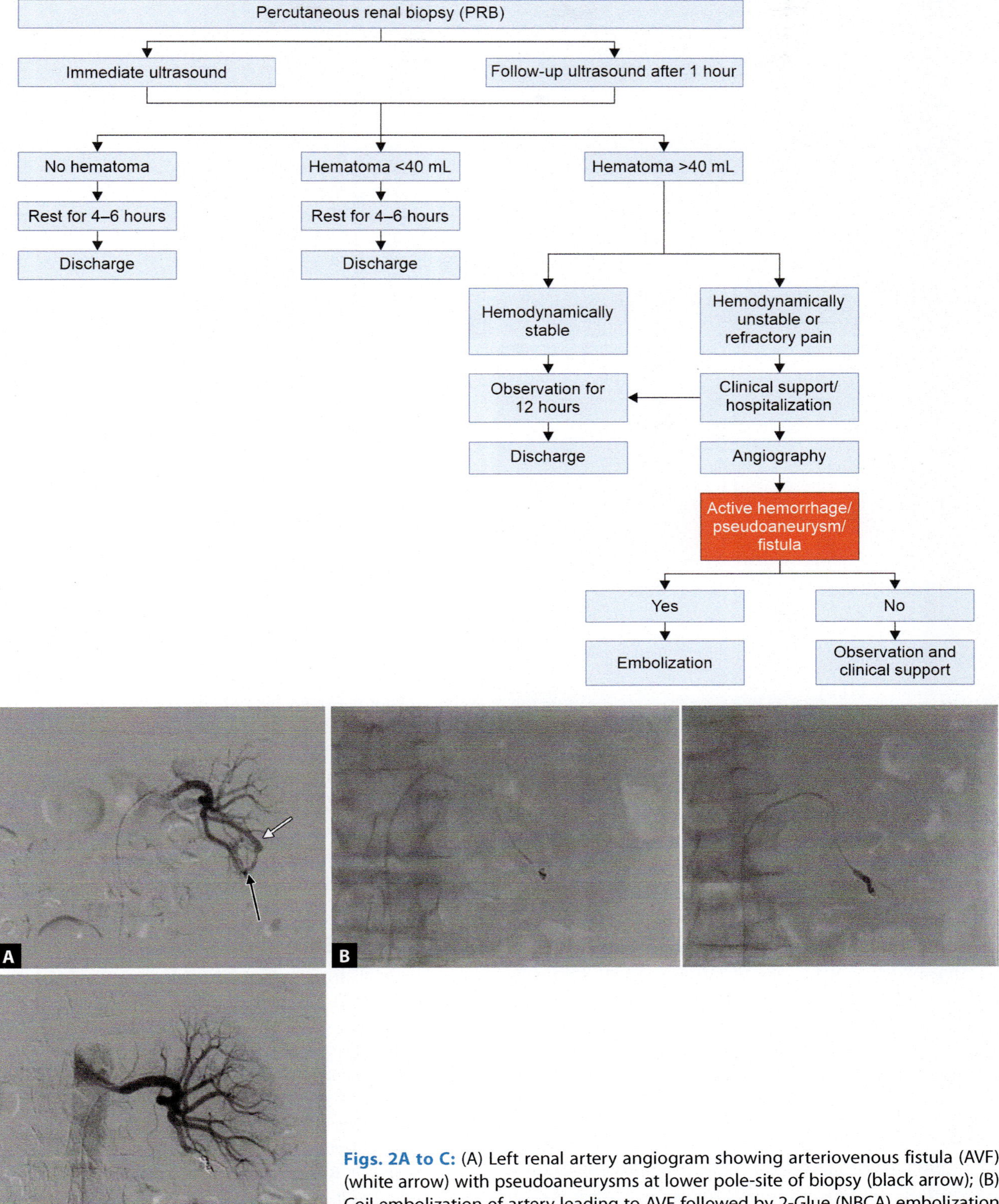

Figs. 2A to C: (A) Left renal artery angiogram showing arteriovenous fistula (AVF) (white arrow) with pseudoaneurysms at lower pole-site of biopsy (black arrow); (B) Coil embolization of artery leading to AVF followed by 2-Glue (NBCA) embolization of residual artery stump; (C) Postembolization left renal angiogram showing absence of flow in AVF.

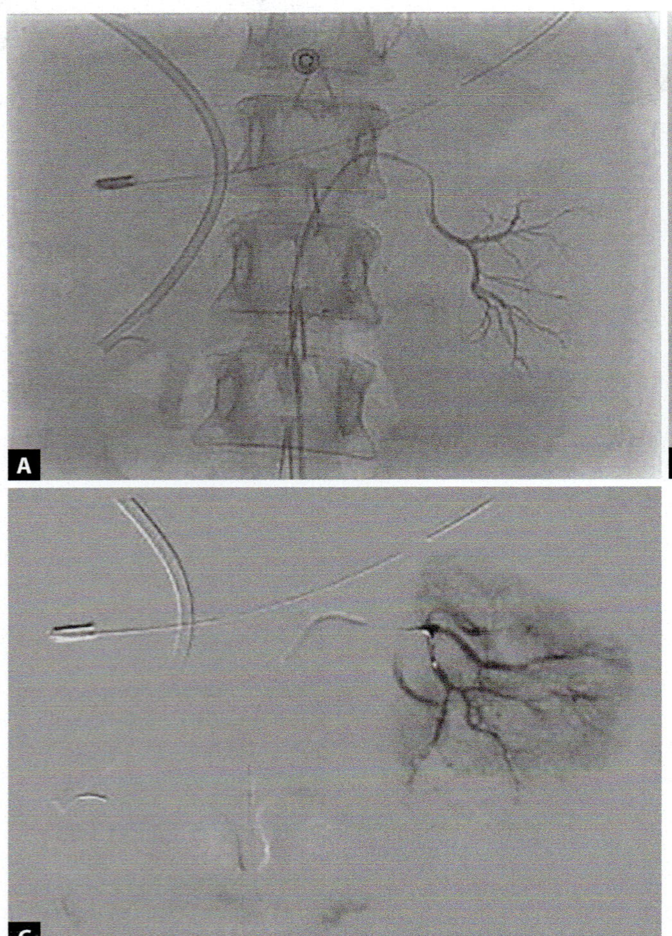

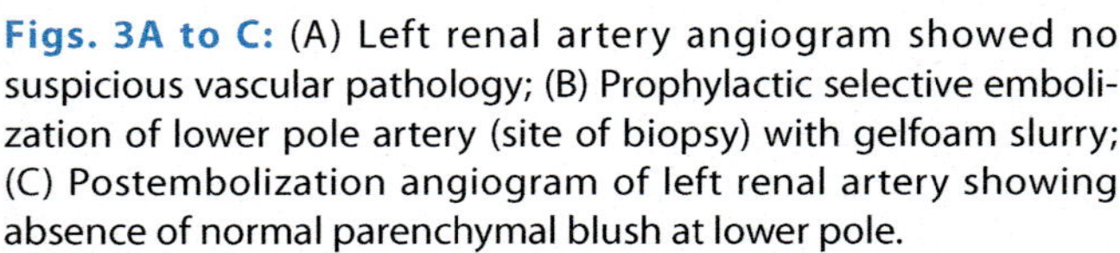

Figs. 3A to C: (A) Left renal artery angiogram showed no suspicious vascular pathology; (B) Prophylactic selective embolization of lower pole artery (site of biopsy) with gelfoam slurry; (C) Postembolization angiogram of left renal artery showing absence of normal parenchymal blush at lower pole.

CASE SCENARIO 3

A 30-year-old female patient presented with persistent lower limb edema and high creatinine levels after few months of normal vaginal delivery. She underwent USG-guided renal parenchymal biopsy from the lower pole of left kidney. After 2 hours, the patient had hypotensive episodes for which she was shifted to ICU. She was later considered for endovascular management; however, no active extravasation/pseudoaneurysm or fistulous communication was seen. Due to persistent hypotensive episodes and mild persistent hematuria prophylactic embolization of lower pole artery was done with gelfoam slurry **(Figs. 3A to C)**.

CONCLUSION

This chapter summarizes the risks, complications, and management of percutaneous renal biopsies which require a comprehensive approach that prioritizes early detection, accurate diagnosis, and timely intervention. By understanding the spectrum of complications, implementing appropriate management strategies, and utilizing advanced endovascular techniques, clinicians can effectively minimize the risk of major complications and optimize patient outcomes.

REFERENCES

1. Iversen P, Brun C. Aspiration biopsy of the kidney. Am J Med. 1951;11:324-30.
2. Kark R M, Muehrcke RC Biopsy of kidney in prone position. Lancet. 1954;266:1047-9.
3. Madaio MP. Renal biopsy. Kidney Int. 1990;38:529-43.
4. McWilliams JP, Kee ST. Native renal biopsy: The perfect storm. J Vasc Interv Radiol. 2015;26:212-3.
5. Lees JS, McQuarrie EP, Mordi N, Geddes CC, Fox JG, Mackinnon B. Risk factors for bleeding complications after nephrologist-performed native renal biopsy. Clin Kidney J. 2017;10:573-7.

6. Whittier WL, Korbet SM. Timing of complications in percutaneous renal biopsy. J Am Soc Nephrol. 2004;15: 142-7.
7. Prasad N, Kumar S, Manjunath R, Bhadauria D, Kaul A, Sharma RK, et al. Real-time ultrasound-guided percutaneous renal biopsy with needle guide by nephrologists decreases post-biopsy complications. Clin Kidney J. 2015;8:151-6.
8. Waldo B, Korbet SM, Freimanis MG, Lewis EJ. The value of post-biopsy ultrasound in predicting complications after percutaneous renal biopsy of native kidneys. Nephrol Dial Transplant. 2009;24:2433-9.
9. Kriegshauser JS, Patel MD, Young SW, Chen F, Eversman WG, Chang YH. Risk of bleeding after native renal biopsy as a function of preprocedural systolic and diastolic blood pressure. J Vasc Interv Radiol. 2015;26:206-12.
10. Shidham GB, Siddiqi N, Beres JA, Logan B, Nagaraja HN, Shidham SG, et al. Clinical risk factors associated with bleeding after native kidney biopsy. Nephrology (Carlton). 2005;10:305-10.
11. Corapi KM, Chen JL, Balk EM, Gordon CE. Bleeding complications of native kidney biopsy: A systematic review and meta-analysis. Am J Kidney Dis. 2012;60:62-73.
12. Xu DM, Chen M, Zhou FD, Zhao MH. Risk factors for severe bleeding complications in percutaneous renal biopsy. Am J Med Sci. 2017;353:230-5.
13. Patel IJ, Davidson JC, Nikolic B, Salazar GM, Schwartzberg MS, Walker TG, et al. Consensus guidelines for periprocedural management of coagulation status and hemostasis risk in percutaneous image-guided interventions. J Vasc Interv Radiol. 2012;23:727-36.
14. Baffour FI, Hickson LJ, Stegall MD, Dean PG, Gunderson TM, Atwell TD, et al. Effects of aspirin therapy on ultrasound-guided renal allograft biopsy bleeding complications. J Vasc Interv Radiol. 2017;28:188-94.
15. Torres Muñoz A, Valdez-Ortiz R, González-Parra C, Espinoza-Dávila E, Morales-Buenrostro LE, Correa-Rotter R. Percutaneous renal biopsy of native kidneys: Efficiency, safety and risk factors associated with major complications. Arch Med Sci. 2011;7:823-31.
16. Manno C, Bonifati C, Torres DD, Campobasso N, Schena FP. Desmopressin acetate in percutaneous ultrasound-guided kidney biopsy: a randomized controlled trial. Am J Kidney Dis. 2011;57:850-5.
17. Whittier WL, Gashti C, Saltzberg S, Korbet S. Comparison of native and transplant kidney biopsies: diagnostic yield and complications. Clin Kidney J. 2018;11:616–22.
18. Hergesell O, Felten H, Andrassy K, Kühn K, Ritz E. Safety of ultrasound-guided percutaneous renal biopsy-retrospective analysis of 1090 consecutive cases. Nephrol Dial Transplant. 1998;13:975–7.
19. Babaei Jandaghi A, Lebady M, Zamani A-A, Heidarzadeh A, Monfared A, Pourghorban R. A randomised clinical trial to compare coaxial and noncoaxial techniques in percutaneous core needle biopsy of renal parenchyma. Cardiovasc Intervent Radiol. 2017;40:106-11.
20. Wang HL, Xu CY, Wang HH, Xu W. Emergency transcatheter arterial embolization for acute renal hemorrhage. Medicine (Baltimore). 2015;94(42):e1667.
21. Ramos Botelho Antunes P, Almeida Araújo S, Maria Carvalho Miranda S, Franco Monteiro Prado F, Felipe França Antunes L, Carvalho de Siqueira E, et al. Post-biopsy complications associated with percutaneous kidney biopsy. In: Edward T Zawadav ET Jr., Salim SA (Eds). Renal Diseases. UK: IntechOpen; 2020.

CHAPTER 36

Renal Artery Angioplasty and Stenting

Raghav Seth, Manish Malik, Tarun Kumar

CASE SCENARIO

A 54-year-old male presented to casualty with recurrent severe headaches along with nausea and vomiting episodes. Past history was nonsignificant. There was no history of alcohol or tobacco use. There was no similar family history. Physical examination revealed a heart rate of 82 beats/min, respiratory rate of 14/min, and blood pressure (BP) of 200/110 mm Hg. The BP recordings were almost the same in both upper limbs. The distal pulses were also symmetrical in all four limbs. The rest of the abdominal, cardiac, and respiratory examinations were within normal limits. He was taking amlodipine 10 mg and enalapril 20 mg for the last 2 months (advised from an outside hospital). His renal function test (RFT) was normal with a serum creatinine of 0.9 mg/dL.

He was admitted and his BP was controlled with intravenous antihypertensive drugs. Renal artery evaluation was performed by renal doppler which revealed normal-sized bilateral kidneys and imaging features consistent with high-grade left renal artery stenosis. Similar findings were confirmed by magnetic resonance angiography, which showed the level of stenosis in the proximal left renal artery **(Fig. 1A)**.

Subsequently, he was planned for renal stenting. Digital subtraction angiography (DSA) showed significant stenosis in the proximal left renal artery **(Fig. 1B)**. The site of stenosis was crossed using an appropriate guidewire **(Fig. 1C)** and the pressure gradient across the site of stenosis was measured, which came out to be 25 mm Hg. The site of stenosis was dilated using a 3.0 mm × 15 mm balloon **(Fig. 1D)**. However, residual stenosis of >60% was still seen. Thus, a 6.0 mm × 15 mm balloon expandable stent was implanted **(Fig. 1E)**. Post-stenting, there was no significant pressure gradient and a good flow across the stent.

The patient is on follow-up for the last 1 year and his BP improved over time (under control with single antihypertensive) with normal RFT.

INTRODUCTION

Renal artery stenosis (RAS) can occur due to multiple reasons. The two most common causes are atherosclerosis and fibromuscular dysplasia (FMD).[1] Atherosclerotic occlusion is the most common cause and is seen in >90% of cases. Other causes are listed in **Box 1**. The clinical features of RAS include hypertension and subsequently renal failure, if untreated.[2]

If we discuss about hypertension, we will find that the majority of population will suffer from primary hypertension, which is also called essential hypertension. This is seen in 95–98% of the cases, and no structural lesion can be identified in these patients.[3] The other type is secondary hypertension. RAS is the most common cause of secondary hypertension and in general accounts for approximately 1–5% of patients with hypertension.[4]

The main mechanism causing hypertension in RAS is the activation of the renin–angiotensin–aldosterone system (RAAS). When the RAS occurs, blood flow and pressure to the kidneys decrease. This stimulates the release of renin, which converts angiotensinogen (released from liver) into angiotensin I which is further converted to angiotensin II in the lung. This causes increased aldosterone secretion which causes sodium and water retention and thus leads to increased blood volume and blood pressure. This RAAS activation and sympathetic overactivity are responsible for cardiovascular and renal morbidity in RAS patients.[5]

Many patients of RAS may be asymptomatic. Studies have shown that approximately 30% of patients with mild atherosclerotic narrowing of renal artery (<50% occlusion) actually have symptoms, which increases to about 50% if there is moderate-to-severe stenosis (>50%).[1]

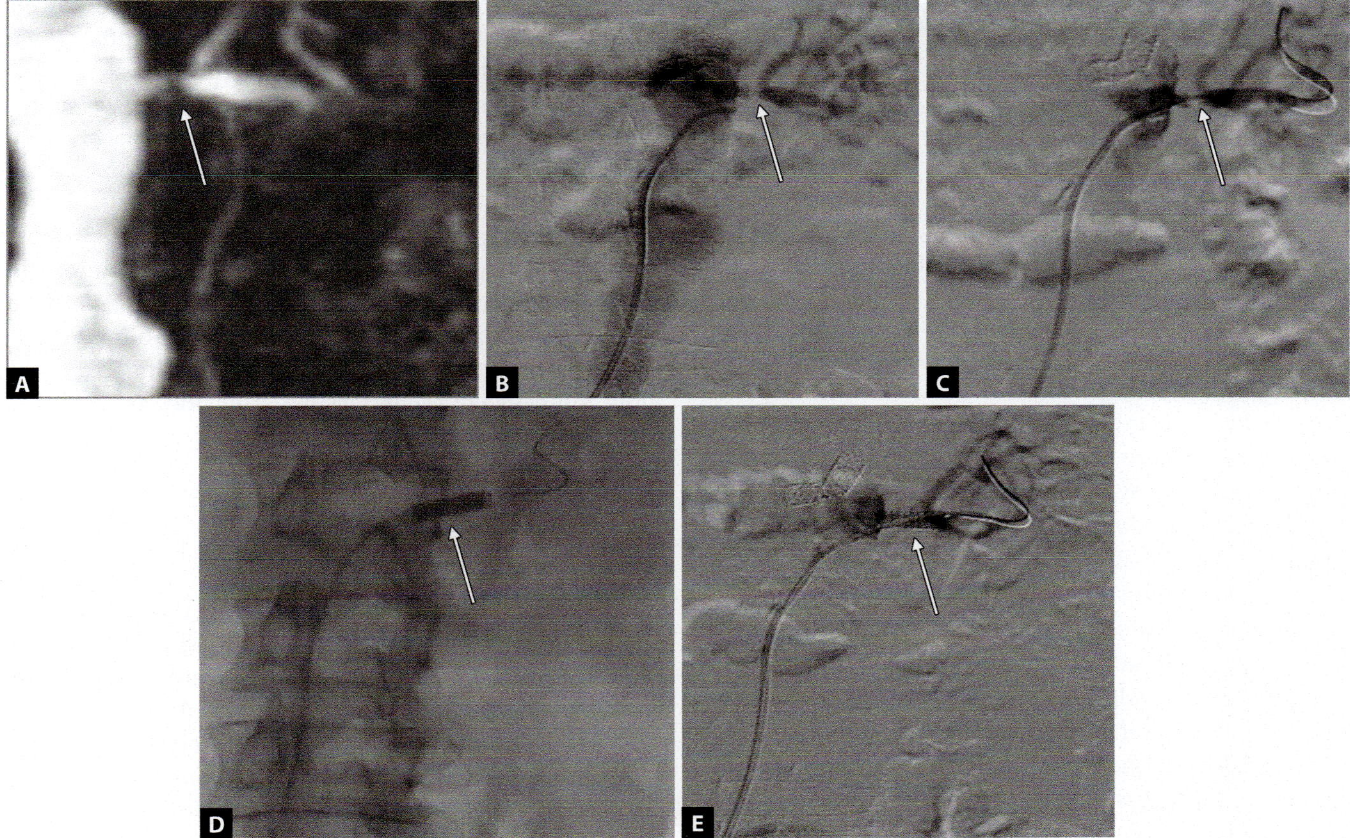

Figs. 1A to E: (A) Coronal magnetic resonance angiography image showing significant stenosis in the proximal left renal artery (arrow); (B) Digital subtraction angiography image showing significant stenosis in the proximal left renal artery (arrow); (C) Digital subtraction angiography image showing successful crossing of the site of stenosis using appropriate guidewire, with the arrow showing the site of stenosis; (D) Digital subtraction angiography image showing dilatation of the site of stenosis using a 3.0 mm × 15 mm balloon (arrow); (E) Digital subtraction angiography image showing poststent (6.0 mm × 15 mm balloon expandable stent) deployment angiogram showing good flow across the stent (arrow).

BOX 1: Causes of RAS.

- Atherosclerosis
- FMD
- Vasculitis:
  - Takayasu arteritis
  - Polyarteritis nodosa
  - SLE
- Coarctation of aorta
- Congenital or traumatic arteriovenous fistulas
- Compression by tumor
- Iatrogenic:
  - Radiation-induced vasculopathy
  - Surgical trauma or prior renal artery instrumentation

(FMD: fibromuscular dysplasia; RAS: renal artery stenosis; SLE: systemic lupus erythematosus)

The clinical features in symptomatic RAS patients include sudden-onset severe hypertension, onset of hypertension at less than 30 years of age or older than 55 years of age, and hypertension that is poorly controlled by multiple drug therapy and renal failure. The clinical features of RAS are summarized in **Box 2**.

ATHEROSCLEROTIC RENAL ARTERY STENOSIS

These patients are generally in their sixth or seventh decade and more common in males. An important point to note here is that stenosis due to atherosclerosis is almost always (more than 90% times) located within the proximal part of

BOX 2: Clinical signs of RAS.

- Sudden-onset severe hypertension
- Onset of hypertension at <30 or >55 years of age
- Hypertension unresponsive to multiple drugs
- Unexplained atrophic kidney
- Unexplained renal failure
- Renal failure in response to ACEIs/ARBs

(ACEIs: angiotensin-converting enzyme inhibitors; ARBs: angiotensin II-receptor blockers; RAS: renal artery stenosis)

renal artery, within the first few centimeters (within 1 cm most commonly) of its origin. These are known as *ostial* stenotic lesions. Only less than 10% of the atherosclerotic stenotic lesions are actually confined to the renal artery proper (>1 cm away from the renal artery ostium). These are known as *proximal* stenotic lesions. Rarely, intrarenal branches may be affected. This is seen in patients with severe atherosclerosis or long-standing hypertension.

In general, atherosclerotic RAS is more likely to be associated with nephropathy than with renovascular hypertension.[1] In addition, atherosclerosis is systemic and not limited to the renal artery in these patients. Thus, this is a progressive disease characterized by worsening stenosis and eventual occlusion with much wider implications in terms of organ dysfunction as well as patient prognosis.

NONATHEROSCLEROTIC RENAL ARTERY STENOSIS

Fibromuscular Dysplasia

In contrast to atherosclerosis, FMD is seen in young patients (third to fifth decade) and is more common in females. Histologically, it may involve the intima, media, or adventitia. The most common pathological type is medial fibroplasia (>80% of FMD cases).[6] There are multiple tiny webs that obstruct the blood flow and thus cause renovascular hypertension.

Another difference from atherosclerotic RAS is that it is usually seen in the distal main renal artery and may extend till the first-order renal branches (one-fourth of cases). About 50% of patients may have bilateral disease and approximately 25–30% of patients may have progressive disease. The presence of renal artery aneurysms may also be seen in up to 10% of patients with FMD.[6] A rare complication of FMD is spontaneous intrarenal dissection in which the patient typically presents with hypertension, acute flank pain, and hematuria.

On DSA, FMD is typically seen as a "beads-on-a-string" appearance due to contrast filling of consecutive aneurysms in the renal artery. A very important point to note here is that although FMD may resemble vasculitis, it is a noninflammatory disease and its actual cause is not known (genetic component may be involved). In general, FMD is associated with a good prognosis.

Other causes of renovascular hypertension are less common. The geographical variation in the etiology of renovascular hypertension is also very interesting. In North America and Europe, FMD is a very common cause of RAS, whereas in Asia, Takayasu's arteritis is a more common cause of secondary hypertension, especially in the pediatric population.[7]

DIAGNOSIS

The choice of the diagnostic modality that is used for diagnosis of renovascular hypertension depends on the clinical history. For the pediatric population presenting with hypertension, careful evaluation for coarctation of aorta, pheochromocytoma, vasculitis, and chronic renal parenchymal injury must be performed. Young adults with normal renal function and suspected RAS based on clinical features should undergo DSA, because subtle or peripheral FMD can be missed by noninvasive imaging tests. In addition, management in the form of balloon angioplasty can also be performed in the same sitting.

Adults with suspected RAS should initially have at least one noninvasive test before DSA is done.

Duplex ultrasonography combines the B-mode imaging for direct visualization of renal arteries with Doppler for velocity measurements of blood flow. It can provide the following information:

- Kidney size
- Location and degree of stenosis
- Visualization of other processes (obstruction or mass)
- Assessment of intrinsic small-vessel renovascular disease

It has a number of advantages:

- Noninvasive
- Not affected by medications
- Least expensive imaging
- No intravenous contrast required
- No radiation exposure
- Particularly useful for follow-up after stenting

It must be performed on a fasting patient in the morning. The criteria for diagnosis are given in the following text.

Proximal Criteria (Direct Evaluation of the Stenosis)

Measurement of a high peak systolic velocity (PSV) of renal artery of >180 cm/s or by renal aortic ratio (RAR), which is calculated by dividing the PSV of renal artery by the PSV of the adjacent aorta. A normal RAR is <3.5. The sensitivity and specificity of RAR of >3.5 are approximately 84% and 97%, respectively. This translates to a positive predictive value (PPV) of approximately 95% for detection of RAS (>60% stenosis).[8]

Distal Criteria (Indirect Evaluation of the Stenosis)

- Loss of early systolic peak
- Acceleration index (AI) <3 m/s^2
- Acceleration time (AT) >0.07 second
- Difference between both kidneys in RI of >5%

The rationale for all these is that the flow in the renal vessels distal to a hemodynamically significant stenosis becomes damped and shows a slow rise to the peak systole. This is called "*tardus-parvus*" effect, meaning that the waveform is smaller with a slower systolic acceleration.[9]

Both *magnetic resonance angiography (MRA) and computed tomography angiography (CTA)* have excellent sensitivity and specificity for detection of RAS (>90%).[10]

Features that indicate hemodynamically significant disease include:

- Reduction in luminal diameter of >75%
- Poststenotic dilatation
- Decrease in renal size

CTA and MRA allow evaluation of the renal artery in multiple planes. This is a significant advantage of cross-sectional imaging that is not seen in DSA. However, a clear evaluation of intrarenal branches is not possible yet with these techniques. In patients with normal renal function, another modality that can be used is *captopril scintigraphy*. It has similar sensitivity and specificity to CTA/MRA but has a big disadvantage of not providing the required anatomical information that is crucial for planning a procedure.[11]

Digital subtraction angiography

The angiographic diagnosis of RAS is suggested by the following points:[12]

- Degree of luminal narrowing
- Poststenotic dilatation
- Slow flow distal to stenosis
- Pressure gradient across the stenotic site
- Presence of collaterals
- Small renal size

The location as well as the extent of the stenosis should be carefully evaluated. As far as pressure gradient is concerned, mean systolic pressure gradient >10 mm Hg or peak systolic gradient >20 mm Hg between the aorta and the renal artery distal to stenosis indicates a hemodynamically significant stenosis.[12,13] In general, the higher the gradient, the more chances are that treating the stenosis will actually resolve the renovascular hypertension.

RENAL VEIN SAMPLING OF RENIN

Blood samples are obtained from both the renal veins and IVC above and below the renal veins. Using a curved angiographic catheter, bilateral renal veins are cannulated and samples are collected within a short period of time. If the renin level from one kidney is more than 1.5 times that of the contralateral kidney, it is indicative of renovascular hypertension. A higher renin value between suprarenal and infrarenal IVC also provides supportive evidence of renovascular hypertension.[14]

INDICATIONS OF INTERVENTION IN RENAL ARTERY STENOSIS

The indications for intervention are different for renovascular hypertension and nephropathy due to RAS. All symptomatic stenoses which are not managed medically require intervention in patients with reasonable life expectancy. Asymptomatic stenoses should not be treated unless the patient has a solitary kidney. The indications of intervention in RAS are summarized in **Box 3**.

BOX 3: Indications for intervention in RAS.

Severe hypertension with:
- Unilateral or bilateral RAS
- Mean pressure gradient >10 mm Hg or peak systolic gradient >20 mm Hg
- Atherosclerosis, FMD, Takayasu's arteritis, dissection

Renal failure with:
- No other explanation for renal failure
- Bilateral stenosis
- Mean pressure gradient >10 mm Hg or peak systolic gradient >20 mm Hg
- Atherosclerosis, dissection

(FMD: fibromuscular dysplasia; RAS: renal artery stenosis)

SURGICAL APPROACHES FOR RENAL ARTERY STENOSIS

Multiple surgical options are available for revascularization of the renal arteries. These include:

- Aortorenal bypass
- Aortorenal endarterectomy
- Ileorenal bypass
- Autotransplantation in pelvis
- Nephrectomy

Ostial and proximal atherosclerotic RAS are easier to manage than distal or segmental RAS. The overall mortality after surgery is approximately 4%. The cure rates for hypertension are 15–20%, improvement is seen in 70–75%, and no change or worse is seen in 10%. For renal failure, improvement is seen in 45–50% of cases, no change in 35–40%, and worsening in 10% of the cases.[15,16]

Angioplasty and Stenting

This is the most commonly used technique for the management of RAS. The basic principle here is that RAS due to atherosclerosis is almost always managed with stenting, whereas nonatherosclerotic FMD almost always responds to angioplasty alone. This is because in ostial lesions, the stenosis is caused by aortic plaque and not by the renal artery plaque.

Preprocedure

Angioplasty and stenting for RAS should be planned in a careful manner, as these can be amongst the most difficult interventions.

Before the procedure, the patients should decrease the dose of long-acting antihypertensive agents. This is because after the angioplasty or stenting, there may be profound hypotension as the drug effects persist even after the renal revascularization. For the same reason, patients are instructed to drink plenty of fluids before the procedure until 2 hours before, when IV fluids are initiated. According to some studies, administration of calcium-channel blockers should be done, before the procedure, to prevent vasospasm.[17] Patients with renal failure can be treated beforehand with a renal protective strategy according to the institutional policy.

Procedure

CO_2 angiography can be considered in patients with azotemia. Most commonly, a femoral access is performed and heparin (5,000–10,000 units) is administered. Next, an aortogram is performed before proceeding. For ostial lesions, the image intensifier is angled in such a way that we can see the ostium of the renal artery in profile. A long curved sheath (6Fr or 7Fr) or a curved guiding catheter (7Fr or 8Fr) is inserted. Utmost care should be taken to minimize any manipulation in the aorta as this may result in cholesterol embolization. Then, an appropriate 5Fr catheter is used to find the renal artery origin and a gentle puff of contrast is injected for confirmation. The renal artery ostium should be probed only with a nontraumatic, steerable guidewire. If the ostial lesion is completely or near-completely stenotic, a microwire should be used to cross it. Once the guidewire has crossed the lesion, the catheter is advanced over it. The guidewire is removed and then blood is aspirated gently, followed by injection of a small amount of contrast for confirmation. Next, nitroglycerin (NTG; 100–200 µg) is injected. An appropriate working wire (moderately stiff 0.035-inch or 0.018-inch guidewire with a short straight floppy tip) is then carefully exchanged.

The sheath or the guiding catheter is brought as close as possible to the renal artery ostium. This helps in added stability as well as a port for contrast injection to monitor the progress of the procedure. Then, predilatation is performed with an undersized balloon. The ideal stent for RAS has not been defined but most commonly, a balloon-expandable metallic stent is preferred. Both bare and covered metallic stents provide similar results. The most commonly used stents for RAS range from a diameter of 5 to 7 mm with a length of 1.2–2 cm. A very important point to consider here is that the stent should protrude into the aorta a few millimeters so that there is adequate displacement of the aortic plaque. Drug-eluting stents can be used when treating smaller (≤3.5–4 mm) renal arteries like in accessory or segmental arteries. This is because data suggests that bare stents in renal arteries <5 mm have poor long-term patency.

Renal artery FMD responds well to simple angioplasty with excellent long-term results. The best results are seen in younger patients (<50 years), with a duration of hypertension that is <8 years and without any evidence of peripheral arterial disease. The technical success rate is >90%, with approximately 50% of patients experiencing complete normalization of BP and approximately 33% experiencing improved BP control with medications. Restenosis may occur in 20–25% of cases, and these should undergo repeat angioplasty. The use of stents should be avoided in FMD. Involvement of the intrarenal branches can occur with FMD. These can be tackled with small-diameter balloons and 0.18-inch guidewires.

Complications

In general, renal angioplasty and stenting is a challenging procedure. The complications generally occur more commonly when stenting is performed (approximately 15%) than with angioplasty alone (5–10%). The highest complication rate is when stenting is performed in cases with diffuse aortic and renal artery atherosclerosis and the least complication rate is for angioplasty for FMD.[18]

The most dreaded complication is renal artery rupture. It is minimized when balloon sizes are carefully selected. Prompt recognition with reinflation of a balloon across the rupture is life-saving followed by placement of a stent graft. Other complications that may occur include stent malposition, significant residual stenosis, renal artery thrombosis, antegrade renal artery dissection, retrograde aortic dissection, and distal embolization. The complications and their incidence are summarized in **Table 1**.[18,19]

Goals of Intervention

Atherosclerotic disease causing RAS can result in hypertension and/or renal failure and there are different goals for management of both. In hypertension, the improvement is proportional to the baseline systolic pressure. The goal is to reduce the BP by 10–15 mm Hg for pretreatment systolic pressure of 155–180 mm Hg. A target of 165 mm Hg is suggested for pretreatment systolic pressures higher than 180 mm Hg after renal artery stenting. The reduction in the number of drugs required to maintain the target BP also indicates clinical success. For patients with advanced renal failure due to atherosclerotic RAS, the improvement in renal function is the goal. In this population, a low resistive index is also a predictor of clinical success.

TABLE 1: Complications of renal artery angioplasty and stenting.

Complication	***Incidence (%)***
Puncture site complications (hematoma, pseudoaneurysm)	5–10
Renal failure	5–7
Flow-limiting dissection	5
Branch artery occlusion	3–5
Renal artery rupture	<1
Renal artery thrombosis	<1
Death within 30 days	<0.5

Many large prospective trials for interventions in atherosclerotic RAS have been conducted. The DRASTIC (Dutch Renal Artery Stenosis Intervention Cooperative) study compared medical therapy and angioplasty for hypertension and found a better and sustained BP control and fewer renal artery occlusions at 1-year postintervention in the angioplasty group.[20]

The ASTRAL (Angioplasty and Stenting for Renal Artery Lesions) trial randomized patients into two groups: Medical therapy alone or medical therapy plus catheter-based intervention.

The primary outcome was improvement in renal function, and BP control was a secondary outcome. It failed to show improved renal function or BP control with stenting. However, major limitations of this study were low technical success rate (80%); approximately 40% of patients had stenosis <70% and the patients in whom the referring clinicians wanted them to be treated with stents were not enrolled.[21]

The CORAL (Cardiovascular Outcomes in Renal Atherosclerotic Lesions) trial evaluated the rate of renal and cardiovascular adverse events in patients with atherosclerotic RAS and raised BP, chronic kidney disease (CKD) or both, by dividing them into two groups: Medical therapy alone or medical therapy plus stenting. A total of 947 patients were randomly assigned to medical therapy group (480) or stenting plus medical therapy group (467). It was found that patients had similar outcomes in both the groups. The urine albumin to creatinine ratio (ACR) may be a factor that may decide which patients will benefit from stent intervention versus whom that are less likely to get any benefit. Very importantly, increased benefit was seen with a higher grade of stenosis. The results of these trials shows the importance of patient selection for interventions in RAS.[22]

The comparison of different landmark trials on outcomes of interventions for RAS are summarized in **Table 2**.

TABLE 2: Comparison of different landmark trials on outcomes of angioplasty/stenting for RAS.

Name of trial	*Year*	*Type*	*Inclusion*	*Intervention*	*Primary outcome*	*Key findings*
DRASTIC	2000	RCT	106 patients with >50% RAS	PTRA vs. medical therapy	Blood pressure control and renal function	No significant benefit of PTRA over medical therapy; high crossover rate (44%); small sample size; inclusion of patients with nonhemodynamically significant lesions
ASTRAL	2009	RCT	806 patients with RAS	Revascularization (angioplasty ± stenting) + medical therapy vs. medical therapy alone	Rate of decline in renal function	No significant difference in renal function, blood pressure control, or cardiovascular events; inclusion criteria led to selection bias; 41% had <70% stenosis
STAR	2009	RCT	140 patients with ≥50% RAS and impaired renal function	Stenting + medical therapy vs. medical therapy alone	≥20% decrease in creatinine clearance	No significant difference in renal function decline; limited sample size; only 46 patients received stents
CORAL	2014	RCT	947 patients with ≥60% RAS and hypertension or CKD	Stenting + medical therapy vs. medical therapy alone	Composite of cardiovascular and renal events	No significant difference in primary outcome; modest reduction in systolic BP (~2 mm Hg) with stenting; no benefit in subgroups with severe stenosis
HERCULES	2010	Prospective, non-randomized	Patients with uncontrolled hypertension and RAS	Stenting	Change in systolic BP	Significant reduction in systolic BP; low in-stent restenosis rate (10.5% at 9 months); low complication rate (1.5% at 30 days)
RENAISSANCE	2008	Prospective, nonrandomized	Patients with RAS	Stenting with duplex ultrasound follow-up	Binary restenosis at 9 months	Technical success rate of 99%; binary restenosis rate of 21.3% at 9 months; duplex ultrasound effective for follow-up

(BP: blood pressure; CKD: chronic kidney disease; PTRA: percutaneous transluminal renal angioplasty; RAS: renal artery stenosis)

CONCLUSION

In general, stenting for atherosclerotic RAS has a very high technical success rate. Approximately 60–65% patients experience improved BP with fewer medications, approximately 30% do not respond and in 5%, the condition may worsen. The restenosis rate of stents is approximately 15% at 1 year. Intimal hyperplasia is the main factor that causes restenosis of stents, whether placed percutaneously or surgically. There is always some degree of intimal hyperplasia that occurs after every intervention; thus, the larger the initial postprocedural lumen of renal artery, the higher will be the long-term patency rate. In addition, it has also been found that the best long-term results are achieved when the final diameter of the renal artery is >6 mm. Finally, multiple techniques like placement of covered stents, drug-eluting stents, and brachytherapy are being evaluated to improve the long-term outcomes in these patients.

REFERENCES

1. Weber BR, Dieter RS. Renal artery stenosis: epidemiology and treatment. Int J Nephrol Renovasc Dis. 2014;7:169-81.
2. Safian RD. Renal artery stenosis. Prog Cardiovasc Dis. 2021;65:60-70.
3. Messerli FH, Williams B, Ritz E. Essential hypertension. Lancet. 2007;370(9587):591-603.
4. Puar THK, Mok Y, Debajyoti R, Khoo J, How CH, Ng AKH. Secondary hypertension in adults. Singapore Med J. 2016;57(5):228-32.
5. Covic A, Gusbeth-Tatomir P. The role of the renin-angiotensin-aldosterone system in renal artery stenosis, renovascular hypertension, and ischemic nephropathy: diagnostic implications. Prog Cardiovasc Dis. 2009;52(3):204-8.

6. Safian RD, Textor SC. Renal-artery stenosis. N Engl J Med. 2001;344(6):431–42.
7. Maritati F, Iannuzzella F, Pavia MP, Pasquali S, Vaglio A. Kidney involvement in medium- and large-vessel vasculitis. J Nephrol. 2016;29(4):495-505.
8. Granata A, Fiorini F, Andrulli S, Logias F, Gallieni M, Romano G, et al. Doppler ultrasound and renal artery stenosis: An overview. J Ultrasound. 2009;12(4):133-43.
9. Li JC, Wang L, Jiang YX, Dai Q, Cai S, Lv K, et al. Evaluation of renal artery stenosis with velocity parameters of Doppler sonography. J Ultrasound Med. 2006;25(6):735-42; quiz 743-4.
10. Marcos HB, Choyke PL. Magnetic resonance angiography of the kidney. Semin Nephrol. 2000;20(5):450-5.
11. Huot SJ, Hansson JH, Dey H, Concato J. Utility of captopril renal scans for detecting renal artery stenosis. Arch Int Med. 2002;162(17):1981-4.
12. Rountas C, Vlychou M, Vassiou K, Liakopoulos V, Kapsalaki E, Koukoulis G, et al. Imaging modalities for renal artery stenosis in suspected renovascular hypertension: prospective intraindividual comparison of color Doppler US, CT angiography, GD-enhanced MR angiography, and digital subtraction angiography. Renal Fail. 2007;29(3):295-302.
13. Tullus K. Renal artery stenosis: is angiography still the gold standard in 2011? Pediatr Nephrol. 2011;26(6):833-7.
14. Rossi GP, Cesari M, Chiesura-Corona M, Miotto D, Semplicini A, Pessina AC. Renal vein renin measurements accurately identify renovascular hypertension caused by total occlusion of the renal artery. J Hypertens. 2002;20(5):975-84.
15. McLaughlin K, Jardine AG, Moss JG. Renal artery stenosis. BMJ. 2000;320(7242):1124-7.
16. Vagaonescu TD, Dangas G. Renal artery stenosis: diagnosis and management. J Clin Hypertens (Greenwich). 2007;4(5):363-70.
17. Jennings CG, Houston JG, Severn A, Bell S, Mackenzie IS, MacDonald TM. Renal Artery Stenosis—When To Screen, What To Stent? Curr Atheroscler Rep. 2014;16(6):416.
18. Ivanovic V, McKusick MA, Johnson CM, Sabater EA, Andrews JC, Breen JF, et al. Renal artery stent placement: complications at a single tertiary care center. J Vasc Interv Radiol. 2003;14(2 Pt 1):217-25.
19. Funaki B. Renal Ostial Angioplasty and Stenting. Part 2: Pitfalls and Complications. Semin Intervent Radiol. 2009;26(2):151-8.
20. van Jaarsveld B, Krijnen P, Bartelink A, Dees A, Derkx F, Man in't Veld A, et al. The dutch renal artery stenosis intervention cooperative (DRASTIC) study: rationale, design and inclusion data. J Hypertens Suppl. 1998;16(6):S21-7.
21. The ASTRAL Investigators. Revascularization versus medical therapy for renal-artery stenosis. New Engl J Med. 2009;361:1953-62.
22. Gupta R, Assiri S, Cooper CJ. Renal Artery Stenosis: New Findings from the CORAL Trial. Curr Cardiol Rep. 2017; 19(9):75.

CHAPTER 37

Renal Denervation Techniques

Kristin George, Ranjan Shetty

CASE SCENARIO

Mr C, a 43-year-old banker, diabetic since 5 years on oral hypoglycemic agents with glycated hemoglobin (HbA1c) of 7.2% and hypertensive since 1 year on telmisartan 40 mg and hydrochlorthiazide 12.5 mg, presented with a recent increase in home as well as office BP readings. He was started on cilnidipine 20 mg/day, and telmisartan was increased to 80 mg/day. But the home BP is still around 150/100 mm Hg and urine albumin creatinine ratio (UACR) is 324 mg/day. He also has dyslipidemia with total cholesterol of 248 mg/dL and high-density lipoprotein (HDL) cholesterol of 32 mg/dL. He has a strong family history of coronary artery disease in father and stroke in mother.

Mr C is concerned about the persistent high blood pressure (BP) readings despite being on three antihypertensives and wants to know if there is any way to improve BP control without increasing his already high pill burden.

INTRODUCTION

Hypertension (HTN) is a leading cause of cardiovascular (CV) morbidity and mortality and of chronic kidney disease worldwide. Despite the availability of effective medical therapy, more than half of patients with HTN do not meet the target blood pressure (BP) goals. In addition to challenges of adherence, drug-related adverse effects, and cost, drug-resistant HTN also contributes to the burden of uncontrolled BP.

Device-based therapies to control HTN have been available for some time.

With advancements in the device design and improved efficacy, there is a renewed interest in this modality of controlling drug-resistant HTN.

RENAL SYMPATHETIC INNERVATION AND HYPERTENSION

The pathogenesis of systemic HTN is multifactorial. In addition to the various inherited and lifestyle-related factors, activation of the sympathetic system is an established factor in the causation of HTN. The renal efferent sympathetic nerves mediate renal arteriolar vasoconstriction and increased renin, angiotensin, and aldosterone stimulation leading to sodium and water retention and high BP. The afferent nerves are stimulated by renal ischemia or stress and in turn lead to stimulation of the hypothalamus and hence the central sympathetic outflow, leading to increased vascular resistance and HTN.

The first successful demonstration of the antihypertensive potential of sympathectomy was done way back in the 1940s and 1950s when there was limited availability of effective oral medications. Subdiaphragmatic lumbodorsal splanchnicectomy was used as a possible treatment for malignant HTN. It was effective but had limited acceptance due to high perioperative morbidity and mortality.

Subsequently, with better understanding of the renal vascular anatomy regarding the close proximity of renal sympathetic nerves and the vessel, intra-arterial catheter-based systems to interrupt the nerve signaling were developed, the principle being that the heat generated is well tolerated by the renal arterial wall but is toxic to the nerves surrounding the vessel. The first proof-of-concept intervention was done by Krum et al.[1] who, by utilizing high focused radiofrequency (RF) energy, could achieve sustained reduction in BP in patients with resistant HTN. This procedure has now been refined with catheters with improvised design aiming at more targeted delivery of RF energy and better conformation to the anatomy of the renal arteries.

In addition, other modalities like ultrasound and ethanol ablation have also been explored.

EVIDENCE

The initial SYMPLICITY HTN 3 trial failed to show definitive benefit of renal denervation (RDN) compared with antihypertensive therapy alone. But further analysis revealed confounders in the selected patient subgroups, related to procedural technique and medication variability.[2]

Subsequent randomized, sham-controlled trials with revised design and conduct have demonstrated significant reductions in BP with RDN in patients across a wide range of HTN severity, in both the presence and absence of antihypertensive drug therapy **(Figs. 1A and B)**.

An important finding in these trials has been a consistent reduction in BP with RDN across all the time points in a 24-hour period in comparison with the control group, a phenomenon described as the "always on" effect of RDN. This provides special benefit to patients with variable BP phenotypes like nocturnal HTN and also eliminates the variability with drug pharmacokinetic profiles, dose timings, and adherence to oral medications.

In addition to immediate efficacy in reducing BP, another important parameter is the durability of BP reduction with RDN. This is a difficult parameter to assess

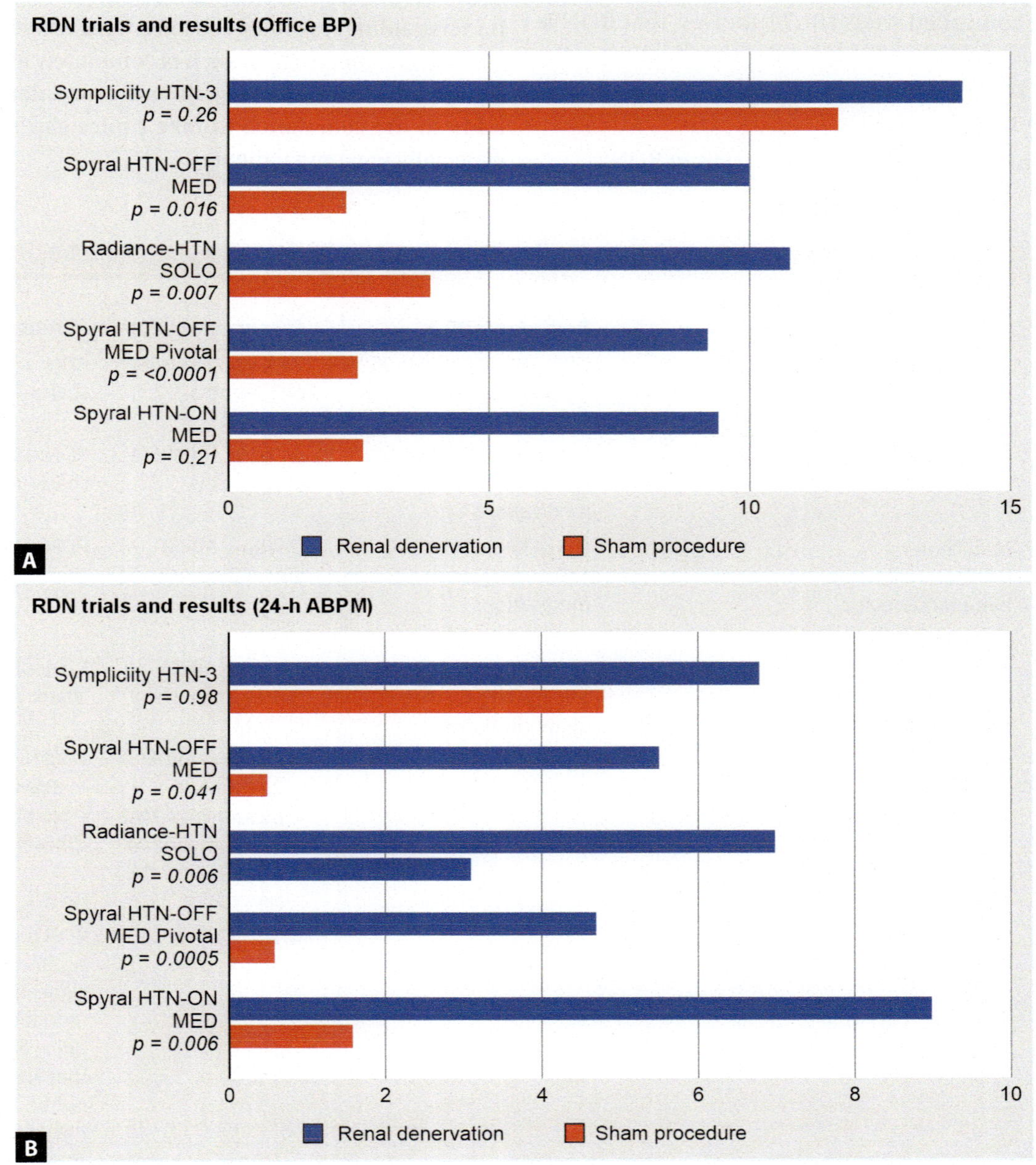

Figs. 1A and B: Reduction in SBP with RDN versus sham in pivotal trials. The x-axis depicts the mean reduction in BP (in mm Hg) in each arm. (ABPM: ambulatory blood pressure monitoring; RDN: renal denervation; SBP: systolic blood pressure)

in trials with added variation in medications, lifestyle, and comorbidities with long-term follow-up. As per data from the Global Symplicity Registry, through 3 years of follow-up, patients who underwent RDN were found to have sustained and significant reductions in both office and ambulatory BP.[3]

Another aspect, which is also an ongoing area of research, is regarding the efficacy across different patient populations. As per Global Symplicity Registry, a similar degree of BP reduction was observed with RDN among patients with a varying CV risk. A recent meta-analysis of randomized controlled trials (RCT) showed that RDN is associated with an estimated 10% relative reduction in the lifetime risk of CV events and 7.5% relative reduction in all-cause mortality.[4]

Table 1 summarizes the landmark trials in RDN.

INDICATIONS

Selecting the ideal patient who would benefit the most from this procedure requires a careful consideration of the risks and benefits involved. To begin with, RDN was offered to patients with uncontrolled BP despite the use of at least three antihypertensive medications including one diuretic. But there may also be other patients who may benefit from this procedure including those who are noncompliant to long-term oral medications due to various reasons. Nonadherence in some may be related to the side effects of the medicines while it might be cost, anxiety, or a lack of understanding regarding the long-term benefits in others.

The fact that HTN as such is completely asymptomatic in almost all the patients till end-organ damage occurs adds to the reluctance to take prolonged medications, especially in young patients.

TABLE 1: Landmark trials in RDN.

Trial	*Design*	*Method used*	*n*	*Patient selection*	*Primary endpoint*	*Results*
SPYRAL HTN-OFF MED	Randomized sham-controlled trial	RFA	331	Office BP 150–179/≥90 mm Hg on no BP medications	24-hour ABPM SBP at 3 months	RDN: ↓5 mm Hg; sham: ↓1 mm Hg
SPYRAL HTN-ON MED	Randomized sham-controlled trial	RFA	80	Office BP 150–179/≥90 mm Hg on 1–3 stable BP medications	24-hour ABPM SBP at 6 months	RDN: ↓9 mm Hg; sham: ↓2 mm Hg
RADIANCE-HTN SOLO	Multicenter international single-blind randomized sham-controlled trial	US	146	Office BP 140–180/90–110 mm Hg on no BP medications	Daytime ABPM SBP at 2 months	RDN: ↓8 mm Hg; sham: ↓2 mm Hg
RADIANCE-HTN TRIO	Multicenter single-blind randomized sham-controlled trial	US	136	Office BP ≥140/≥90 mm Hg on three stable BP medications	Daytime ABPM SBP at 2 months	RDN: ↓8 mm Hg; sham: ↓3 mm Hg
RADIANCE II (pivotal)	Randomized sham-controlled trial	US	224	Stage 2 HTN on 0–2 medications	• Daytime ABPM at 2 months • Incidence of MAE from baseline to 30 days after the procedure	• RDN: ↓7.9 mm Hg; sham: ↓1.8 mm Hg • No MAEs from baseline to 30 days
Global SIMPLICITY Registry	Prospective open-label single-arm multicenter observational study	RFA	>3,000		N/A	RDN resulted in significant and clinically meaningful reductions in both office and 24-hour BP that were sustained out to 3 years after the procedure

(ABPM: ambulatory blood pressure measurement; BP: blood pressure; HTN: hypertension; RFA: radiofrequency ablation; RDN: renal denervation; SBP: systolic blood pressure; US: ultrasound)

In 2021, the Society for Cardiovascular Angiography & Interventions (SCAI), along with the National Kidney Foundation (NKF), published an expert consensus roundtable statement on multidisciplinary evaluation and decision-making considerations for potential patients who may benefit from catheter-based RDN.[5]

Firstly, accurate measurement of BP is crucial to assess the efficacy of antihypertensive medications and for risk assessment. Office BP has numerous limitations like white-coat effect, masked HTN, and nocturnal HTN being missed. Home BP and ambulatory BP monitoring (ABPM) are more reliable and can circumvent the limitations of office BP measurement.

It is important to have a detailed assessment of risk-benefit balance for each patient and focus on shared decision-making with the patient and family.

Patient selection criteria for RDN:

- Patients with resistant HTN defined as office BP ≥140/90 mm Hg (24-hour ambulatory BP ≥130/80 mm Hg) despite being on maximally tolerated doses of three antihypertensive medications (like angiotensin-converting enzyme inhibitors or angiotensin II receptor blockers, calcium channel blockers, thiazide diuretics, and beta blockers), one of them being a diuretic
- Resistant HTN to be confirmed by out-of-office BP measurement techniques like ABPM or home BP
- RDN can be offered to patients with uncontrolled BP due to nonadherence or intolerant to medications.
- Secondary causes of HTN should be excluded.
- RDN should be offered on priority to patients with elevated CV risk, established CV event, diabetes, prior transient ischemic attack/cerebrovascular accident, or chronic kidney disease (end-organ damage).
- Estimated glomerular filtration rate (eGFR) >40 mL/min/1.73 m^2

In addition to the above-mentioned factors, patient preference is increasingly being recognized as an important factor to be considered while selecting patients for RDN.

Although this factor is inadequately studied in the trials, data based on surveys among hypertensive patients suggest that approximately one third of patients prefer catheter-based intervention for uncontrolled BP over further addition of medications.[6]

Patient's age may also affect the choice of therapy, as adherence rates to lifelong medications tend to be low in young individuals with HTN, who may benefit from a one-time procedure like RDN.

Another important factor while considering RDN is evidence of end-organ damage as a result of HTN like albuminuria, left ventricular hypertrophy, declining eGFR, established coronary artery disease, and CV disease risk.

In addition to the patient selection criteria and contraindications mentioned in the beginning, it is important to have endorsement regarding the procedure by at least two specialists from cardiology, nephrology, and internal medicine. The procedure should be performed by an experienced interventional specialist with appropriate equipment and laboratory setting.

PROCEDURE

Two systems currently available for RDN are Paradise® Ultrasound RDN system from RECOR and Symplicity Spyral™ RDN system from Medtronic. The former uses ultrasonic energy while the latter uses RF energy to the renal nerves.

Preprocedure imaging to rule out renal artery stenosis is of paramount importance. As per the European Society of Cardiology/European Association of Percutaneous Cardiovascular Interventions (ESC/EAPCI) recommendations:

- Selective renal angiography immediately before RDN remains the gold standard because computed tomography (CT) angiography or magnetic resonance angiography (MRA) may miss some renal artery abnormalities
- If invasive renal artery imaging is not an option, CT or MRA is preferential to duplex ultrasound.

The procedure of performing RDN using the Symplicity Spyral™ system which is more widely used is described subsequently.

The procedure is done under sedation or short general anesthesia (GA). The process of securing vascular access is similar to renal angiography and angioplasty. Femoral artery is accessed using standard techniques with a 6F sheath. Anticoagulation is administered during the procedure, usually with unfractionated heparin (UFH) with an activated clotting time (ACT) goal of >250 seconds. A loading dose of aspirin is also recommended. Continuous monitoring of vital parameters is done throughout the procedure.

Once the renal artery is cannulated, an angiography with diluted contrast is performed to evaluate the anatomy of the renal arteries. It is also important to delineate the outline of the kidneys to decide how deep to go with the catheter. The ablation catheter is subsequently placed in the distal segment of the renal artery under fluoroscopic guidance. The branches are ablated first and then the main renal artery.

The Medtronic G3 generator algorithm controls the RF energy delivery. One ablation run lasts for 60 seconds and one can achieve four RF ablations with one run.

The catheter is retracted by at least 5 mm and the tip rotated by 90 after each RF ablation application, starting from the distal branch of the main renal artery to the ostium. Multiple (four to six) RF applications are used depending on the length of the artery to provide circumferential disruption of sympathetic nerves. The same procedure is then repeated on the other renal artery.

Figure 2 is a diagrammatic representation of the Symplicity Spyral™ catheter within a renal artery and **Flowchart 1** shows a summary of the procedure steps as described above.

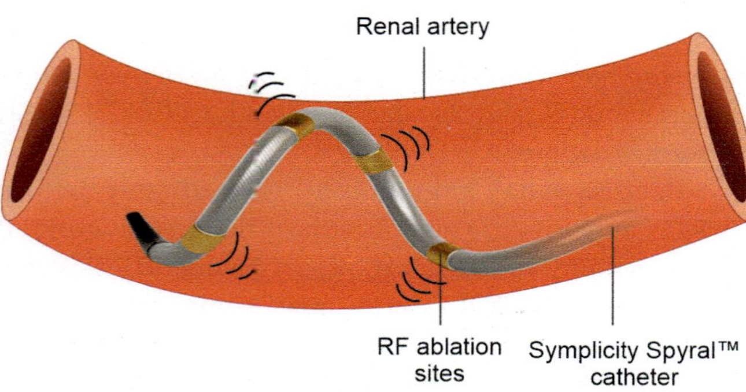

Fig. 2: Diagrammatic representation of the Symplicity Spyral™ catheter within a renal artery. (RF: radiofrequency)

Flowchart 1: Steps involved in renal denervation (RDN).

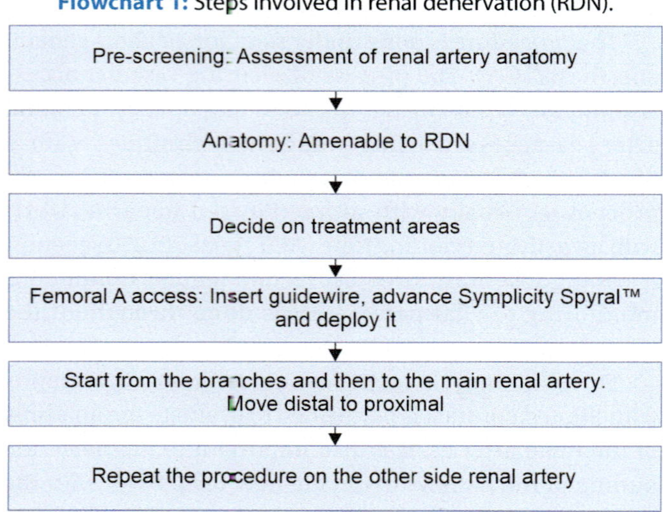

Postprocedure care:
- Patients are observed for any local complications at the groin access. This may involve overnight stay.
- Patients should maintain their existing antihypertensive medications. They should be informed that BP will not come down immediately but over the next 2–3 months.
- Regular follow-up at 1, 3, 6, and 12 months post procedure
- Regular monitoring of office as well as home BP
- Ultrasound screening at 6 months and 1 year to check for renal artery stenosis

The ultrasound RDN system involves a set of ultrasound emitting sources that are mounted on a catheter with an inflatable balloon system allowing irrigation of the portion in contact with the arterial wall.

The third approach involves using a small catheter with three concentrically placed microneedles embedded in it. After positioning the catheter appropriately, the microneedles are extended, thereby penetrating the renal artery wall and a small amount of neurotoxin (usually around 0.6 mL of absolute ethanol) is injected around the sympathetic nerves in the perivascular space.

COMPLICATIONS

Although the overall rates of complications are low, some of the described complications with RDN are as follows:

Immediate complications:[7]
- Bradycardia during the application of RF energy
- Postprocedure vasovagal syncope, hypotension
- Renal artery vasospasm
- Renal artery thrombosis (usually microthrombus)
- Access-site vascular injury, access site hematoma, femoral pseudoaneurysm
- Renal artery dissection/perforation

Late complications:
- Renal artery stenosis
- Acute kidney injury
- Failure to achieve BP reduction

Nonresponder rate with RDN is around one third as per the RCT data. But predicting who would and who would not benefit from the procedure is difficult. Patients with higher systolic BP tend to respond better to therapy (Wilder's principle).

In addition, as RDN targets the sympathetic system, some markers of higher sympathetic activity may suggest better response to therapy. These include higher resting heart rate, orthostatic HTN, and higher nocturnal BPs. Some studies have also shown association with sleep apnea, obesity, and plasma renin activity.

CONTRAINDICATIONS

Some patients may be unsuitable for RDN. Some of the relative and absolute contraindications are as follows:

- Patients with eGFR <40 mL/min/1.73 m^2. Most of the trials have used eGFR between 45 and 40 mL/min/1.73 m^2 as the cutoff.
- Patients requiring dialysis
- HTN secondary to renal artery stenosis and those with renal artery diameter <3 mm (although the trials performed with the Symplicity Spyral system did not exclude patients with smaller vessel sizes)
- Secondary HTN from causes such as pregnancy, primary aldosteronism, or valvular heart disease (therefore a thorough workup of secondary causes is mandatory)
- Structural abnormalities of the kidney
- Renal transplant recipients
- Patients with fibromuscular dysplasia
- Single functioning kidney

The overall rates of renal artery-related complications post RDN are low as seen in a meta-analysis of 50 trials that included a total population of 5,769 patients and 10,249 patient-years of data, wherein the annual incidence of renal artery stenting following RF RDN was 0.20%, which is comparable to the reported natural incidence of events in an untreated hypertensive population.[8]

GUIDELINES

As per the European Society of Cardiology (ESC) guidelines 2024, RDN can be considered as an additional treatment option in patients with resistant HTN with BP uncontrolled on three drugs or with increased cardiovascular disease (CVD) risk and uncontrolled BP or fewer than three antihypertensives (Class IIB and IIA indications, respectively) provided the patients express a desire for the procedure after a shared risk-benefit discussion and multidisciplinary assessment.[9]

CONCLUSION

With an increasing burden of poorly controlled HTN globally, RDN has emerged as an important modality in the treatment armamentarium of HTN. It is important to have a shared decision-making, taking into account the perspectives of patients and a multidisciplinary team of healthcare professionals while selecting candidates for RDN.

As healthcare professionals treating HTN and interventionalists, it is important to be familiar with the procedure, to provide the maximum benefit to the right patient.

REFERENCES

1. Krum H, Schlaich M, Whitbourn R, Sobotka PA, Sadowski J, Bartus K, et al. Catheter-based renal sympathetic denervation for resistant hypertension: a multicentre safety and proof-of-principle cohort study. Lancet. 2009;373:1275-81.
2. Kandzari DE, Mahfoud F, Bhatt DL, Böhm M, Weber MA, Townsend RR, et al. Confounding factors in renal denervation trials: revisiting old and identifying new challenges in trial design of device therapies for hypertension. Hypertension. 2020;76:1410-7.
3. Mahfoud F, Mancia G, Schmieder R, Narkiewicz K, Ruilope L, Schlaich M, et al. (2020). Three-year safety and efficacy in the Global Symplicity Registry: Impact of anti-hypertensive medication burden on blood pressure reduction. [online] Available from https://media.pcronline.com/diapos/PCReCourse2020/172-20200625_1611_Abstracts_and_Cases_Corner_Mahfoud_Felix_0000_(672)/Mahfoud_Felix_20200625_1600_Community_channel_4.pdf [Last accessed June, 2025].
4. Ahmad Y, Kane C, Arnold AD, Cook CM, Keene D, Shun-Shin M, et al. Randomized blinded placebo controlled trials of renal sympathetic denervation for hypertension: a meta-analysis. Cardiovasc Revasc Med. 2022;34:112-8.
5. Kandzari DE, Townsend RR, Bakris G, Basile J, Bloch MJ, Cohen DL, et al. Renal denervation in hypertension patients: proceedings from an expert consensus roundtable cosponsored by SCAI and NKF. Catheter Cardiovasc Interv. 2021;98(3):416-26.
6. Schmieder RE, Högerl K, Jung S, Bramlage P, Veelken R, Ott C. Patient preference for therapies in hypertension: a cross-sectional survey of German patients. Clin Res Cardiol. 2019;108:1331-42.
7. Reyes KRL, Rader F. Long-Term Safety and Antihypertensive Effects of Renal Denervation: Current Insights. Integr Blood Press Control. 2023;16:59-70.
8. Townsend RR, Walton A, Hettrick DA, Hickey GL, Well J, Sharp ASW, et al. Review and metaanalysis of renal artery damage following percutaneous renal denervation with radiofrequency renal artery ablation. EuroIntervention. 2020;16:89-96.
9. McEvoy JW, McCarthy CP, Bruno RM, Brouwers S, Canavan MD, Ceconi C, et al.; ESC Scientific Document Group. 2024 ESC guidelines for the management of elevated blood pressure and hypertension: Developed by the task force on the management of elevated blood pressure and hypertension of the European Society of Cardiology (ESC) and endorsed by the European Society of Endocrinology (ESE) and the European Stroke Organisation (ESO). Eur Heart J. 2024;45(38):391218.

SECTION 9

Point-of-Care Ultrasound

CHAPTER 38

Point-of-Care Ultrasound for Fluid Status Assessment

ET Arun Thomas

POINT-OF-CARE ULTRASOUND FOR FLUID STATUS ASSESSMENT IN ACUTE KIDNEY INJURY

Fluid management in critically ill patients with acute kidney injury (AKI) has traditionally relied on clinical assessment. However, clinical signs alone can be misleading, particularly in complex scenarios such as sepsis-related AKI. Hypoalbuminemia and increased capillary permeability in sepsis often result in edema and third-space fluid accumulation. Despite the apparent fluid overload, intravascular volume depletion may persist, leading to worsening AKI and uncorrected hypotension. Acute respiratory distress syndrome (ARDS), commonly seen in sepsis, can further complicate the clinical picture. Crepitations and hypoxia on examination may be misinterpreted as pulmonary edema, prompting undue fluid restriction. This can exacerbate hypovolemia and worsen outcomes. These challenges in clinical assessment necessitate precise tools for evaluating fluid status, and point-of-care ultrasound (POCUS) emerges as an invaluable modality for this purpose. The advent of portable ultrasound devices and the relatively short learning curve for POCUS have revolutionized bedside fluid management. POCUS provides real-time, noninvasive, and repeatable insights into fluid status, aiding in the development of tailored treatment strategies.

KEY POCUS TECHNIQUES FOR FLUID ASSESSMENT

Inferior Vena Cava Assessment

The inferior vena cava (IVC) is a central vein that reflects intravascular volume status and right atrial pressure, making it a vital parameter in fluid assessment. Ultrasound evaluation of the IVC is noninvasive, readily available, and easy to perform at the bedside, especially in critically ill patients.[1] For assessment, a curvilinear or cardiac (phased-array) probe can be used. The probe should be placed just below the xiphisternum, angled slightly upward to visualize the right atrium, and slightly toward the right side, as the IVC lies to the right of the midline, while the aorta lies to the left **(Fig. 1)**.

At times, obtaining a clear view of the IVC from the subxiphoid window may be challenging; in such cases, the IVC can be visualized from the mid-axillary line as an alternative. The IVC diameter should be measured at the point where the hepatic vein joins the IVC, or approximately 2 cm below the right atrium, to ensure standardization and consistency **(Fig. 2)**.

An IVC diameter >2 cm is generally considered indicative of a higher volume status. One key limitation in IVC assessment is the cylinder tangential effect, which

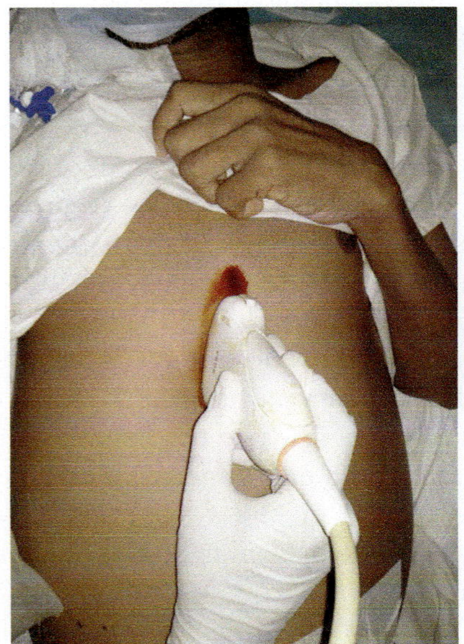

Fig. 1: Positioning of ultrasound probe for inferior vena cava (IVC) assessment.

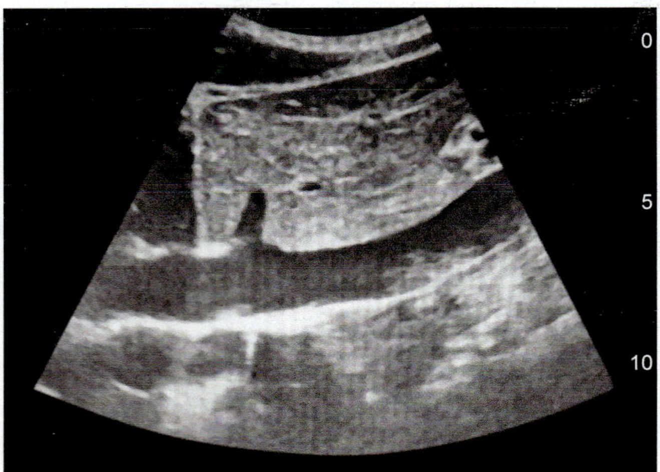

Fig. 2: Inferior vena cava (IVC) imaging showing the hepatic vein joining the IVC.

refers to the geometric distortion that occurs when a cylindrical structure like the IVC is imaged off-axis. This can lead to underestimation or overestimation of the true diameter. This issue is further compounded by operator dependency and variable patient anatomy.

The Inferior Vena Cava Collapsibility Index (IVCCI) offers an improvement by integrating multiple measurements—namely the maximum and minimum diameters during respiration—and standardizing the approach to reduce tangential error, thereby providing a more reliable assessment of dynamic changes. IVCCI is calculated as: IVCCI = [(Maximum diameter – Minimum diameter)/Minimum diameter] × 100.[2]

In spontaneously breathing patients, the maximum diameter is typically seen during expiration and the minimum diameter during inspiration. In mechanically ventilated patients, this pattern is reversed, with the maximum diameter observed during inspiration. Therefore, in ventilated patients, the index is more appropriately referred to as the IVC distensibility index.

To calculate IVCCI, once the IVC is clearly visualized, M-mode should be employed. The M-mode cursor line is placed at the point where the hepatic vein joins the IVC. This provides a one-dimensional image over time (with time plotted on the *x*-axis), allowing accurate measurement of the maximum and minimum diameters at that location.

An IVCCI >50% in the setting of critical illness, especially sepsis, is considered indicative of volume depletion and may necessitate fluid resuscitation. If the index is <30%, the IVC is considered adequately filled, and a restrictive fluid strategy should be considered. Decisions in cases where the index falls between 30 and 50% should be individualized.

However, IVC measurements alone may lead to errors in volume status assessment due to inherent limitations. These include reduced reliability in conditions such as right heart failure, presence of a kinked IVC, cylinder tangential effect, difficulty in IVC visualization, and tachypnea, where respiratory fluctuations make IVCCI measurement challenging and less dependable.

Case 1: A 38-year-old renal allograft recipient with a baseline serum creatinine of 1.0 mg/dL was admitted with a 3-day history of fever, chills, lethargy, and decreased urine output, progressing to anuria at the time of admission. On presentation, his blood pressure was 90/60 mm Hg, heart rate was 112/min, and there was no peripheral edema. Graft site tenderness was noted, but the chest was clear on auscultation. Laboratory investigations revealed a serum creatinine of 5.7 mg/dL, blood urea of 186 mg/dL, sodium of 128 mEq/L, and potassium of 4.2 mEq/L. POCUS showed a fully collapsing IVC **(Fig. 3)**. The patient was started on piperacillin-tazobactam, and fluid resuscitation was initiated with hourly monitoring of IVC parameters. In the first 6 hours, the patient received 8 L of crystalloids, with a total of 14 L administered over the first 24 hours. Following this, the IVC became less collapsible **(Fig. 4)**, urine output improved to 100 mL/h, and renal function began to recover. Dialysis was not required. Administering 14 L of fluids to an anuric patient with AKI would have been difficult to justify based solely on clinical assessment a couple of decades ago. In this case, objective assessment using IVC measurements via POCUS provided the treating team with the confidence to proceed with aggressive fluid resuscitation.

Carotid Artery Flow Assessment

Carotid artery peak systolic velocity (PSV) variability is a dynamic marker of fluid responsiveness, particularly in mechanically ventilated patients. During positive-pressure ventilation, intrathoracic pressure fluctuations influence venous return, stroke volume, and, consequently, carotid artery flow. These changes manifest as variations in carotid PSV, which can be measured using Doppler ultrasound. A significant variation in PSV during the respiratory cycle suggests that cardiac output is sensitive to preload changes, indicating fluid responsiveness.

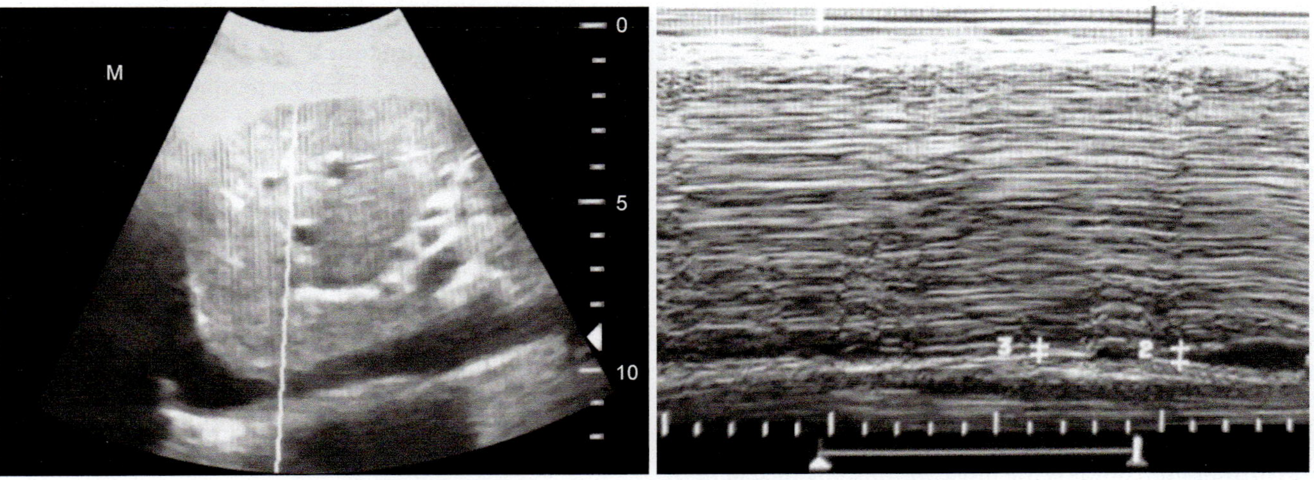

Fig. 3: Fully collapsing inferior vena cava (IVC) before fluid resuscitation.

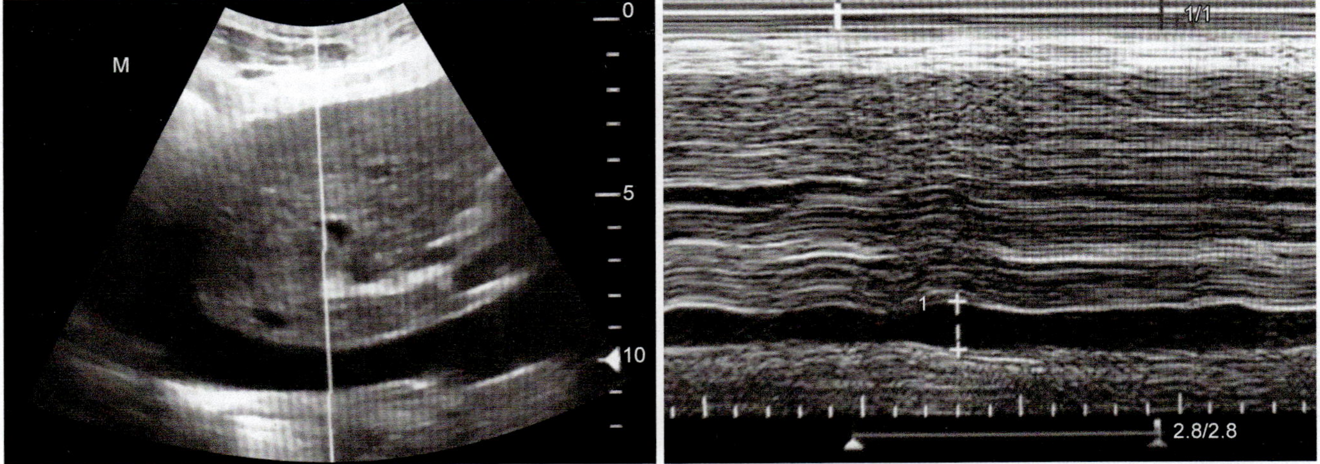

Fig. 4: Inferior vena cava (IVC) after 14 L of crystalloid administration.

The ease of accessing the carotid artery and the reproducibility of Doppler measurements make this an attractive tool for bedside assessment, especially in hemodynamically unstable patients.[3]

Passive leg raise (PLR) is a reversible maneuver that mimics a fluid bolus by transiently increasing venous return and preload. A rise in carotid PSV and a reduction in its variability following PLR confirm fluid responsiveness, guiding the clinician to administer fluids only when necessary. This dynamic assessment reduces the risks associated with blind fluid administration, such as volume overload and tissue edema—both detrimental in conditions like sepsis and AKI.[4] Moreover, unlike central venous pressure (CVP) or other static preload measures, carotid PSV variability provides real-time, actionable insights, making it a critical component of modern fluid management strategies.

Carotid PSV variability is measured using Doppler ultrasound, with the probe placed on the neck to visualize the common carotid artery. The clinician positions the probe at an appropriate angle to ensure an optimal Doppler signal, taking care to avoid excessive pressure that could distort the measurements. PSV is recorded during both inspiration and expiration over three consecutive respiratory cycles to account for variability. The percentage variation is calculated using the formula: PSV variability (%) = [(PSVmax − PSVmin)/PSVmean] × 100, where PSVmax is the peak velocity during expiration, PSVmin is the peak velocity during inspiration, and PSVmean is the average of both. A threshold value, typically around 10–15%, is used to identify significant variability indicative of fluid responsiveness.

Case 2: A 65-year-old female with long-standing diabetes was under care in the medical intensive care unit (ICU) for urosepsis and oliguric AKI. During her ICU stay, her blood pressure dropped suddenly. The IVCCI was 30%. There was uncertainty about whether to initiate noradrenaline or administer a fluid bolus. The hesitation in giving a fluid bolus stemmed from the patient's oliguric state and relatively low IVCCI, raising concerns about the risk of pulmonary edema. To aid decision-making, carotid artery PSV variability was assessed and found to be 16% **(Fig. 5)**. This indicates that the hypotension is preload responsive, and further fluid bolus is the most appropriate next action.

Lung Ultrasound

Lung ultrasound (LUS) has become a vital tool in the point-of-care evaluation of fluid status, particularly due to its ability to detect B-lines—vertical, hyperechoic artifacts that arise from the pleural line and extend to the bottom of the ultrasound screen without fading. These artifacts move synchronously with lung sliding and are generated by the interaction of ultrasound waves with fluid-filled or thickened interlobular septa. The presence of B-lines serves as an indirect but reliable marker of pulmonary interstitial fluid accumulation, making them especially useful in detecting pulmonary congestion, alveolar edema, and various interstitial lung processes.[5]

Lung ultrasound for B-line assessment can be performed using a linear, curvilinear, or phased-array probe, selected based on the patient's body habitus and the depth of the target structures. The probe is typically placed in an intercostal space with a perpendicular orientation to obtain a clear view of the pleural line and the underlying lung parenchyma. B-lines appear as vertical, laser-like, hyperechoic artifacts that obliterate the normally seen horizontal A-lines and move with respiration. Their appearance and distribution provide valuable information regarding lung aeration and fluid status.

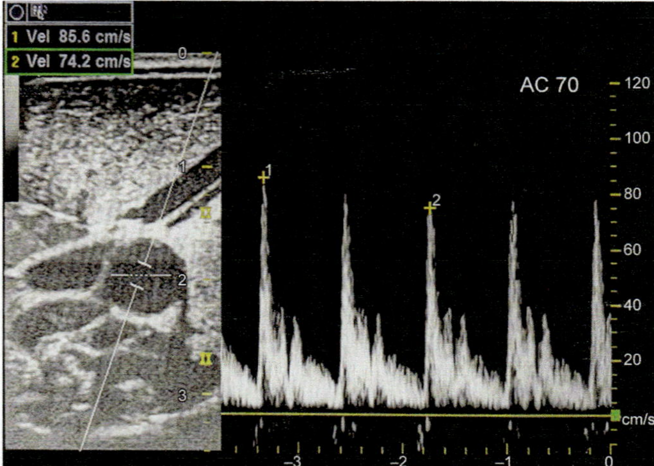

Fig. 5: Doppler ultrasound image showing carotid artery peak systolic velocity (PSV) variability. The measured PSV variability is 16%.

Several scanning protocols are available to standardize the assessment of B-lines. The eight-zone protocol is commonly used for rapid bedside evaluations and involves scanning two anterior and two lateral zones on each hemithorax. See **Figure 6A to H**, which demonstrates significant lung congestion with a notable number of B-lines in an eight-zone LUS. This protocol offers a balance between speed and clinical utility. In contrast, the 28-zone protocol includes anterior, lateral, and posterior lung fields for a more comprehensive evaluation and is often utilized in research settings or when detailed quantification of pulmonary involvement is required.

Quantifying B-lines allows clinicians to stratify the severity of pulmonary congestion. A scoring system that can be used for routine practice assign:

- 0 for no B-lines
- 1 for 1–5 B-lines (mild congestion)
- 2 for six or more B-lines in a zone (moderate congestion)
- 3 for coalescent B-lines or a "white lung" pattern (severe congestion)

Summing the scores across all scanned zones yields a total congestion score, which can be tracked over time to monitor fluid status and guide therapy.

Despite its utility, B-line assessment has limitations and potential pitfalls. It is highly operator-dependent, with variability in probe handling and image interpretation affecting diagnostic accuracy. The choice of probe also influences findings: Low-frequency probes may miss subtle B-lines, while high-frequency probes can exaggerate artifacts. Additionally, in conditions such as pneumothorax or pleural adhesions, where lung sliding is absent, B-lines may not be visualized—even in the presence of interstitial fluid. Patient positioning, particularly in obese or supine individuals, can also alter fluid distribution and affect B-line detection. Importantly, the presence of B-lines is not specific to pulmonary congestion. They may also be observed in several other conditions:

- Pulmonary fibrosis, where thickened interlobular septa create diffuse B-lines

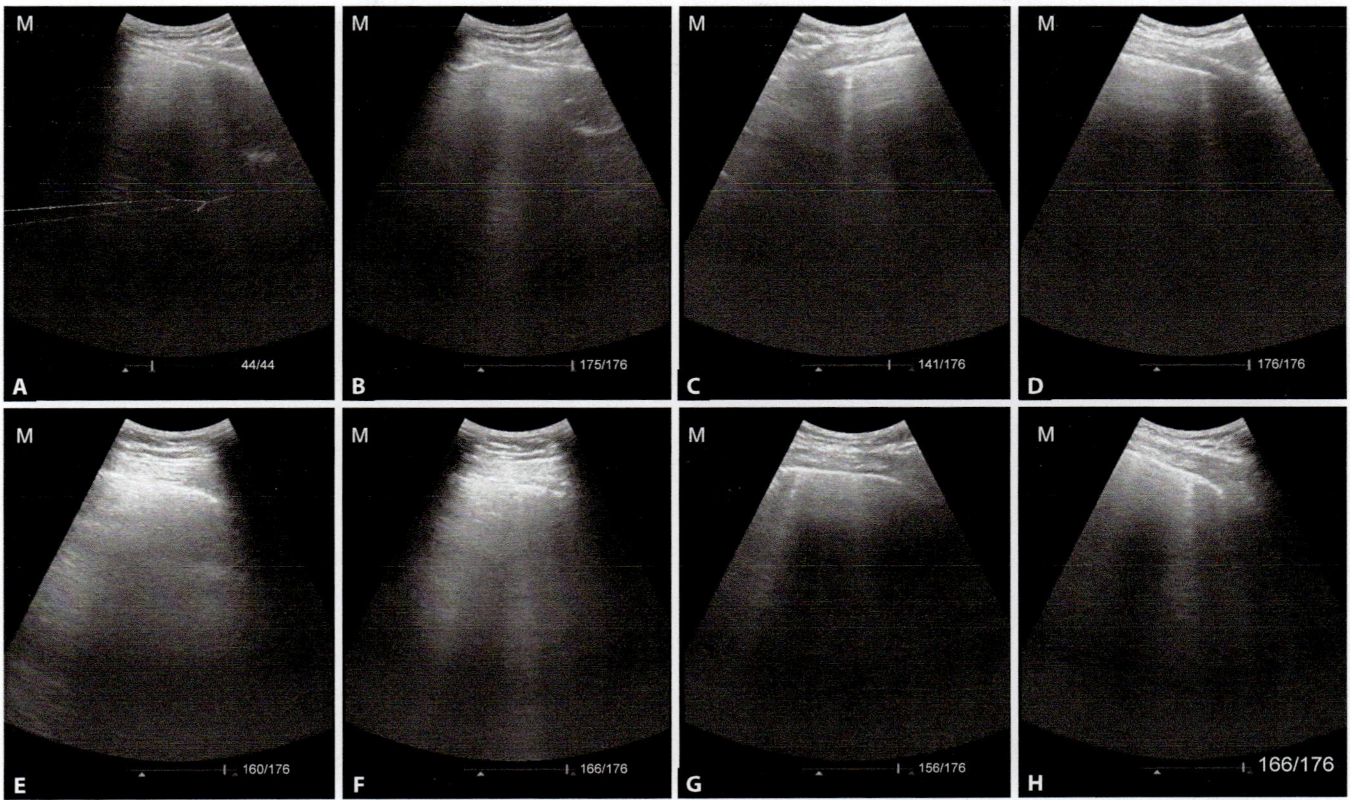

Figs. 6A to H: Lung ultrasound image demonstrating multiple B-lines in anterior and lateral lung zones, consistent with significant pulmonary congestion.

- ARDS, which often shows heterogeneous distribution
- Infectious pneumonia, where localized B-lines appear adjacent to areas of consolidation
- Pulmonary contusion, from post-traumatic interstitial edema
- Elderly or obese individuals, where mild B-lines may occur without significant pathology

Therefore, the clinical context and distribution pattern of B-lines are critical for accurate interpretation.

From a fluid management perspective, B-lines provide dynamic insights that inform clinical decisions. In hypovolemic patients, the absence or minimal presence of B-lines suggests preserved lung aeration and supports safe fluid resuscitation. However, serial assessments are necessary to detect early signs of pulmonary congestion. In contrast, numerous or coalescent B-lines indicate interstitial or alveolar fluid accumulation, warranting fluid restriction and consideration of diuretic therapy. This is particularly relevant in patients with heart failure or AKI, where fluid overload can worsen respiratory compromise.

One of the greatest strengths of LUS in fluid status assessment lies in its utility for serial, dynamic monitoring. Following a fluid challenge, a sudden increase in B-lines may signal emerging congestion and prompt reassessment of the fluid strategy. Conversely, a reduction in B-lines after diuretic therapy supports the effectiveness of decongestive treatment and informs decisions about continuing or adjusting therapy.

Venous Excess Ultrasound Score

The Venous Excess Ultrasound Score (VExUS) is an ultrasound-based tool designed to assess systemic venous congestion and its effects on end-organ perfusion, particularly in critically ill patients. By examining venous Doppler flow patterns in the hepatic, portal, and renal veins, VExUS provides insight into elevated right atrial pressure and its downstream consequences. This scoring system helps identify venous congestion that may compromise kidney function, liver perfusion, or gastrointestinal integrity, allowing clinicians to tailor fluid therapy accordingly.[6]

VExUS is performed using a low-frequency curvilinear or phased-array probe. The hepatic vein and IVC are visualized from a subxiphoid view **(Fig. 7)**, the portal vein is imaged from the right mid-abdomen, where a glistening white halo can be seen around the portal vein for identification **(Fig. 8)**, and the renal veins are typically assessed from the flank, depending on the patient's anatomy and acoustic windows. Doppler interrogation of these vessels is central to the VExUS protocol. In the hepatic vein, normal triphasic waveforms progressively become biphasic or monophasic as venous congestion increases. The portal vein, which normally exhibits continuous forward flow, becomes pulsatile or phasic in the setting of elevated right-sided pressures. Similarly, the renal vein normally shows continuous forward flow, but with worsening congestion, the waveform may become biphasic or even show flow reversal. As the renal vein always accompanies the renal artery, the measurement is usually taken at the site of the artery, with the waveform below the baseline being taken from the renal vein, as arterial and venous flow are in opposite directions **(Fig. 9)**. VExUS is graded based on IVC diameter and the severity of abnormal Doppler patterns **(Table 1)**.

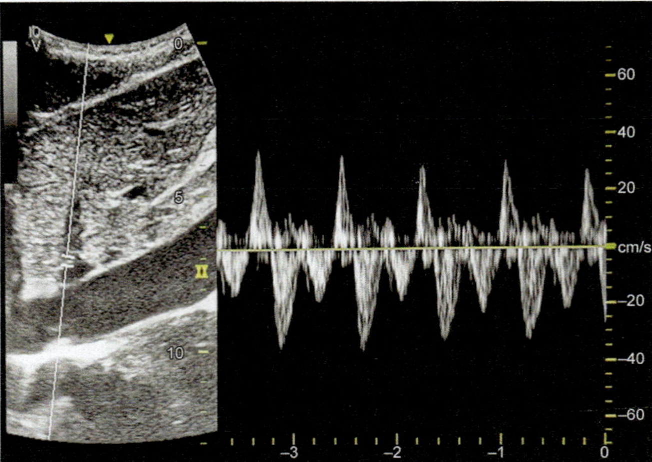

Fig. 7: Subxiphoid view of the hepatic vein and inferior vena cava (IVC) using Doppler ultrasound. The IVC diameter is assessed to evaluate venous congestion.

In fluid management, VExUS serves as a valuable guide. A high VExUS reflects advanced systemic venous congestion and signals the need to avoid further fluid loading, as continued fluid administration may exacerbate organ dysfunction. In such cases, fluid restriction or active decongestive measures—such as diuretics or ultrafiltration—may be warranted. Conversely, a low VExUS indicates minimal congestion, suggesting that fluid resuscitation can be considered safer in the appropriate clinical context. Thus, VExUS helps clinicians decide when to halt or escalate fluid therapy based on the patient's current hemodynamic state.[7]

Beyond guiding fluid administration, VExUS enables ongoing monitoring of treatment responses. Serial assessments allow for dynamic evaluation of venous

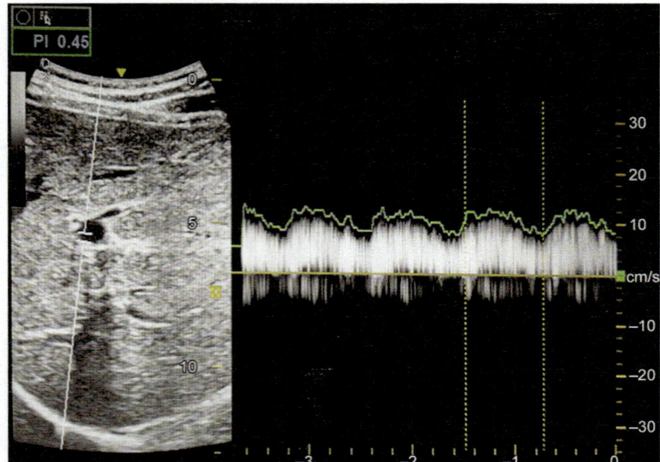

Fig. 8: Doppler ultrasound of the portal vein in the right mid-abdomen, with a glistening white halo around the portal vein for identification. Pulsatile or phasic flow indicates elevated right-sided pressures.

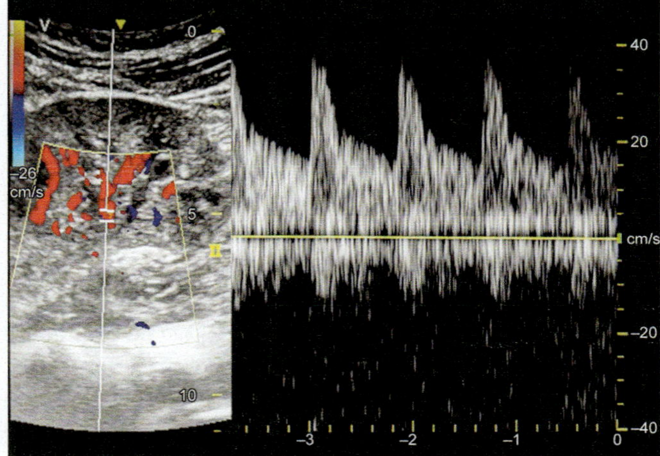

Fig. 9: Doppler ultrasound of the renal veins, with measurement taken at the site of the renal artery. The waveform below the baseline represents venous flow, as arterial and venous flow move in opposite directions.

TABLE 1: Venous Excess Ultrasound Score grading integrates inferior vena cava (IVC) size with Doppler patterns from the hepatic, portal, and renal veins to assess the degree of systemic venous congestion.

IVC findings	*Hepatic vein Doppler*	*Portal vein Doppler*	*Renal vein Doppler*	*Interpretation*
IVC <2 cm or collapsible	Not assessed or normal	Not assessed or normal	Not assessed or normal	No venous congestion
IVC >2 cm with minimal respiratory variation	Normal triphasic waveform	Continuous monophasic flow	Continuous flow	Mild congestion
IVC >2 cm	S wave < D wave (dampened biphasic)	Pulsatile flow, pulsatility index >30%	Biphasic or mildly discontinuous flow	Moderate congestion
IVC >2 cm	Reversed S wave (retrograde systolic flow)	Markedly pulsatile or biphasic, pulsatility index >50%	Monophasic or absent diastolic flow	Severe congestion

Note: Pulsatility index for portal vein is calculated as (Vmax – Vmin)/Vmax × 100. The VeXUS score grades venous congestion from 0 to 3, where Grade 0 indicates an IVC <2 cm (no congestion), Grade 1 indicates an IVC ≥2 cm with only normal or mildly abnormal Doppler patterns (mild congestion), Grade 2 indicates an IVC ≥2 cm with one severely abnormal Doppler pattern (moderate congestion), and Grade 3 indicates an IVC ≥2 cm with two or more severely abnormal Doppler patterns (severe congestion).

congestion, facilitating the fine-tuning of fluid and diuretic therapy to maintain optimal volume status. This is particularly relevant in patients with conditions such as AKI, heart failure, or sepsis, where both over- and under-resuscitation can have significant consequences. VExUS can detect early signs of venous congestion, enabling prompt intervention to prevent complications such as worsening renal function, hepatic congestion, or bowel wall edema.

Despite its benefits, VExUS has limitations. Technical challenges may arise in obese patients or those with suboptimal acoustic windows, making it difficult to obtain clear Doppler signals. As with many ultrasound techniques, VExUS is operator-dependent, requiring experience and attention to technique for accurate interpretation. Additionally, certain cardiovascular conditions—such as tricuspid regurgitation, atrial fibrillation, or chronic venous insufficiency—can alter Doppler waveforms independent of fluid status, potentially leading to misinterpretation. VExUS findings may also be influenced by rapidly changing hemodynamic states, such as during dialysis or after fluid boluses, necessitating careful correlation with the overall clinical picture.

Nonetheless, VExUS offers several compelling advantages. It provides a comprehensive and noninvasive assessment of systemic venous congestion and can be easily repeated at the bedside. By integrating VExUS into routine critical care practice, clinicians can move beyond static volume assessments to gain a more nuanced understanding of venous hemodynamics. This enables individualized fluid strategies aimed at ensuring adequate perfusion while avoiding the detrimental effects of venous congestion, ultimately improving patient outcomes in complex fluid management scenarios.

CONCLUSION

An ideal approach to fluid status assessment in clinical practice should not rely solely on a single modality. Instead, it should be multifaceted and dynamic, integrating thorough clinical evaluation with multiple POCUS techniques, each complementing the limitations of the other. Incorporating additional physiological markers—such as pulse pressure variation from arterial line monitoring, serum lactate levels, and capillary refill time—can further enhance accuracy. Most importantly, real-time trends and changes in these parameters should be prioritized over isolated values, as they offer a more accurate reflection of the patient's evolving hemodynamic status. This comprehensive and integrative strategy supports more precise and individualized fluid management, ultimately improving patient outcomes.

Point-of-Care Ultrasound for Dry Weight Assessment for Hemodialysis Patients

Accurate assessment of dry weight in patients undergoing hemodialysis (HD) remains a critical yet often imprecise aspect of volume management. Achieving optimal dry weight is essential to avoid both hypovolemia and fluid overload—conditions that can not only impair patient well-being but also contribute to long-term cardiovascular complications. Traditionally, dry weight is defined as the lowest postdialysis weight that is well tolerated and not associated with symptoms or signs of either volume depletion or excess. This estimation is generally based on clinical judgment and a trial-and-error approach, which can be subjective and prone to error.

In recent years, a variety of techniques have been explored to refine dry weight estimation, including online blood volume monitoring, bioimpedance spectroscopy, natriuretic peptide levels, IVC diameter measurements, and LUS. However, none of these methods have seen widespread adoption in routine clinical practice. Among patients with chronic kidney disease (CKD), asymptomatic pulmonary congestion—undetectable through standard clinical examination—is not uncommon. This subclinical congestion has been linked to increased cardiovascular morbidity and mortality, independent of traditional risk factors or CKD-specific contributors. LUS, by detecting interstitial fluid in the lungs, offers a promising solution to identifying this hidden congestion.

Combining lung and IVC ultrasound provides a more comprehensive evaluation of a patient's fluid status by assessing both extravascular and intravascular compartments. Performing this integrated POCUS assessment approximately 30 minutes post dialysis allows clinicians to evaluate the adequacy of fluid removal during the HD session. If signs of residual fluid overload persist, ultrafiltration can be increased in the subsequent session. Conversely, evidence of hypovolemia may warrant reducing fluid removal to avoid adverse effects.[8]

For this integrated assessment, a curvilinear probe (3–5 MHz) is suitable for imaging both lung fields and the IVC. LUS is performed at four points on each hemithorax—specifically, the upper and lower anterior chest along the midclavicular and midaxillary lines. The number of B-lines is counted at each site, providing a quantifiable measure of pulmonary congestion. To assess the IVC, the probe is positioned subxiphoidally, and M-mode is used to measure both maximum and minimum IVC diameters. The IVCCI is then calculated using the formula:

IVCCI = (maximum diameter – minimum diameter)/ maximum diameter, with measurements taken during a normal spontaneous respiratory cycle.

The target ultrasonographic dry weight is defined as the weight at which the total number of B-lines is fewer than four across the eight lung zones and the IVCCI falls between 50 and 75%. To achieve this target, patient dry weight is titrated by 0.5–1.0 kg across dialysis sessions based on ultrasound findings. In patients who continue to exhibit a high B-line burden (>4) despite an IVCCI of 75% or more, further evaluation with echocardiography is recommended to assess cardiac function and to rule out an underlying parenchymal lung disease.[8]

This integrated POCUS approach offers a practical, repeatable, and noninvasive method to refine dry weight estimation in HD patients. It supports individualized fluid management strategies that improve patient safety and may reduce the risk of fluid-related complications.

REFERENCES

1. Di Nicolò P, Tavazzi G, Nannoni L, Corradi F. Inferior vena cava ultrasonography for volume status evaluation: An intriguing promise never fulfilled. J Clin Med. 2023;12(6):2217.
2. Karacabey S, Sanri E, Guneysel O. A non-invasive method for assessment of intravascular fluid status: Inferior vena cava diameters and collapsibility index. Pak J Med Sci. 2016;32(4):836-40.
3. Roy A, Pachisia AV, Govil D, Kn J, Patel S, Harne R, et al. Fluid responsiveness in critically ill patients using carotid peak systolic velocity variability: A new frontier. Cureus. 2023;15(7):e42083.
4. Monnet X, Marik P, Teboul JL. Passive leg raising for predicting fluid responsiveness: a systematic review and meta-analysis. Intensive Care Med. 2016;42(12):1935-47.
5. Ciumanghel A, Siriopol I, Blaj M, Siriopol D, Gavrilovici C, Covic A. B-lines score on lung ultrasound as a direct measure of respiratory dysfunction in ICU patients with acute kidney injury. Int Urol Nephrol. 2018;50(1):113-9.
6. Longino A, Martin K, Leyba K, Siegel G, Thai TN, Riscinti M, et al. Prospective evaluation of venous excess ultrasound for estimation of venous congestion. Chest. 2024;165(3):590-600.
7. Rihl MF, Pellegrini JAS, Boniatti MM. VExUS score in the management of patients with acute kidney injury in the intensive care unit: AKIVEX Study. J Ultrasound Med. 2023;42(11):2547-56.
8. Arun Thomas ET, Mohandas MK, George J. Comparison between clinical judgment and integrated lung and inferior vena cava ultrasonography for dry weight estimation in hemodialysis patients. Hemodial Int. 2019;23(4): 494-503.

CHAPTER 39

Renal Allograft Complications and Their Management

Vel Arvind, Karthik Balasubramaniam

INTRODUCTION

Renal transplantation remains the definitive therapy for patients with end-stage kidney disease (ESKD), offering superior survival and quality of life compared to dialysis.[1] However, despite advances in surgical techniques, immunosuppression, and postoperative care, a variety of complications can compromise the function and survival of the renal allograft. Among these, vascular and urological complications are particularly significant due to their potential to cause graft dysfunction, hypertension, and even graft loss.[2-4]

The traditional management of post-transplant complications has often involved transplant surgeons and interventional radiologists. However, with the evolution of interventional nephrology as a subspecialty, nephrologists are increasingly capable of diagnosing and managing many of these complications using minimally invasive, image-guided techniques.[2,5] These procedures not only enable timely intervention but also reduce dependence on surgical solutions, particularly in resource-limited or remote settings.

This chapter focuses on transplant-related complications that can be addressed by interventional nephrologists. It excludes surgical interventions and instead emphasizes on minimally invasive approaches that can be performed by nephrologists with appropriate training. Emphasis is placed on diagnostic imaging—point-of-care ultrasound (POCUS), endovascular techniques, percutaneous procedures, and safe biopsy practices.[6] A sound understanding of transplant anatomy, imaging interpretation, and access techniques is essential to this role.[3]

ANATOMY

Most kidney transplants are placed in the right or left iliac fossa **(Figs. 1A to C)**. The right iliac fossa is preferred because of the superficial position of the iliac vessels for anastomosis. In the case of vascular irregularities, like stenosis, calcification, or other anatomical variants of the bilateral pelvic vessels, the kidney transplant can be placed in an intraperitoneal position for the anastomosis.

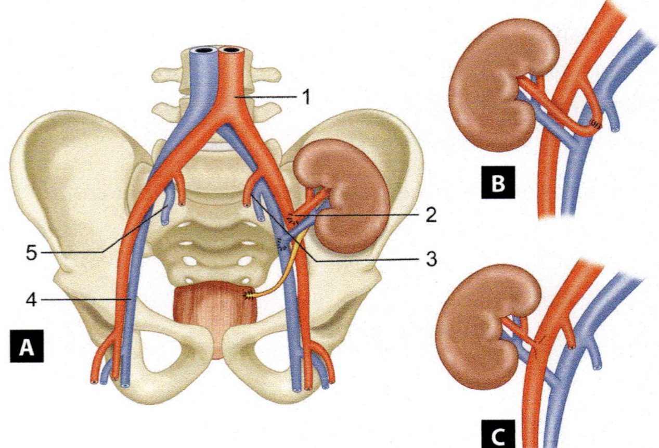

Figs. 1A to C: Anastomotic techniques for renal allograft. (A) Arterial and venous anatomy of the pelvis. 1. Aorta; 2. External Iliac artery (EIA); 3. Internal iliac artery (IIA); 4. External iliac vein; 5. Internal iliac vein (IIV); (B) End-to-end anastomosis of the internal iliac artery to renal artery; (C) End-to-side anastomosis of the external iliac artery to renal artery.

The anastomosis of the transplant renal artery is end-to-side anastomosis between the transplant artery and the external iliac artery of the recipient, or end-to-end anastomosis between the transplant artery and the internal iliac artery is used.[2] In the case of organs from deceased donors, the renal artery of the donor together with part of the aorta (Carrel patch) is typically connected to the external iliac artery of the recipient in an end-to-side anastomosis.[3]

The venous anastomosis is usually made end to side between the transplant renal vein and the external iliac vein of the recipient.[2] The ureteral anastomosis is typically made by implanting the transplant ureter in the bladder through a muscle tunnel in the bladder wall (ureteroneocystostomy).[1,2]

IMAGING AND INTERPRETATIONS

POCUS plays a crucial role in monitoring renal transplant (Tx) recipients to promptly assess potential complications at the bedside. It offers a noninvasive and easily accessible way to provide immediate and real-time information on both immediate postoperative concerns and long-term issues.

It enables swift diagnosis, guides interventions, and allows for dynamic monitoring of complications.[7] However, it is operator dependent, has depth limitations, and may require additional imaging or procedures for confirmation of findings.[8] Types of perinephric collection are shown in **Figures 2A to D**.

Applications of POCUS in renal transplant complications:

- Collection around the graft
- Ureteric complications
- Graft rejection
- Perfusion-related complications
    - Transplant renal artery stenosis (TRAS)
    - Renal artery kinking/torsion
- Infection
- Chronic graft dysfunction

Approach to Perinephric Collection

Approach to perinephric collection is shown in **Figures 2A to D**.

Progressive increase in the size of the collection or any suggestion of infection, like fever and pain over a graft site, warrants intervention. Drainage is the best option. Mere needle aspiration is not recommended, especially repeated drainage. Continuous and complete drainage with indwelling catheters is the right way. It is prudent to take surgical help. The nature of perinephric collection is shown in **Flowchart 1**.

Ureteric Complications[1,2,9]

Urine leak: Focal or perigraft fluid collection, hypoechoic, often increasing in size on serial imaging associated with reduced urine output and signs of infection.

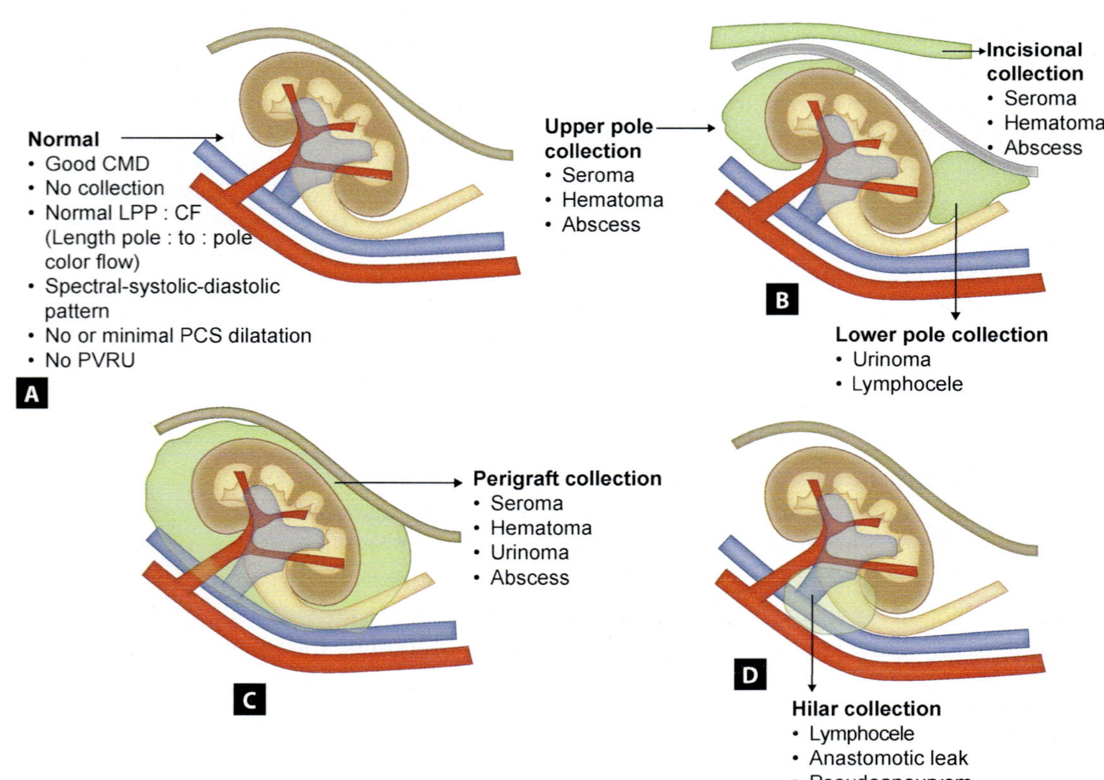

Figs. 2A to D: Types of perinephric collection.
(CMD: corticomedullary differentiation; PCS: pelvicalyceal system; PVRU: post-void residual urine)

Flowchart 1: Nature of collection.

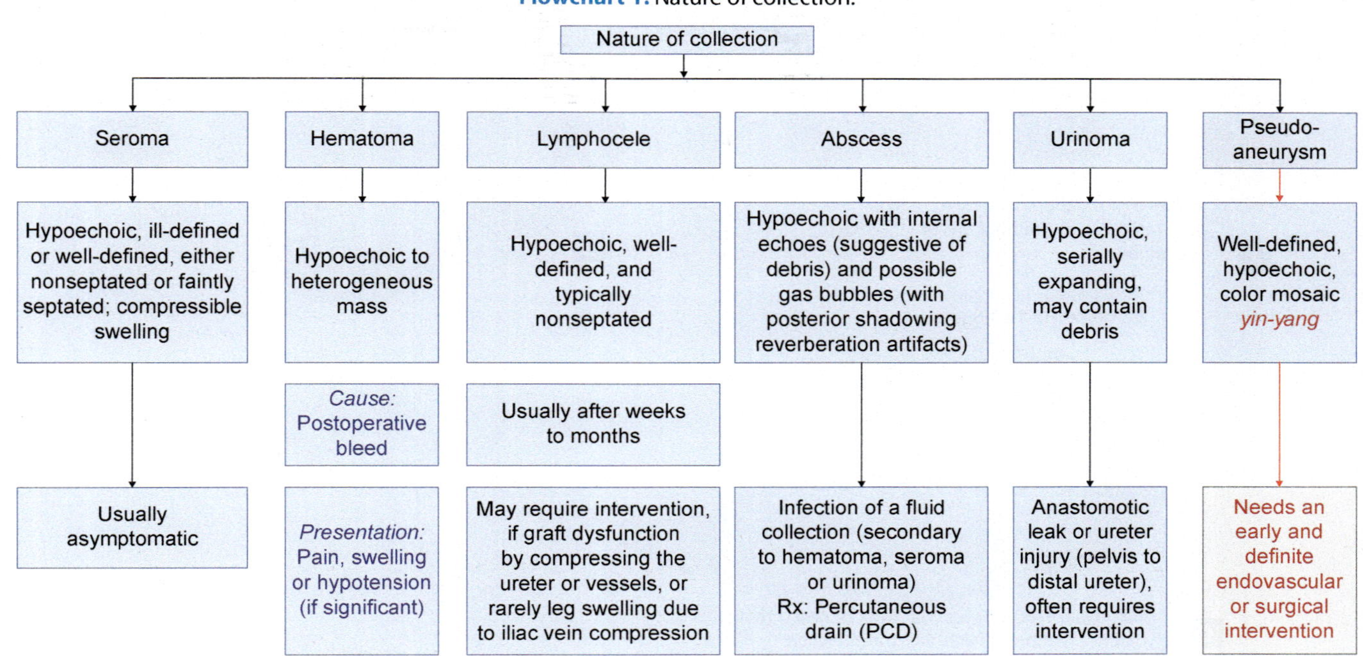

Ureteral obstruction: Hydronephrosis (dilated renal pelvis and calyces) with thinning of the renal cortex.

Ureteric complications **(Figs. 3A to C)** can be suspected and diagnosed early by interventional nephrologists given their skills in imaging by an ultrasonogram. However, the cause of obstruction is better managed by urologists.

Rejection

Diagnosing and managing rejections are the responsibility of nephrologists. Although renal biopsy is the "gold standard" for diagnosing and managing rejection, early diagnosis by various imaging methods can lead to better outcome. An interventional nephrologist, who is well trained in ultrasonogram/Doppler examination, can give a head start for early management. The various Doppler patterns seen in normal and abnormal conditions have been well observed. We prefer to describe them with names from structures and images from real life for better understanding and remembering. Studying the systolic and diastolic phases of the Doppler graph sets apart various disease states from normal. The normal pattern is described as "Nandhi pattern" **(Figs. 4A to C)**.

Acute cellular rejection:

- *Enlarged kidney:* Increased graft size due to interstitial edema and inflammation
- Increased cortical echogenicity
- Loss of corticomedullary differentiation
- Resistive index (RI) >0.8[10]

Antibody-mediated rejection:

- Enlarged kidney and increased echogenicity[11]
- *Patchy hypoechoic areas:* May indicate cortical infarcts due to microvascular injury
- *Reduced perfusion:* Indicates decreased flow in small cortical vessels
- RI >0.8

POCUS in rejection generally involves two key points:

1. Systolic phase
2. Early diastolic reversal

Contrast USG: Evaluating and fixing the cause for renal graft dysfunction continues to be a vexing problem **(Figs. 5A to C)**. Renal biopsy continues to be the gold standard.[2,12] This is a new emerging imaging modality which is a noninvasive, non-nephrotoxic, repeatable, reproducible method which can contribute to the early diagnosis.[13] Up to 50% of all rejection episodes are subclinical and occur without changes in standard parameters, such as creatinine or blood urea nitrogen. Most of these vascular insults affect small parenchymal arteries and arterioles, which cannot be assessed by conventional Doppler ultrasound.[12]

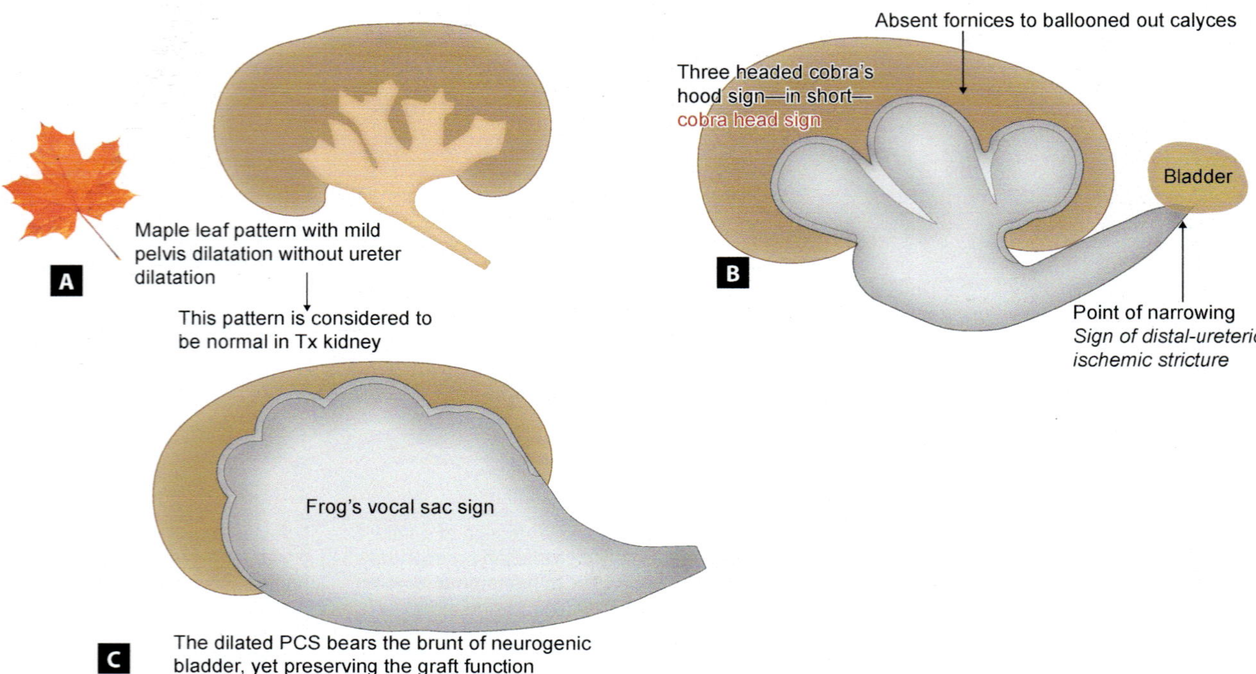

Figs. 3A to C: Ureteric dilations. (A) Maple leaf pattern: Innocent—needs only observation; (B) Cobra hood pattern: Distal ureteric stenosis—intervention is urgent; (C) Bush Frog's vocal sac sign: Gross refluxing ureter—Rx: CIC/double voiding/cholinergics.[1,2] (PCS: pelvicalyceal system)

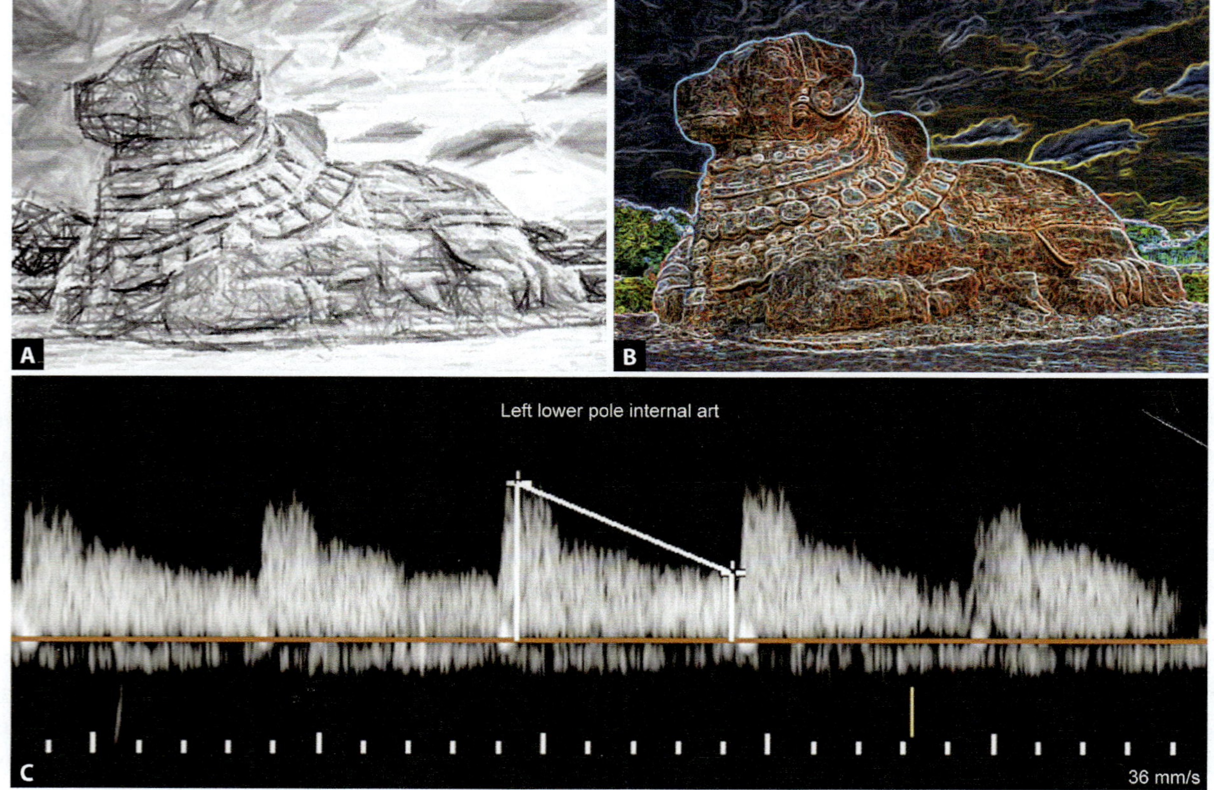

Figs. 4A to C: Nandhi patterns of normal graft.

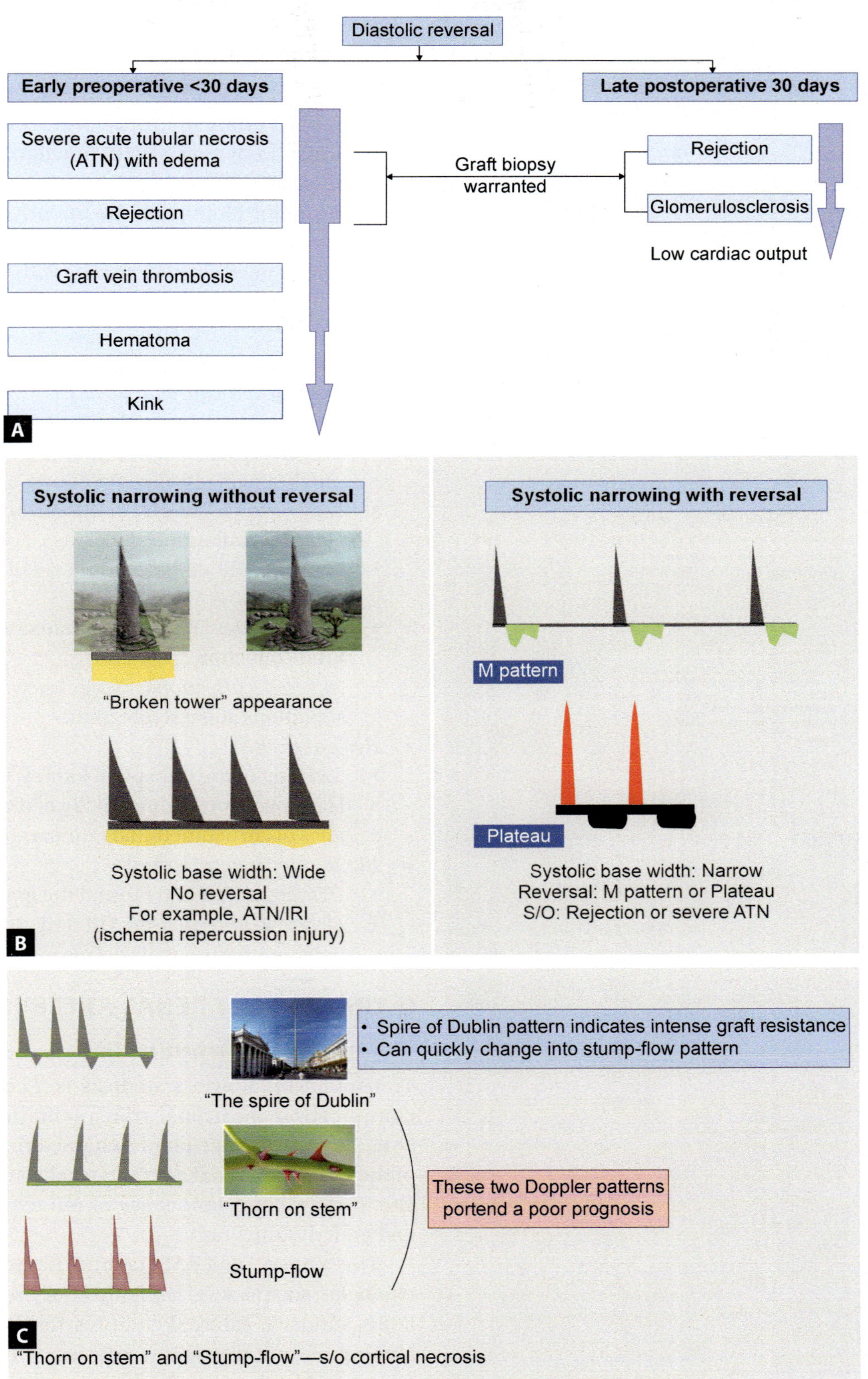

Figs. 5A to C: Doppler findings in graft dysfunction.

It might be helpful to derive early changes and evidence by evaluating renal allograft microperfusion by contrast USG. Microbubble-based contrast agents **(Fig. 6)** have lowered the detection threshold and now allow detection of blood in vessels as small as capillaries **(Video 1; Figs. 7A and B)**.

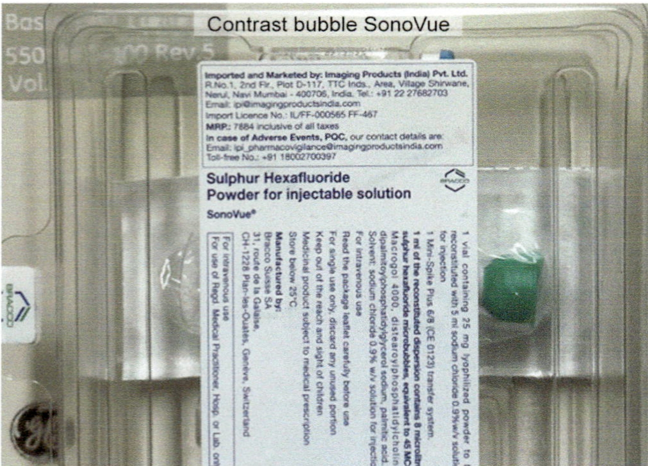

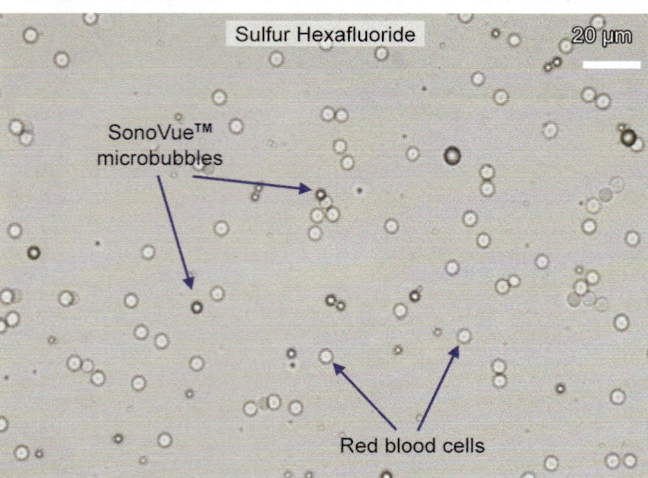

Fig. 6: Contrast agents for contrast-enhanced USG.

Advantages:
- Contrast-enhanced ultrasound clearly identifies abnormal from normal graft function.
- It appears useful to identify graft dysfunction early.
- It is used for identifying the underlying cause for the dysfunction although suggestive patterns have been noticed. It needs further studies with larger numbers.

Graft Infection

Role of POCUS in kidney transplant infection:
- *Perinephric or intrarenal abscess:*
  - Hypoechoic or complex fluid collections around the kidney or within the graft
  - Thick irregular walls, septations, or internal debris[1]
  - Increased vascularity in the surrounding tissues on Doppler (inflammation)
  - Lymphocele or hematoma turning into infected collections
  - *Lymphocele:* Hypoechoic, anechoic well-defined fluid collection
  - *Infected collections:* Irregular walls, debris, and septations suggest infection.
- *Pyelonephritis:*
  - Swelling of the transplant kidney
  - Heterogeneous echogenicity of renal parenchyma
  - Loss of corticomedullary differentiation
- *Bladder or ureteral issues:*
  - *Urinary leak:* Fluid around the graft or pelvis
  - *Ureteral obstruction:* Dilated ureter +/- dilated pelvis with echogenic debris indicating infection

TRANSPLANT RENAL ARTERY STENOSIS

Definition and Significance

Transplant renal artery stenosis is a common vascular complication[2] postrenal transplantation occurring in 3–12.5% of renal transplants, characterized by narrowing of the transplant renal artery, typically at the anastomotic site. It is an important cause of refractory hypertension and graft dysfunction.

The cause of TRAS is multifactorial, including etiologies, such as surgical clamp injury, intimal dissection, faulty suturing, external compression from fibrosis, and kinking of long transplant arteries. Other predisposing factors include increased cold ischemia time, cyclosporine toxicity, acute cellular rejection, and cytomegalovirus

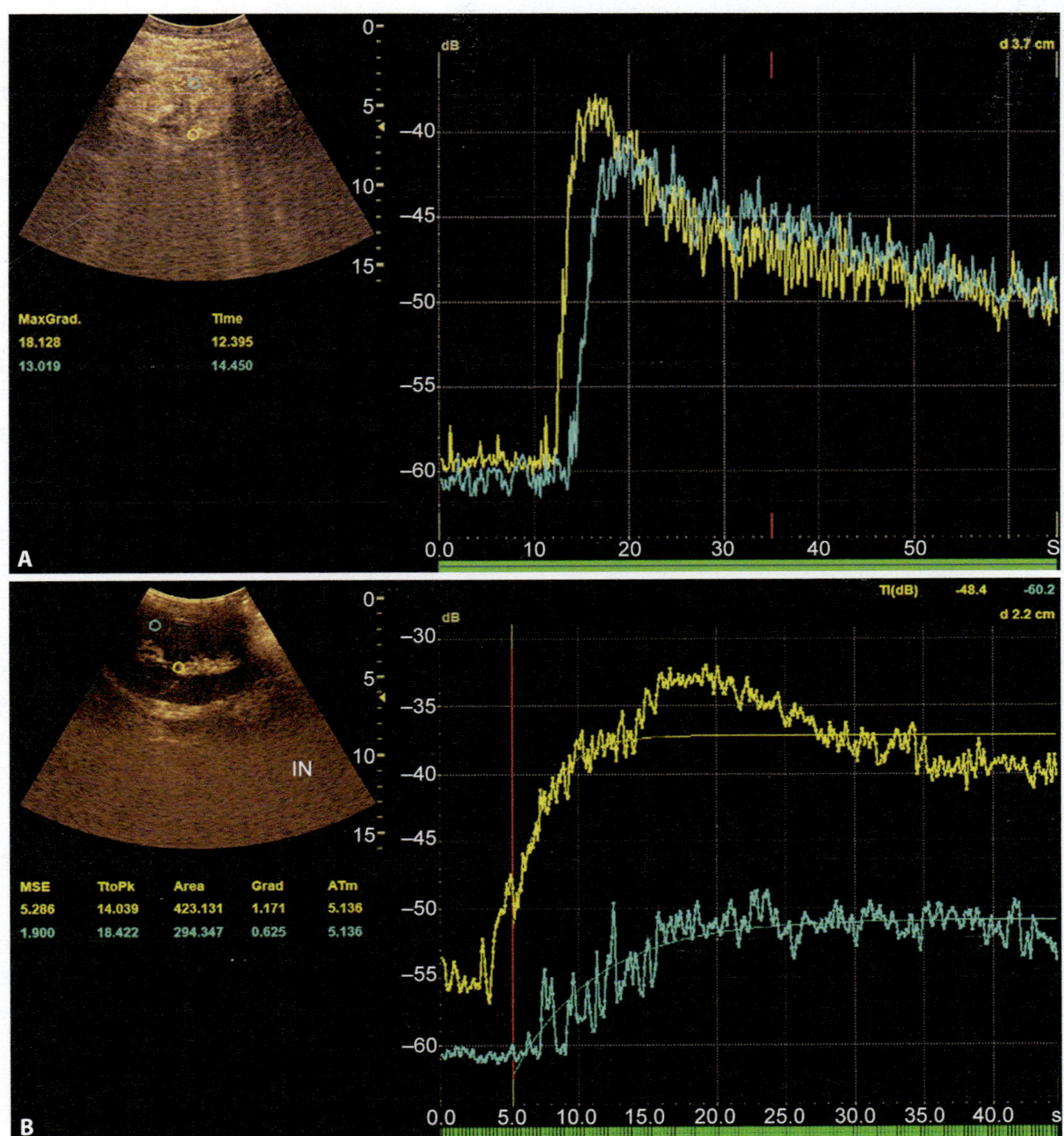

Figs. 7A and B: Normal versus abnormal contrast-enhanced USG.

(CMV) infection. Proximal TRAS refers to preexisting or developing atherosclerotic inflow stenosis in the native iliac arteries (aortoiliac atherosclerotic disease) of the transplant recipient.

Postanastomotic lesions may be related to accelerated atherosclerosis or immune-mediated vascular injury and intimal hyperplasia and may occur later after transplantation. Preanastomotic aortoiliac lesions are most commonly due to progression of occlusive atherosclerotic disease and diagnosed later after transplantation, but can also represent vessel clamp injuries, and therefore be diagnosed early.

Diagnostic Criteria for Transplant Renal Artery Stenosis

Doppler ultrasound criteria **(Fig. 8)**:

- *Peak systolic velocity (PSV) at the stenotic segment:* PSV >180–200 cm/s is suggestive of significant stenosis.
- *Renal artery velocity ratio (RAR):* RAR >3.5: Ratio of PSV in the renal artery to PSV in the external iliac artery or aorta
- *Tardus-parvus waveform:* Low-velocity, dampened waveforms in the intrarenal arteries distal to the stenosis.[8,14] Reflects delayed acceleration (upstroke)

due to proximal obstruction. Acceleration time <100 ms/s^2 and time to peak >100 ms/s^2 can be taken as practical limits to diagnose parvus tardus objectively.[8] Doppler study with these criteria not only is diagnostic of TRAS but would also indicate good reversibility following intervention.[2]

- *Poststenotic turbulence:* Increased turbulent flow seen distal to the site of narrowing

Clinical features supporting diagnosis:

- *Resistant hypertension:* Hypertension that is difficult to control despite multiple antihypertensives
- *New-onset hypertension:* Development of hypertension weeks to months after transplant
- *Graft dysfunction:* Rising serum creatinine without other clear causes + peripheral edema
- *Audible bruit:* Over the graft site, indicating turbulent blood flow[15]

Confirmatory imaging:

- CT angiography (CTA)
- MR angiography (MRA)
- *Digital subtraction angiography (DSA):* The gold standard for diagnosing TRAS
- Allows for simultaneous diagnosis and treatment via angioplasty or stenting

Diagnostic Angiography

Ipsilateral femoral access usually affords optimal lines of force for endovascular interventions when the transplant renal artery is anastomosed to the external iliac artery. Conversely, contralateral femoral access is preferred when anastomosis is between the internal iliac artery and the transplant renal artery. Either femoral access site can be used if the arterial anastomosis has been created with the abdominal aorta.

Initial angiography may be performed using carbon dioxide as a contrast agent to minimize the risk of iodinated contrast-induced nephropathy. A 4 or 5 Fr marking pigtail is advanced to the infrarenal aorta. Angiography is then repeated with iodinated contrast material in this projection.

Transplant renal artery stenosis more than 50% is considered significant and subsequent endovascular intervention is usually pursued. The *kink* acts as an elastic stenosis when treated with percutaneous transluminal angioplasty (PTA), returning to its former configuration after balloon dilation. Placement of a stent across the kink usually results in propagation of the kink to the distal or proximal edge of the stent, or worse can be complicated by incomplete expansion of the stent and worsening of preexisting obstruction. Thus, patients in whom an arterial kink is identified are referred for consideration of surgical correction.

INTERVENTIONAL MANAGEMENT

Percutaneous transluminal angioplasty: First-line minimally invasive treatment. Balloon angioplasty is performed to dilate the stenotic segment, ideally using a

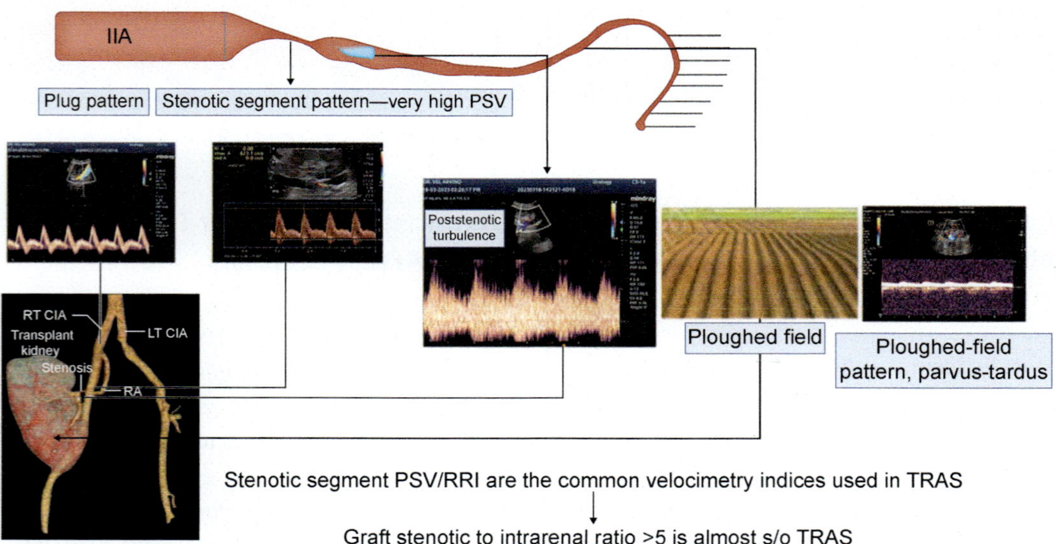

Fig. 8: Doppler findings in TRAS. (RRI: renal resistive index; PSV: peak systolic velocity; TRAS: transplant renal artery stenosis)

balloon size equal to or slightly smaller than the adjacent normal vessel segment.

Stent placement: Indicated when PTA yields suboptimal results—such as residual stenosis, vessel recoil, or recurrent narrowing. Balloon-expandable bare-metal or drug-eluting stents are deployed to maintain vessel patency.

Outcomes:

- PTA +/– stenting leads to significant improvement in blood pressure and graft function.
- Stenting achieves better long-term patency than PTA alone.
- Complications such as arterial dissection, thrombosis, or restenosis are possible but infrequent with experienced operators.
- Robust data comparing these treatment strategies in matched patients are lacking; however, lower rates of restenosis have been reported with primary stenting.

Role of an Interventional Nephrologist

Nephrologists trained in interventional techniques can perform angioplasty and stenting, often collaborating with radiology or vascular specialists. Early detection and timely intervention are critical for graft preservation.

Endovascular Intervention Procedure

Primary stent placement is technically straightforward. The patient is given 3,000–5,000 units of heparin intravenously to prevent intervention-related arterial thrombosis. Nitroglycerin is prepared at a concentration of 10 μg/mL. Vasospasm of the renal artery and its branches is not uncommon during instrumentation; nitroglycerin may be administered as needed during the procedure in aliquots of 50 μg (5 mL) to treat vasospasm.

Angioplasty balloon and stent diameters are chosen to be equal to or more than 1 mm the diameter of the normal portion of the renal artery adjacent to the stenosis. A balloon angioplasty catheter with a high-rated burst pressure and short balloon length are chosen. Balloon-expandable stents are preferable to self- expanding stents because of their greater radial force and more precise deployment mechanisms. Vascular access sheath size is chosen to accommodate the angioplasty balloon catheter or stent delivery catheter; a 5 Fr sheath is usually sufficient.

A 5 Fr angiographic catheter and a 0.035 inch hydrophilic guidewire are used to carefully cross the stenosis.

Completion angiography is performed. If necessary, PTA can be repeated to adequately oppose the stent to the vessel wall. If the translesional pressure gradient was previously measured, this should be repeated after stent deployment and completion angiography, aiming to achieve a reduction in the peak trans-lesional pressure gradient to <20 mm Hg or in the mean translesional pressure gradient to <10 mm Hg.

Primary PTA with provisional stenting or primary stenting with bare-metal or covered stents are viable treatment strategies with good long-term primary and secondary patency rates. The optimal initial management of these lesions remains debated.

Follow-up

Patients are observed overnight in the hospital following endovascular intervention. A Doppler ultrasound study is performed before discharge to document the new baseline appearance of the renal artery waveform. If PTA alone has been performed, indefinite therapy with aspirin 75 mg daily is instituted immediately following intervention. If a bare-metal stent or drug-eluting stent has been placed, dual-antiplatelet therapy begun immediately with aspirin 75 mg and clopidogrel 75 mg and continued for 6 months, after which clopidogrel is discontinued and the patient remains on indefinite aspirin therapy alone. Serum creatinine levels are followed up frequently by the kidney transplant service. A Doppler ultrasound study is repeated at any time following intervention if renal transplant function or blood pressure control worsens, raising the possibility of restenosis or in-stent stenosis.

Case 1: Stenting for TRAS

A 28-year-old renal transplant recipient had a history of creeping creatinine with rising blood pressure for 3 months post transplant. There was no proteinuria, no fever, and no graft tenderness. CMV and BK virus serology were all negative. Insignificant protein was found with bland sediments. Renal Doppler showed a typical parvus-tardus pattern in the segmental and interlobar arteries. As the creatinine was 2.4 mg/dL, CT angiogram was not done. The patient was taken for cathlab renal angiogram where a left femoral (contralateral) puncture with a 6 Fr sheath was placed. The guidewire was taken across the bifurcation of aorta to the right common iliac artery and into the internal iliac artery. There guiding catheter, passed up to the common iliac, angiogram done. Significant (85%) stenosis at the internal iliac renal anastomotic area is noticed. PTA passed and crossed the collection and the tip part in the segmental artery. The size was measured and a 5 × 15 mm bare-metal stent was deployed. Good result was achieved and brisk perfusion of the kidney was noticed. Over the next 4 weeks, serum creatinine settled down to 1.4 mg/dL.

TRANSPLANT RENAL ARTERY KINKS

Arterial kinks are formed due to arterial redundancy or due to a shift in the graft and/or pelvic contents with time that causes torquing of the artery. By angiography, a transplant arterial kink is defined as an eccentric narrowing on the concavity of a sharp arterial turn due to coaptation of the arterial wall on the concavity of the turn. It is important to identify an arterial narrowing to be a kink and not a simple stenosis. However, it is not always easy to do so, particularly if the stenosed anastomosis is at a hairpin turn or with suboptimal visualization of the narrowing due to vessels' tortuosity, overlapping vessels, and/or use of suboptimal contrast (CO_2 or gadolinium) **(Fig. 9; Video 2)**.

Surgery remains the primary treatment for arterial kinks. In cases where surgery is not feasible or patients refuse surgery, higher risk endoluminal management can be resorted to. Kinks are notorious for being refractory to balloon angioplasty and may increase the risk of arterial vasospasm and/or dissection. In addition, placing stents across kinks can be technically challenging and when deployed, self-expanding stents with low hoop strength can still be kinked or short balloon expandable stents with higher hoop strength may lead to propagation of the kink to one end, if not both ends, of the stent. Because of this, the current authors prefer to place both stents (a self-expanding and a balloon-expandable stent) coaxially to minimize their individual disadvantages. First, a relatively long self-expanding stent is placed to buttress the artery with its proximal limb (proximal to the kink) and its distal limb (distal to the kink). A short balloon-expandable stent is then deployed right at the apex of the kink. Its high hoop strength opens the kink, and the longer self-expanding stent reduces the risk of kink propagation.

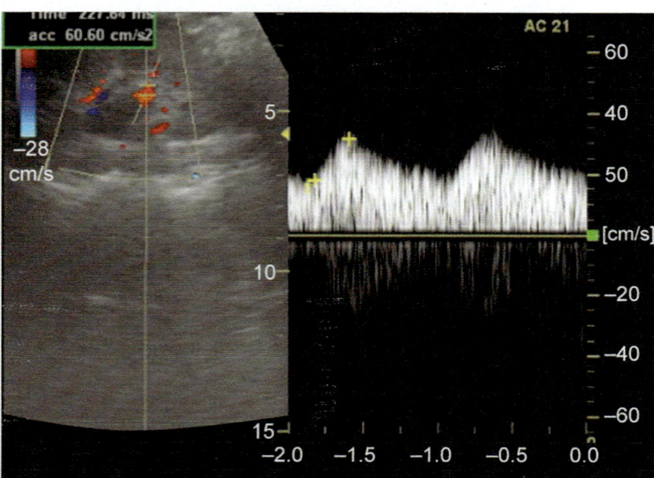

Fig. 9: Typical parvus-tardus pattern.

Case 2: Stenting for Transplant Renal Artery Rotation/Kinking

A 46-year-old female teacher, who was on maintenance hemodialysis for 4 years, had cadaver transplantation. During transplant, when the clamp was released, there was incomplete filling of the kidney. On rotating/changing the position of the kidney, the blood flow seemed to improve, indicating that there was a kink in the artery. As the ischemia time was getting prolonged and as the blood flow improved following rotating the kidney (nearly 260°), redo of anastomosis was not done. The graft function recovered well and the nadir creatinine 1.2 mg was achieved by the end of 5 days. Things seem to go well for the next 4 months when the creatinine started creeping up. As there was no obvious immunological drug or infective problem, TRAS was suspected by picking up the parvus-tardus pattern in renal Doppler. This was confirmed by MRA. She was taken for cathlab intervention. Hence, it was an unusual case of delayed TRAS caused by rotation and kinking of the renal vessel during engrafting. A 5 × 15 mm bare-metal stent was placed uneventfully by contralateral puncture in the left femoral artery. There was good recovery of renal function. Contrary to expectations, the graft is functioning well even now after 5 years.

Transplant Kidney Biopsy

Renal allograft biopsy remains the gold standard for diagnosing the etiology of graft dysfunction in kidney transplant recipients. It provides crucial histological information to differentiate rejection, drug toxicity (e.g., calcineurin inhibitor nephrotoxicity), infection, recurrence of native kidney disease, or other causes of injury. This allows for tailored and timely management, ultimately impacting graft and patient survival.

Renal transplant (allograft) biopsy is generally safe when performed under ultrasound guidance, but it is associated with both minor and major complications.

Prebiopsy Evaluation

- Review the patient's history, current medications, and the specific indication for biopsy.

- *Coagulation profile:* International normalized ratio (INR) <1.5, activated partial thromboplastin time (aPTT) within normal limits
- *Platelet count:* >50,000/μL, ideally >100,000/μL.
- *Hemoglobin:* Stable hemoglobin
- *Blood pressure:* Control hypertension to target <140/90 mm Hg, ideally <130/80 mm Hg, before the procedure to minimize bleeding risk.
- *Informed consent:* Thoroughly explain the procedure, potential risks (especially bleeding), benefits, and alternatives to the patient.

Ultrasound Guidance and POCUS

Real-time ultrasound guidance is mandatory for all renal allograft biopsies. This ensures precision, minimizes complications, and increases diagnostic yield.

POCUS is increasingly utilized by nephrologists for prebiopsy planning, real-time needle guidance, and immediate postbiopsy assessment. It adds to the safety of the procedure. Real-time visualization of the needle path prevents injury to adjacent organs and major vessels. Postbiopsy assessment helps immediate detection of complications like hematoma or arteriovenous fistula (AVF).

Choosing the Biopsy Site (Poles of the Kidney)

The lower pole of the transplant kidney is the preferred biopsy site. This is due to its more superficial location, ease of access, and lower risk of injury to the hilar vessels, renal pelvis, and ureter compared to the upper pole.

The biopsy needle should ideally enter the cortex tangentially, avoiding a perpendicular approach which may increase the risk of capsular tearing and injury to larger vessels. Typically, a 22–25-gauge needle is used for local anesthetic infiltration.

Biopsy needle: Automated, spring-loaded core biopsy needles (often referred to as "biopsy guns") are standard. These devices allow for rapid, controlled cutting and retrieval of tissue. Commonly, 16-gauge or 18-gauge needles are used. While 14-gauge needles can obtain larger samples, they are associated with a higher risk of bleeding. The choice depends on operator preference and the need for diagnostic tissue (e.g., 18-gauge needle for children or when minimal passes are desired; 16-gauge needle for routine adult biopsies). The length varies based on the depth of the kidney; common lengths are 10–15 cm.

Hemostasis: Apply manual compression to the biopsy site immediately after each pass and after needle withdrawal.

Postbiopsy Management and Monitoring

- Perform a rapid postbiopsy ultrasound or Doppler study to check for perinephric hematoma or active bleeding at the biopsy site.
- Pressure dressing
- Advise bed rest for 4–6 hours.
- Closely monitor vital signs, complete blood count, and urine output. Watch for signs of bleeding (flank pain, gross hematuria, hypotension, tachycardia, dropping hemoglobin).

What if the patient is on anticoagulants?

Antiplatelet agents (e.g., aspirin, clopidogrel): Generally, aspirin is continued if the patient is on it for cardiovascular protection. Clopidogrel (and other P2Y12 inhibitors) should ideally be held for 5–7 days before biopsy.

Oral anticoagulants [e.g., warfarin, direct oral anticoagulants (DOACs)] must be withheld and INR normalized (for warfarin) or sufficient washout period observed. Bridging anticoagulation [e.g., with heparin or low molecular weight heparin (LMWH)] is usually avoided for renal biopsy due to increased bleeding risk, unless medically imperative.

Absolute Contraindications

- *Uncontrolled hypertension:* Blood pressure >160/100 mm Hg significantly increases bleeding risk
- *Uncorrectable coagulopathy or severe thrombocytopenia:* INR >1.5 or platelet count <50,000/μL.
- *Active bleeding diathesis:* For example, hemophilia, severe von Willebrand disease
- *Severe hydronephrosis:* Can alter renal architecture and increase risk
- *Active infection at biopsy site:* Increases risk of spreading infection
- *Patient noncooperation:* Inability to lie still or follow instructions

Relative Contraindications

- Multiple cysts or large perinephric fluid collections obscuring the biopsy path
- Very deep or awkwardly located allograft
- Single functioning kidney (though often performed if no alternative)
- Uncontrolled diabetes mellitus (may impair healing)

Common Complications

- *Hematuria (blood in urine):* The most frequent complication, seen in up to 12% of cases, usually presents as gross or microscopic hematuria and is mostly self-limiting. Rarely, it can cause urinary tract obstruction.
- *Perinephric hematoma:* Blood collection around the graft, seen in up to 24% of biopsies, but most are small and asymptomatic. Larger hematomas may require intervention.
- *Pain*: Mild pain at the biopsy site is common and transient.
- *AVF:* Occurs in up to 5–10% detected by ultrasound, often resolves spontaneously but rarely can cause ongoing hematuria, hypertension, or graft dysfunction, and may then require coil embolization
- *Pseudoaneurysm:* Rare, but significant if it occurs, as it can cause delayed bleeding and requires intervention
- *Need for blood transfusion:* Seen in approximately 0.2–1% of biopsies, usually for significant bleeding
- *Major bleeding or surgical intervention:* Very rare (under 1%); may require angiographic embolization or, in extremely rare cases, surgical exploration or even nephrectomy
- *Infection:* Infection at the biopsy site or perinephric abscess is rare (<0.1%).

Mortality is exceedingly low, estimated at 0.01–0.5% in large series.

Using real-time ultrasound guidance, minimizing the number of biopsy passes, and careful patient selection further reduce risk.

INTERVENTIONS/COIL EMBOLIZATION FOR BIOPSY BLEEDING IN RENAL ALLOGRAFT

When postbiopsy bleeding in a renal allograft is significant—marked by ongoing hematuria, large or expanding perinephric hematoma, hemodynamic instability, or vascular complications (such as AVF or pseudoaneurysm)—minimally invasive endovascular interventions, especially coil embolization, become the treatment of choice.

Procedure Overview

- Access the arterial system (commonly via the femoral artery) using fluoroscopy to navigate a catheter to the transplant renal artery.
- A microcatheter is then steered superselectively into the small branch feeding the bleeding site or AVF.
- Through this microcatheter, one or more detachable platinum microcoils—sized appropriately to exceed the vessel diameter—are deployed, physically occluding the culprit vessel and halting blood flow to the site of bleeding.
- Postdeployment angiography confirms cessation of bleeding, closure of the fistula or pseudoaneurysm, and preservation of flow to the remaining allograft tissue.

Efficacy and Safety

- Coil embolization is highly effective, with technical and clinical success rates exceeding 90% for controlling postbiopsy bleeding and AVFs, while preserving graft function.
- The use of microcatheters and superselective technique ensures maximal parenchymal preservation and minimizes the risk of nontarget embolization.
- Complications are uncommon but can include coil migration, local infarction, or rarely contrast-induced nephropathy.

Careful patient selection, timely imaging, and prompt access to interventional procedures are essential for optimal outcomes.

Postbiopsy Arteriovenous Fistula

Arteriovenous fistulas in transplant kidneys are usually related to percutaneous needle biopsy resulting in simultaneous laceration of arterial and venous branches and occur in 1–18% of renal allograft biopsies. Most AVFs are asymptomatic and resolve spontaneously within 1–2 years. About 30% persist and become symptomatic, causing hematuria, hypertension, and graft dysfunction due to intrarenal arteriovenous shunting creating a steal phenomenon.

Risk factors for AVF formation include hypertension, multiple needle passes, central renal biopsies, and renal medullary disease. AVFs may be symptomatic and cause steal syndrome by creating relative ischemia of the renal parenchyma outside the lesion. This may result in secondary hypertension, decline in allograft function, or heart failure due to high-flow shunting. AVFs may also result in bleeding and hematuria and enlarge to cause rupture.

Asymptomatic AVFs are typically treated non-operatively with observation and serial imaging to the usual spontaneous resolution in 70% of cases.

Postbiopsy Ultrasonography

Ultrasonography is a very sensitive means of detecting postbiopsy vascular complications. Characteristic findings include Doppler identification of a focal pool of color representing venous and arterial components, increased systolic and diastolic flow on spectral analysis, and detection of turbulent venous flow and a large draining vein. Three-dimensional ultrasonography may be helpful for precisely identifying the location of the fistula. Occasionally, AVF is missed on ultrasound evaluation.

Open surgical treatment is associated with the loss of significant amounts of renal parenchyma, and endovascular treatment has become the preferred method of addressing symptomatic AVFs. Symptomatic AVFs can be treated with superselective transcatheter embolization of the feeding vessels **(Figs. 10A to D)**. Percutaneous transarterial superselective embolization with the use of microcatheters is safe and has been shown not to result in the loss of transplant kidney parenchyma.

Microcatheters

Microcatheters are extremely thin, flexible tubes designed to be navigated through tortuous and small blood vessels to deliver embolic agents precisely at the target site.

- *Function:* Their primary role is to provide a stable conduit from a larger guide catheter in the main renal artery to the very small segmental or subsegmental artery that is feeding the AVF.
- *Sizing (outer diameter):* Microcatheters are measured in French sizes, where 1 Fr equals 0.33 mm. For renal AVF embolization, very small catheters are used to minimize vascular trauma.

Embolization Coils

Coils are soft, platinum or stainless-steel wires that are pushed through the microcatheter and assume a pre-set, complex shape upon deployment in the vessel, forming a metallic scaffold that promotes thrombosis and occlusion **(Videos 3A and B)**.

- *Composition:*
  - *Material:* Most modern coils are made of *platinum* because it is soft, malleable, and highly visible on X-ray (radiopaque).
  - *Coatings:* Coils can be bare metal or feature enhancements to increase their effectiveness. *Fibered coils* have synthetic fibers (like Dacron or nylon) to promote faster clot formation. *Hydrogel-coated coils* expand in contact with blood, allowing for a more complete mechanical blockage, which is particularly useful in patients with clotting disorders.
- *Sizing principle:*
  - The most critical rule in coil selection is *oversizing.* The coil's deployed diameter should be *20% to 50% larger* than the target vessel's diameter. This ensures that the coil anchors securely and does not migrate downstream, which is especially important in high-flow AVFs.
- *Dimensions:* Coils have two main size specifications:
  - *Wire diameter:* This refers to the diameter of the platinum wire itself and determines compatibility with the microcatheter. Common systems are *0.018* and *0.035 inch.* Smaller systems (e.g., 0.010 inch) exist for finer applications.
  - *Deployed diameter and length:* This is the diameter of the loop the coil forms when it exits the catheter. The range is vast to match vessel anatomy.

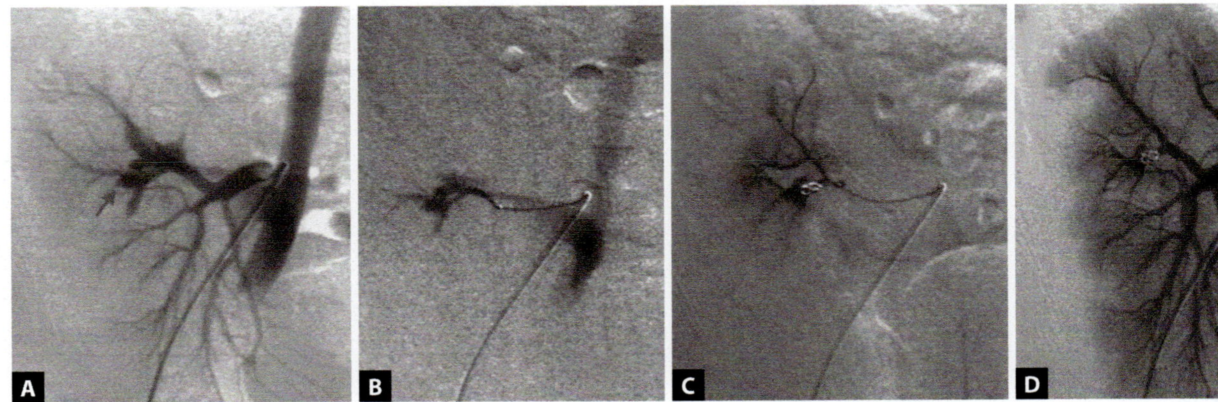

Figs. 10A to D: Superselective transcatheter embolization.

- *Diameter:* Can range from *1 to 2 mm* for tiny vessels to over *20 mm* for large feeding arteries or aneurysmal sacs
- *Length:* Can range from *1 to >60 cm.*

- *Types and shapes:*
  - *Framing coils:* The first coil deployed is often a stiffer, complex 3D-shaped coil that creates a stable "frame" or "basket" within the vessel.
  - *Filling/packing coils:* Softer, helical-shaped coils are then packed densely inside the framing coil to achieve complete occlusion.

Detachable Coils

Modern coils are almost exclusively detachable. This allows the interventionalist to deploy, assess the position, and even retract the coil if its placement is not perfect before committing to final detachment, greatly increasing the safety and precision of the procedure.

CONCLUSION

Interventional nephrologists are at the frontline of minimally invasive management for a broad range of renal transplant complications, particularly those involving vascular and urinary tract pathology. Their expertise in both the diagnostic and therapeutic aspects of these disorders is indispensable for improving graft survival, reducing morbidity, and limiting healthcare costs. As technology advances and more nephrologists acquire intervention skills, their role will expand further, reinforcing the nephrologist's position as a central figure in comprehensive renal transplant care.

REFERENCES

1. Verloh N, Probst U, Wiggermann P, Stroszczynski C, Jung EM. Interventional Management of vascular complications after renal transplantation. Rofo. 2023;195(3):233-41.
2. Iezzi R, Posa A, Merlino B, Salvatori FM, Bonomo L. Interventional radiological treatment of renal transplant complications. Biomed Res Int. 2015;2015:825025.
3. Inci MF, Savran B, Inci E, Ozkan F. Renal Transplant Complications: Diagnostic and Interventional Radiology. Journal of Radiology. 2014.
4. Christopher N, Kumar S, Ananthakrishnan R. Renal transplant complications—A pictorial review. Journal of Clinical and Diagnostic Research. 2022;16(2):TE01-TE06.
5. Sugi MD, Joshi G, Maddu KK, Dahiya N, Menias CO. Imaging of renal transplant complications throughout the life of the allograft : Comprehensive Multimodality Review. Radiographics. 2019;39(5):1320-43.
6. Ghodsipour E, Lee T, Ghahramani N. Transplant renal artery stenosis: clinical manifestations, diagnosis and therapy. Journal of Nephrology. 2014;27(5):499-508.
7. Duty BD, Barry JM. Diagnosis and management of ureteral complications following renal transplantation. Asian J Urol. 2015;2(4):202-7.
8. Al-Geizawi SMT, Al-Mousawi F, Bakr MA, Donia F. Evaluation of the Graft Kidney in the Early Postoperative Period. J Ultrasound Med. 2021.
9. Heckemann R, Rehwald U, Jakubowski HD, Donhuijsen K. Sonographic criteria for renal allograft rejection. Urol Radio. 1982.
10. Mayo Clinic. Renal artery stenosis - Diagnosis and treatment. 2025.
11. Kolli KP, Stauf F, Kohi MP, et al. Interventional Management of Nonvascular Renal Transplant Complications. Techniques in Vascular and Interventional Radiology. 2016.
12. Rosenblatt R, Horrow MM, Muallem G, et al. Screening for Transplant Renal Artery Stenosis: Ultrasound-Based Criteria Revisited. American Journal of Roentgenology. 2017.
13. Garg M, Kumar A, Prakash G, Kumar J. Urologic complications in renal transplants. Urol Ann. 2018.
14. Al-Adra D, Al-Shehri M, Al-Qahtani M. Renal transplant ultrasound: The nephrologist's perspective. Saudi J Kidney Dis Transpl. 2016.
15. Köhnke R, Görg C, Klose K-J, Lauenstein TC. Update on imaging-based diagnosis of acute renal allograft rejection. Der Radiologe. 2019.

SECTION 10

Future Directions and Innovations in Vascular Access

CHAPTER 40

Artificial Intelligence for Vascular Access in Hemodialysis

Priti Meena, Ashwani Gupta

INTRODUCTION

Vascular access (VA) is a critical component of hemodialysis, enabling effective removal of toxins and excess fluids from the bloodstream. Ensuring optimal functionality and longevity of arteriovenous fistulas (AVFs), grafts, and catheters is essential for improving patient outcomes and reducing healthcare costs. Despite advances in surgical techniques and management strategies, challenges such as stenosis, thrombosis, and nonmaturation persist. The integration of artificial intelligence (AI) into vascular access management offers innovative solutions to these challenges, leveraging advanced analytics, machine learning (ML), and automation to enhance diagnostic accuracy, predictive capabilities, and clinical decision-making.

OVERVIEW OF ARTIFICIAL INTELLIGENCE

Machine learning, a branch of AI, involves developing algorithms that learn from data to make predictions or decisions autonomously, without being explicitly programmed.[1] It incorporates various approaches, including supervised learning, which uses labeled datasets for training, and unsupervised learning, where models discover patterns within unlabeled data. Another specialized method is reinforcement learning, where models optimize actions through iterative trial-and-error interactions with their environment. In nephrology, ML holds significant potential for processing extensive clinical datasets to forecast disease progression, identify high-risk individuals, and suggest tailored treatment strategies. These algorithms typically draw on diverse data sources, such as patient demographics, laboratory findings, and imaging studies, to produce highly accurate predictions. Deep learning (DL), a specialized area within ML, relies on multilayered neural networks to model complex relationships in data. This approach excels at interpreting unstructured data formats, such as medical images.[2] Inspired by the structure and functioning of the human brain, DL utilizes artificial neural networks composed of interconnected layers of "neurons" to extract meaningful features from raw inputs. Common DL architectures include convolutional neural networks (CNNs), which are adept at image processing, and recurrent neural networks (RNNs), designed for sequential data analysis. Moreover, DL models can integrate multimodal inputs—such as images, genetic profiles, and clinical metrics—to offer a holistic understanding of patient conditions.

Natural language processing (NLP) is another pivotal AI discipline that facilitates interaction between machines and human language.[3] Combining ML, DL, and linguistic insights, NLP enables computers to interpret, analyze, and generate human language. In nephrology, NLP tools extract valuable information from unstructured text sources such as electronic health records (EHRs), academic publications, and clinical notes. These tools can identify and categorize critical clinical entities, such as diseases, symptoms, and treatments, as well as elucidate relationships between them. By automating the extraction of relevant patient data, NLP significantly aids in managing kidney diseases.

In the realm of hemodialysis, AI applications span from automated ultrasound imaging to predictive analytics for vascular access outcomes **(Fig. 1)**.

APPLICATIONS OF ARTIFICIAL INTELLIGENCE IN VASCULAR ACCESS MANAGEMENT

- *Preoperative mapping and planning:* AI-powered tools such as the Vexev Access System offer preoperative mapping solutions. The Vexev Ultrasound Imaging System is a robotic solution combining ultrasound imaging with advanced software,

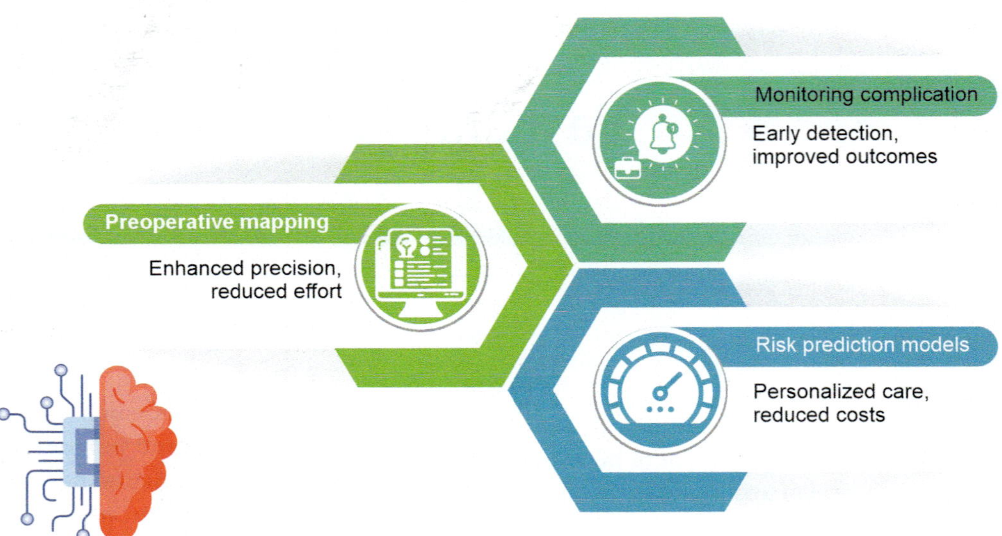

Fig. 1: Application of artificial intelligence (AI) in vascular access for hemodialysis.

enabling semi-autonomous scanning of the upper limb.[4] It is specifically designed for use at points of care, such as dialysis centers or physician offices, providing immediate results for attending clinicians. This innovative system allows for "hands-free" limb scanning, termed robotic tomographic ultrasound (RTU), a novel modality/RTU captures comprehensive B-Mode and Doppler data, akin to a full peripheral vascular ultrasound examination, and integrates probe location information to create a cohesive "digital tissue block". This enables the generation of detailed three-dimensional (3D) structural and flow data comparable to CT or MRI scans but without exposure to radiation or nephrotoxic contrast agents. Once the data is collected, it is processed and transferred to vxView, a cloud-based reporting and analysis platform. Accessible via web browsers on any internet-enabled device, vxView supports remote analysis and annotation by accredited vascular sonographers. These experts label and confirm vascular structures and identify pathologies such as stenosis, aneurysms, or thrombosis within the 3D vascular model.

- *Prediction of AVF maturation:* Machine learning models such as k-Nearest Neighbors (k-NN) have demonstrated high accuracy in predicting AVF maturation, blood flow velocities, and diameters. These models can guide surgical planning, reducing the rate of nonmaturation and optimizing resource utilization. Doneda et al. used parametric and nonparametric ML approaches to predict AVF maturation and postoperative blood flow velocities (BFVs), achieving high prediction accuracy (96.8%) with low computational effort.[5]
- *Monitoring and early detection of complications:* AI applications in VA monitoring include:
  - *DeepVAQ* combines photoplethysmography (PPG) sensors with deep learning to predict VA quality with over 92% accuracy.

    PPG sensors are noninvasive devices designed to measure variations in blood volume within the vascular system. These sensors work by detecting changes in how light is absorbed or reflected, enabling the estimation of vital physiological parameters such as pulse rate, blood flow, and oxygen levels. Julkew et al. proposed using cost-effective PPG sensors, which are efficient in capturing biosignals, alongside a deep learning model optimized with convolutional neural network architecture, termed "DeepVAQ".[6] The DeepVAQ system exhibited exceptional accuracy in predicting and assessing vascular access quality in hemodialysis patients, offering a reliable method for early detection.

    In another investigation involving 398 hemodialysis patients, a one-dimensional convolutional neural network (CNND) outperformed other models in accuracy.[7] The use of a SelectKBest-based feature selection technique further enhanced its performance, achieving an accuracy of 92.05% compared to 90.79% with the full dataset. These findings suggest that the new feature selection strategy can significantly improve the prediction of vascular access quality, contributing to the development of advanced diagnostic tools. Such advancements may improve the identification and management of vascular complications such as stenosis.

- *Mel Spectrogram analysis:* A recent research involved the use of Mel spectrograms, which provide a two-dimensional visual representation of audio signals and are widely employed in audio recognition tasks. This technique extracts features from audio recordings by applying a frequency-domain filter bank to signals segmented in time, effectively filtering out background noise. By doing so, it enables deep learning models to identify both physiological and pathological characteristics with greater precision.[8] Studies have explored the use of Mel spectrograms in analyzing arteriovenous access bruit sounds.[9] For example, convolutional neural networks have been developed to classify these sounds into various categories. One study utilized a CNN model to detect significant AVF stenosis and predict 6-month primary patency, demonstrating promising results.[10] Chung et al. recorded AV access bruits using an electronic stethoscope and transformed the audio data into Mel-scaled spectrograms.[11] They developed and compared three deep learning models: A CNN, a convolutional recurrent neural network (CRNN), and a vision transformer-GRU (ViT-GRU). Among these, the CNN model outperformed the others in the test set with an F1 score of 0.7037 and an AUROC of 0.7112. The ViT-GRU model performed well in out-of-fold predictions but demonstrated lower generalization on the test set. The authors concluded that the CNN model, leveraging Mel spectrograms, could effectively predict malfunctioning AV access requiring intervention within 10 days, offering a valuable screening tool for high-risk patients.

- *Risk prediction models:* AI-based predictive models such as AVF-FM (XG-Boost) and PREDICT-AVF utilize patient-specific data to estimate the likelihood of complications such as thrombosis and the need for reintervention. These tools enhance shared decision-making and personalized surveillance strategies.[12,13]

Prediction of recurrent intervention: Heindel et al. introduced the PREDICT-AVF web application, a machine learning-based tool aimed at predicting recurrent interventions following radiocephalic AVF creation.[12] This tool was developed based on data collected from a prospective cohort study involving 914 adults across the United States and Canada, all of whom underwent radiocephalic AVF creation as part of the PATENCY-1 or -2 trials.

The study utilized clinical data, including patient demographics, comorbidities, prior access history, anatomical details, and postoperative ultrasound measurements taken at 4–6 weeks and 12 weeks, to forecast the likelihood of recurrent interventions within 1 year. Multiple machine learning models, including Cox proportional hazards, random survival forest, pooled logistic regression, and elastic net recurrent event survival prediction models, were employed to analyze these factors. The random survival forest model, based on baseline characteristics alone, demonstrated the best performance with an area under the receiver operating characteristic curve (AUROC) of 0.75 (95% CI 0.67–0.82) for predicting 1-year outcomes. Incorporating ultrasound data did not markedly enhance model accuracy; however, standalone Cox models using ultrasound data from either 4–6 or 12 weeks yielded slightly higher AUROCs of 0.77 (0.70–0.85) and 0.76 (0.70–0.83), respectively. The authors emphasized that this tool can support patient counseling, facilitate shared decision-making, and align treatment plans with patient-centered goals in end-stage kidney disease management.

- *Fistula failure model:* Peralta et al. developed and validated a ML model, the Arteriovenous Fistula Failure Model (AVF-FM), designed to predict the risk of AVF failure within 3 months in patients undergoing in-center dialysis.[13] This model, based on the XGBoost algorithm, was trained using 70% of the initial cohort, leveraging data routinely collected in the Nephrocare European Clinical Database (EuCliD®). The remaining 30% of the cohort was used to assess the model's performance through concordance statistics and calibration charts. The SHAP method was employed to determine feature importance. The AVF-FM achieved an Area Under the ROC Curve (AUC-ROC) of 0.80 (95% CI 0.79–0.81) and demonstrated excellent calibration, accurately reflecting observed failure risks. The key variables influencing risk predictions included a prior history of AVF complications, access recirculation, and other functional parameters such as trends in dialysis dose, blood flow, and dynamic venous and arterial pressures. This model shows promise for enabling personalized, risk-based strategies for AVF monitoring and management.

- *Postoperative monitoring and optimization:* AI-based solutions improve postoperative outcomes by enabling real-time assessment of VA functionality. Tools such as lightweight CNN models have demonstrated exceptional accuracy (up to 100%) in classifying AVF conditions before and after angioplasty, aiding timely clinical interventions. Wang et al. highlighted that lightweight CNN models outperform traditional ones while being computationally efficient.[14]

A study by Grochawina aimed to create an affordable tool for monitoring AVF using the phonoangiography method.[15] The system comprises three main components: (1) AVF signal acquisition, (2) data processing and classification, and (3) a module for displaying results. This approach is both noninvasive and cost-effective, designed to analyze the sound patterns of bruit generated by AVF. A specialized sensor with higher sensitivity than a traditional stethoscope was employed to capture sound signals from the fistula. Signal acquisition was conducted using custom-designed software developed specifically for the study. The phonoangiogram produced 23 features, which were analyzed in a decision-making algorithm. Of these, six features were derived from the time-domain waveform, while 17 were extracted from the frequency spectrum. The final feature vector composition was determined using various selection techniques, including feature-class correlation, forward search, Principal Component Analysis (PCA), and the Joined-Pairs method. A supervised ML approach was subsequently utilized to develop the most effective classification model.

CHALLENGES AND FUTURE DIRECTIONS

- Implementing AI in nephrology faces challenges such as regulatory barriers, data biases, and the need for large, high-quality datasets. Integrating diverse data sources, ensuring generalizability across patient populations, and addressing ethical concerns are important. Explainability and interpretability are essential to maintain transparency, accountability, and patient trust. Explainability refers to the model's ability to justify decisions, while interpretability focuses on understanding overall behavior and cause-effect relationships. Regulatory frameworks such as GDPR underscore the need for ethical handling of health data. While AI has shown immense promise in VA management, challenges remain:
- *Data quality and availability:* Large, annotated datasets are essential for training robust models.
- *Integration into clinical workflows:* Ensuring seamless adoption of AI tools without disrupting existing workflows.
- *Ethical and regulatory considerations:* Addressing patient privacy and algorithmic transparency.

Adopting best practices, such as standardizing electronic health records (EHRs) and addressing biases—selection, measurement, algorithmic, confirmation, and cultural biases—is crucial. Strategies include diversifying data collection, using bias detection tools, and continuous model monitoring. AI deployment requires multidisciplinary collaboration, clinician input feedback loops, and workflows supporting interpretability. Together, these steps ensure reliable, ethical, and effective AI integration into clinical practices.

CONCLUSION

Artificial intelligence has revolutionized vascular access management for hemodialysis, offering innovative solutions for preoperative planning, complication monitoring, and risk prediction. By enhancing diagnostic accuracy and enabling personalized care, AI can improve patient outcomes and streamline clinical workflows. As research advances, AI's integration into vascular access management holds the potential to redefine standards of care in hemodialysis.

REFERENCES

1. Matsuo Y, LeCun Y, Sahani M, Precup D, Silver D, Sugiyama M, et al. Deep learning, reinforcement learning, and world models. Neural Netw. 2022;152:267-75.
2. Shickel B, Bihorac A. The dawn of multimodal artificial intelligence in nephrology. Nat Rev Nephrol. 2024;20:79-80.
3. Kufel J, Bargieł-Łączek K, Kocot S, Koźlik M, Bartnikowska W, Janik M, et al. What is machine learning, artificial neural networks and deep learning?-examples of practical applications in medicine. Diagnostics (Basel). 20233;13(15):2582.
4. Carroll J, Colley E, Cartmill M, Thomas SD. Robotic tomographic ultrasound and artificial intelligence for

management of haemodialysis arteriovenous fistulae. J Vasc Access. 2023:11297298231210019.
5. Doneda M, Poloni S, Bozzetto M, Remuzzi A, Lanzarone E. Surgical planning of arteriovenous fistulae in routine clinical practice: A machine learning predictive tool. J Vasc Access. 2024;25(4):1170-9.
6. Julkaew S, Wongsirichot T, Damkliang K, Sangthawan P. DeepVAQ: An adaptive deep learning for prediction of vascular access quality in hemodialysis patients. BMC Med Inform Decis Mak. 2024;24:45.
7. Julkaew S, Wongsirichot T, Damkliang K, Sangthawan P. Improving accuracy of vascular access quality classification in hemodialysis patients using deep learning with K highest score feature selection. J Int Med Res. 2024;52(4):3000605241232519.
8. Cheng J, Sun K. Heart sound classification network based on convolution and transformer. Sensors (Basel). 2023;23:8168.
9. Ota K, Nishiura Y, Ishihara S, Adachi H, Yamamoto T, Hamano T. Evaluation of hemodialysis arteriovenous bruit by deep learning. Sensors (Basel). 2020;20:4852.
10. Park JH, Park I, Han K, Yoon J, Sim Y, Kim SJ, et al. Feasibility of deep learning-based analysis of auscultation for screening significant stenosis of native arteriovenous fistula for hemodialysis requiring angioplasty. Korean J Radiol. 2022;23:949-58.
11. Chung TL, Liu YH, Wu PY, Huang JC, Tsai YC, Wang YC, et al. Prediction of arteriovenous access dysfunction by Mel spectrogram-based deep learning model. Int J Med Sci. 2024;21(12):2252-60.
12. Heindel P, Dey T, Fitzgibbon JJ, Mamdani M, Hentschel DM, Belkin M, et al. Predicting recurrent interventions after radiocephalic arteriovenous fistula creation with machine learning and the PREDICT-AVF web app. J Vasc Access. 2025;26(1):202-10.
13. Peralta R, Garbelli M, Bellocchio F, Ponce P, Stuard S, Lodigiani M, et al. Development and validation of a machine learning model predicting arteriovenous fistula failure in a large network of dialysis clinics. Int J Environ Res Public Health. 2021;18(23):12355.
14. Wang JJ, Sharma AK, Liu SH, Zhang H, Chen W, Lee TL. Prediction of vascular access stenosis by lightweight convolutional neural network using blood flow sound signals. Sensors (Basel). 2024;24(18):5922.
15. Grochowina M, Leniowska L, Gala-Błądzińska A. The prototype device for non-invasive diagnosis of arteriovenous fistula condition using machine learning methods. Sci Rep. 2020;10(1):16387.

CHAPTER 41

Emerging Techniques for Vascular Access Creation, Maintenance, and Device Innovations

Suresh Kumar Margassery, Vijayaprakash Sreenarasimhaiah

INTRODUCTION

Since the major breakthrough in developing a functioning hemodialysis access occurred in 1966 with the surgical creation of an autologous radiocephalic (R-C) arteriovenous fistula (AVF) by Brescia-Cimino-Appel-Hurwich,[1] the AVF remains the preferred access for hemodialysis due to higher long-term patency, lower infection rate, and lower occurrence of thrombosis **(Fig. 1)**. Many patients do not have the optimal vascular real estate for the creation of AVF, thereby requiring alternative but less desired forms of vascular accesses like the implantation of arteriovenous graft (AVG) and tunneled catheter-related access for hemodialysis.[2]

Despite more than 5 decades of surgical experience in the creation of AVF, the primary maturation failure rate of surgically created AVF continues to remain as high as 20–60%.[4] The AVG has lower primary 1-year patency of about 51% compared to about 86% for the AVF, and the least desirable central venous catheter (CVC) has higher complications like increased morbidity as well as mortality related to the occurrence of infections or development of central venous stenosis.[5] Due to the limitations in the functioning survival of vascular access, various innovations have been sorted out and progressively developed with promising outcomes in the surgical techniques, devices, and technology for the hemodialysis vascular access care.

This chapter provides insight and description of various newer (novel) devices, techniques, and technologies that are currently available to provide a longer functionally lasting hemodialysis vascular access. The novel approaches in vascular access creation include newer techniques

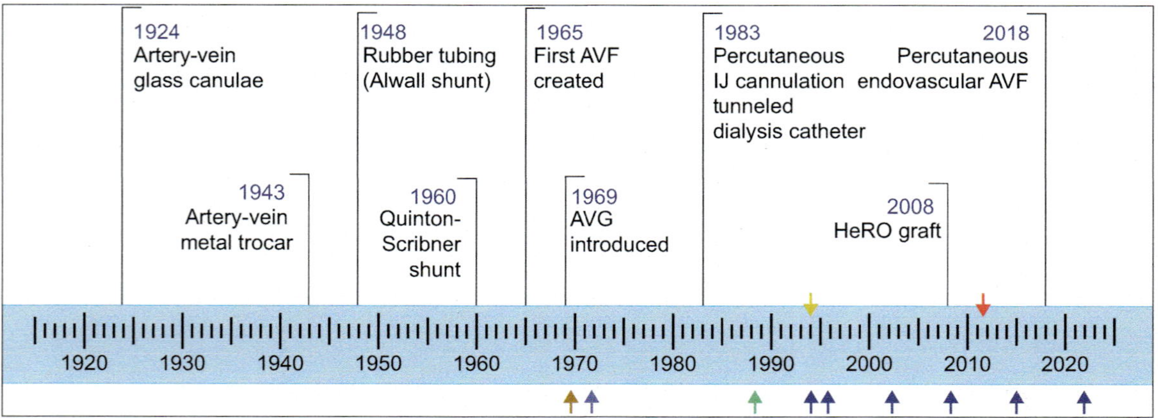

Fig. 1: Timeline for vascular access development over the past 80 years. Dark blue arrows represent the timing of NKF-KDOQI vascular access clinical practice guidelines. Brown arrow reflects the formation of National Medical Care, the first for profit dialysis provider. Light blue arrow points to passage of 1972 Public Law 92-603, section 2991 authorizing medicare payments for treatment of patients with kidney failure. Green arrow reflects the establishment of the USRDS. Yellow arrow reflects the establishment of ESRD Clinical Performance Measures Project. Red arrow reflects the onset of bundled payment for dialysis. (AVF: arteriovenous fistula; AVG: arteriovenous graft; USRDS: United States Renal Data System).
Source: Adapted from Hassanein et al.[3]

and devices used to create AVF by applying nonsurgical methods, using devices during the surgical creation to prevent the occurrence of access inflow segment stenosis due to the development of neointimal hyperplasia, using newer designed sturdy grafts that can be cannulated early after surgery and currently developed immune-negative bioengineered graft for AVG construction. Newer devices have also been developed for the long-term maintenance of AVF and AVG patency, thereby prolonging the access survival.

INNOVATIONS IN ARTERIOVENOUS FISTULA CREATION

The open surgical technique remains the gold standard in the AVF creation since the initial Brescia-Cimino-type AVF creation in 1966.[1] Despite the improvement in the surgical techniques and more than 50 years of experience in creating the surgical AVF (sAVF), the primary maturation failure of AVF continues to be significantly high, varying from 20 to 60%.[6] Many factors can play a role in the occurrence of primary maturation failure including surgery-related factors like arterial anastomosis, fibroblastic stenosis related to the application of suture, and access stenosis due to the development of neointimal hyperplasia resulting from the flow turbulence at the access inflow segment (juxta-arterial anastomosis venous segment) as a result of the acute angulation of the target vein to the feeding artery as well as the mobilization of the target vein from the venous bed resulting in venous wall ischemia.[7] Various device innovations and newer techniques have been developed in the recent past to counter these negative factors and facilitate the progressive maturation of the AVF.

Few of the newer techniques and approved innovations include the following:

- Constructing the arterial anastomosis with surgical technique to minimize the hemodynamic flow turbulence—pSLOT technique
- Mobilizing the feeding artery to create the arterial anastomosis to the target vein with end-to-side anastomosis—RADAR (Radial Artery Deviation and Reimplantation) technique
- Adjuvant technique by applying a structural scaffold at the time of sAVF creation to maintain the optimal angle of the target vein at the anastomosis site and maintain the laminar flow—VasQ external support brace
- Nonsurgical creation of AVF—endoAVF

RADAR Technique

This novel sAVF creation approach was designed to inhibit or prevent the occurrence of venous juxta-anastomosis stenosis (JAS) and increase the primary patency of the R-C AVF. The main principle behind this technique compared to the conventional AVF surgical creation is to avoid mobilization and minimize the dissection around the target vein to avoid devascularization of the venous wall in the juxta-anastomosis segment. The RADAR surgical technique study has shown an increased maturation rate in comparison with the traditional R-C AVF surgery (75% vs. 45% at 6 weeks; 92% vs. 71% at 3 months), decreased incidence of JAS (2% vs. 41%), increased primary patency rates (93% vs. 53%) at 6 months, increased secondary patency rates (100% vs. 89%) at 6 months, decreased incidence of reintervention (10% vs. 74%), and no occurrence of hand steal syndrome,[8] the main limitation being that the RADAR technique can be performed only to create a R-C AVF **(Figs. 2A to D)**. In addition to meeting the basic surgical requirement of having ≥2 mm diameter involving the cephalic vein as well as the radial artery in the distal forearm region, the patients should have fully patent radial and ulnar arteries without heavy calcification and fully patent palmar arterial arches. In the primary study, the RADAR technique was not performed in patients if the cephalic vein and radial artery were in close proximity (<4 mm), in which case a lateral-lateral anastomosis was performed.

Procedure

The RADAR surgery is performed by applying tourniquet on the upper arm, which needs to be inflated at the time of creating the anastomosis. After making the skin incision of about 5 cm at the distal forearm-wrist region, the inner aspect of a 1.5-cm long cephalic venous segment needs to be exposed by cautiously dissecting the surrounding tissues without mobilizing or clamping the vein. The radial artery distal segment pedicle of about 5 cm is dissected free and ligated distally by applying two clips after inflating the tourniquet to 250 mm Hg. Next, the distal end of the artery immediately proximal to the ligation is skeletonized, gently turned with a smooth loop toward the minimally dissected medial aspect of the cephalic vein. A 1-cm long venotomy is in an end-to-side fashion using a continuous suturing with 8-0 polypropylene followed by the deflation of the tourniquet and appropriate closure of the skin incision **(Fig. 3)**.

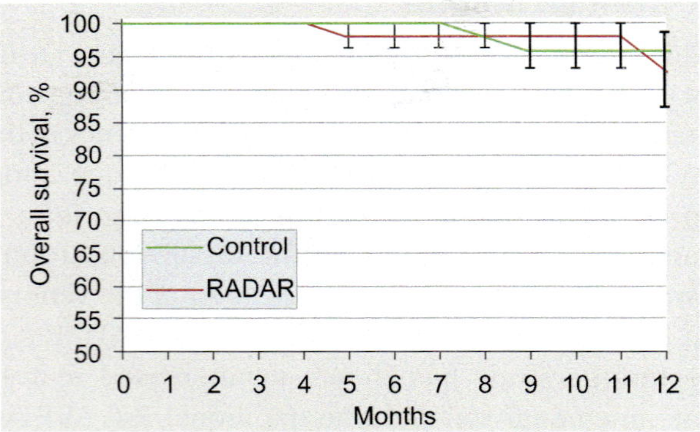

A

Overall survival	Time in months	0	1	3	6	9	12
Control	Number at risk	73	72	67	57	41	32
RADAR	Number at risk	53	53	53	49	31	16

B

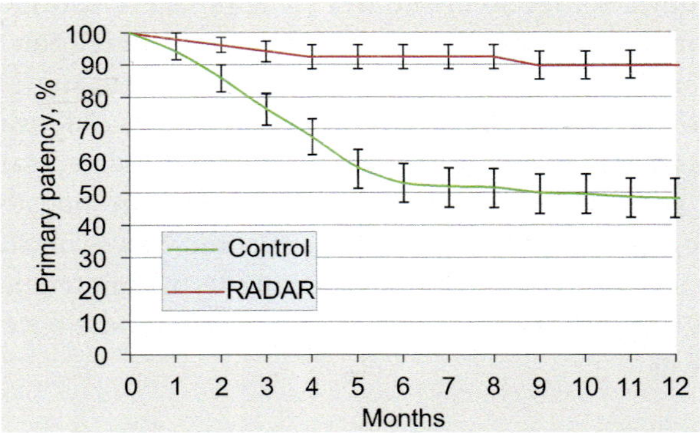

Primary patency	Time in months	0	1	3	6	9	12
Control	Number at risk	73	67	54	33	28	23
RADAR	Number at risk	53	52	50	45	28	14

C

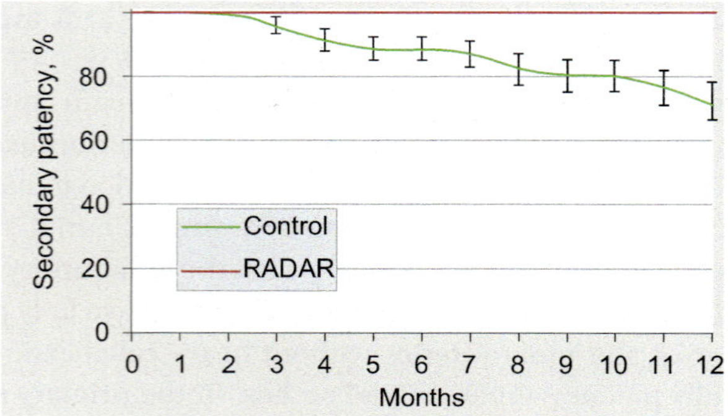

Secondary patency	Time in months	0	1	3	6	9	12
Control	Number at risk	73	72	67	57	41	32
RADAR	Number at risk	53	53	53	49	31	16

D

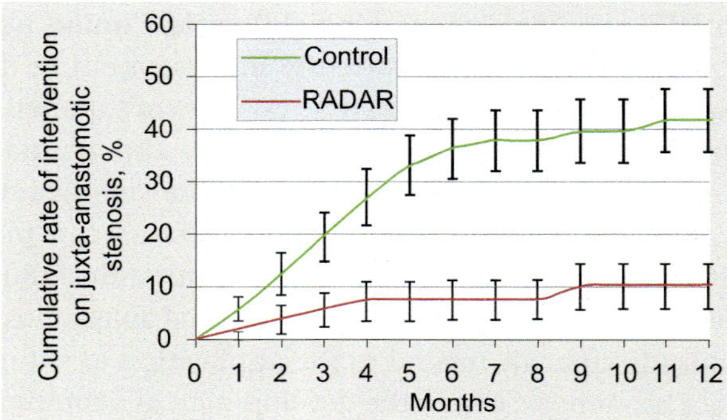

Interventions	Time in months	0	1	3	6	9	12
Control	Number at risk	73	67	55	39	31	25
RADAR	Number at risk	53	52	50	45	28	14

Figs. 2A to D: Kaplan–Meier curves and Breslow analysis for comparison between the radial artery deviation and reimplantation (RADAR) group and the historical control group. (A) Estimation of the overall survival ($p = 0.90$); (B) Estimation of the primary patency ($p < 0.00001$); (C) Estimation of the secondary patency ($p = 0.0003$); (D) Estimation of the cumulative rate of reintervention in the juxta-anastomotic segment ($p = 0.0002$).
Source: Sadaghianloo et al.[8]

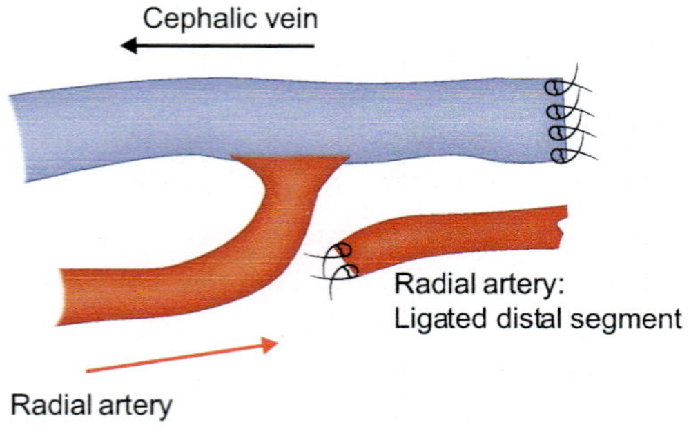

Fig. 3: Classical RADAR surgery.

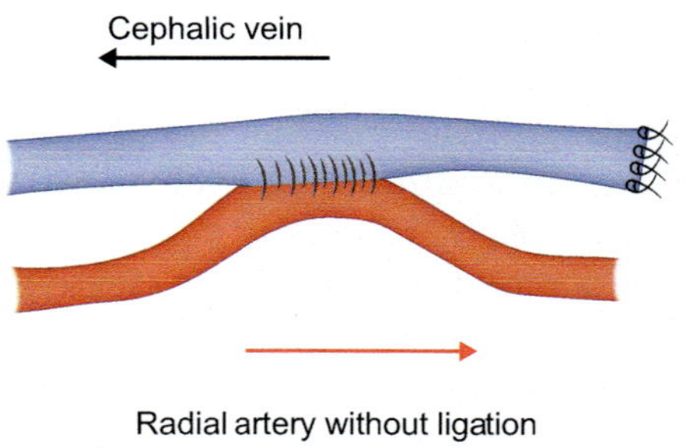

Fig. 4: Modified RADAR surgery.

The originally described RADAR technique can be modified by mobilizing the radial artery distal segment near the wrist region toward the minimally dissected cephalic venous segment and creating a side-to-side anastomosis without ligating the radial artery distal to the anastomosis **(Fig. 4)**.

DISTAL FOREARM RADIOCEPHALIC AVF

Adjuvant Arteriovenous Fistula Creation Technique Using Innovative Device (VasQ External Support Brace)

The primary failure of AVF occurred mostly in the first 6 weeks following the surgical creation due to the dysfunctional remodeling of the juxta-anastomosis venous segment (inflow segment) resulting in JAS. Mechanical and hemodynamic factors play a major role in the development of JAS. The target vein mobilized during surgery loses the structural support of the surrounding tissues resulting in torsion and altered angulation of the inflow venous segment to the feeding artery at the level of arterial anastomosis, which perpetuates hemodynamic changes in the form of flow turbulence causing abnormal stretch, shear stress, and development of JAS with neointimal hyperplasia.[9] These negatively influencing factors cannot be controlled to a great extend at the time of AVF creation surgery. In order to counter the negative mechanical and hemodynamic factors, a nitinol-based mesh support device called VasQ (Laminate Medical Technologies) was developed to provide external structural reinforcement to the mobilized target vein **(Fig. 5)**. The external supporting VasQ thereby maintains the optimal support angle of the inflow venous segment to the feeding artery at the arterial anastomosis as well as preserve an optimal geometric tapered configuration for a stable flow transition from the feeding artery to the target vein at the juxta-anastomosis segment. A 2-year prospective, multicenter, single-arm, open-label (VasQ US pivotal) study evaluated the safety, durability, effectiveness, and outcome of the VasQ device implantation for the surgical creation of brachio-cephalic (B-C) and R-C AVF.[10] The vascular anatomical criteria of study cohorts remained similar to the traditional AVF surgery with the adequate size of the feeding artery ≥2 mm and the target vein size ≥2.5 mm. The major drawback of the study being the use of the device for AVF requiring transposition (brachio-basilic AVF) is not known at this point, since these cohorts were excluded from the study. The study revealed that the VasQ device did not inhibit the ability to use standard percutaneous interventions or surgical procedures when required to maintain or restore the AVF patency. Mandatory X-ray evaluation of the VasQ AVF at 12 and 24 months showed the device fracture incidence of 6.9% with the device implanted within the elbow crease region. The fractured device caused no clinical sequelae or impediment to the function of AVF.

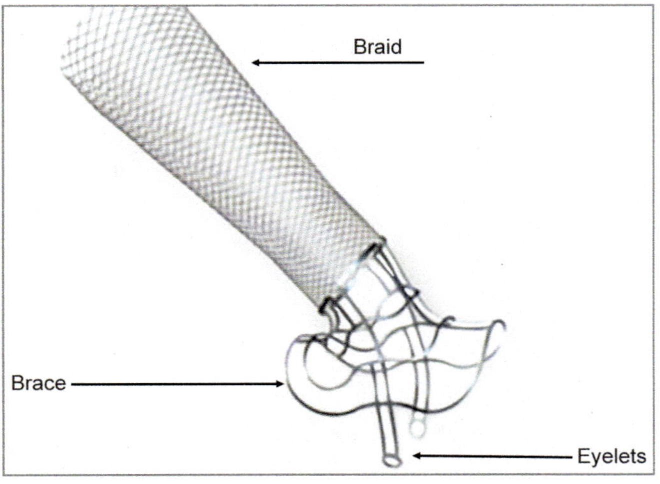

Fig 5: VasQ.
Courtesy: Laminate Medical Technology, Tel Aviv, Israel.

The pivotal study[10] revealed a superior primary patency for VasQ at 6 months post-AVF creation—67% for B-C AVF and 66% for the total cohorts (combined B-C and R-C AVF), the primary failure at 6 months being 7.9% with no difference in the two VasQ AVF cohorts and the physiological maturation being 73.8% at 1.5 months, 82.1% at 3 months, total maturation of 93.5% at 24 months, and cumulative patency of 76.6% in 24 months with the maturation criteria of AVF being ≥500 mL/min flow and the target vein diameter of ≥5 mm. The cumulative rate of intervention to maintain or restore patency was low at 1.07 per patient-year over the full 24-month study follow-up period compared to 1.8 for the traditional AVF. The steal-syndrome rate over long term is shown to be low at 4.2%. The aneurysm formation requiring intervention of the VasQ AVF appeared to be relatively low at 0–2% in the 1st year and increased to 7–14% at 2-year follow-up.

The recently completed prospective, single-arm, multicenter VasQ pivotal study was designed to assess the functional outcome of AVF created with VasQ device and compare it with the unsupported AVF in patients with end-stage kidney disease (ESKD).[11] A total of 104 ESKD patients eligible for R-C and B-C AVF creation were enrolled in the study with 52 patients in the VasQ arm and 52 patients in the control arm across six study sites. VasQ AVFs experienced a significant reduction in median time to first use compared to the standard AVFs (56 vs. 85 days; $p = 0.04$) and fewer interventions to support maturation (0.25 vs. 0.63 per patients; $p = 0.002$). More VasQ AVFs achieved functional success without the assistance of interventions to support maturation at 3 months (46% vs. 23%; $p = 0.013$) and at 6 months (65% vs. 45%; $p = 0.03$). VasQ implantation was significantly associated with greater odds for 3- and 6-month unassisted functional success after AVF creation [adjusted odds ratio 2.95 (95% CI 1.23–7.43) $p = 0.018$ and 2.44 (95% CI 1.09–5.61) $p = 0.031$, respectively] and lower odds for needing reinterventions [adjusted odds ratio 0.40 (95% CI 0.16–0.96) $p = 0.045$]. The pivotal study revealed the clear benefit of using the VasQ support device while creating the AVF compared to the standard unsupported AVF surgical creation, with the VasQ AVFs being associated with more unassisted functional success, an overall lower maturation procedure rate, and shorter time to first use.

Procedure

The surgery involves the traditional technique of end-to-side anastomosis of B-C and R-C AVF creation. During the surgery, application of clips for anastomosis creation or side branch ligation needs to be avoided at the level of the device to prevent interference with the device performance. After exposing the feeding artery and preparing the target vein in the traditional surgical fashion, the dilated target vein as well as the feeding artery diameter are measured by using the device model size selection tool **(Fig. 6)**, and the target vein is inserted into the VasQ device of appropriate size. After creating the AVF anastomosis, the device is gently pulled down around the anastomosis as well as the feeding artery segment and finally, the two clips of the device are secured around the artery using a nonabsorbable suture **(Figs. 7 and 8)**.

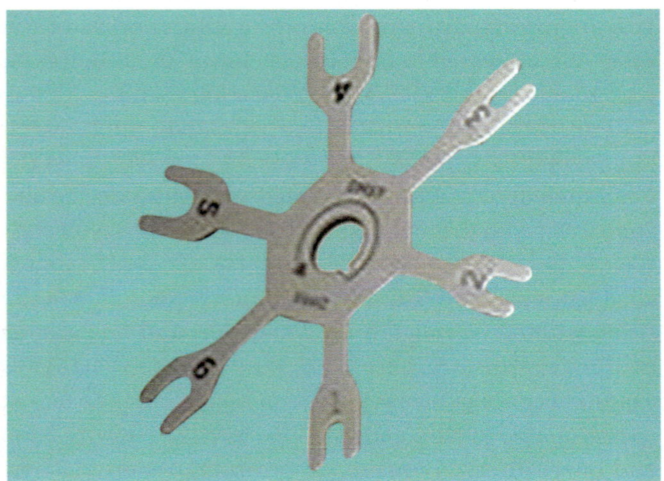

Fig. 6: VasQ device selection tool.
Courtesy: Laminate Medical Technology, Tel Aviv, Israel.

Novel EndoAVF Techniques

Two novel percutaneous endovascular devises with the innovative techniques had been approved by the US Food and Drug Administration (FDA) in 2018 for the nonsurgical creation of AVF exclusively in the upper extremity. The endoAVF creation procedure irrespective of the device technique is performed using local anesthesia with or without sedation, and the additional use of regional anesthesia with brachial plexus nerve block provides the greatest advantage of having the vessels optimally dilated during the entire procedure. The newer endoAVF creation technique includes the following:

- Angiography and fluoroscopy-guided technique using a magnetic catheter-based radiofrequency

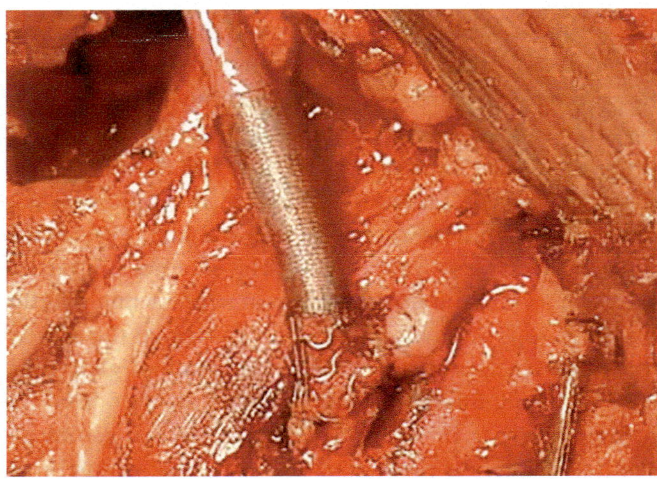

Fig. 7: Arteriovenous (AV) fistula with VasQ device attached.

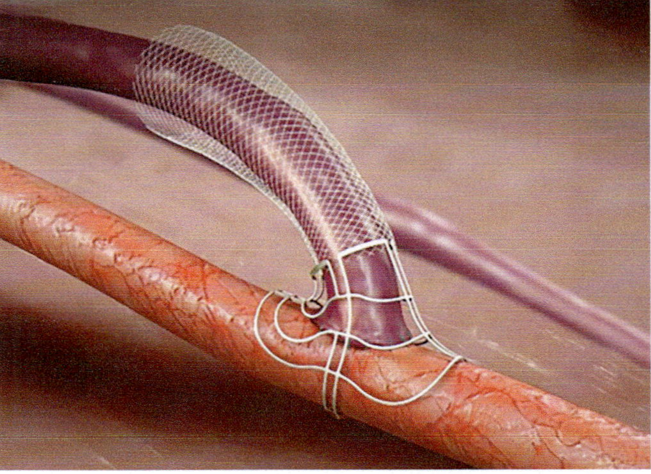

Fig. 8: VasQ device.
Courtesy: Laminate Medical Technology, Tel Aviv, Israel.

(RF) anastomosis device called *WavelinQ* (Becton Dickinson, NJ, USA)

- Ultrasound-guided technique using a thermal resistance anastomosis device called *Ellipsys* (Medtronic, MN, USA)

WavelinQ Device

The device consists of two 4 Fr rapid-exchange-based magnetic catheters (arterial and venous catheters) and a preset RF generator that delivers 60 W RF burst for 0.7 seconds. The arterial catheter contains a ceramic backstop cradle and the venous catheter contains the convex-shaped cutting electrode, which will align appropriately to the ceramic backstop cradle on positioning the catheters optimally within the respective vessels across the site of the anastomosis creation. In addition, both catheters have rotational indicator windows that help to guide the catheters into the correct orientation with fluoroscopic guidance. The device is used to create endoAVF between the feeding artery and the target vein by delivering burst of RF energy.

Procedure: WavelinQ device is used to create endoAVF anastomosis within the proximal forearm region between the proximal segment of the ulnar artery (common ulnar artery—before it divides into the distal ulnar artery segment and the interosseous arteries) and preferably the adjacent lateral ulnar vein called the ulnar-ulnar endoAVF or the proximal segment of the radial artery and preferably the adjacent medial radial vein called the radial-radial endoAVF. The lateral ulnar and medial radial target veins are preferred in creating the respective endoAVF due to the communication of the perforator veins commonly to these target veins, thereby creating the endoAVF with effective venous flow diversion and facilitating optimal arterialization of the superficial veins for the hemodialysis cannulation. In addition to the basic vascular criteria, with the WavelinQ technique the distance between the target artery and vein should be <1 mm.

Initially, the target vein, either the brachial vein in the upper arm region or the radial or ulnar vein in the distal forearm region, is cannulated using a 21-gauge introducer needle with ultrasound guidance after applying a tourniquet around the proximal upper arm region and a 5 Fr slender sheath inserted into the vein, with the brachial vein cannulated retrograde and the radial or ulnar vein being cannulated antegrade. The target vein with a larger size and its close proximity alignment to the target artery determines the venous access. Next, a 4 Fr angled vascular guiding catheter is advanced cautiously through the target vein via the sheath over a 0.014" guidewire under fluoro guidance toward the cubital fossa, and the venogram is performed through the catheter. The purpose of the venogram is to delineate the venous anatomy, the position of the perforator vein in the cubital fossa with its close proximity to the deep target vein, and the superficial venous system to plan the location of the fistula creation as well as to determine the patency of the upper arm superficial veins (cephalic and basilic veins). The cannulation of the appropriate artery with ultrasound guidance is determined based on the predominant target vein visualized during the venogram along with the position of the perforator vein. Either the brachial artery is cannulated antegrade in the upper arm region avoiding the adjoining nerve bundle or the radial or ulnar artery cannulated retrograde in the distal forearm region using the 21-gauge introducer needle and a 5 Fr slender sheath inserted into the cannulated artery. The 4 Fr guiding vascular catheter is advanced through the cannulate artery via the sheath over a 0.014" or 0.018" guidewire and the arteriogram is performed after positioning the catheter tip within the distal segment of brachial artery in the upper arm region. The arteriogram will help to determine the close alignment of the target artery to the target vein in the proximal forearm region within few centimeters, ideally within 1 cm distal to the position of the perforator vein. After the initial insertion of the venous and arterial sheaths, a single dose of heparin either 3,000–5,000 units or weight based (50 units/kg body weight) is given systemically; other medications like nitroglycerine or verapamil can also be given with appropriate dilutions into the access vessel to counteract any occurrence of vasospasms. The final step involves the positioning of the appropriate magnetic catheter within the respective target artery and vein at the planned site for the fistula creation. First, the arterial catheter is advanced through the arterial sheath over the 0.014" guidewire to position the ceramic backstop at the location of fistula creation, followed by the advancement of the venous catheter through the venous sheath to position the electrode opposite to the ceramic backstop. Both the catheters are advanced into the appropriate target vessels over the guidewires following the rapid-exchange technique. Next, the catheters are carefully rotated under fluoro guidance until the rotational indicator windows could be visualized to confirm the optimal positioning of the catheter at the site of the fistula creation. At this point, the magnets of the catheters will be attracted coaptating the target vein with the artery to close proximity with a distance of <1 mm between the two vessels and ensuring that the cutting electrode on the venous catheter is aligned with the ceramic backstop indentation of the arterial catheter. At this point, the venous catheter attached to the RF generator followed by the release of tourniquet from the upper arm and guidewires is also removed from the respective vessels. Finally, the electrode is activated to the preset levels of the generator while the patient's arm is fully restrained, since the RF energy during the electrode activation will cause arm jerks with involuntary muscle contractions. During the energy activation, the electrode should visibly advance and touch the arterial backstop. If the fistula creation failed during the RF activation, the position of catheters should be confirmed and the device can be reactivated for a total of three attempts.

After the creation of endoAVF, the venous catheter is removed followed by the arterial catheter via the respective sheaths and the brachial arteriogram is performed to confirm the target arterial flow into the superficial venous system across the anastomosis through the perforator vein. Finally, the respective brachial venous segment in the distal arm region communicating with the target vein of the endoAVF is coil embolized using the vascular catheter via the venous sheath to channelize the maximum target arterial flow diversion into the superficial vein (without the need for the complete exclusion of flow through the brachial vein), which will facilitate progressive maturation of the fistula. At this point, the sheaths from the access vessels are removed with hemostasis being obtained by following the local protocol (applying optimal manual pressure might suffice to obtain hemostasis).

(An animation video of WavelinQ Procedure is available in https://youtu.be/3ACf6Yx39u0. *Courtesy:* BD, USA.)

Ellipsys Device

The device consists of a single 6 Fr catheter with an elliptical shaped closing tip and the catheter is connected to a thermal energy delivering power controller **(Fig. 9)**. The Ellipsys system uses thermal energy and pressure to create the specific endoAVF.

Procedure: The Ellipsys technique creates anastomosis using ultrasound guidance without the need for fluoroscopy and is used to create the endoAVF involving only one set of vascular real-estate, it being the proximal

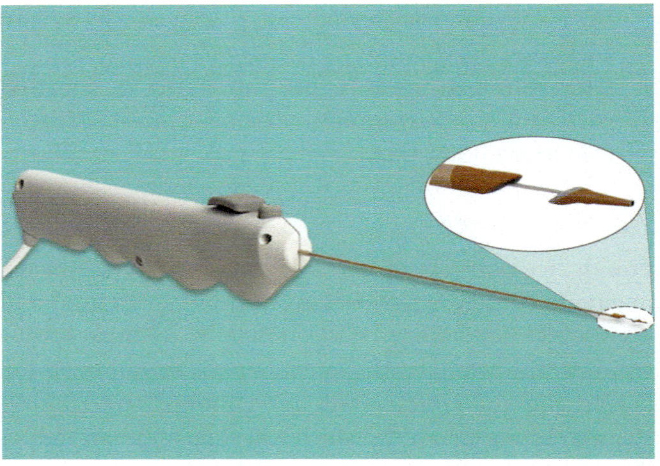

Fig. 9: Ellipsys 6 Fr catheter.

radial artery segment in the cubital fossa with the perforator vein. The Ellipsys endoAVF also provides dual superficial venous outflow through the cephalic and basilic veins like the WavelinQ endoAVF. Using real-time ultrasound guidance, the median cephalic or median basilic vein that drains the perforating vein is accessed in the retrograde direction using a 21-gauge introducer needle about 3–4 cm proximal to the intended site of the anastomosis. The needle is carefully guided in the retrograde direction with ultrasound through this vein and possibly through the median cubital vein into the perforator vein (target vein). The needle is further advanced cautiously with slow movements through the target vein with the ultrasound preferably maintained in the transverse view until the needle tip reaches the point of crossing of the perforator vein to the proximal radial artery segment, which is the expected anastomosis site of the AVF. During this slow distal movement, keeping the needle tip within the center of the target vein and always visualizing the location of the needle tip while maintaining the ultrasound in the transverse view cannot be overemphasized in order to prevent an inadvertent penetration of the venous wall causing hematoma or inducing venospasm by disturbing the venous wall. At this point, the needle is firmly but slowly pushed through the venous wall into the proximal radial artery segment along with the simultaneous gentle maneuver of the ultrasound probe in the transverse direction. The entry of the needle into the artery could be visualized in the ultrasound image and also by the free arterial blood flow through the needle. After achieving the arterial penetration, a 0.018" or 0.021" guidewire is inserted into the radial artery through the needle and advanced into the distal radial artery segment with the intra-arterial position of the guidewire confirmed by ultrasound. At this point, one-time dose of systemic heparin is given (either 2,000–3,000 units or weight-based dose of 50 units/kg body weight) and vasodilating medications like nitroglycerine or verapamil can also be given optionally for occurrence of severe vasospasm of the target vessels. A 6 Fr slender sheath is advanced over a guidewire into the radial artery after removing the access needle and a 0.014" guidewire is exchanged into the artery through the sheath. The Ellipsys catheter is next advanced over the guidewire through the sheath with ultrasound guidance and carefully positions the distal part of the open jaw at the catheter tip within the radial artery across the crossing point and the proximal segment of the open jaw within the perforator vein. The sheath is pulled back into the perforator vein, and the jaws of the catheter are closed, compressing the arterial and venous walls together within the device followed by connecting the device to the power generator. The sensors in the device indicate when there is appropriate coaptation of tissue and also provide the distance between the target vessels, which should be ideally <1.5 mm. At this point, the device is activated so that the generator delivers thermal energy in three rapid circles of heat and pressure, creating the elliptical anastomosis of 5 mm × 1 mm by fusing the vascular tissues. The device disengages at this point after the creation of anastomosis, which is removed from the target vein while maintaining the sheath as well as the guidewire within the target vessels. The ultrasound color doppler evaluation immediately confirms the successful creation of the anastomosis with target arterial flow directed into the perforator vein. An angioplasty of the anastomosis is performed immediately with a 5 × 20 mm balloon over the guidewire with ultrasound guidance, which facilitates the maturation process of AVF and also to avoid any occurrence of thrombosis. Finally, the sheath is removed and hemostasis obtained by applying gentle pressure. Following a successful creation of endoAVF, increased flow can be detected with ultrasound through the brachial artery. Ultimately, the arterial flow into the AVF will be directed through the perforator vein into the superficial veins of the arm (cephalic and basilic veins), which will facilitate the arterialization of the veins for hemodialysis **(Fig. 10)**.

(An animation video of the Ellipsys procedure is available at https://youtu.be/E0NXZ3O6-wY. *Courtesy*: Medtronic, USA.)

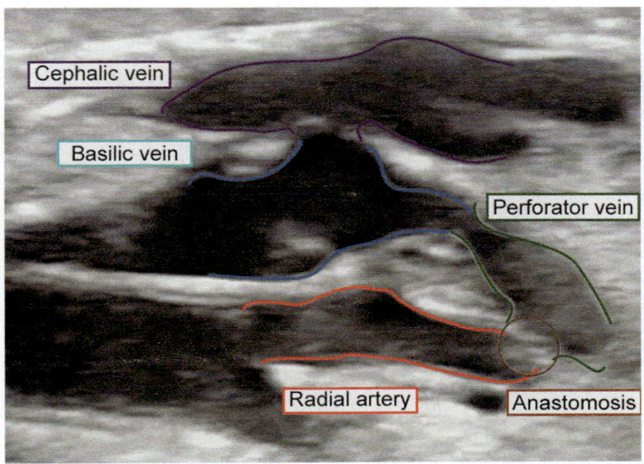

Fig. 10: Ultrasound image of an Ellipsys radial artery to perforator vein endoAVF with dual venous outflow.

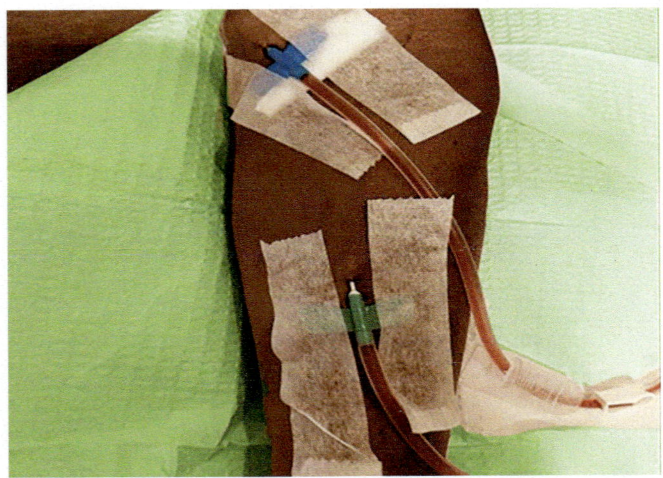

Fig. 11: WavelinQ Ulnar endoAVF—median basilic vein return cannulation (top) and cephalic vein draw cannulation (bottom).

Advantages of EndoAVF

When compared to the sAVF, creation of endoAVF appears to have many advantages **(Figs. 11 to 14)**:

- EndoAVF is a viable minimally invasive alternative to the age-old sAVF without the need for surgical incisions and dissection and is cosmetically appealing due to the absence of scars.
- EndoAVFs are moderate flow and low-pressure access system resulting in decreased flow-related complications like access aneurysm formation and high output cardiac dysfunction.
- EndoAVF creation seems to be safe with high maturation and long-term patency rates.

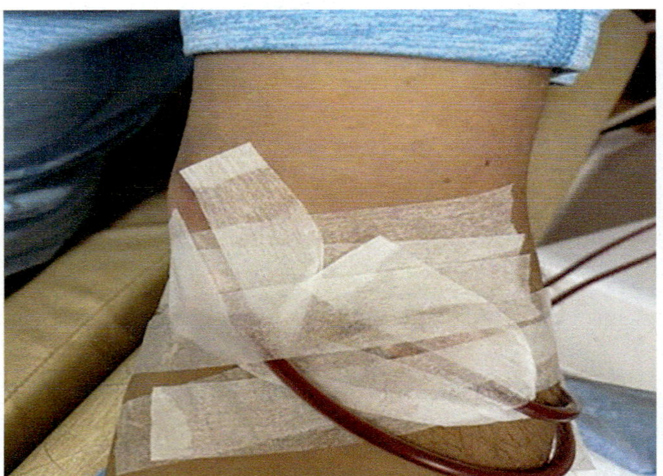

Fig. 12: WavelinQ Ulnar endoAVF—median basilic vein cannulation with two needles.

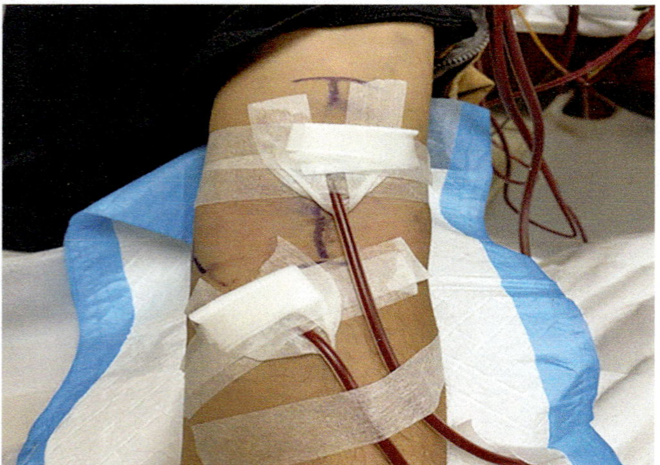

Fig. 13: Ellipsys endoAVF—median basilic vein draw cannulation (bottom) and cephalic vein return cannulation (top).

- EndoAVF provides extended, multiple, and unconventional target areas for cannulation. The target zones can extend down into the forearm region unlike the sAVF and more than one zone can be used for cannulation. The target veins include arm and forearm cephalic veins, distal upper arm region basilic to the median basilic vein across the elbow, median cephalic vein segment across the elbow, median cubital vein, and forearm cephalic vein.
- Short procedure times for the endoAVF that are statistically significant compared with those with the sAVF
- Relatively lower rate of complications
- EndoAVF outcomes appear to be noninferior to the sAVF.

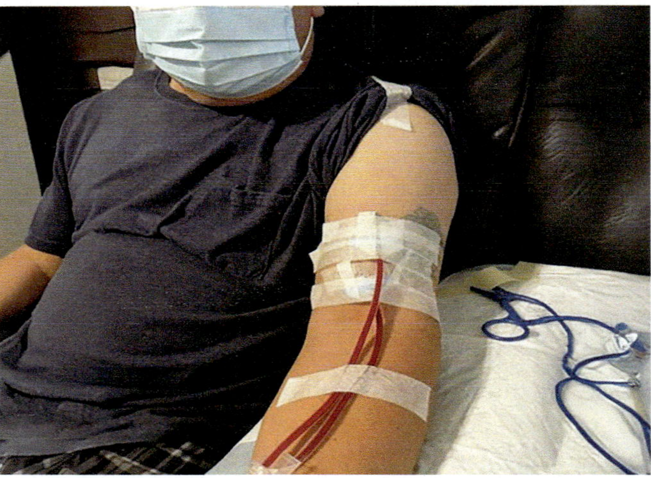

Fig. 14: WavelinQ Ulnar endoAVF—cephalic vein cannulation with two needles.

Literature Review and Outcome of EndoAVF

Multiple clinical studies, observational data, and narrative real-world experiences have provided a favorable outcome for the endoAVF created using the two novel devices. The current knowledge of the WavelinQ endoAVF outcomes are available from the three landmark trials—FLEX and NEAT trials used the earlier 6 Fr WavelinQ system and the EASE trial used the upgraded 4 Fr WavelinQ system. The pivotal multicenter trial, midterm results of pAVF creation, and the maturation for hemodialysis study from the postmarket registry provided outcome data for the Ellipsys device technique of creating the endoAVF.

NEAT Trial: The initially published single-center FLEX trial[12] enrolled only 33 patients using the 6 Fr WavelinQ system to create the ulnar-ulnar endoAVF, which revealed a technical success rate of 97%. In the subsequent NEAT[13] multicenter, single-arm prospective trial using the 6 Fr WavelinQ system to create ulnar and radial endoAVFs that included 80 patients with 57% in the predialysis stage, the reported technical success rate was 98%. The primary endpoint of the trial defined as clinical (successful two-needle dialysis) or physiological (brachial artery flow >500 mL/min and target vein diameter ≥4 mm) was achieved in 87%. The reported 12-month primary patency rate was 69%, cumulative patency was 84%, and functional usability of the AVF was 64%. The secondary procedures performed included transposition, coil embolization, ligation, angioplasty, thrombectomy, surgical artery repair, and new access creation at a reported rate of 0.46 per patient-year.

WavelinQ 4 Fr System Trial: The aggregated study of three trials[14] involving 120 patients that analyzed the use of 4 Fr WavelinQ endoAVF system included the EASE trial (32 patients), EASE-2 trial (24 patients) and EU postmarketing clinical follow-up study (64 patients) revealed a technical success rate of 96.7%. The primary, assisted primary, and 6-month secondary patency rates were 71.9% ± 4.5%, 80.7% ± 4.1%, and 87.8% ± 3.3%, respectively. The average time to the maturation of endoAVF was 41 ± 17 days and the time to successful cannulation averaged at 68 ± 51 days. The device- and procedure-related adverse events were 2.5% and 5.8%, respectively. The reintervention rate of 19.2% was split between 10.8% for maturation and 9.2% for maintenance.

WavelinQ endoAVF versus sAVF: A single-center observational study[15] conducted in the UK compared the outcome of WavelinQ endoAVF created in 30 patients versus surgically created distal forearm R-C AVF (RC sAVF) in 40 patients. The procedural success rate was 96.7% for WavelinQ and 92.6% for sAVF. The primary patency rates for WavelinQ were 65.5% and 56.5% at 6 and 12 months, respectively, and for the sAVF were 53.4% and 44%, respectively. The mean primary patency for WavelinQ was significantly higher at 362 ± 240 days compared to 235 ± 210 days for the sAVF. The secondary patency rates were superior for WavelinQ at 75.8% and 69.5% compared to the sAVF at 66.7% and 57.6% in 6 and 12 months, respectively. The investigators reckoned the superiority of WavelinQ to the surgical distal R-C AVF in their center, especially in patients with lower quality vessels in the distal forearm region. WavelinQ may be considered as the first choice for the AVF creation.

Ellipsys Pivotal Multicenter Trial: The early prospective single-arm trial[16] evaluated the achievement of primary endpoints of brachial artery flow >500 mL/min and target vein ≥4 mm diameter in >49% of 107 intent-to-treat patient and absence of device-related complications at 90 days. The AVF was created in 95% of patients with primary flow and diameter endpoints achieved in 86%, performance goal was >49% and encountered no adverse event. The maturation procedures performed in these patients included anastomosis angioplasty in 72%, brachial vein coil embolization in 32%, cubital vein ligation in 31%, and surgical transposition in 26%. The target veins used for hemodialysis included cephalic vein in 74%, basilic vein in 24%, and brachial vein in 2%. The cumulative patency rates were 91.6%, 89.3%, and 86.7% at 90, 180, and 360 days, respectively **(Fig. 15)**. The two-needle dialysis was achieved in 88% of patients at a mean 114.3 days ± 66.2 days. The functional patency rates were 98.4%, 98.4%, and 92.3% at 90, 180, and 360 days, respectively **(Fig. 16)**.

Ellipsys midterm results: The midterm results of pAVF creation using the Ellipsys vascular access system involved a total of 234 patients[17] with a technical success rate of 99% and the average procedure duration of creating the AVF was shown to be 15 minutes (7–15 minutes). The 1-year

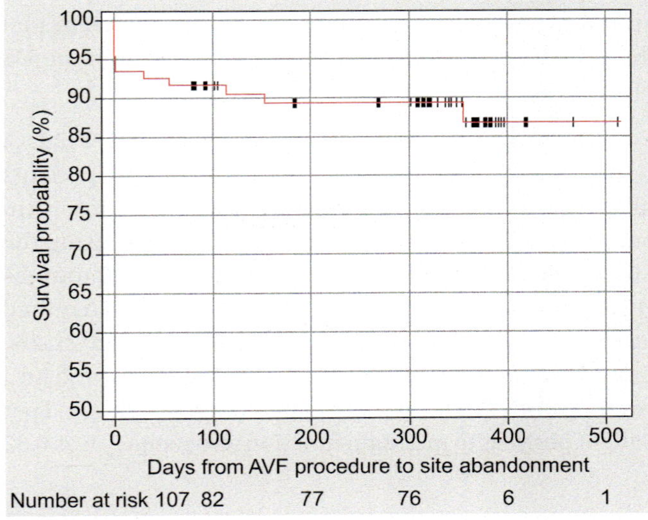

Fig. 15: Cumulative patency of fistulas in the ITT population. (AVF: arteriovenous fistula; ITT: intent to treat)

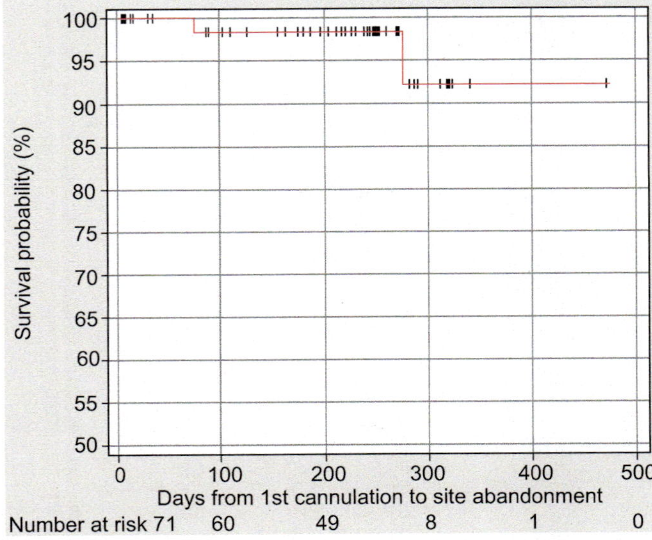

Fig. 16: Functional patency of fistulas from two-needle dialysis to abandonment.
Source: Hull et al.[16]

primary patency, primary-assisted, and secondary patency rates were 54%, 85%, and 96%, respectively **(Fig. 17)**. The average pAVF flow rate was 923 mL/min, average maturation time was 4 weeks (1–12 weeks), there was 6% early cannulation of <2 weeks, and there was no occurrence of any significant adverse event. It is conceivable from the data that the Ellipsys device allows rapid and safe creation of reliable endoAVF with an excellent rate of technical success, patency, and maturation. For patients without a viable surgical option for creation of distal forearm AVF, the Ellipsys technique should be considered as the primary option for AVF creation. Hence, the Ellipsys system met the primary safety and efficacy endpoint goal in the US pivotal trial.

Long-term Results from the Ellipsys Pivotal Trial: A retrospective review of the 107 intent-to-treat patients from the initial pivotal trial provided the long-term outcome of 85 patients with endoAVF created using the Ellipsys system,[18] with a median follow-up of 50 months (12–60 months range). The AVF maintenance was required in 31.8% of patients for fistula dysfunction in 21.2%, thrombosis in 5.9%, cannulation injury in 12.9%, and arm swelling in 4.7%. The number of procedures performed per patient per year to maintain function and patency was 0.32 for years 2–5. The cumulative patency rates were 89.5%, 88.4%, 88.4%, 85.6%, and 82.0% for years 1, 2, 3, 4, and 5, respectively. The functional patency was 91.8% at the end of the study **(Fig. 18)**. There were no major complications related to the AVF during the long-term follow-up.

Following the high technical and clinical success rates of creating the pAVF, it is conceivable from the long-term follow-up trial that pAVF provided effective and durable dialysis with low rates of access maintenance procedures without major complications.

Comparison of Ellipsys Percutaneous AVF with Proximal Forearm Gracz Surgical AVF: The retrospective study[19] reviewed a prospectively maintained database of all dialysis vascular access cases from a single center with a single operator, which compared 89 cases of pAVF created using the Ellipsys system to 69 cases of proximal forearm region surgically created Gracz AVF (same anatomical location). The inflow artery in the pAVF involved the proximal radial artery segment and that of the sAVF involved proximal radial artery 30%, proximal ulnar artery 12%, and distal brachial artery 58%. The technical success rate was 100% in both the groups, and the average procedure time was 14 minutes for pAVF and 74 minutes for sAVF. The access flow volumes, times to maturation,

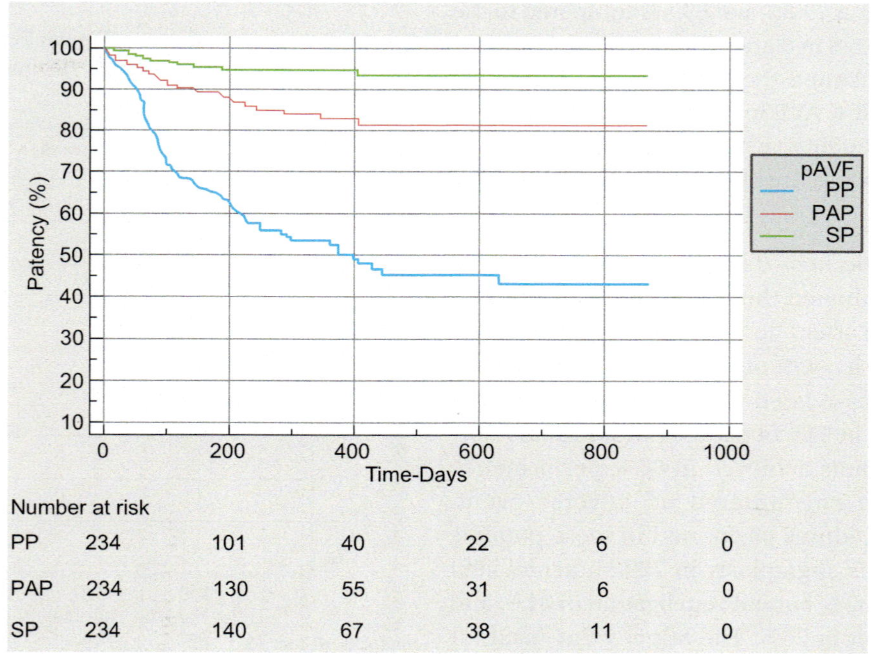

Number at risk						
PP	234	101	40	22	6	0
PAP	234	130	55	31	6	0
SP	234	140	67	38	11	0

Fig. 17: Kaplan–Meier analysis for patency rates, Paris Series. (pAVF: percutaneous arteriovenous fistula; PAP: primary-assisted patency; PP: primary patency; SP: secondary patency)
Source: Mallios et al.[17]

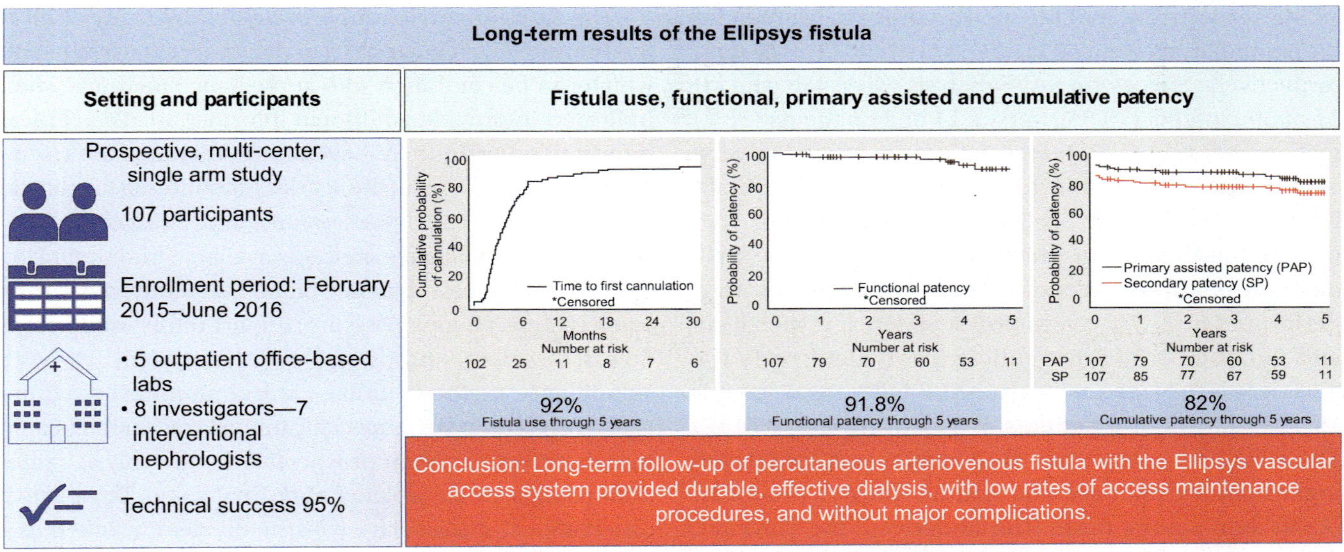

Fig. 18: Graphical abstract of the long-term outcomes of the pivotal multicenter trial.
Source: Hull et al.[18]

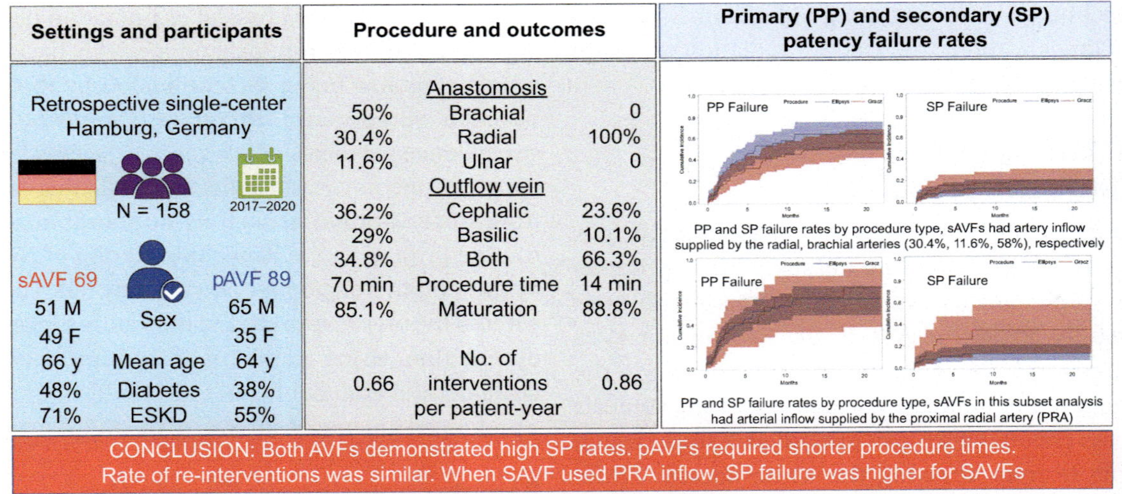

Fig. 19: Graphical abstract comparing Ellipsys percutaneous and proximal forearm Gracz-type surgical arteriovenous fistulas.
Source: Shahverdyan et al.[20]

and overall numbers of interventions per patient-year were not significantly different. The cumulative incidence of primary patency failure at 12 months was lower for sAVF (47% vs. 64%; $p = 0.1$), but secondary patency failure was not different between groups (20% vs. 12%; $p = 0.3$). PRA sAVFs had similar primary patency (65% vs. 64%; $p = 0.8$) but higher secondary patency failure rates than pAVFs at 12 months (34% vs. 12%; $p = 0.04$) **(Fig. 19)**.

Comparison of outcomes of percutaneous arteriovenous fistulae creation by Ellipsys and WavelinQ devices: The retrospective review with prospectively collected data of 100 patients who underwent pAVF creation by Ellipsys and WavelinQ techniques done by a single operator between December 2017 and December 2019 at a single center evaluated the primary endpoints of technical success, time to maturation, functional patency, and time to first clinical use.[20] Comparing Ellipsys to the WavelinQ technique, the technical success rate was 100% versus 97%, respectively, with the median procedure times being 14 versus 63 minutes, respectively ($p < 0.001$), with 183 (1–487) versus 185 (0–760) days follow-up, respectively. The pAVF maturation rate at 4 weeks was 68.3% versus

54.3%, respectively, and the median times to cannulation for hemodialysis were 60 (1–164) versus 90 (1–180) days, respectively. Successful pAVF dialysis was established in 31 of 39 patients (79.5%) versus 14 of 24 patients (58%), respectively ($p = 0.071$), and the access-related adverse events were observed in four individuals (one Ellipsys vs. three WavelinQ). Six patients (five vs. one) with matured outflow from previous AVFs underwent first-day cannulations. Access-related interventions were performed in 27.7% versus 26.5% patients, respectively, and the number of interventions per patient-years was 0.96 versus 0.46, respectively. pAVF failure was seen in 15.4% versus 37.1% patients, respectively ($p = 0.0137$). The secondary patency rate at 12 months was significantly higher among patients who had an Ellipsys procedure (82%) than among those who underwent the WavelinQ procedure (60%). It is conceivable from this study data that pAVFs were created using both devices with high technical success and low complication rates, with the Ellipsys technique demonstrating significantly shorter procedure times without the need for radiation exposure and revealed superior secondary patency rates.

MAINTENANCE OF ARTERIOVENOUS FISTULA

Maintenance of a functionally patent AVF for hemodialysis assisted with clinical monitoring and surveillance program is equally important as executing various techniques to successfully create the AVF itself. Most of the AVFs with dysfunction have an anatomic problem due to the development of neointimal hyperplasia causing stenosis in the access circuit, which can present as a single lesion or multiple lesions affecting the same access. These stenotic lesions commonly involve the access circuit at the inflow segment (arterial anastomosis and juxta-arterial anastomosis venous segment), the venous outflow segment of the AVF due to the disruption in the laminal flow resulting from anatomical variations (cephalic venous arch segment and swing segment angulation involving the transposed basilic venous segment), and the access cannulation sites due to abnormal remodeling with fibrotic transformation. Being a well-known fact that vascular access dysfunction leads to increased patient morbidity as well as mortality, early detection of AVF dysfunction due to stenosis and timely intervention will help to maintain the access functional patency and also prevent the occurrence of access failure with thrombosis.

The AVF function can be evaluated by using clinical monitoring on a regular basis to detect access dysfunction, which can be combined with surveillance methods when indicated to provide additional information. The clinical monitoring used for AVF evaluation includes the use of physical examination of the access,[21] monitoring for clinical problems during dialysis sessions, and monitoring Kt/V values. The surveillance methods available for monitoring include intra-access dynamic blood flow study, measuring static dialysis venous pressure, duplex ultrasound access flow assessment, and using Vasc Alert system. The AVF surveillance methods unlike clinical monitoring require specialized equipment, specially trained staff, and repeated measurement to obtain prospective trend analysis rather than using a single isolated abnormal value. Prospective observational studies have consistently demonstrated that physical examination performed by trained personnel is an accurate method for the diagnosis of fistula stenosis.[22] The KDOQI clinical practice guideline for vascular access recommends that the physical examination be performed on all mature AVFs routinely on a weekly basis, with such monitoring also being recommended by the Society for Vascular Surgery and, therefore, should be part of all surveillance protocols of the vascular access.[23] Due to the paucity of unequivocal benefits and conflicting data available from observational as well as nonrandomized studies, routine primary surveillance monitoring of AVF followed by pre-emptive angioplasty is currently not recommended without the presence of clinical indicators suggestive of AVF dysfunction. Using a systematic multipronged approach facilitates the evaluation and timely intervention to ensure a prolonged functional survival of the AVF.

Percutaneous Innovations in the Management of Arteriovenous Fistula Dysfunction due to Stenosis

Arteriovenous fistula flow dysfunction is a common problem due to the occurrence of neointimal hyperplasia resulting in the development of stenosis, which can result in the failure of the AV access due to thrombosis and contribute significantly to the patients' morbidity. Endovascular intervention using angioplasty with various compliant and noncompliant plain balloons has been the treatment of choice for AV access stenosis that causes abnormal access blood flow parameters associated with abnormal symptoms as well as clinical findings. The balloon angioplasty of the AV access stenosis causes a spectrum of vessel wall changes from simple stretching at the angioplasty site to significant anatomic disruption varying from dissection, tears, elastic recoil, or in various combinations. Plain balloon angioplasty (PBA) continues to be the standard treatment for significant stenotic lesions in the hemodialysis access circuit, with the angioplasty outcomes being more favorable in AVF compared to the AVG. The primary patency for AVF circuit stenosis at 6 and 12 months from cohort studies ranges between 42 and 63% and 23 and 50.5%, respectively.[24] Failure of angioplasty using plain balloons is known to occur at varying rates with highly resistant stenotic lesions or from elastic recoil at the site of angioplasty despite using high-pressure noncompliant plain angioplasty balloon catheters. Higher rates of AVF circuit restenosis have been reported in association with lesions at specific sites like the cephalic venous arch segment, juxta-anastomosis venous segment, or the angle of transposition of the AVF. Using intravascular ultrasound (IVUS) after the angioplasty, restenosis due to vascular wall rupture has been reported at a relatively higher rate of 18% or elastic recoil occurring within 5–10 minutes after the angioplasty at a rate that could be as high as 50%.[25,26] In these cases with angioplasty failure or rapid recurrence, alternative newer approaches to salvage therapy are currently available. Endovascular approach with angioplasty using newer balloon and technical innovations continues to be the primary option for AVF salvage before considering any surgical revision.

Innovations extending beyond the use of plain balloons for the angioplasty of AVF circuit-resistant stenotic lesions or stenosis with marked elastic recoils prior to the consideration of stent deployment include the use of cutting balloons, drug-coated (drug-eluting) balloons, and vessel preparation device followed by balloon angioplasty.

Cutting Balloon Angioplasty

Cutting balloon used for angioplasty is a special balloon catheter with three to four microsurgical cutting blades or atherotomes incorporated longitudinally to the balloon surface **(Fig. 20)**, which on inflation creates discrete longitudinal incisions through the resistant fibrous stenotic lesions at a lower inflation pressure. Cutting balloon angioplasty under low pressure can reduce the inflammatory response and the risks of cell proliferation at the angioplasty site.[27] These balloons can be used to treat resistant or elastic recoiling stenotic lesions in the hemodialysis access sites as an alternative to the high-pressure balloons, thereby delaying the occurrence of restenosis caused by neointimal hyperplasia.

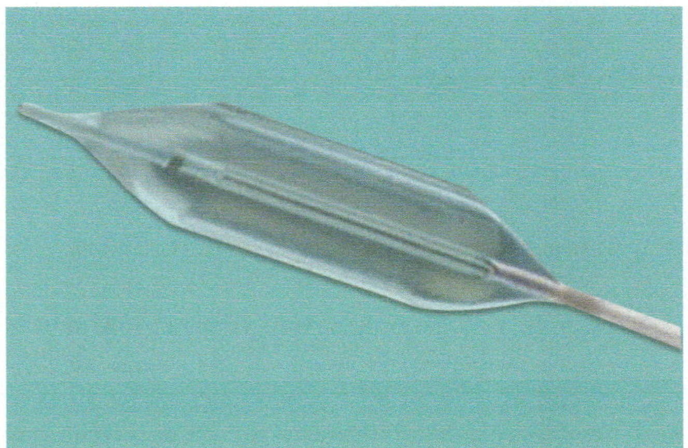

Fig. 20: Angioplasty balloon with microcutting blades (atherotomes).

A systematic review and meta-analysis of three studies compared 90 patients in the cutting balloon angioplasty group with 90 patients in the high-pressure balloon angioplasty group.[28] The results of the meta-analysis suggested that compared with high-pressure balloon angioplasty, cutting balloon angioplasty can improve primary lesion patency rates of AVFs at 6 months [relative risk, 1.45; 95% confidence interval (CI) 1.08–1.96; $p = 0.01$] **(Fig. 21)**.

However, the meta-analysis showed no significant differences between the technical and clinical success rates. The use of cutting balloon to angioplasty AVF circuit stenosis is likely to increase primary lesion patency rates at 6 months, but a large sample of randomized controlled trials is obviously needed for absolute validation.

Another meta-analysis involving three studies with 1,034 participants,[29] with 525 in the cutting balloon group and 509 in the plain balloon control arm, showed no immediate difference in the procedural success rates between the two groups. The 6-month target lesion patency was significantly higher in the cutting balloon angioplasty arm [67.2% vs. 55.6%; risk difference (RD) 0.12; 95% CI 0.05–0.19; $p < 0.05$] with a number needed to treat (NNT) of 9. The device-related complications were not statistically significant between the two groups (RD 0.03; 95% CI –0.02 to 0.07; $p = 0.26$).

Drug-Coated (Drug-Eluting) Balloon Angioplasty

Endovascular intervention with percutaneous transluminal angioplasty continues to remain the common

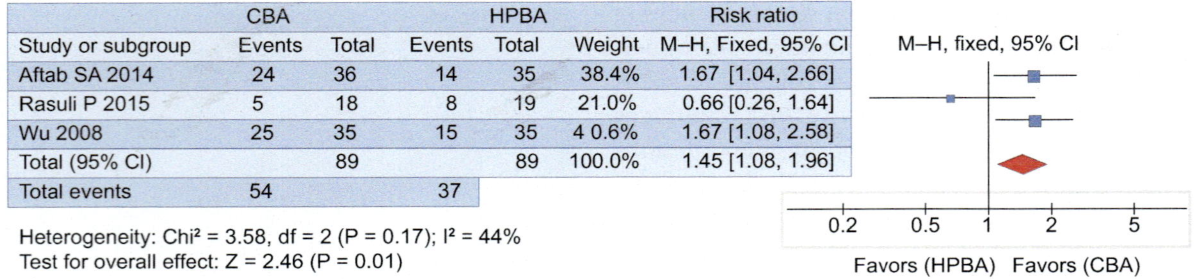

Study or subgroup	CBA Events	CBA Total	HPBA Events	HPBA Total	Weight	Risk ratio M–H, Fixed, 95% CI
Aftab SA 2014	24	36	14	35	38.4%	1.67 [1.04, 2.66]
Rasuli P 2015	5	18	8	19	21.0%	0.66 [0.26, 1.64]
Wu 2008	25	35	15	35	4 0.6%	1.67 [1.08, 2.58]
Total (95% CI)		89		89	100.0%	1.45 [1.08, 1.96]
Total events	54		37			

Heterogeneity: Chi² = 3.58, df = 2 (P = 0.17); I² = 44%
Test for overall effect: Z = 2.46 (P = 0.01)

Fig. 21: Forest plot of primary lesion patency rates at 6 months.
Source: Pang et al.[28]

and primary mode of therapy for stenosis causing hemodialysis vascular circuit dysfunction due to the instantaneous benefit and procedural convenience compared to the surgical intervention. Unfortunately, the primary patency rate at 1 year following angioplasty with conventional plain balloons including the use of high-pressure noncompliant balloons remains at a relatively lower variable rate of 26–58%[30,31] and the patients undergoing repeat interventions for restenosis within 6 months have been estimated to be approximately 50% in systematic reviews and metanalysis.[29,32-34] The idea of using an innovative approach to the angioplasty of vascular stenosis and prevent or prolong the patency of vascular circuit blossomed from the antiproliferative properties of chemotherapeutic agents, which can be applied directly to the target lesions by using drug-coated balloons (DCBs). The locally applied antiproliferative agents will in turn prevent neointimal hyperplasia by causing cellular apoptosis and inhibiting smooth muscle cell migration. The two drugs currently approved for coating the angioplasty balloons, which shares the property of inhibiting cell proliferation and prevention of vascular restenosis includes Paclitaxel and Sirolimus. Early studies using angioplasty balloon coated with Paclitaxel have been shown to be effective and safe with femoral-popliteal artery stenosis in reducing restenosis caused by neointimal hyperplasia, thereby improving primary patency as well as reducing the need for clinically driven target lesion revascularization.[35]

The idea behind the use of antiproliferative agents for treating vascular circuit stenosis is based on the scientific fact that T-cell activation, increase in the regulatory T cells, or proliferation of dendritic cells occurs locally in the vascular circuit resulting in the immune vessel wall injury, which in turn facilitates the migration as well as growth of smooth muscle cells with eventual transformation to neointimal hyperplasia causing stenosis.[36-38] The vascular circuit target site activation of neutrophilic leukocytes is also known to facilitate restenosis.[39] The DCB technology involves the antiproliferative pharmacological agent loaded on the semicompliant carrier balloon with polymeric coating or added with a hydrophilic excipient, which on inflation will quickly and efficiently transfer the agent to the vessel wall at the target stenotic lesion. The agent with high lipophilic property or the use of phospholipid encapsulation of the carrier helps to deliver the agent at the target site with maximum effective lower dose to reduce toxicity, obtain minimal loss in the circulation during device delivery, and also facilitate the agent to remain within the vessel wall of the target lesion to provide the antiproliferative effect for an extended period.

Paclitaxel is an antiproliferative chemotherapy drug, which stabilizes microtubules by binding to the cellular beta subunit of tubulin, thereby preventing their disassembly and suppressing mitotic division resulting in cellular apoptosis.[40] The drug has a dose-dependent effect with the lower concentrations having the ability to trigger programmed cell death.[41] The high lipophilic property of the drug facilitates efficient passive absorption through the cell membrane and prolonged retention within the vessel wall to provide the local target site pharmacodynamic effects. The Paclitaxel dose loaded in the carrier angioplasty balloons ranges from 2.0 to 3.5 $\mu g/mm^2$.

Sirolimus is an immunosuppressant drug that modulates the activity of mammalian target of rapamycin (mTOR) by binding to the cytosolic protein FKBP12 and thereby causing the cell-cycle blockage in G1-S phase by inhibiting the IL-2-mediated signal transduction.[42] Sirolimus inhibits smooth muscle cell proliferation and migration without inducing apoptosis. Sirolimus in comparison with Paclitaxel exhibits anti-inflammatory properties and has a broader therapeutic window, increased safety margin and negligible effect on the endothelial cellular function.[39] The low lipophilic property of Sirolimus can cause higher washout during deployment of carrier balloon, slower local penetration rate, and decreased retention within the vessel wall, compromising the bioavailability of this drug at the vascular target site. The bioavailability of Sirolimus in DCBs can be enhanced to a great extent with controlled drug delivery by using absorption enhancers like encapsulation in a phospholipid carrier with Nanolute technology (MagicTouch PTA, Concept Medical, Gujarat, India) or using biodegradable polymer as the drug carrier that facilitates increased uptake into the vessel wall through microreservoirs (SELUTION SLR, MedAlliance, Nyon, Switzerland, now marketed by Cordis, Miami Lakes, USA). Once the antiproliferative drug is delivered effectively to the vascular circuit target site, Sirolimus has a theoretical advantage of a longer therapeutic effect due to the longer half-life of around 90 days compared to that of Paclitaxel which is to around days to week.[43]

Sirolimus DCBs are currently approved for use in coronary and peripheral artery disease, whereas the two approved DCBs currently used for treating hemodialysis vascular access circuit stenosis are the Lutonix (CR Bard, Providence, NJ, USA) and IN.PACT Admiral (Medtronic, Minneapolis, MN, USA). The Lutonix DCB delivers a dose of 2 μg/mm^2 of Paclitaxel with the excipient being polysorbate/sorbitol and the IN.PACT Admiral DCB delivers a dose of 3 μg/mm^2 of Paclitaxel with urea as the excipient. The DCB angioplasty procedure for the dialysis vascular circuit stenosis involves the initial preparation of the target lesion with primary angioplasty followed by the use of DCB at the primed stenosis site. The proper primary preparation of the stenotic lesions is essential to obtain optimal peri- and postprocedural clinical outcomes. The primary angioplasty should be initially performed with any kind of balloons (plain semicompliant/noncompliants as well as cutting or scoring balloons) according to the severity of the lesion to obtain the maximum dilatation benefit with a minimal postangioplasty residual lesion of less than 30%. After the priming or vessel preparation angioplasty, a DCB of appropriate diameter and length (same diameter of the priming balloon or 1 mm greater and length of the balloon to exceed the stenotic lesion by 0.5–1.0 cm at proximal as well as distal to the lesion) is used to complete the procedure by quickly deploying the DCB and maintaining the balloon at the target site in the recommended nominal inflation pressure for a duration of 2.5–3 minutes.

Various single-center studies have shown the benefit of angioplasty using DCB for access circuit stenosis. The randomized investigational-device-exemption controlled trial with 285 enrolled patients having access circuit stenosis did not meet the target lesion primary patency (TLPP) at 180 days (showed similar patency) with DCB (Lutonix balloon with Paclitaxel 2 μg/mm^2 and Sorbitol excipient) angioplasty compared to the standard balloon angioplasty, and the primary safety endpoint did not differ between groups.[44]

The prospective, single-blinded, multicenter (29 international sites), 1:1 randomized trial enrolled 330 participants with upper extremity AVF stenosis to evaluate the effect of angioplasty using DCB (IN.PACT Admiral Balloon with Paclitaxel 3.5 μg/mm^2 and urea excipient) in 170 participants compared to the standard balloon in 160 participants. During the 6 months' period after the index procedure, the target-lesion primary patency was maintained more often in participants treated with DCB angioplasty than in those treated with a standard balloon (82.2% vs. 59.5%; difference in risk, 22.8 percentage points; 95% CI 12.8–32.8; $p < 0.001$). DCB was noninferior to standard balloon with respect to the primary safety endpoint within 30 days (4.2% and 4.4%, respectively; difference in risk, –0.2 percentage points; 95% CI –5.5 to 5.0; $p = 0.002$ for noninferiority). The study outcome showed DCB angioplasty to be superior to standard angioplasty **(Figs. 22A and B)** for the treatment of stenotic lesions in dysfunctional hemodialysis AVFs during 6 months after the index procedure.[45]

A meta-analysis of 18 randomized controlled trials compared 877 patients in the DCB group and 875 patients in the PBA group for TLPP, circuit patency, target lesion revascularization, and mortality. The TLPP was higher in the DCB group (OR 2.93; 95% CI 2.13–4.03; $p < 0.001$) at 6 months and (OR 2.47; 95% CI 1.53–3.99; $p < 0.001$) at 1 year. The DCB group had a higher dialysis circuit patency at 6 months (OR 2.42; 95% CI 1.56–3.77; $p < 0.001$) and (OR 1.91; 95% CI 1.22–3.00; $p = 0.005$) at 1 year. Compared with the PBA group, the DCB group had lower odds of target lesion revascularization during follow-up (OR 0.43; 95% CI 0.23–0.82; $p = 0.001$) at 6 months and (OR 0.74; 95% CI 0.32–1.73; $p = 0.490$) at 1 year. The OR of mortality was comparable between 2 groups at 6 months (OR 1.18; 95% CI 0.42–3.33; $p = 0.760$) and 1 year (OR 0.93; 95% CI 0.58–1.48; $p = 0.750$).[46] Based on the meta-analysis, the DCB angioplasty appeared to be superior to PBA in maintaining TLPP and dialysis circuit patency among

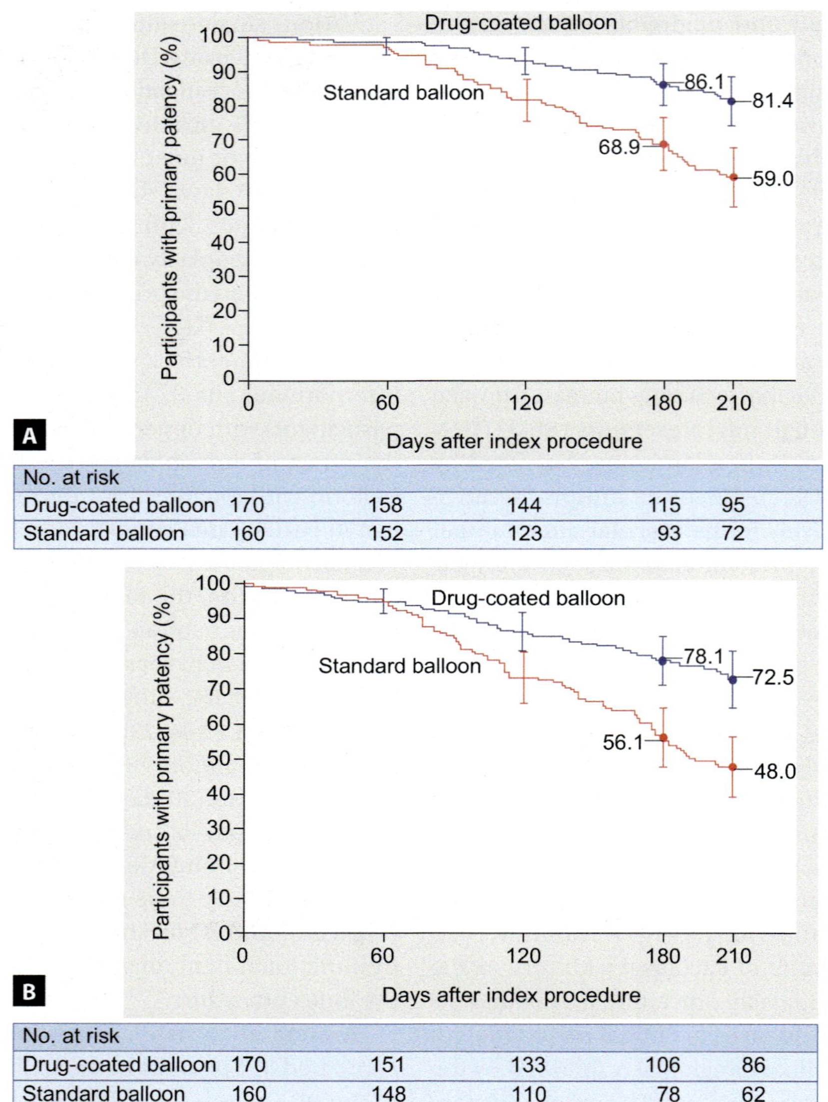

No. at risk					
Drug-coated balloon	170	158	144	115	95
Standard balloon	160	152	123	93	72

No. at risk					
Drug-coated balloon	170	151	133	106	86
Standard balloon	160	148	110	78	62

Figs. 22A and B: Kaplan–Meier analysis of primary patency during the 6 months after the index procedure. (A) Target-lesion primary patency; (B) Access-circuit primary patency.
Source: Lookstein et al.[45]

patients with dialysis circuit stenosis. DCB angioplasty also reduces target lesion revascularization with a similar risk of mortality compared with PBA.

The clinical trials using DCB appear to be heterogenous with variable outcomes, probably related to the difference in the carrier balloon brand that has variable drug dose along with different excipients. At this point, the DCB can be used as an adjunct to the standard balloon for treating high-risk or recurring access circuit stenosis to improve access patency by reducing neointimal hyperplasia. Appropriate patient selection, adequate preparation of the stenotic lesions, and following the proper DCB procedural technique are the key factors that can help to realize the maximum benefit of using DCB to treat stenosis causing access circuit dysfunction.

Vascular Preparation Technique for Access Circuit Stenosis Prior to Angioplasty—FLEX VP

Angioplasty remains the standard of care in treating stenotic lesions causing access circuit dysfunction, and high- or ultra high-pressure balloons are frequently required to treat resistant lesions. Even though the angioplasty provides immediate success, the long-term patency rates continue to be variable and many times discouraging due to the recurrence of stenosis. The use of high-pressure balloons for angioplasty can result in the occurrence of acute complications like vessel rupture, formation of aneurysm or pseudoaneurysm, etc. Newer devices and techniques are being developed with the goal to provide long-term effective patency outcomes for hemodialysis access with dysfunction due to stenosis. In addition to the cutting as well as scoring balloon technology used to provide effective angioplasty with resistant stenotic lesions, an innovative approach has been developed to prepare the site of the target stenotic lesions prior to the angioplasty by the newer device called the FLEX Vessel Prep System (FLEX VP - VentureMed Group, Minneapolis, MN). The FLEX device **(Fig. 23)** is a dynamic, self-sizing, nonballoon over-the-wire sheathed catheter device with a three-strut treatment element at the distal tip **(Fig. 24)**. The device is 6-Fr sheath as well as a 0.014" or 0.018" guidewire compatibility system and available in two working lengths (40 or 120 cm). The proximal portion of each treatment element strut includes a 0.010" microsurgical blade. Upon releasing the three struts from the catheter sheath within the access circuit at the target lesion, the struts expand and the microsurgical blades will independently engage the stenotic lesion and create three parallel longitudinal microincisions of depth about 250 μm along the entire length of the target lesion while the device is pulled back over the guidewire. The blades of the device exert a consistent opposed radial force of approximately 1 atm. on the vessel well to deliver the precise microincisions at the lesions with neointimal hyperplasia. The microincisions applied by rotating the device multiple times in turn improve acute luminal gain and vessel compliance by releasing circumferential tension in the lesion.

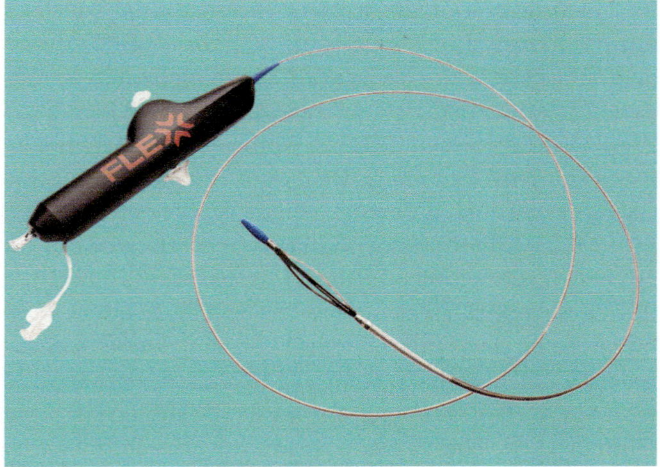

Fig. 23: FLEX VP device.
Courtesy: VentureMed, MN, USA

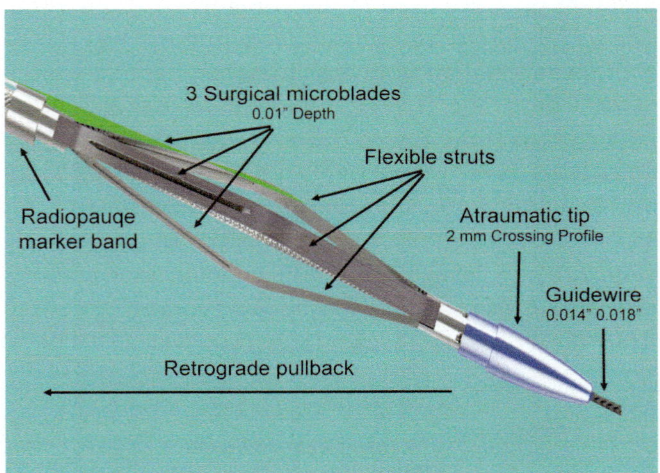

Fig. 24: Distal segment of device.
Courtesy: VentureMed, MN, USA.

FLEX VP device procedure: The FLEX device catheter is advanced through the hemodialysis access via a sheath of minimal 6 Fr size over a 0.018" guidewire. After crossing the target stenosis with the device, the treatment element at the distal segment of the catheter is unsheathed and expanded. Next, the catheter is slowly drawn back allowing the microsurgical blades on the proximal end of each treatment element strut to independently engage in the lesion and create three parallel continuous microincisions along the entire length of the lesion. Once the lesion is crossed back, the treatment element is resheathed and advanced again across the lesion with the device rotated approximately 30–90° before the treatment element is re-deployed and the retrograde pullback as described above is repeated. This process is repeated, as required, based on operator preference to create multiple longitudinal microincisions across the target lesion. After completing the endovascular primary vessel preparation with this device, traditional angioplasty can be performed with a relatively lower inflation pressure at the target site by using a standard balloon or DCB.

(An animation video of FLEX VP device procedure is available at https://youtu.be/bY0EBUrYXLw. *Courtesy:* VentureMed Group, MN, USA.)

The multicenter, prospective, observational registry[47] enrolled hemodialysis patients scheduled to undergo angioplasty of their AVF or graft due to clinical or hemodynamic abnormalities for treatment with FLEX Vessel Prep System followed by an appropriate angioplasty using standard balloon or DCB. A primary endpoint was anatomic success, defined as angiographic confirmation of <30% residual stenosis post procedure without an adverse event, and additional assessments included device technical success, clinical success, freedom from target lesion revascularization, TLPP, and circuit primary patency at 6 months. A total of 148 lesions were treated with FLEX VP prior to angioplasty in 114 subjects at eight clinical sites. The vessel preparation was followed by plain balloon angioplasty in 82 of 114 subjects (71.9%) and plain balloon + DCB angioplasty in 32 of 114 subjects (28.1%). The maximum average angioplasty inflation pressure used in the study was 15.2 ± 5.9 atm. The TLPP across all subjects at 6 months was 62.2% with mean freedom from target lesion revascularization of 202.7 days. The TLPP and freedom from target lesion revascularization for AVF cases ($n = 72$) were 67.5% and 212.9 days, respectively **(Fig. 25A)**. The TLPP and freedom from target lesion revascularization for AVGs ($n = 42$) were 52.4% and 183.3 days, respectively **(Fig. 25B)**. In cases treating AVF cephalic arch stenosis ($n = 25$), 6-month TLPP was 70.6% and freedom from target lesion revascularization was 213.4 days. Five procedural complications were recorded in the study without any serious adverse events.

Despite several limitations, especially with the lack of a matched cohort, the use of FLEX VP device prior to angioplasty of access circuit stenosis appeared to be safe and effective, notably with the lesions presenting in the cephalic venous arch and the AVGs. The postpreparation angioplasty with either plain balloon or DCB appeared to be safe without requiring higher balloon inflation pressure to obtain target lesion effacement target and patency (effacement could be mostly obtained with subnominal inflation pressure).

The AVAFLEX Prospective Observational Study **(Fig. 26)** compared FLEX prior to Lutonix DCB with Lutonix IDE treated cephalic venous arch stenoses in 53% of enrolled patients. The study excluded patients with residual stenosis ≥30% following PTA to open the stenosis (e.g., vessel prep).

The FLEX VP system seems to be an interesting novel and safe device available for the treatment of difficult or recurrent access circuit stenosis, more specifically the lesions involving cephalic venous arch as well as AVG without compromising procedural safety. This device has the potential to obtain effective and longer lasting access circuit patency, especially when combined with DCB angioplasty. The early promising results with the use of FLEX VP innovation device needs further authentication with additional larger randomized cohort matched control studies.

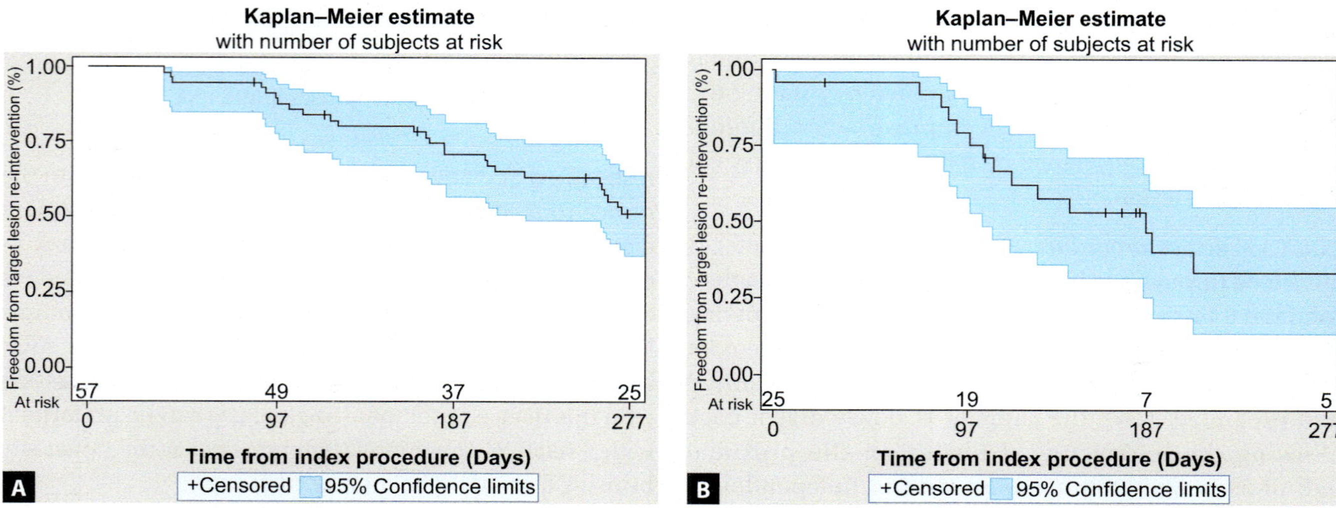

Figs. 25A and B: Kaplan–Meier estimates of (A) 6-month functional patency FLEX + PTA in AVF and (B) 6-month functional patency FLEX + PTA in AVG. (AVF: arteriovenous fistula; AVG: arteriovenous graft; PTA: percutaneous transluminal angioplasty)
Source: Aruny et al.[47]

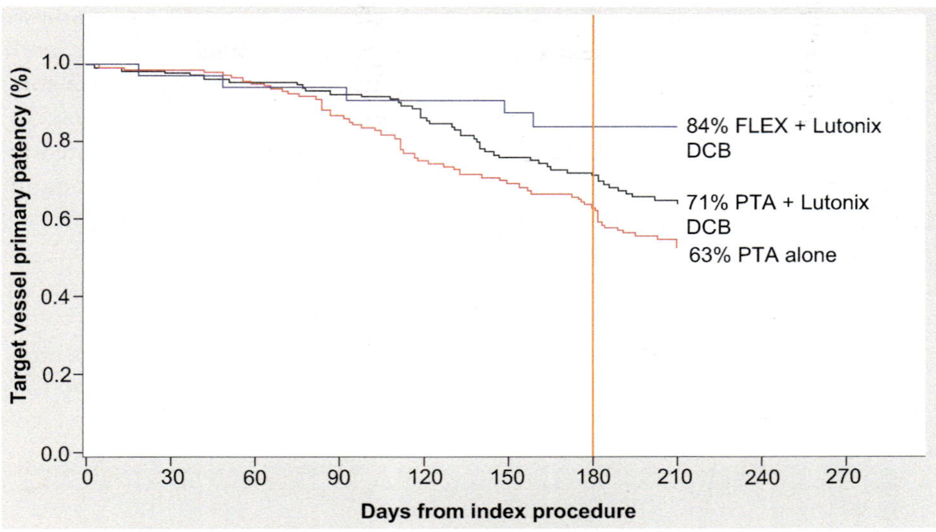

Fig. 26: Kaplan–Meier analysis of target lesion patency during the 6 months.
Source: Ross et al.[60]

STENT GRAFTS FOR ARTERIOVENOUS FISTULA PATENCY

The development of neointimal hyperplasia causing hemodialysis vascular access circuit stenosis continues to be a nemesis hindering the efficiency of dialysis treatment provided to the patient and thereby significantly increasing morbidity as well as mortality. Percutaneous balloon angioplasty intervention continues to be the standard first-line treatment for access circuit stenosis. The intermediate and long-term access circuit patency outcomes remain suboptimal despite various innovations in the angioplasty balloons used for the endovascular treatment of access circuit stenosis. Stents have been used for the management of stenosis and salvage access for providing hemodialysis that has failed angioplasty or developed complications like vessel rupture or extravasation during angioplasty. Early use of uncovered stents like the bare metal (stainless steel) and self-expanding (nitinol) smart stents showed no significant advantage or benefit in the patency rates compared to the standard angioplasty.[48-51] The access with stents developed dysfunction due to neointimal growth into the stent causing in-stent stenosis, stenosis occurring at the ends of the stents in contact with the vessel wall, and also due to the fracture of stent struts. Innovation to overcome the limitations of uncovered stents lead to the development of covered stents called stent grafts. These stents are made of nitinol struts and covered with a fabric coat of graft material, either expanded polytetrafluorethylene (ePTFE) or Dacron, which will provide the biocompatible barrier to prevent tissue (smooth muscle cell) in-growth into the stent that causes the restenosis. Various stent grafts with ePTFE lining available for clinical use include Flair, Fluency Plus, Covera (BD, USA), and Viabahn (Gore, USA) stents. In addition to the ePTFE fabric coat, the configuration of Flair, Fluency Plus, and Covera stents may have either straight ends or flared leading end to an additional 4 mm size along with a carbon-impregnated luminal surface, whereas the Viabahn stent has straight-end configuration and is also available with the luminal surface modified with heparin bioactive surface.

Various landmark clinical trials (FLAIR, Viabahn Stent, RENOVA, RESCUE, REVISE trials) have shown a clear benefit of using stent grafts compared to the uncovered stents or balloon angioplasty alone with significant improvement in the primary access circuit as well as target lesion patency of failing dialysis access grafts and also significantly reduced the number of reinterventions. The data regarding the use of stent graft in dysfunctional AVFs due to stenosis are limited except for recurring or resistant stenosis occurring at specific anatomical locations like the cephalic venous arch segment, basilic angle of transposition, and in-stent stenosis occurring within previously existing access circuit stent.

The prospective randomized trial[52] comparing the Fluency (BD, US) stent graft (BD, US) with Luminex (BD, US) bare metal stent showed recurrence of stenosis in the cephalic arch segment within 3 months following a successful angioplasty. The restenosis rate in stent grafts was 18% as compared with 70% restenosis in the bare metal stent group. The primary patency rates of the 13 stent grafts were 82, 82, and 32% after 3, 6, and 12 months, respectively, while the 12 bare metal stents had primary patency rates of 39, 39, and 0% at the same time intervals **(Figs. 27 and 28)**.

A systematic review and meta-analysis[53] of endovascular treatment of cephalic arch stenosis in B-C AVF included 11 studies with a total of 457 patients, demonstrated a significant benefit in using stent grafts in cephalic arch stenosis compared to bare metal stents or percutaneous transluminal angioplasty with higher primary and secondary patency rates at 6- and 12-month post-treatment.

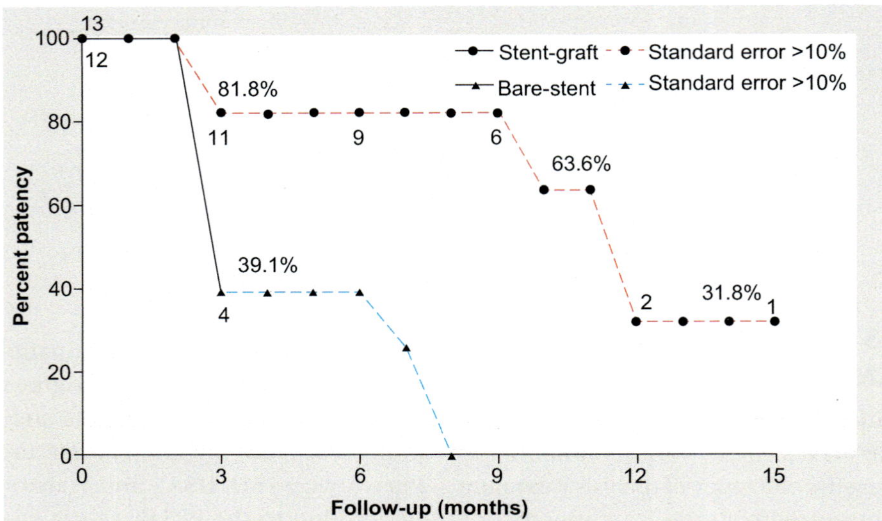

Fig. 27: Lifetable analysis of primary patency rates for 25 consecutive angioplasties of cephalic arch using bare stents (circles) or stent grafts (triangles).

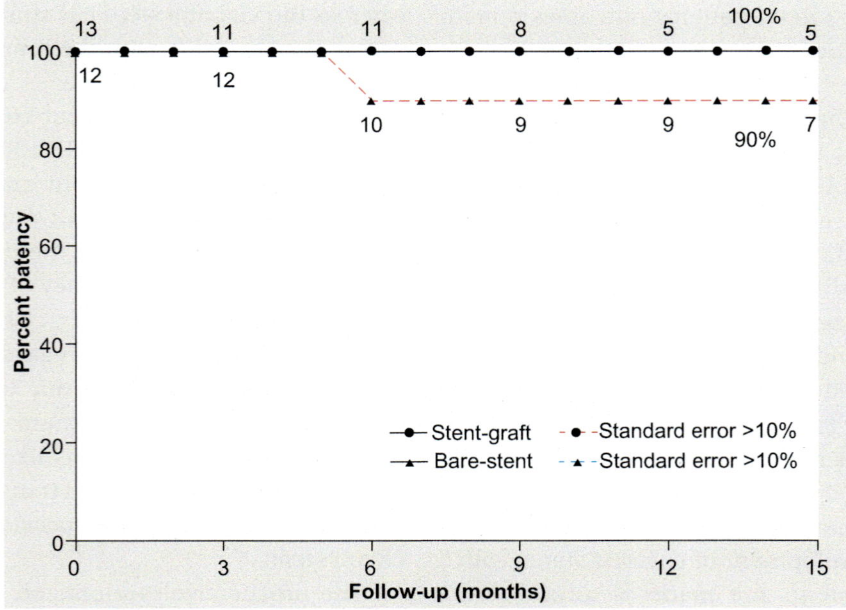

Fig. 28: Life-table analysis of functional patency rates for 25 consecutive angioplasties of cephalic arch using bare stents (triangles) or stent grafts (circles).

Despite the use of stent grafts instead of bare metal stents in the treatment of access circuit stenosis, the primary patency rates of the access circuit appear to decrease after 12 months with data showing a variable decreased patency rate ranging from 29 to 32%[54] and up to 70% of patients require reintervention within 12 months.[55,56] The mechanisms that interplay in developing stenosis after treatment with stent graft includes neointimal hyperplasia with blood interactions within the device surface, tissue interaction with hyperplasia occurring at the peri-stent area (inflow and outflow end of the stent) and transmural cell growth through the porous polymer covering leading to neointimal hyperplasia.[57] The aforementioned limitations in achieving long-term durable patency of access circuit with the use of currently available stent grafts and continued innovations seeking to overcome the setbacks resulted in the development of a novel cell impermeable endoprosthesis device (stent graft) called WRAPSODY Endoprosthesis (Merit Medical Systems, Inc.; South Jordan, Utah, USA), which is currently approved by FDA for treating vascular access circuit stenosis of both AVG and AVF morphology.

NOVEL VASC-ALERT MONITORING SYSTEM

Vasc-Alert (VA) is a novel FDA-approved device, which can be used for dialysis access dysfunction surveillance. VA utilizes the readily available intradialytic pressures, blood flow readings standardized to hematocrit, and blood pressure and provides a derived static venous pressure in the form of a ratio to mean arterial pressure. A vascular access risk score ranging from 1 to 10 (low-risk to high-risk score, respectively) is obtained by using the novel risk stratification algorithm that analyzes various VA measurements, including the rate of change in derived venous pressure, the number of recently derived venous pressure readings above threshold (alerts), inability to reach prescribed blood flow, and arterial pressure alerts.

The risk score obtained showed an increased incidence of intervention with high-risk scores with the odds of intervention increased by two-fold between the lowest and highest scores. A single-center prospective observational proof-of-concept validation trial was conducted, with the primary aim being to analyze the association between VA scores and stenosis detection in dialysis accesses and the secondary aim being to determine the alignment between VA scores and clinical monitoring findings. The scores were generated for each dialysis session and reported weekly based on the three-dialysis sessions.

There were 38 patients enrolled in the study, with the patients being categorized into two groups based on VA scores and assigned a probability risk for stenosis detection as a low-risk group of 18 patients (scores 1–3) and a high-risk group of 20 patients (scores 8–10). All enrolled patients received a physical examination, and POCUS was performed by an interventional nephrologist prior to the dialysis session. There were 24 AVFs in the cohort: 13 (72%) in the low-risk group and 11 (52%) in the high-risk group ($p=0.27$); among the 14 arteriovenous grafts, 9 were in the high-risk group and 5 in the low-risk group. Clinical monitoring was positive in 37% of the low-risk group and 63% of the high-risk group ($p=0.19$). Of all 38 subjects, 16 (42%) patients had significant stenosis. The high-risk group had more significant stenosis than the low-risk group (81% vs. 19%; $p=0.003$). History of stenosis was present in 20 (53%) patients: 8 (44%) in the low-risk group and 12 (60%) in the high-risk group ($p=0.15$). The sensitivity and specificity of identifying stenosis in the high-risk group were 81% and 68%, respectively. The positive predictive value in the high-risk group was 65% and the negative predictive value was 80%. A total of 19 patients had positive clinical monitoring results, and only 11 of the 19 patients (58%) with positive clinical monitoring had significant stenosis: 2 (11%) in the low-risk group and 9 (47%) in the high-risk group ($p=0.05$). Among 19 patients with no positive clinical monitoring findings, 5 (26%) patients had significant stenosis: 1 (5%) in the low-risk group and 4 (21%) in the high-risk group ($p=0.05$). Of the 24 patients who had an AVF dialysis access, 8 (33%) had significant stenosis: 2 (8%) in the low-risk and 6 (25%) in the high-risk group ($p=0.04$). Of the 14 patients who had arteriovenous graft dialysis access, 8 (57%) had significant stenosis: 1 (7%) in the low-risk and 7 (50%) in the high-risk group ($p=0.04$). Adjusted for risk score, a positive clinical monitoring finding and prior stenotic history were not significantly associated with significant stenosis. While the positive predictive value was 65% for VA high-risk score and the clinical monitoring was only 58%, the negative predictive value was 83% for VA high-risk score and only 74% for clinical monitoring.

The study highlighted with statistical significance that a high VA risk score could identify four of the five accesses that were false negatives by clinical monitoring with every unit increase in the score being associated with 34% higher odds of stenosis; a high-risk score was

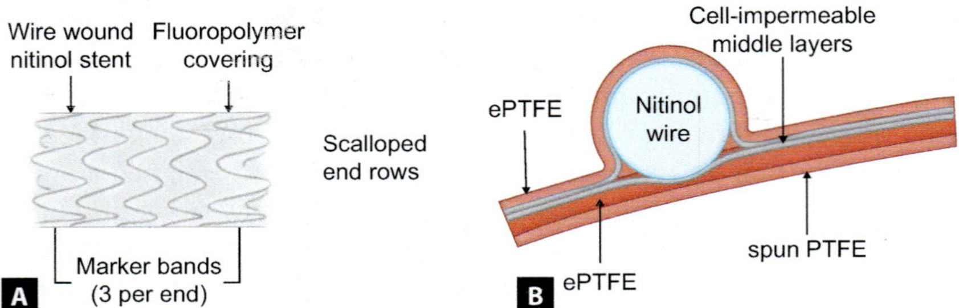

Figs. 29A and B: (A) Representative image of a 14 mm diameter × 30 mm device; (B) Cross-sectional schematic surrounding a single nitinol wire illustrating the organization of the multilayer graft covering. (PTFE: polytetrafluoroethylene)
Courtesy: Merit Medical System, USA.

associated with seven-fold higher odds of stenosis after adjusting for other variables included in the model and 83% negative predictive value for the presence of stenosis. The study investigators concluded that the vascular access risk stratification score may be an excellent, reliable, and efficient tool for identifying dialysis accesses that have significant stenosis. The study also suggested that it may be comparable to or even better than clinical monitoring alone. The VA risk score provides an automated, simple-to-use, repeated, and reliable objective measure for risk stratification, even for patients without positive clinical monitoring findings.

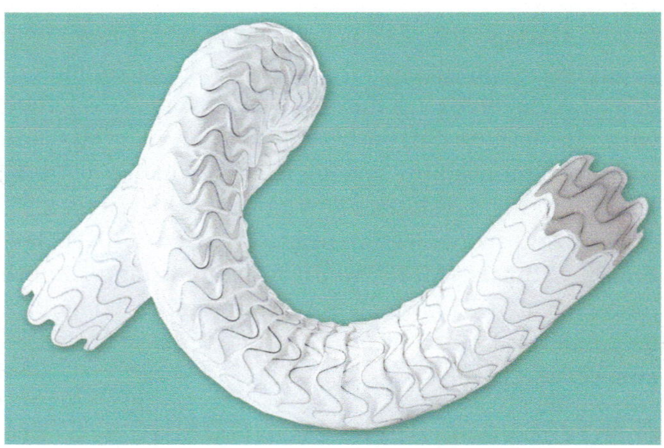

Fig. 30: WRAPSODY stent with softened end rows.
Courtesy: Merit Medical, USA

Novel Cell-impermeable Stent Graft—WRAPSODY Endoprosthesis

WRAPSODY stent is a self-expanding and cell-impermeable endoprosthesis, which has innovative covering with trilayered microstructure designed to maintain long-term vessel patency. The endoprosthesis is composed of a helically wound nitinol wire (struts) stent fully encapsulated in a multilayer fluoropolymer covering **(Figs. 29A and B)**. The covering's luminal layer is composed of a spun polytetrafluoroethylene (spun PTFE) designed to limit fibrin deposition and thrombus formation. The cell-impermeable middle layer is designed to prevent transmural cell growth. The outer layer is made of a traditional expanded polytetrafluoroethylene (ePTFE), permitting cell ingrowth for device anchoring.

The prospective, observational first in human study[58] evaluated the safety and effectiveness of WRAPSODY cell-impermeable Endoprosthesis (Merit Medical Systems, Inc.) in the treatment of AVF and AVG access circuit stenosis **(Figs. 30 and 31)**. Investigators conducted a prospective analysis of 46 patients with access circuit stenosis from three centers, which consisted of 11 patients with central venous stenosis. Device- or procedure-related adverse

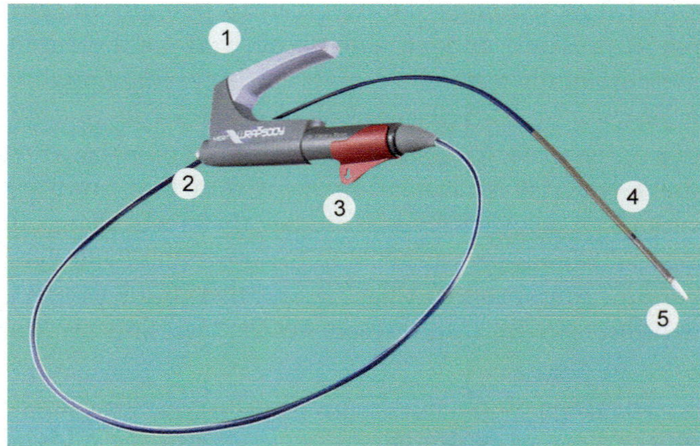

Fig. 31: WRAPSODY stent catheter. (1) Ratcheted deployment handle: For one-handed accurate and controlled cell-impermeable stent graft placement; (2) Single port: For flushing guidewire lumen and cell-impermeable stent graft pod; (3) Safety clip: To prevent inadvertent deployment; (4) Radiopaque marker bands: for enhanced visualization; (5) Soft atraumatic tip: For a seamless transition over a 0.035" guidewire.
Courtesy: Merit Medical, USA

events and TLPP were assessed at 3, 6, and 12 months. Assisted TLPP, access circuit primary patency (ACPP), and access circuit secondary patency were evaluated at 1, 3, 6, and 12 months. The device appeared to be safe and effective for treatment of stenoses in the peripheral and central veins of arteriovenous access circuits and all initial procedures were successful. The TLPP rates at 6 and 12 months were 97.7% (42/43) and 84.6.% (33/39), respectively **(Figs. 32A and B)**. The ACPP rates at 6 and 12 months were 84.4% (38/45) and 65.9% (29/44), respectively **(Figs. 33A and B)**.

After the initial human study of the novel device, WRAPSODY Arteriovenous Access Efficacy (WAVE) pivotal large-scale trial[59] was designed to assess the outcome of WRAPSODY endoprosthesis as compared to PTA of access circuit stenosis. This prospective, randomized, multicenter study enrolled 245 patients with AVF peripheral venous circuit outflow stenosis requiring intervention from

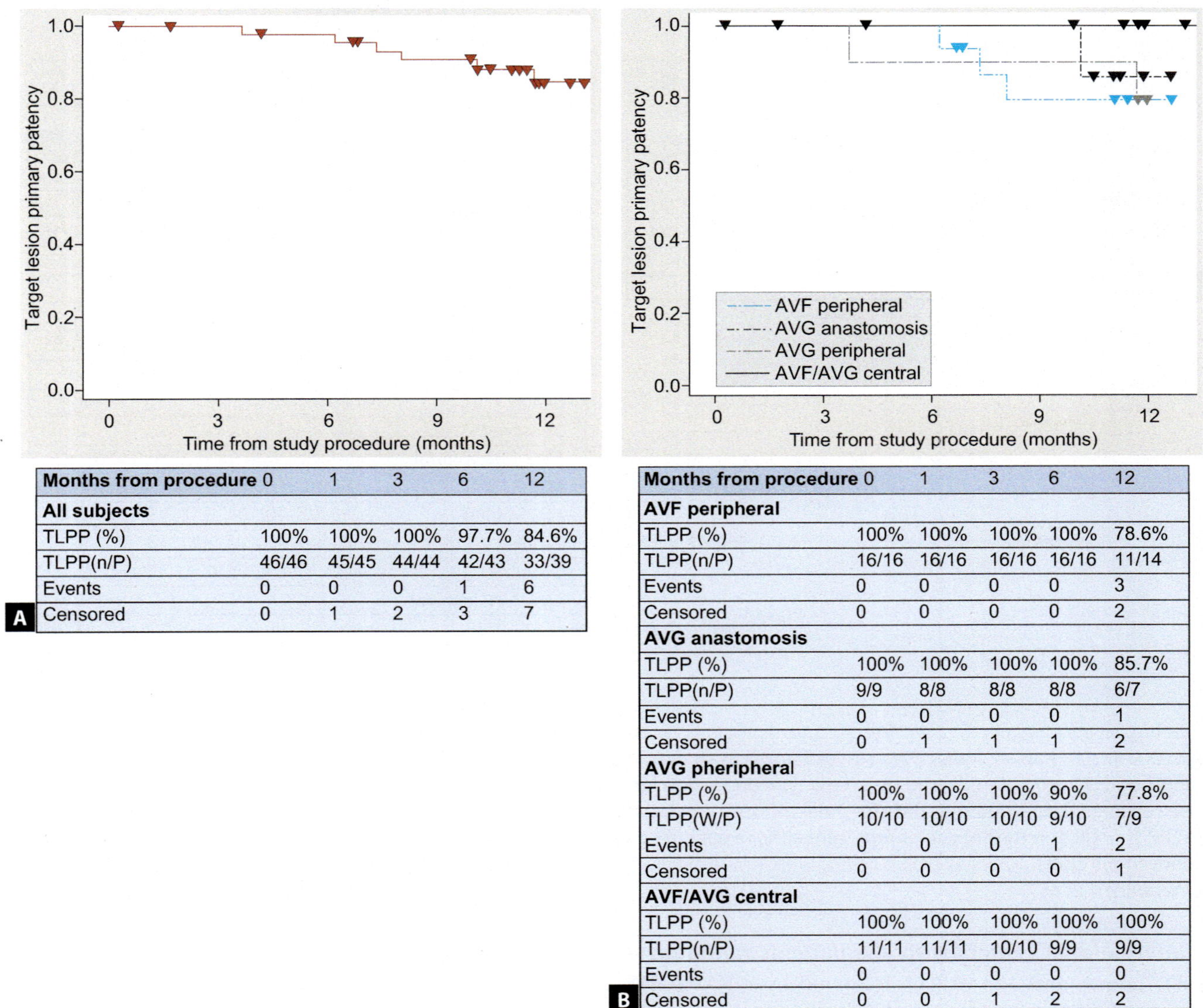

Months from procedure	0	1	3	6	12
All subjects					
TLPP (%)	100%	100%	100%	97.7%	84.6%
TLPP(n/P)	46/46	45/45	44/44	42/43	33/39
Events	0	0	0	1	6
Censored	0	1	2	3	7

Months from procedure	0	1	3	6	12
AVF peripheral					
TLPP (%)	100%	100%	100%	100%	78.6%
TLPP(n/P)	16/16	16/16	16/16	16/16	11/14
Events	0	0	0	0	3
Censored	0	0	0	0	2
AVG anastomosis					
TLPP (%)	100%	100%	100%	100%	85.7%
TLPP(n/P)	9/9	8/8	8/8	8/8	6/7
Events	0	0	0	0	1
Censored	0	1	1	1	2
AVG pheripheral					
TLPP (%)	100%	100%	100%	90%	77.8%
TLPP(W/P)	10/10	10/10	10/10	9/10	7/9
Events	0	0	0	1	2
Censored	0	0	0	0	1
AVF/AVG central					
TLPP (%)	100%	100%	100%	100%	100%
TLPP(n/P)	11/11	11/11	10/10	9/9	9/9
Events	0	0	0	0	0
Censored	0	0	1	2	2

Figs. 32A and B: Target lesion primary patency (TLPP) through 12 months. Kaplan–Meier (KM) curves for (A) all patients and (B) subcohorts based on access type and lesion location. The tables below each graph list the number of patients at risk, those censored (i.e., exited the study for renal transplant or loss to follow-up), and those who experienced an event leading to the loss of TLPP. Triangles on the KM curves represent either a patient's date of censoring or final follow-up visit. (AVF: arteriovenous fistula; AVG: arteriovenous graft)
Source: Gilbert et al.[58]

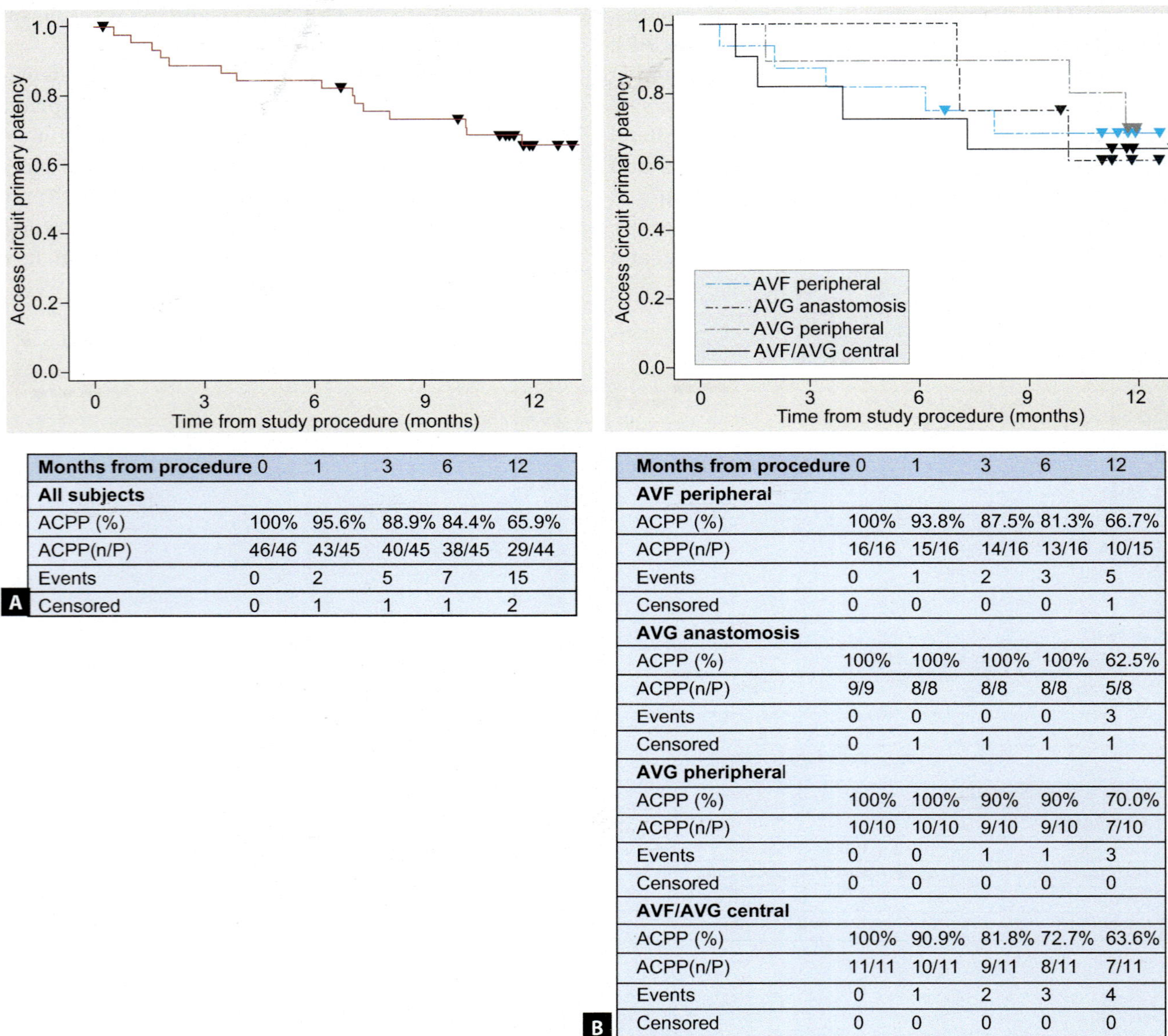

Months from procedure	0	1	3	6	12
All subjects					
ACPP (%)	100%	95.6%	88.9%	84.4%	65.9%
ACPP(n/P)	46/46	43/45	40/45	38/45	29/44
Events	0	2	5	7	15
Censored	0	1	1	1	2

Months from procedure	0	1	3	6	12
AVF peripheral					
ACPP (%)	100%	93.8%	87.5%	81.3%	66.7%
ACPP(n/P)	16/16	15/16	14/16	13/16	10/15
Events	0	1	2	3	5
Censored	0	0	0	0	1
AVG anastomosis					
ACPP (%)	100%	100%	100%	100%	62.5%
ACPP(n/P)	9/9	8/8	8/8	8/8	5/8
Events	0	0	0	0	3
Censored	0	1	1	1	1
AVG pheripheral					
ACPP (%)	100%	100%	90%	90%	70.0%
ACPP(n/P)	10/10	10/10	9/10	9/10	7/10
Events	0	0	1	1	3
Censored	0	0	0	0	0
AVF/AVG central					
ACPP (%)	100%	90.9%	81.8%	72.7%	63.6%
ACPP(n/P)	11/11	10/11	9/11	8/11	7/11
Events	0	1	2	3	4
Censored	0	0	0	0	0

Figs. 33A and B: Kaplan–Meier (KM) curves for access circuit primary patency (ACPP). ACPP through 12 months. KM curves for (A) all patients and (B) subcohorts based on access type and lesion location. The tables below each graph list the number of patients at risk, those censored (i.e., exited the study for renal transplant or loss to follow-up), and those who experienced an event leading to the loss of ACPP. Triangles on the KM curves represent either a patient's date of censoring or final follow-up visit. (AVF: arteriovenous fistula; AVG: arteriovenous graft)
Source: Gilbert et al.[58]

43 international centers with 123 patients randomized to PTA alone and 123 to PTA followed by WRAPSODY. The study results presented on September 16, 2024, at the Cardiovascular and Interventional Radiology Society of Europe (CIRSE) annual congress revealed that the TLPP in patients treated with WRAPSODY was 27% higher than that in patients in the PTA cohort—89.8% vs. 62.8% ($p < 0.0001$), ACPP higher at 72.6% vs. 57.9% ($p < 0.015$) and the proportion of patients who experienced an adverse event was similar between cohorts. The novel WRAPSODY cell-impermeable endoprosthesis showed promising outcome in the first human trial followed by superior 6-month efficacy data revealed by the pivotal study. Further extended follow-up observation of these

cohorts or comparison study with other stent grafts with extended follow-up will eventually provide the most needed data regarding the utility of a cell-impermeable device in prolonging the patency of dialysis access.

CONCLUSION

Optimally functioning access for dialysis is the linchpin of the survival of patients with end-stage kidney disease who are also not eligible candidates for renal transplantation. Various innovative techniques and novel devices have been developed since the initial creation of the Cimino-type AVF in 1996 to prolong the functional patency of the dialysis access. Unfortunately, a perfectly functioning long-term access for dialysis remains elusive despite the current progress. Many more innovations are being developed for the foreseeable future to obtain the ultimate goal of providing long-term dialysis treatments with a perfectly functioning dialysis access.

REFERENCES

1. Brescia MJ, Cimino JE, Appel K, Hurwich BJ. Chronic hemodialysis using venipuncture and a surgically created arteriovenous fistula. N Engl J Med. 1966;275(20):1089-92.
2. Besarab A, Frinak S, Margassery S, Wish JB. Hemodialysis Vascular Access: A Historical Perspective on Access Promotion, Barriers, and Lessons for the Future. Kidney Med. 2024;6(9):100871.
3. Hassanein M, Radhakrishnan Y, Garcilazo NH, Yuan Khor S, Norouzi S, Anvari E, et al. Global hemodialysis vascular access care: three decades of evolution. J Vasc Access. 2023;26(1):5-14.
4. Dember LM, Imrey PB, Beck GJ, Cheung AKC, Himmelfarb J, Huber TS, et al. Objectives and design of the hemodialysis fistula maturation study. Am J Kidney Dis. 2014;63(1):104-12.
5. Harms JC, Rangarajan S, Young CJ, Barker-Finkel J, Allon M. Outcomes of arteriovenous fistulas and grafts with or without intervention prior to successful use. J Vasc Surg. 2016;64(1):155-62.
6. Al-Jaishi AA, Oliver MJ, Thomas SM, Lok CE, Zhang JC, Garg AX, et al. Patency rates of the arteriovenous fistula for hemodialysis: a systematic review and meta-analysis. Am J Kidney Dis. 2014;63(3):464-78.
7. Gorecka J, Fereydooni A, Gonzalez L, Lee SR, Liu S, Ono S, et al. Molecular Targets for Improving Arteriovenous Fistula Maturation and Patency. Vasc Investig Ther. 2019;2(2):33-41.
8. Sadaghianloo N, Declemy S, Jean-Baptiste E, Haudebourg P, Robino C, Islam MS, et al. Radial artery deviation and reimplantation inhibits venous juxta-anastomotic stenosis and increases primary patency of radial-cephalic fistulas for hemodialysis. J Vasc Surg. 2016;64(3):698-706.e1.
9. Quencer KB, Arici M. Arteriovenous Fistulas and Their Characteristic Sites of Stenosis. Am J Roentgenol. 2015;205(4):726-34.
10. Dillavou ED, Lucas JF, Woodside K, Burgess J, Farber A, Hentschel D, et al. VasQ U.S. pivotal study demonstrates the safety and effectiveness of an external vascular support for arteriovenous fistula creation. J Vasc Surg. 2023;78(5):1302-12.e3.
11. Hussain MA, Keith Ozaki C, Nation D, Burgess J, Hentschel DM, Settle CS, et al. Extravascular supported arteriovenous fistulas reduced the need for interventions to support maturation and time to achieve two-needle cannulation for end-stage kidney disease patients in a multicenter US study. J Vasc Surg Vascular Insights (JVS-VI). 2025;3:100205.
12. Rajan DK, Ebner A, Desai SB, Rios JM, Cohn WE. Percutaneous Creation of an Arteriovenous Fistula for Hemodialysis Access. J of Vascular and Interventional Radiology. 2015;26(4):484-90.
13. Lok CE, Rajan DK, Clement J, Kiaii M, Sidhu R, Thomson K, et al.; NEAT Investigators. Endovascular Proximal Forearm Arteriovenous Fistula for Hemodialysis Access: Results of the Prospective, Multicenter Novel Endovascular Access Trial (NEAT). Am J Kidney Dis. 2017;70(4):486-97.
14. Berland T, Clement J, Inston N, Kreienberg P, Ouriel K, on behalf of the WavelinQ 4 French Investigators. Percutaneous arteriovenous fistula creation with the 4F WavelinQ EndoAVF System. J Vasc Surg. 2022;75(3):1038-46.e3.
15. Inston N, Khawaja A, Tullett K, Jones R. WavelinQ created arteriovenous fistulas versus surgical radiocephalic arteriovenous fistulas? A single-centre observational study. J Vasc Access. 2020;21(5):646-51.
16. Hull JE, Jennings WC, Cooper RI, Waheed U, Schaefer ME, Narayan R. The pivotal multicenter trial of ultrasound-guided percutaneous arteriovenous fistula creation for hemodialysis access. J Vasc Interv Radiol. 2018;29(2):149-58.e5.
17. Mallios A, Bourquelot P, Franco G, Fonkoua H, Hebibi H, Allouache M, et al. Midterm results of percutaneous arteriovenous fistula creation with the Ellipsys Vascular Access System, technical recommendations, and an algorithm for maintenance. J Vasc Surg. 2020;72(6):2097-106.
18. Hull JE, Jennings WC, Cooper RI, Narayan R, Mawla N, Decker MD. Long-Term Results from the Pivotal Multicenter Trial of Ultrasound-Guided Percutaneous Arteriovenous Fistula Creation for Hemodialysis Access. J Vasc Interv Radiol. 2022;33(10):1143-50.
19. Shahverdyan R, Beathard G, Mushtaq N, Litchfield TF, Vartanian S, Konner K, et al. Comparison of Ellipsys Percutaneous and Proximal Forearm Gracz-Type Surgical Arteriovenous Fistulas. Am J Kidney Dis. 2021;78(4):520-9.e1.
20. Shahverdyan R, Beathard G, Mushtaq N, Litchfield TF, Nelson PR, Jennings WC. Comparison of Outcomes of Percutaneous Arteriovenous Fistulae Creation by Ellipsys and WavelinQ Devices. J Vasc Interv Radiol. 2020;31(9):1365-72.

21. Salman L, Beathard G. Physical examination as a tool for surveillance for the hemodialysis arteriovenous access. Clin J Am Soc Nephrol. 2013;8(7):1220-7.
22. Coentrão L, Turmel-Rodrigues L. Monitoring dialysis arteriovenous fistulae: it's in our hands. J Vasc Access. 2013;14:209.
23. Beathard GA. An algorithm for the physical examination of early fistula failure. Semin Dial. 2005;18:331.
24. Ratnam L, Karunanithy N, Mailli L, Diamantopoulos A, Morgan RA. Dialysis Access Maintenance: Plain Balloon Angioplasty. Cardiovasc Intervent Radiol (CIR). 2023;46(9):1136-43.
25. Davidson CJ, Newman GE, Sheikh KH, Kisslo K, Stack RS, Schwab SJ. Mechanisms of angioplasty in hemodialysis fistula stenoses evaluated by intravascular ultrasound. Kidney Int. 1991;40(1):91-5.
26. Higuchi T, Okuda N, Aoki K, Ishii Y, Matsumoto H, Ohnishi Y, et al. Intravascular ultrasound imaging before and after angioplasty for stenosis of arteriovenous fistulae in haemodialysis patients. Nephrol Dial Transplant. 2001;16(1):151-5.
27. Song X, Adachi T, Kawase Y, Kimura T, Saito N. Efficacy of the Wolverine cutting balloon on a circumferential calcified coronary lesion: Bench test using a three-dimensional printer and computer simulation with the finite element method. Cardiovasc Interv Ther. 2022;37(1):78-88.
28. Pang S, Chang T, Chang M, Huang X, Wang X, Song M, et al. Efficacy of cutting balloon angioplasty versus high-pressure balloon angioplasty for the treatment of arteriovenous fistula stenoses in patients undergoing hemodialysis: Systematic review and meta-analysis. PLoS One. 2024;19(1): e0296191.
29. Agarwal SK, Nadkarni GN, Yacoub R, Patel AA, Jenkins JS, Collins TJ, et al. Comparison of Cutting Balloon Angioplasty and Percutaneous Balloon Angioplasty of Arteriovenous Fistula Stenosis: A Meta-Analysis and Systematic Review of Randomized Clinical Trials. J Interv Cardiol. 2015;28:288.
30. Clark TW, Hirsch DA, Jindal KJ, Veugelers PJ, LeBlanc J. Outcome and prognostic factors of restenosis after percutaneous treatment of native hemodialysis fistulas. Journal of vascular and interventional radiology: JVIR. 2002;13(1):51-9.
31. Maeda K, Furukawa A, Yamasaki M, Murata K. Percutaneous transluminal angioplasty for Brescia-Cimino hemodialysis fistula dysfunction: technical success rate, patency rate and factors that influence the results. Eur J Radiol. 2005;54(3):426-30.
32. Kennedy SA, Mafeld S, Baerlocher MO, Jaberi A, Rajan DK. Drug-coated balloon angioplasty in hemodialysis circuits: a systematic review and meta-analysis. J Vasc Interv Radiol. 2019;30(4):483-94.e1.
33. Kitrou P, Spiliopoulos S, Karnabatidis D, Katsanos K. Cutting balloons, covered stents and paclitaxel-coated balloons for the treatment of dysfunctional dialysis access. Expert Rev Med Devices. 2016;13:1119-26.
34. Hu H, Wu Z, Zhao J, Wang J, Huang B, Yang Y, et al. Stent graft placement versus angioplasty for hemodialysis access failure: a meta-analysis. J Surg Res. 2018;226:82-8.
35. Tepe G, Laird J, Schneider P, Brodmann M, Krishnan P, Micari A, et al. Drug-coated balloon versus standard percutaneous transluminal angioplasty for the treatment of superficial femoral and popliteal peripheral artery disease: 12-month results from the IN.PACT SFA randomized trial. Circulation. 2015;131:495-502.
36. Vicari AP, Luu R, Zhang N, Patel S, Makinen SR, Hanson DC, et al. Paclitaxel reduces regulatory T cell numbers and inhibitory function and enhances the anti-tumor effects of the TLR9 agonist PF-3512676 in the mouse. Cancer Immunol Immunother. 2009;58(4):615-28.
37. Ferrer IR, Araki K, Ford ML. Paradoxical aspects of rapamycin immunobiology in transplantation. Am J Transplant. 2011;11(4):654-9.
38. Maga P, Mikolajczyk TP, Partyka L, Siedlinski M, Maga M, Krzanowski M, et al. Involvement of CD8+ T cell subsets in early response to vascular injury in patients with peripheral artery disease in vivo. Clin Immunol. 2018;194:26-33.
39. Wessely R, Blaich B, Belaiba RS, Merl S, Görlach A, Kastrati A, et al. Comparative characterization of cellular and molecular anti-restenotic profiles of paclitaxel and sirolimus. Implications for local drug delivery. Thromb Haemost. 2007;97:1003-12.
40. Long BH, Fairchild CR. Paclitaxel inhibits progression of mitotic cells to G1 phase by interference with spindle formation without affecting other microtubule functions during anaphase and telophase. Cancer Res. 1994;54:4355-61.
41. Giannakakou P, Robey R, Fojo T, Blagosklonny MV. Low concentrations of paclitaxel induce cell type-dependent p53, p21 and G1/G2 arrest instead of mitotic arrest: Molecular determinants of paclitaxel-induced cytotoxicity. Oncogene. 2001;20:3806-13.
42. Wang D, Eisen HJ. Mechanistic Target of Rapamycin (mTOR) Inhibitors. Handb Exp Pharmacol. 2022;272:53-72.
43. Cortese B, Caiazzo G, Di Palma G, De Rosa S. Comparison Between Sirolimus- and Paclitaxel-Coated Balloon for Revascularization of Coronary Arteries: The SIRPAC (SIRolimus-PAClitaxel) Study. Cardiovasc Revasc Med. 2021;28:1-6.
44. Trerotola SO, Lawson J, Roy-Chaudhury P, Saad TF. Drug coated balloon angioplasty in failing AV fistulas: a randomized controlled trial. Clin J Am Soc Nephrol. 2018;13:1215-24.
45. Lookstein RA, Haruguchi H, Ouriel K, Weinberg I, Lei L, Cihlar S, et al.; for the IN.PACT AV Access Investigators. Drug-Coated Balloons for Dysfunctional Dialysis Arteriovenous Fistulas. N Engl J Med. 2020;383:733-42.

46. Liu C, Wolfers M, Awan BZ, Ali I, Lorenzana AM, Smith Q, et al. Drug-Coated Balloon Versus Plain Balloon Angioplasty for Hemodialysis Dysfunction: A Meta-Analysis of Randomized Controlled Trials. J Am Heart Assoc. 2021;10(23): e022060.
47. Aruny JE, FLEX Vessel Prep System AV Registry Clinical Trial Results. Presented in 2022 Vascular Access for Hemodialysis Symposium. [online] Available from VASA-ARUNY-2022-Symposium-Aruny-AV-Reg-data-53122-updates.pdf [Last accessed June, 2025].
48. Beathard GA. Gianturco self-expanding stent in the treatment of stenosis in dialysis access grafts. Kidney Int. 1993;43(4):872-7.
49. Quinn SF, Schuman ES, Demlow TA, Standage BA, Ragsdale JW, Green GS, et al. Percutaneous transluminal angioplasty versus endovascular stent placement in the treatment of venous stenoses in patients undergoing hemodialysis: intermediate results. J Vasc Interv Radiol. 1995;6(6):851-5.
50. Hoffer EK, Sultan S, Herskowitz MM, Daniels ID, Sclafani SJ. Prospective randomized trial of a metallic intravascular stent in hemodialysis graft maintenance. J Vasc Interv Radiol. 1997;8(6):965-73.
51. Kariya S, Tanigawa N, Kojima H, Komemushi A, Shomura Y, Shiraishi T, et al. Peripheral stent placement in hemodialysis grafts. Cardiovasc Intervent Radiol. 2009;32(5):960-6.
52. Shemesh D, Goldin I, Zaghal I, Berlowitz D, Raveh D, Olsha O, et al. Angioplasty with stent graft versus bare stent for recurrent cephalic arch stenosis in autogenous arteriovenous access for hemodialysis: A prospective randomized clinical trial. J Vasc Surg. 2008;48(6): 1524-31.e2.
53. D'cruz RT, Leong SW, Syn N, Tiwari A, Sannasi VV, Singh Sidhu HR, et al. Endovascular treatment of cephalic arch stenosis in brachiocephalic arteriovenous fistulas: A systematic review and meta-analysis. J Vasc Access. 2019;20(04):345-55.
54. Rajan DK, Falk A. A Randomized Prospective Study Comparing Outcomes of Angioplasty versus VIABAHN Stent-Graft Placement for Cephalic Arch Stenosis in Dysfunctional Hemodialysis Accesses. J Vasc Interv Radiol. 2015;26(9):1355-61.
55. Haskal ZJ, Trerotola S, Dolmatch B, Schuman E, Altman S, Mietling S, et al. Stent graft versus balloon angioplasty for failing dialysis-access grafts. N Engl J Med. 2010;362(6):494-503.
56. Schmelter C, Raab U, Lazarus F, Ruppert V, Vorwerk D. Outcomes of AV fistulas and AV grafts after interventional stent-graft deployment in haemodialysis patients. Cardiovasc Interv Radiol. 2015;38(4):878-86.
57. Dolmatch BL, Hall JW, Mower WL, Rousselle SD. Evaluation of a novel spun polytetrafluoroethylene stent graft in an ovine external iliac artery model. J Vasc Interv Radiol. 2020;31(3):494-502.
58. Gilbert J, Rai J, Kingsmore D, Skousen J, Ptohis N. First Clinical Results of the Merit WRAPSODY™ Cell-Impermeable Endoprosthesis for Treatment of Access Circuit Stenosis in Haemodialysis Patients. Cardiovasc Intervent Radiol. 2021;44(12):1903-13.
59. Razavi MK, Jones RG. Wrapsody Arteriovenous Access Efficacy (WAVE) pivotal large-scale trial. The data were delivered in a First@CIRSE presentation during the Cardiovascular and Interventional Radiological Society of Europe's CIRSE 2024 held September 14-18 in Lisbon, Portugal. Interv News Issue. 2024;96.
60. Ross J. Does Vessel Prep Make a Difference? Presented during CIDA 2019; San Diego, CA.

SECTION

11 Ethical and Legal Considerations in Intervention for Nephrologist

CHAPTER 42

Patient Consent and Shared Decision-making

Manisha Sahay, AK Bhalla, Shyam B Bansal

INTRODUCTION

Patients with chronic kidney disease (CKD) are required to make difficult decisions, negotiating between the risks, burdens, and benefits for any treatment or procedure. This process can be extremely challenging, since these decisions involve inherent risks, which can impact survival and quality of life. Informed consent is the process in which a healthcare professional educates a patient about the risks, benefits, and alternatives of a given procedure or intervention.[1] The patient has a legal right to autonomy and self-determination enshrined within Article 21 of the Indian Constitution, and hence informed consent from the patient is essential regarding his or her treatment. Consent is a legal requirement of medical practice and not a procedural formality.

HISTORY

In the earlier years of practice of medicine, all medical decisions were made by the physicians on behalf of their patients. The patients were not informed about the details of their treatment. However, several medical cases were reported where unethical medical treatment was undertaken. Some examples are the Tuskegee Study of Untreated Syphilis in the Negro Male and the Nazi human experiments during World War II. In 1914 in the landmark case of *Schloendorff vs. Society of New York Hospital*, the court ruled that "every adult human being of sound mind has a right to determine what shall be done with his own body." This marked the beginning of the concept that patients must agree to medical procedures. Subsequently, the Nuremberg Code and the Declaration of Helsinki came into existence. Thus, the informed consent became an ethical requirement in both research and clinical practice.[2]

TYPES OF INFORMED CONSENT

To standardize the practice, the Medical Council of India (MCI) has laid down guidelines that are issued as regulations. A patient who comes to a doctor for treatment implies that he is agreeable to general physical (not intimate) examination. This is *implied consent*. When a patient specifically states his consent (verbal/written), it is called *informed consent*. *Verbal consent* may be obtained for relatively minor examinations or procedures in the presence of a witness. *Informed written consent* must be obtained before all major diagnostic, anesthesia, and surgical procedures as it is the most undisputable form of consent (prior informed consent).

HOW TO WRITE AN INFORMED CONSENT IN CLINICAL PRACTICE?

Components of an Informed Consent

The components of an informed consent include the following:

- Name of the procedure, description, and reasoning for the procedure
- Risks and benefits of the procedure
- Reasonable alternatives for the procedure if these exist. However, informed consent does not require the presence of another choice; it has to be taken even if there is only one option (unlike in shared decision-making where at least two options are required)
- Risks and benefits of alternatives
- Assessment of the patient's understanding of the process
- Assessment of the decision-making capacity or competency of the patient. Technically, a person can only be declared "incompetent" by a court of law.
- The consent form may express no guarantees that the proposed procedure will cure the problem being addressed.
- The consent form should be signed and dated by both the competent doctor and the patient. A nephrologist (DM/DNB Nephrology) is required to be competent in performing kidney biopsies, central line insertions,

percutaneous peritoneal dialysis catheter insertions, hemodialysis, and peritoneal dialysis and should be trained in handling medical aspects of transplantation. AVATAR is coming out with core curriculum and guidelines for interventional nephology on lines with American Society of Diagnostic and Interventional Nephrology (ASDIN).

- It is important to have witness signature on the consent form. The parent can sign for their child.
- The form should mention that the informed consent is voluntary, i.e., it is being given by the patient without coercion. The clinician must avoid making the patient feel forced to agree with the clinician. The patient has the autonomy to choose even a "bad decision" that may result in serious disability or even death. If the patient has been given the option of obtaining a recommended treatment or test and has chosen not to undergo the test or the treatment, the patient may be asked to sign an Against Medical Advice (AMA) form to protect the healthcare provider from legal liability for not providing the recommended treatment.

The entire process should be documented.[2,3] The patient may ask for a copy of the signed consent form.

Table 1 shows the risks of various nephrology procedures and the alternative therapies available. **Table 2** shows a sample informed consent form for hemodialysis.

TABLE 1: Risks of various nephrology procedures and the alternative therapies available.

Procedure	*Alternative*	*Risks*
Central catheter	AV fistula AV graft CAPD	• Risk of bleeding during the procedure or with accidental removal of catheter • As the catheter is a foreign body that comes in contact with blood directly, it can lead to local infection or spread of infection in blood • Disfiguring scar can be there at the insertion site of dialysis catheter. Damage to surrounding structures such as blood vessels, organs, and muscles, requiring further treatment • Injury to blood vessel during procedure or narrowing of vein over a period of time can occur • Catheter may kink or block and that can become the reason for removal or replacement of catheter • Pneumothorax, a collection of air around the lining of the lungs, this usually resolves by itself but sometimes may require a tube to be inserted into the chest • Tachycardia or arrhythmias beat can occur. This usually resolves on its own but sometimes it may need further treatment • An air bubble enters the bloodstream. This can cause air embolism • Failure to gain access to the vein can occur. This may require a second attempt from a different location. The procedure may not be possible due to medical and/or technical reasons • Blood clot blocking the vein, may require medication to treat • Loose end of catheter needs to be taken care so that it does not get entangled with cloths which can lead to accidental removal and/or severe bleeding
AV fistula	Catheter CAPD	• Failure of fistula to work • Bleeding may require further surgery • Thrombosis/blood clotting issues can lead to failure of AVF/AVG and for that need for some intervention or medication will require. If presentation to the doctor is late, then new fistula creation will require • Stenosis/abnormal narrowing of veins generally presents with persistently swollen extremity with access and difficulty in needle placement • Failure of veins to dilate sufficient for hemodialysis use can occur • Infection requiring antibiotics • Blackening of fingers can occur • Nerve damage may occur • Aneurysm formation requiring further surgery • A blood transfusion may be required during procedure
CAPD	Hemodialysis transplant	• Bleeding from the operation site, but this usually stops after a short while • In a small number of surgeries, the wound bleeds under the skin and this causes swelling and bruising (hematoma) • Rarely, bleeding may continue and a further intervention may be needed but usually the swelling and bruising subside over time

Contd...

Contd...

Procedure	*Alternative*	*Risks*
		• The position of the CAPD catheter is close to the bowel and bladder and on extremely rare occasions these may be punctured. This could require emergency surgery • Infection of the wound may occur following surgery. On very rare occasions, peritonitis may occur. Antibiotics would be needed on both occasions
Kidney biopsy	• Empirical treatment • Serology if available for the disease	• Pain mild • Hematuria 10% of biopsies and usually clears on its own within 1–2 days, but in rare instances, it may persist for 2–3 weeks. In approximately 1% of cases, bleeding may be severe to cause a drop in blood pressure and that will need blood transfusion • Surgery, to repair a tear or to stop persistent or massive bleeding, is required in less than 1 per 500 biopsies and in less than 1 per 2,000 cases. Very rarely, it becomes necessary to remove the kidney • Most patients describe soreness rather than pain • Other uncommon complications that can happen are puncture of other organs of abdominal cavity (liver, spleen, bowel) or the fistula creation (a connection between an artery and vein). Fistulas rarely cause any symptoms and generally disappear without treatment
Kidney transplantation	Maintenance hemodialysis or CAPD	• Body may not accept the donor kidney (rejection) • Delayed function, need for dialysis • Need for biopsy of kidney • Infections, urine leak, lymphocele • Artery clot/block/thrombus • Need for mechanical ventilation post transplant • Need for continuous dialysis if kidney does not function • Side effects of medicines • Diabetes, bone disease, CMV, BKV infection, malignancy • Death

(AV: arteriovenous; BKV: BK virus; CAPD: continuous ambulatory peritoneal dialysis; CMV: cytomegalovirus)

TABLE 2: Informed consent for hemodialysis.

I,______________________**(name of patient)** have been informed that my kidneys are not functioning and that I need hemodialysis to sustain my life **(reasoning for procedure)**. I understand that while hemodialysis is a life-sustaining procedure, it is not a cure for kidney failure **(no guarantee)**.

The procedure necessary to treat my condition that has been explained to me by my physician is as follows: Hemodialysis will clean my blood by pumping it through a device that will remove wastes and excess fluids. I understand that hemodialysis involves, among other things, the insertion of tubes and/or needles into my veins or fistula or through a catheter and the use of artificial kidneys to filter my blood. I also understand that, along with the hemodialysis treatment, I may need laboratory tests, radiology and surgical procedures to assure adequate function of the equipment and effectiveness of the treatment. I understand that it will be necessary for me to follow certain dietary restrictions. It will be my responsibility to follow these dietary restrictions and failure to do so can cause bone disease, calcification of my heart, blood vessels and skin, heart failure, and even sudden death. In addition, I understand that it will be my responsibility to take my medication as prescribed by my physician. The success of hemodialysis also depends upon my agreeing to remain on the machine for the prescribed length of time so that my blood can be adequately cleansed. I will immediately notify my physician of any adverse reactions or problems I may have with regard to these hemodialysis treatments.

(Description of the procedure)

I have been informed that the following risks are associated with hemodialysis and that while such risks are not common, one or more can occur and be potentially life-threatening **(risks of procedure)**:

- Bacterial and/or viral (e.g., Hepatitis B or C) contamination of my blood which may cause infection or bacterial infection of the blood called sepsis
- Bleeding due to blood clotting problems or disconnection of blood tubing
- "Destruction" or the breakdown of red blood cells, known as hemolysis
- Internal bleeding or bleeding from the access site
- Infections of my access site (catheter or fistula infections)

Contd...

Contd...

- Introduction of air into my bloodstream
- Shock or cardiac arrest
- Allergic and toxic reactions to drugs, solutions, artificial kidneys or other equipment used during the hemodialysis treatment
- Clotting of my access or infiltration of my access

I have also been informed that there may be some side effects associated with hemodialysis related to fluid and chemical changes during or after the hemodialysis treatment. Some of the side effects are osteoporosis, electrolyte imbalance, headache, nausea, dizziness, fainting, irregular heartbeats, decrease in blood pressure, muscle cramping, and mild confusion

The hemodialysis procedure and the alternatives to hemodialysis have been explained to me. I understand the alternatives to hemodialysis to be peritoneal dialysis, or transplantation, and that I may be evaluated for whenever I choose. Transplantation provides cure, but there may be possibility of rejection while peritoneal dialysis is home-based therapy though peritonitis infection and procedure failure may occur **(alternate options and risks of benefits of these)**

I authorize repeated hemodialysis treatments, unless I specifically revoke this consent **(repeat consent)**

I have read this consent and fully understand its contents **(understanding)**. I have had a chance to have my questions answered in words I can understand **(patient competency)**

I hereby execute this consent form freely and with full acceptance and know of the contents in it **(voluntary)**. I also understand that this is a legal document

______________________________ Date __________ Time: __________

Patient or Legally Authorized Representative

______________________________ Date __________ Time: __________

Physician Signature

______________________________ Date __________ Time: __________

Witness Signature

Thus, informed consent is the legal process used to promote patient autonomy. Use of multimedia and technology can enhance understanding.[4]

PRACTICAL IMPLICATIONS OF INFORMED CONSENT: WHAT A NEPHROLOGIST SHOULD KNOW

It is preferable to take written consent in a patient's vernacular language. It may be better to make the patient write down his consent in the presence of a witness.[5] It is desirable to use short and simple sentences and nonmedical terminology that is written/typed legibly.[6] Alterations or additions should not be made in the consent form without a patient's signed authorization. No one can consent on behalf of a competent adult. If the consent of a relative is taken instead of the patient, even when patient is a competent adult it is not valid.

Consent should be procedure specific: As per the law, if the consent of the patient is taken for diagnostic procedure/surgery, such consent cannot be considered as authorization to perform therapeutic surgery except in a life-threatening emergent situation. In addition, if the consent by the patient is for a particular operative surgery, it cannot be treated as consent for an unauthorized additional procedure involving removal of an organ only on the ground that it is beneficial to the patient or is likely to prevent some danger from developing in the future. An additional procedure may be performed without consent only if it is necessary to save the life or preserve the health of the patient and it would be unreasonable to delay, until the patient regains consciousness and takes a decision. In addition, this decision curtails the scope of proxy consent from the person having parental authority or an attendant. An all-encompassing consent to the effect "I authorize so and so to carry out any test/procedure/surgery in the course of my treatment" is not valid.[7]

Consent in emergency: In case of emergency, a doctor is duty-bound to treat a patient, without waiting for any formalities. Hypothetically, if a patient in an emergency resists taking treatment, what shall be the way out? Indian courts are not very clear on that. When a surgeon or medical man advances a plea that the patient did not give his consent for the surgery or the course of treatment advised by him, the burden is on him to prove that the nonperformance of the surgery or the nonadministration of the treatment was on account of the refusal of the patient to give consent thereto. Thus, refusing treatment in life-threatening situations due to nonavailability of consent may hold the doctor guilty, unless there is a documented refusal to treatment by the patient.

Period of validity of consent: Consent remains valid for an indefinite period, provided there is no change in the patient's condition or proposed intervention. It should be confirmed at the time of surgery.

Children: A child >12 years of age can give a valid consent for physical/medical examination[8] (Indian Penal Code, Section 89). This is not termed "informed consent" but "informed permission or assent." However, prior to performing any procedure on a child <18 years of age, the consent of a person with parental responsibility, e.g., parents or legal guardians, should be taken. Legislation regarding minors and informed consent varies across the world. In some countries, minors who are under 18 years of age and married, those serving in the military, those who are financially independent, and mothers of children (married or not) are allowed to provide informed consent.

Extent of information provided to patient during the consent process: If the possibility of a risk, including the risk of death, due to the performance of a procedure or its refusal, is remote or only theoretical, it need not be explained. Exceptions to a physician's duty to disclose include the following: (1) Patient's refusal to be informed; this should be documented. (2) If the doctor feels that providing information to a patient who is anxious or disturbed would not be processed rationally by him and is likely to psychologically harm him, the information may be withheld from him (therapeutic privilege); he should then communicate with the patient's close relative, family doctor, or both.

Consent for blood transfusion: When blood transfusion is anticipated, a specific written consent should be taken, exception being an emergency situation where blood transfusion is needed to save life and consent cannot be attempted.[9]

Consent for repeat procedure: A fresh written informed consent must be obtained prior to every surgical procedure that includes a re-exploration procedure.[10]

Consent for anesthesia: Informed consent for anesthesia must be taken by the anesthesia provider as only he can impart anesthesia-related necessary information and explain the risks involved. It may be documented by the anesthesiologist on the surgical consent form by a hand-written note or on a separate anesthesia consent form.[11]

Can a patient refuse to consent? Competent patients have the legal and moral right to refuse treatment, even in life-threatening emergency situations.[11] In such cases, informed refusal must be obtained and documented, over the patient's witnessed signature.[12] It may be advisable that two doctors document the reason for nonperformance of life-saving surgery or treatment as express refusal by the patient or the authorized representative and inform the hospital administrator about the same. To detain an adult patient against his will in a hospital is unlawful.[13] If a patient demands discharge from the hospital against medical advice, this should be recorded and his signature obtained.

Role of witness in consent: Witnessed consents are legally more dependable. The role of a witness is even more important in instances when the patient is illiterate and one needs to take his/her thumb impression.[5]

Documentation of consent: Consent should be properly documented. Video-recording of the informed consent process may also be done but with a prior consent for the same. This should be documented. It is commonly done for organ transplant procedures.

Consent for illegal procedures is invalid. There can be no valid consent for operations or procedures which are illegal. Consent for an illegal act such as criminal abortion is invalid. Consent is no defense in cases of professional negligence.[13]

Special situations: Patients with impaired decision-making capacity: Informed consent can be challenging in patients who have impaired decision-making capacity due to cognitive impairments or mental illness. However, these medical conditions do not revoke an individual's right to provide informed consent as long as they have the capacity to understand, evaluate, and communicate his/her decisions. In case this capacity is lost, the following options are available:

- In some cases, patients may give advance directives and living will before losing decision-making capacity. These legal documents direct doctors and other healthcare providers as to what the patient wants.
- If a patient has not given advance directives, then involvement from surrogates may be needed as per the hierarchy of decision-makers, determined by

the state's laws. Proxy consent can be taken from a surrogate/proxy decision maker who is the next of kin (spouse/adult child/parent/sibling/lawful guardian).

- If this is not possible, a legal guardian may need to be appointed by the court.

MEMBERS INVOLVED IN INFORMED CONSENT PROCESS

Apart from the physician and the patient, physician assistants and nurses play a critical role in reinforcing and clarifying the information provided by the physician. Skilled social workers, patient advocates, and care coordinators can provide additional support, especially in complex cases involving vulnerable populations or challenging decision-making scenarios. Thus, informed consent is a team effort, where each professional's expertise contributes to a comprehensive understanding for the patient. Members of the team may also serve as witnesses to the consent. There should be a regular communication among the care team members to ensure that no conflicting messages are provided to the patients and all aspects of care including medical, social, emotional, etc., are covered. Follow-up interaction with the patient is also important to address any further questions or concerns the patient might have. The patient has a right to reconsider or change his/her decision anytime which should again be documented. The legal term for failing to obtain informed consent before performing a test or procedure on a patient is called battery (a form of assault).

FUNCTION/PURPOSE OF INFORMED CONSENT

Informed consent serves both ethical and legal purposes.

- It helps the patients as informed consent ensures that patients understand the risks, benefits, alternatives, and potential consequences of medical interventions, allowing them to weigh their options and participate actively in their treatment plans. It, thus, safeguards a patient's rights. It ensures patient autonomy and allows patients to make decisions aligned with their values, beliefs, and preferences. It enhances patient-centered care.
- Also, the informed consent protects clinicians by documenting that patients were adequately informed, reducing legal liability in case of adverse outcomes. It strengthens the physician–patient relationship and trust through open and honest communication.

SCENARIOS IN MEDICINE WHICH REQUIRE INFORMED CONSENT

Tests:

- Some blood tests like HIV testing
- Testing for genetic disorders
- Some advanced medical tests, like a biopsy

Interventions:

- Most surgeries
- Blood transfusions
- Anesthesia
- Radiation
- Chemotherapy

Medical interventions: Permacath, hemodialysis, peritoneal dialysis, kidney transplantation.

Most vaccinations

CHALLENGES IN INFORMED CONSENT

- *Lack of training of medical professionals:* There is a dearth of teaching and training about informed consent in the medical curriculum. A chapter on this important topic should be included in the course right from the entry of student into medical profession.
- *Language barriers:* The patients may come from diverse populations and may not be fluent in the language spoken by the healthcare provider. In such cases, medical interpreter services can be utilized. Sign language medical interpreters should be made available for deaf patients.[2]
- *Lack of patient comprehension:* The health literacy of patients may be variable. Even if the communication is imparted in the language understood by the patient, the use of complex medical jargon by the medical professionals may make it difficult for the patient to understand the procedure. It is recommended to use everyday language instead of medical jargon when communicating with patients. There are several tools like the teach-back method or test/feedback method which can be used to assess whether patients understand the risks, benefits, and alternatives of their treatment. Patients should be encouraged to ask questions. Open-ended questions may be used to understand patients' needs and preferences. Patient's comprehension can be improved by interactive media and graphical tools.
- *Cultural differences:* It is crucial to be aware of cultural differences in the informed consent process. In certain

cultures, decisions are made collectively by a group rather than by individuals. Some patients may consider written consent as a sign of mistrust. In some cultures, the decisions are made by the family patriarch or a male representative designated by the family. This should be respected at the same time maintaining the autonomy of the patient.

- *Patient-physician relationship:* Patients may feel inhibited to express their opinion as they may feel intimidated by the physicians due to the unequal power relationship. This is especially seen in vulnerable populations, such as elderly, patients with special needs, or individuals with acute medical conditions.
- *Inadequate time spent with the patient by the physician:* The healthcare professionals might not spend sufficient time to discuss all aspects of the procedure. The decision-making process should allow patients some time to discuss with family and reflect. The consent process should occur in a clinic or office setting with adequate time prior to the procedure where patients have ample time to ask questions and process their emotions, rather than 15 minutes before the procedure.
- *Evolving/new diseases:* New medical conditions, such as the COVID-19 pandemic, need updating of consent forms to include new risks, treatment protocols, and uncertainties related to the condition.
- *Incomplete disclosure:* Sometimes, the information is not disclosed completely by the doctor, either intentionally or unintentionally. The treating doctor may downplay certain risks or may not present all available treatment options, including the option of nontreatment. This occurs as clinicians may assume what is "best" for the patient without involving them in the decision-making process. In order to decide how much information to disclose to the patient, it is suggested to use the "reasonable patient standard" which focuses on *What would the average patient need to know to be able to make an informed decision?*
- *Inadequate documentation:* The healthcare professionals may be vulnerable to legal action if the documentation of informed consent is inadequate as the patients may claim later that they were not fully informed. All required elements of informed consent **(Fig. 1)** should be documented. Training sessions should be carried out for educating the medical professionals including the residents and physicians who most often obtain consent.

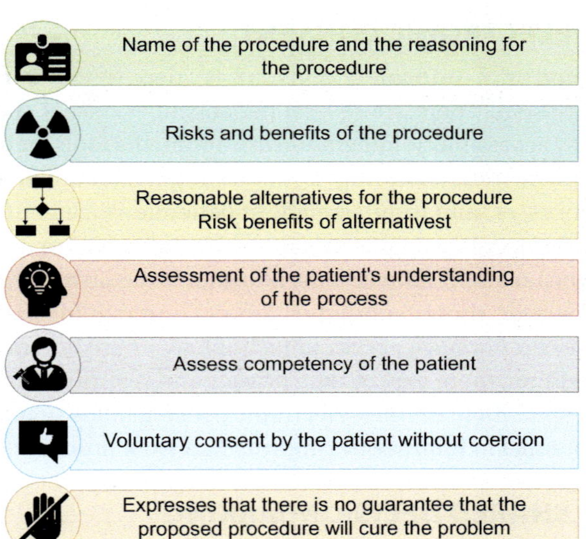

Fig. 1: Essential elements of informed consent.

PENALTIES

The consequences of not taking a consent would be payment of compensation (in civil) and imprisonment (in criminal). The patient may sue the medical practitioner in tort for trespass to person. Alternatively, the health professional may be sued for negligence. In certain extreme cases, there is a theoretical possibility of criminal prosecution for assault or battery. The traditional definition of battery is an act that directly and either intentionally or negligently causes some physical contact with another person without that person's consent. A doctor may be held liable for criminal breach if there is gross disrespect to the patient's bodily autonomy, for instance, if a patient's organs are taken without his consent.

INFORMED CONSENT IN RESEARCH—HUMAN CLINICAL STUDIES

Informed consent is mandatory for all clinical trials involving human beings.

Adherence to ethical standards in study design and execution is usually monitored by an Institutional Review Board (IRB). The IRB was established in the United States in 1974 by the National Research Act. An IRB may waive informed consent if certain conditions are met. One example of minimal risk research is the assessment of interventions that generally occur in emergency situations. Examples include studying medications used for intubation in the emergency department or conducting a retrospective chart review.[14]

ELECTRONIC CONSENT

Electronic informed consent is also referred to as eConsent. There are several benefits of eConsent such as easy accessibility, integration of multimedia tools for better patient understanding, streamlining of documentation processes, and improvement of patient engagement. The latter occurs as patients can review information at their own pace and can access the information again if they want. However, these techniques are not suitable for patients who do not have access to technology or are illiterate. In addition, there may be data privacy and security concerns. Despite these hurdles, electronic consent holds significant potential to improve the informed consent process.

SHARED DECISION-MAKING

Shared decision-making is a collaborative process where healthcare professionals and patients work together to make informed decisions.

Advantages

- Shared decision-making offers a patient-centered approach in partnering with patients to make decisions about their treatment, which reflect their values and preferences. Even for the same disease, different patients may have different preferences.
- Shared decision-making prepares the patient and helps in adherence to the treatment agreed upon. It contributes to the patient's satisfaction. SDM is not "another thing clinicians must do", but it is a method of care and is as essential to the clinician's art as history taking, physical examination, selection and interpretation of diagnostic tests, and patient education and counseling.[3]

Process of Shared Decision-making

Shared decision-making recognizes the importance of both the clinician and the patient. The clinician is an expert in understanding medical evidence and treatment options, while the patients are the best to decide their preferences, values, and unique circumstances. Both clinician and patient have *open dialogue* and share information. The clinician explains the various options, risks, benefits, and uncertainties of each of the options, while the patient expresses his/her goals, concerns, and priorities. This helps in decisions which are more aligned with the patient's values and improves satisfaction, adherence to treatment plans, and overall health outcomes. SDM is thus a more patient-centered and holistic approach and empowers patients to take an active role in their health management. SDM is the standard of care for patients and their clinicians to arrive at a medical decision.

The discussion may be between the physician and the patient. Other team members can include a multidisciplinary team as required and other relatives of the patient. Translators may also be used as needed.

Aids can be used to improve a patient's understanding of the various options available.

DIFFERENCE BETWEEN INFORMED CONSENT AND SHARED DECISION-MAKING

Informed consent is the legal process used to promote patient autonomy, while SDM is an ethical approach.[15] SDM is most appropriate in situations of uncertainty, in which two or more clinically reasonable alternatives exist.[16]

Shared Decision-making in Dialysis

Dialysis patients often report the perception that they were passive participants in the decision to start dialysis. SDM indicators mainly involve three items:

1. *Kidney replacement therapy (KRT) which includes dialysis or transplant:* SDM for CKD patients is mainly used in the selection of KRT.
2. *Dialysis methods including hemodialysis and peritoneal dialysis:* The process of SDM helps patients decide the method of dialysis in the future.
3. Timing of creation of dialysis access

Shared decision-making for KRT for CKD patients should be initiated during a visit to the nephrologist in CKD stage 5 if the patient has a risk of kidney failure within 1 year. The decision time is defined as the number of days from when the physician started KRT SDM until the patient made a decision for modality of dialysis.

Shared Decision-making Needs to be Individualized

There is a tremendous variation among patients in their willingness to take part in their medical decisions. The highly educated and opinionated patient may want to dictate exactly what tests and treatments to receive. Here, the physician's role is to listen to the patient, determine if the patient has understood the disease and treatment options correctly, and if so the physician can assume the role of a medical advisor and facilitator of the patient's wishes. However, in other sicker, less educated or more dependent patients who trust the physician to make all medical decisions, the physician has to be the leader. The physician may try to elicit the patient's preferences. In case the patient wishes the physician to make the choice for him/her, the physician can offer the option which he/she considers the best under the circumstances. Most patients fall between these two extremes. Thus, shared decision-making is not only science but also an art and the final goal is to achieve patient satisfaction.[17]

Challenges

Challenges to SDM include caring for patients who want an unproved therapy or one that conflicts with the physician's expertise or ethics.

- Some patients elect not to follow a physician's recommendation and choose a disproportionately risky or less effective therapy; e.g., a young patient with stage V CKD may not want transplantation but may opt for lifelong hemodialysis. The role of the physician here is to inquire about why the patient chose that particular course. If the patient offers adequate reasons, understands the risks and benefits, and if the choice is an accepted therapy for the condition, the physician generally should accede to the patient's choice.
- However, there are times a physician may find a patient's choice to be ethically unacceptable.[18] One such example is a young CKD5 patient who is oliguric and azotemic but does not wish to go on hemodialysis or register for transplant. Here, shared decision-making requires the physician to explore the reasons for the patient's choice, offer acceptable alternatives such as peritoneal dialysis, and compassionately explain why the physician cannot agree to the patient's wishes.

CONCLUSION

Informed consent is an important legal document and the medical fraternity should be well acquainted with the nitty-gritties of an informed consent process. Shared decision making is equally important where the doctor and patient make informed choices about their treatment.

REFERENCES

1. Hariri E, Al Hammoud M, Donovan E, Shah K, Kittleson MM. The role of informed consent in clinical and research settings. Med Clin North Am. 2022;106(4):663-74.
2. Shah P, Thornton I, Turrin D, Kopitnik NL, Hipskind JE. NCBI Bookshelf. A Service of the National Library of Medicine, National Institutes of Health. StatPearls [Internet]. Treasure Island (FL): StatPearls Publishing; 2024 Jan-.
3. Montori VM, Ruissen MM, Hargraves IG, Brito JP, Kunneman M. Shared decision-making as a method of care. BMJ Evid Based Med. 2023;28(4):213-7.
4. Glaser J, Nouri S, Fernandez A, Sudore RL, Schillinger D, Klein-Fedyshin M, et al. Interventions to Improve Patient Comprehension in Informed Consent for Medical and Surgical Procedures: An Updated Systematic Review. Med Decis Making. 2020;40(2):119-43.
5. Bastia BK. Consent to treatment: Practice vis-à-vis principle. Indian J Med Ethics. 2008;5:113-4.
6. Kaushik JS, Narang M, Agarwal N. Informed consent in pediatric practice. Indian Pediatr. 2010;47:1039-46.
7. Satyanarayana Rao KH. Informed consent: An ethical obligation or legal compulsion? J Cutan Aesthet Surg. 2008;1:33-5.
8. Kumar A, Mullick P, Prakash S, Bharadwaj A. Consent and the Indian medical practitioner. Indian J Anaesth. 2015;59(11):695-700.
9. Kekre NS. Medical law and the physician. Indian J Urol. 2008;24:135-6.
10. Dr Shailesh Shah v. Aphraim Jayanand Rathod, FA No. 597 of 1995 (NCDRC, 2003). Retrieved from http://www.ncdrc.nic.in/fa59795.html [Last accessed June, 2025].
11. Waisel DB. Legal aspects of anesthesia care. In: Miller RD, Eriksson LI, Fleisher LA, Wiener-Kronish JP, Young WL (Eds). Miller's Anesthesia, 7th edition. Philadelphia: Churchill Livingstone Elsevier; 2010. pp. 221-33.
12. Tewari A, Garg S. Informed consent and anaesthesia. Indian J Anaesth. 2003;47:311-2.
13. Reddy KS, Murty OP. Medical law and ethics. In: The Essentials of Forensic Medicine and Toxicology, 32nd edition. Hyderabad: K Suguna Devi; 2013. pp. 22-55.
14. New Drugs and Clinical Trials Rules, 2019, Ministry of Health and Fam. Welfare, Notification, GSR. 227(E), (March 19, 2019). [online] Available from "https://cdsco.gov.in/opencms/opencms/system/modules/CDSCO.WEB/elements/download_file_division.jsp? [Last accessed August, 2025].
15. Whitney SN, McGuire AL, McCullough LB. A typology of shared decision making, informed consent, and simple consent. Ann Intern Med. 2004;140(1):54-9.
16. Bernat JL, McQuillen MP. On Shared Decision-making and Informed Consent. Neurol Clin Pract. 2021;11(2):93-4.
17. Quill TE, Brody H. Physician recommendation and patient autonomy: finding a balance between physician power and patient choice. Ann Intern Med. 1996;125:763-9.
18. Bernat JL, McQuillen MP. Physician-assisted death in chronic neurological diseases. Neurology. 2017;88:1488-9.

CHAPTER 43

Legal Aspects and Liability Issues in Vascular Access for Interventional Nephrologists in India

Narinder Pal Singh, Urmila Anandh

INTRODUCTION

As the management of chronic kidney disease (CKD) becomes more complex, the patient often has to meet many members of the healthcare system for his overall care. It is thus important that the nephrologist is in the forefront in the care of this vulnerable individual. Even 25 years back, arteriovenous shunts were successfully converted into arteriovenous fistulas (AVFs) and were an important aspect in nephrology training.[1] A major nephrology center in west India was doing pioneering work in treating atherosclerotic renal artery stenosis.[2] Over the years, unfortunately many aspects of this care have moved out of the purview of the nephrologist. The kidney biopsies are being done by the radiologists, and establishing a vascular access for dialysis (temporary or permanent) is now in the domain of the interventional radiologists, intensivists, and anesthesiologists. Even though less utilized as a modality of renal replacement therapy (RRT), peritoneal dialysis catheters are inserted by surgeons. This often leads to lack of ownership of the overall care of the patient at the expense of the patient (literally and figuratively). To facilitate care of CKD, the nephrologist should take up the role of an interventional nephrologist.

THE NEPHROLOGIST AS AN INTERVENTIONALIST

Chronic kidney disease is a burgeoning problem worldwide and is a major issue in a vast country like ours where tertiary health care has not reached all nooks and corners of the country. It is in the remote and inaccessible parts of the country that nephrologists have started to develop comprehensive systems of care where they are managing the vascular access of their patients. This has become a necessity, and reports presented in conferences in India have emphasized that the nephrologists trained in interventions can improve care as follows:

- Nephrologist–patient ratio is low in India and the nephrologists are concentrated in large metropolitan cities.
- Delivery of kidney care is better in districts with interventional nephrologists, in spite of fewer nephrologists.
- Promoting interventional nephrology among nephrologists and trainees can enhance delivery of renal care delivery to the rising number of populations with renal disease in developing countries.

Also, the involvement of nephrologists in creation of AVFs will decrease the number of patients initiating dialysis with temporary catheters.[3] As we get overwhelmed with rising numbers of CKD patients, more and more nephrologists will need to hone their skills in interventional nephrology and the scope of work will be immense and not just restricted to establishing vascular access for dialysis.

Nephrologist and Vascular Access

The major area of concern is the establishment of a hemodialysis vascular access as it is an essential component in the treatment of patients with end-stage renal disease. Individuals with end-stage kidney disease (ESKD) should have access to the best available care in RRT. There are data from various parts of the world that prove that access established by nephrologists is no way inferior.[4,5] Venous puncture and catheterization have always been done by nephrologists; putting in a tunneled permcath is often left to the interventional radiologist. Now the trend is changing with more and more nephrologists undertaking this procedure. Live workshops and demonstrations have kindled an interest and have instilled confidence into many young nephrologists. Over the last few years, permcaths are becoming increasingly popular as they become a bridge to transplantation. With the incidence of elderly and diabetic CKD patients increasing, nephrologists often prefer a permcath as fistula maturation takes longer.[6]

As a young qualified nephrologist ventures into the field of interventions, he is faced with ambivalence (turf wars) from many of his colleagues which is understandable. He needs to assure himself that what he is doing is for the overall betterment of his patients. Also, vascular access creation has and is part of the nephrology core curriculum. There is a growing interest in the involvement of nephrologists in creation of AVFs. In Singapore, a 2-month elective program in interventional nephrology is offered to junior nephrologists to equip them with fundamental endovascular interventional skills.[7] The International Society of Nephrology publishes a list of specialized centers for interventional nephrology worldwide. The Indian Society of Nephrology is also offering postdoctoral fellowships in interventional nephrology. As the subspeciality matures and the awareness improves, legal hassles hopefully will reduce in the future.[8,9]

Despite the improving scenario, in India, interventional nephrologists face many legal and liability challenges that are associated with vascular access creation and maintenance of AVFs, grafts, and central venous catheters (CVCs). In the chapter, we explore the legal framework, liability issues, and strategies to mitigate risks in the context of vascular access for interventional nephrologists in India.[10]

LEGAL FRAMEWORK GOVERNING VASCULAR ACCESS

Regulatory Standards

In India, interventional nephrology practices including vascular access procedures are mainly regulated by ethical and medical guidelines. The National Medical Council (Ethics, Professional Conduct, and Etiquette) Regulation Act provides regulatory standards for medical practices in India.[11] Additionally, Kidney Disease Outcomes Quality Initiative (KDOQI) clinical practice guidelines for vascular access, the Indian Society of Critical Care Medicine, and the Indian Society of Nephrology provide regulatory instructions and recommendations on best practices for vascular access. These societies help develop a statutory framework and adhering to their guidelines avoid legal issues while practicing interventional nephrology.

Informed Consent

Before performing any clinical procedure, the nephrologists should obtain the signed documented informed consent of the patient. The name of the operating surgeon nephrologist must be mentioned in the medical records. The necessary information such as the procedure's nature, potential risks/benefits, and alternative options available must be informed and documented. These procedures ensure that the patients have informed decisions about their standard of care and secure the nephrologists from legal claims related to lack of consent.[11]

Documentation and Record Keeping

Accurate documentation and record-keeping are crucial for legal protection. There must be detailed documented records of patient assessments, procedural details, complications, and follow-up care of each patient. These documents can serve as evidence in case of any legal disputes or allegations of negligence. All signatures in the notes, prescriptions, certificates, orders, referral summaries, etc., should carry the nephrologist's name and medical registration number.[11]

Confidentiality

Every communication between healthcare workers and patients shall be kept confidential. Such communication, whether personal or related to health and treatment, shall not be revealed unless required by the laws of the state, or if nondisclosure may itself be detrimental to the health of the patient or another human being.[11]

LIABILITY ISSUES IN VASCULAR ACCESS

Medical Negligence

Complications associated with vascular access procedures can be the main origin of medical negligence claims. Common issues that could be involved are infections, stenosis/thrombosis, and mechanical complications at the time of catheterization procedures or AVF creation. Nephrologists must adhere to the established protocol to minimize these risks.[12]

- *Standard of care:* The standard of care is a "legal term" that refers to what a competent nephrologist would do under similar conditions. It can help determine whether the professional obligations to the patients have been met by the clinicians. Deviations from this standard of care procedure can originate in medical negligence claims.[13]

- *Complication management:* It is essential to recognize the potential complications of the vascular access procedures and their prompt management. For example, failure to manage catheter-related bloodstream infections (CRBSIs) can lead to liability.[12]

Vicarious Liability

Hospitals are also held vicarious liability for the actions of their employed nephrologists. This can be extended to procedural errors or omissions which occur within the scope of employment. The hospitals need to ensure that their staff is adequately trained and supervised. At the time of employment, a thorough check of the nephrologists' subspeciality training in interventional nephrology should be done and appropriate credentialling and privileges should be offered to the employee. For instance, the hospital management may allow the nephrologist to perform routine permcath insertions but may withhold the privileges of allowing the physician to create AVFs. The hospital management should also help the nephrologist in doing interventional procedures to attend/participate in regular workshops/demonstrations in various conferences.

Ethical Considerations

Patient Autonomy

Respecting patient autonomy is the main integral part of ethics in medical sciences and contributes to vascular access decisions. Based on the principle of autonomy, patients should be involved in choosing the type of vascular access as per their lifestyle, medical history, and preferences. There should be an ethical practice that balances between medical recommendations and patient choice.

Equity in Access

Access to vascular access procedures should be equitable. It is a vital ethical obligation. Geographic location or socioeconomic factors can influence the disparities in access to care. Nephrologists should advocate for policies that promote equitable healthcare delivery.

Risks and Benefits Assessment

The choice of vascular access/procedure should lead to a favorable outcome and benefit the patients. Nephrologists must provide information about the risks and benefits of vascular access procedures and support patients or their surrogate decision-makers in the evaluation of available choice of vascular access. It is mandatory to justify the risk, which is the probability of causing discomfort or any anticipated physical, psychological, social, economic, and/or legal adversity. Healthcare professionals should always attempt to maximize benefits and minimize risk/discomfort to patients.

Besides the patient-centric approach, nephrologists involved in creating AVFs should be aware of the policies of the insurance providers and third-party administrators. The legal aspects of AVF creation are summarized in **Table 1**.

CASE STUDIES HIGHLIGHTING LEGAL CHALLENGES

Case Study 1: Infection Control Lapses

A case of legal action came out against a hospital where multiple patients developed catheter-related bloodstream infections following CVC placement. Multiple lapses in infection control protocols were observed. In this case, strict aseptic techniques were not followed up during catheter insertion.[12]

Case Study 2: Consent Issues

A case was filed against a nephrologist for performing an AVF procedure without adequate informed consent. The patient and his relative claimed that they were not informed about alternative available options and anticipated potential complications related to the procedures. This highlights the necessity of comprehensive consent processes.

PRACTICE RECOMMENDATIONS FOR INTERVENTIONAL NEPHROLOGISTS INVOLVED IN VASCULAR ACCESS PROCEDURES

Risk Management Strategies

Training and Competency

Continuous training programs ensure that nephrologists are up to date with current practices and technologies related to vascular access. Nephrologists should be well trained in decision-making procedures and develop multidisciplinary teams. Competency assessments can help maintain high standards of care. Healthcare professionals should receive education about shared decision-making, advance care planning, counseling, and communication.

TABLE 1: Legal aspects that a nephrologist should be aware of while creating an arteriovenous fistula (AVF).

Legal issues	*Comments*
Patient selection and referral	• *Patient selection:* Carefully select patients and often avoid difficult complex procedures with higher risks of failure • *Referral to vascular surgeon:* Low threshold of referral, especially if a complex procedure is required and if the nephrologist has less experience in that procedure
Scope of practice and credentialling	• *Scope of practice:* Must operate within their capabilities—level of training and expertise • *Credentialing and privileging:* Must meet the standards of privileging and credentialling of their institution in order to perform vascular access procedures/surgeries
Medical malpractice and liability	• *Standard of care:* – Must adhere to stand of care which is applicable to vascular surgeons and members of other surgical specialties involved in creating AV fistulas – Patients must provide informed consent before the procedure as per the guidelines • *Complications and adverse events:* Nephrologists should be aware that they may be liable for complications like bleeding, infection, and nerve damage. They should ask for help at the earliest instance when they are aware of such complications
Documentation	• *Reimbursement and billing:* The nephrologist should be aware of the standard coding and billing for the AVF creation. Incorrect or overcharging can lead to liability damages • *Informed consent documents:* Besides information about the procedure, the document should also contain information about the patient's rights and their independence to choose an alternate option (a vascular surgeon for the procedure)
Regulatory compliance	• *NMC guidelines:* The practicing physician should uphold all values and principles enshrined in the NMC while performing vascular access procedures • *Local hospital guidelines:* The nephrologist should follow all guidelines pertaining to requirements while performing the procedure (i.e., infection control guidelines, operation theater protocols, radiation exposure regulations, etc.)

Protocol Development

A standardized protocol for medical clinical decision-making, specifically concerning the choice of vascular access and vascular access procedures, should be developed; where the protocol has been implemented, sharing of best outcomes/practices is essential across the jurisdiction. It can reduce variability in practice and improve patient outcomes. The protocol should include guidelines for infection prevention, complication management, and follow-up care.

Additionally, policies and guidelines governing access to vascular access procedures should strive to:

- Avoid futile procedures for vascular access
- Confirm a minimum anticipated benefit threshold
- Promote equality of opportunity
- Maximize utilization of the existing resources
- Exclusion should be made for the criteria that are not morally justifiable concerning allocation decisions, such as gender, ethnicity, religion, and socioeconomic status
- Ensure transparency of policies

Quality Improvement Initiatives

Implementing quality improvement initiatives focused on reducing complications associated with vascular access can enhance patient safety. Regular audits and feedback mechanisms help identify areas for improvement.[14]

Cost of Vascular Access Procedure

Interventional nephrologists should strive to reduce the costs involved in the creation of vascular access procedures using simple, safe, and affordable options for vascular access choice without compromising the quality of care provided to patients.

Multidisciplinary Action

Nephrologists and renal care nurses should collaborate with other health professionals, microbiologists, pathologists, senior management officials, legal experts, and ethicists to investigate specific ethical issues at various levels. Professional societies and medical councils should ensure that healthcare professionals working with patients with ESKD are familiar with their responsibilities for patient care, including their obligations to provide care to those who might be perceived to pose risks to care providers (e.g., from infectious disease). Encourage a patient referral system for better quality services.[15]

CONCLUSION

In India, interventional nephrologists must handle a complex landscape of legal responsibilities and potential liabilities related to vascular access procedures. By understanding the legal framework, adhering to ethical standards, and implementing robust risk management strategies, nephrologists can minimize liability risks while providing high-quality care to their patients.

REFERENCES

1. Murthy ML, Niyamathullah MM, Hariharan S, Kirubakaran MG, Shastry JC. Conversion of arteriovenous shunts to fistulae for maintenance haemodialysis: its applicability in a developing country. J Assoc Physicians India. 1989;37(3):220-1.
2. Hegde U, Rajapurkar M, Sishir Gang, Khanapet M, Durugkar S, Gohel K, et al. Fifteen Years' Experience of Treating Atherosclerotic Renal Artery Stenosis by Interventional Nephrologists in India. Semin Dial. 2012;25(1):97-104.
3. Asif A, Leclercq B, Merril D, Bourgoigne JJ, Roth D. Fistula Creation: Should US Nephrologists Get Involved? Am J Kid Dis. 2003;42:1293-300.
4. Mahapatra HS, Binoy R, Inamdar NA, Kumar DPK, Kaur A. Continuing arteriovenous fistula creation by nephrologist and its outcome during COVID pandemic-analysis of 376 cases. Semin Dial. 2022;35(1):3-5.
5. Nguyen B, Duong MC, Tran HND, Do KQ, Ng KTT. Arteriovenous fistula creation by nephrologist and its outcomes: a prospective cohort study from Vietnam. BMC Nephrol. 2023;24:88.
6. Sampathkumar K, Ramakrishnan M, Sah AK, Sooraj Y, Mahaldhar A, Ajeshkumar R. Tunneled central venous catheter - Experience from a single center. Indian J Nephrol. 2011;21:107-11.
7. Pang SC, Tan RY, Kwek JL, Lee KG, Foo MWY, Choong LHL, et al. Current state of vascular access in Singapore. J Vasc Access. 2020;21(5):582-8.
8. https://www.theisn.org/in-action/grants/isn-interventional-nephrology-training/
9. International Society of Nephrology. [online] Available from https://www.theisn.org/in-action/grants/isn-indian-society-of-nephrology-grant-programs/ [Last accessed July, 2025].
10. Ramachandran R, Bhargava V, Jasuja S, Gallieni M, Jha V, Sahay M, et al. Interventional nephrology and vascular access practice: A perspective from South and Southeast Asia. J Vasc Access. 2022;23(6):849-60.
11. National Medical Commission. (2012) [online] Available from https://www.nmc.org.in/rules-regulations/national-medical-commission-registered-medical-practitioner-professional-conduct-regulations-2023-reg/ [Last accessed July, 2025].
12. Jha V, Martin DE, Bargman JM, International Society of Nephrology Ethical Dialysis Task Force. Ethical issues in dialysis therapy. Lancet. 2017;389(10081):1851-6.
13. Vali PS, Parikh N, Mohan K, Anandh U. The changing landscape in nephrology education in India. Front Nephrol. 2023;3:1110704.
14. Javeri Y, Jagathkar G, Dixit S, Chaudhary D, Zirpe KG, Mehta Y, et al. Indian Society of Critical Care Medicine Position Statement for Central Venous Catheterization and Management 2020. Indian J Crit Care Med. 2020;24(Suppl 1):S6-S30.
15. Crews DC, Bello AK, Saadi G; World Kidney Day Steering Committee. Burden, Access, and Disparities in Kidney Disease. Kidney Int Rep. 2019;4(3):372-9.

SECTION 12

Peritoneal Dialysis

CHAPTER 44

Anatomy and Physiology of Peritoneum

Anirudha Datta, Pratik Das, Upal Sengupta

CASE SCENARIO

A 60-year-old diabetic male, on continuous ambulatory peritoneal dialysis (CAPD) for a duration of 10 years, presented with complaints of nausea vomiting, abdominal pain, distention, and progressive weight loss. He gives history of multiple episodes of peritonitis in the past. Presently, he has noticed that his net daily ultrafiltration has reduced from 800–900 to 200–300 mL/day over the last 3–4 months. He switched to 4.5% solution, but it has not been of much help. There is no history of constipation or diarrhea. Abdominal X-ray shows the presence of dilated bowel loops. What could be the possible cause?

Encapsulating peritoneal sclerosis is a dreaded complication which results due to long-term exposure to high concentrations of glucose and advanced glycation end products along with repeated infections. The anatomical modification results in ultrafiltration failure as well as features of bowel obstruction.

INTRODUCTION

Peritoneum is the largest serous membrane in the human body, which essentially is composed of thin layers of connective tissue covered by sheets of mesothelium. This membrane folds to form the omentum, mesentery, and various organ-specific ligaments.

"More than a century ago, Robinson, after summarizing more than two centuries of research, defined the diverse natural functions of the peritoneum as follows:

- To regulate fluid for nutrient and mechanical purposes
- To facilitate motion
- To minimize friction
- To conduct vessels and nerves to the viscera"[1]

The evolutionary development of the celomic cavity can be traced from lower life forms to higher vertebrates, showcasing its roles as an excretory organ, part of the reproductive system, and a lymph reservoir. In humans, the peritoneal cavity, when provided with an artificial pore (peritoneal catheter), can recapitulate its original excretory function.[2]

The peritoneum has two layers, the visceral peritoneum which covers the intra-abdominal organs and the parietal peritoneum which covers the intra-abdominal wall and the abdominal surface of the diaphragm. The anatomical surface area of the peritoneum for an adult human varies from 1.72 to 2.08 m^2 with an area:body weight ratio of 0.284.[3] For infants having a body weight of 2,700–2,900 g, the total peritoneal surface varied between 0.106 and 0.151 m^2, with a higher area:body weight ratio of 0.383 to 0.522.[4,5]

The visceral peritoneum makes up 80% of the surface area, while the parietal peritoneum accounts for the remaining 20%. However, the effective surface area is substantially lower than the total anatomical surface area as the peritoneal area in contact with the dialysate fluid is significantly lower. Studies have shown that the effective surface area is about one-third of the total anatomical surface area.[6-8]

MICROSCOPIC STRUCTURE

Structurally, the peritoneal membrane is a tissue comprising three different compartments, the vasculature, interstitium, and mesothelium, each consisting of different types of cells as their principal component, endothelial cells in the vasculature, fibroblasts in the interstitium and the mesothelial cells, a layer of epithelial cells of mesenchymal origin in the mesothelium **(Fig. 1)**.[9]

Mesothelial Cells

Mesothelial cells are the lining epithelium of the peritoneum. They are derived from the mesenchymal cells that get flattened and develop their own basement membrane and intercellular junctional complexes as

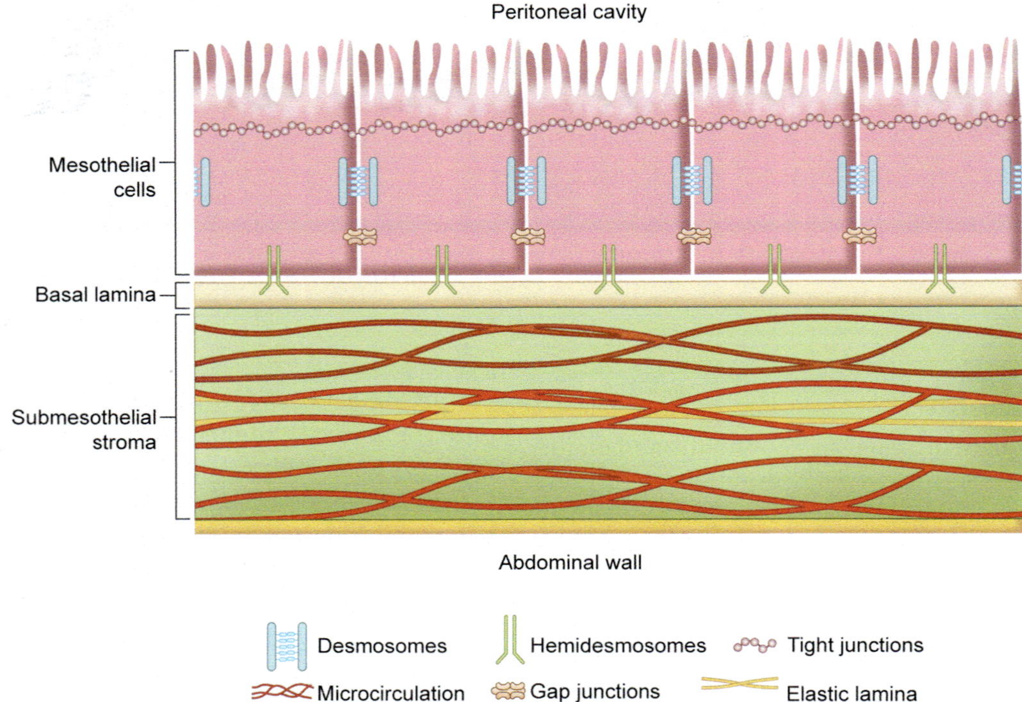

Fig. 1: Schematic diagram of the peritoneum.
Source: Kastelein AW, Vos LMC, de Jong KH, van Baal JOAM, Nieuwland R, van Noorden CJF, et al. Embryology, anatomy, physiology and pathophysiology of the peritoneum and the peritoneal vasculature. Semin Cell Develop Biol. 2019;92:27-36.

tight junction (TJ) and desmosomes. Under the light microscope, these cells appear as flat sheets of polygonal cells having tortuous and overlapping boundaries. The apical surfaces have multiple cytoplasmic projections called microvilli. The distribution and density of the microvilli vary according to the location. These are very sensitive to minor injury and the loss of microvilli, as seen in continuous ambulatory peritoneal dialysis (CAPD) patients, signifies impending apoptosis.

The apical surface of the mesothelium including the microvilli are covered with a layer of negatively charged glycocalyx.[10]

The mesothelium contains multiple cell membrane-based vesicles which conduct various transcellular pathways of molecular transport. It also expresses aquaporin (AQP) channels, their density being a function of various osmotic and nonosmotic modulators. The mesothelial cell borders contain various cellular junctional complexes as TJs [zonula occludens (ZO)], intermediate junctions (zonula adherens), desmosomes, and gap junctions (GJs).[11]

In addition to the commonly seen flattened epithelial-like mesothelial cells, a cuboidal variant of mesothelial cells can also be found. They are found adjacent to parenchymal organs and near lymphatic stomata which are gaps opening into submesothelial lymphatic channels and contain actin-like microfilaments in the mesothelium as well as endothelium conferring it contractile properties **(Fig. 2)**.[12,13]

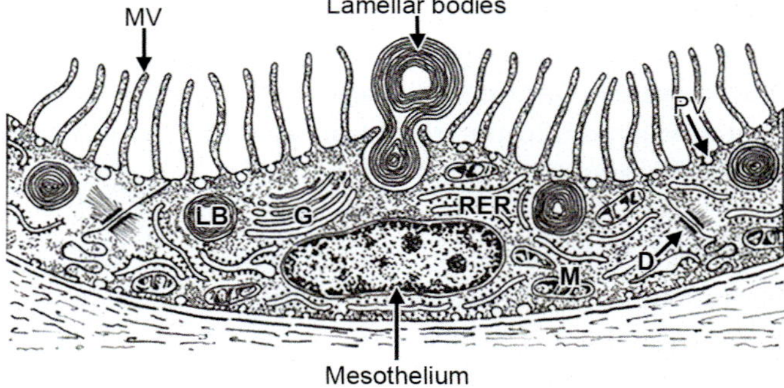

Fig. 2: Schematic representation of the ultrastructure of the mesothelial cell with flattened/reniform nuclei. (D: desmosomes; G: Golgi body; LB: lamellar body; M: mitochondria; MV: microvilli; PV: plasmalemmal vesicles; RER: rough endoplasmic reticulum)

Greater details on cell junctions' transcellular transport and lymphatic stomata are discussed in the following text.

Submesothelial Basement Membrane/Basal Lamina

It is a thin (<100 nm) dense matrix of fibers lying between the mesothelial cells and the submesothelial stroma. Its main components are collagen IV and glycoproteins (laminin, perlecan, entactin). The collagen type IV fiber network acts as a skeleton of the basal lamina, whereas laminin provides binding sites for adhesion of mesothelial cells via hemidesmosomes.

It is visualized as a homogeneous, continuous structure under the electron microscope; however, reduplication of the basement membrane has been seen in case of diabetics and uremic patients treated with maintenance peritoneal dialysis (PD). Studies using cationic tracers have shown the presence of anionic charges through the lamina.[14-16]

Submesothelial Stroma/Interstitium

Originating from the mesenchyme, this layer contains multiple cellular elements like mast cells, macrophages, monocytes, few adipocytes, and principally the fibroblasts, embedded in an amorphous gel-like substance consisting of collagen type I fibers, laminin, fibronectin, glycosaminoglycans, and proteoglycans (heparan sulfate, chondroitin sulfate, and keratan sulfate) through which the vascular, lymphatic, and nerve bundles are interspersed.[17]

The fibroblast is a spindle-shaped cell having a dynamic and heterogeneous population with a diverse functional and phenotypic variety. The quiescent fibroblasts express CD34, a marker common in hematopoietic stem cells, and its expression varies inversely with the presence of inflammation and appearance of myofibroblastic phenotypes.[18,19]

The thickness of the interstitium is variable, and it is an important determinant of molecular movement through the interstitial stroma, to and from the microvasculature. Other important denominators are the size, molecular weight, and electrical charge of the molecule.[20-22]

The interstitium is negatively charged at physiological pH due to polyanionic glycosaminoglycans which influence the distribution and movements of the plasma proteins coming out through the vessels.[21]

Another important factor is the presence of an extremely low to slightly negative pressure (0 to –4 mm Hg) through the interstitium which modulates plasma to lymphatics transfer as well as prevents development of interstitial edema. During clinical PD, the intra-abdominal pressure increases up to 4–10 cmH_2O, creating a pressure gradient that facilitates solute as well as fluid clearance thorough the peritoneal membranes.[23-27]

Vascular System

Blood Vascular System

The main blood supply of the peritoneum differs between the parietal and the visceral parts. The parietal peritoneum receives blood supply from the lumbar, intercostal, and epigastric arteries and drains into the inferior vena cava. The visceral peritoneum receives blood supply from the mesenteric artery and drains into the portal system.

Depending on the anatomical structure, the vasculature of the peritoneum consists of small artery → arteriole → precapillary arteriole → capillary → postcapillary venule (PCV) → muscular venule → small vein → vein.[28]

The small artery and arteriole differ in the number of smooth muscle cells in the tunica media, with the small arteries (ϕ 100–2 mm) having several smooth muscle cell layers with internal elastic membrane between the intima and media, whereas the arterioles (ϕ 10–100 μm) have one of two layers without the internal elastic membrane. The arterioles control the blood flow through the capillary networks.

Capillaries have the smallest diameter (ϕ 4–0 μm) and consist of a single layer of endothelial cell and basement membrane. In some areas of the capillaries, pericytes are associated with the endothelial cells which are surrounded by the basal lamina shared by the endothelial cells and have TJ and GJ with the endothelial cells. They allow gases, electrolytes, metabolites, and small and large molecules to pass through their thin walls transcellularly and paracellularly.

Postcapillary venules (ϕ 10–50 μm) collect blood from the capillary network and deliver it to downstream muscular venules (ϕ 50–100 μm) which are distinguished by the presence of layers of smooth muscle cells forming the tunica media instead of the pericytes seen in PCV along with a thin layer of tunica adventitia.[29]

Postcapillary venules act as an important site of substance exchange as well as a site for interaction and migration of the inflammatory cells and vasoactive substances. It is also the principal affected site during long-term PD-related hyalinizing vasculopathy, and the dysfunction of the PCV is intimately related to the increased permeability of the peritoneum and PD-associated complications, such as ultrafiltration failure (UFF) and encapsulating peritoneal sclerosis (EPS).[30,31]

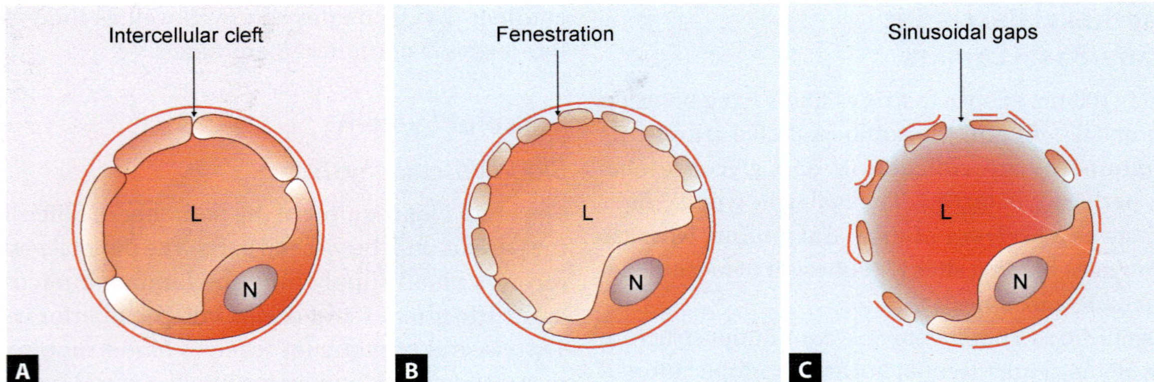

Figs. 3A to C: Types of capillaries: (A) Continuous nonfenestrated; (B) Continuous fenestrated; (C) Discontinuous/sinusoidal.
Source: Cleaver O, Melton DA, Endothelial signaling during development. Nat Med. 2003;9(6):661-8.

Based on the classification by Majno, there are mainly three types of capillaries **(Figs. 3A to C)**:[29]

1. Continuous
2. Fenestrated
3. Discontinuous or sinusoidal

The continuous type is mainly seen in the peritoneum with few fenestrated capillaries.

The continuous capillaries have endothelial cells connected to each other via TJs, adherent junctions (AJs), and GJs. TJs predominate in the arteries and the arterioles, whereas the AJs are more abundant in the capillaries and the PCVs.[32]

Typically found in kidneys and various endocrine glands, the fenestrated capillaries are comparatively low in number (1.7% of the total number of capillaries) in the human parietal peritoneum. The diameter of the fenestrae ranges between 60 and 90 nm. These are static structures and can be increased in number or induced even on continuous capillaries under the influence of vascular endothelial growth factor (VEGF) released by inflammatory cells.[33]

The fenestrae permit movement of the small to large solutes; however, they restrict movement of large plasma proteins by the virtue of the electronegative diaphragm and the glycocalyx.

Overall, the fenestrated capillaries have higher hydraulic conductivity and permeability in comparison to the continuous endothelium.[34,35]

In the mesothelial as well as the endothelial cell lining, there are mainly two transport routes: Intercellular or paracellular and transcellular **(Flowcharts 1A and B)**.

Transcellular transport: The intercellular route is mediated via gaps or clefts where the intercellular junctional complexes as TJs, AJs, GJs, or desmosomes become loose.

The transcellular pathways are mediated via vesicles (endocytosis), directly via the membrane by simple diffusion (lipid-soluble small uncharged molecules) or by carrier or transporter proteins (water-soluble molecules via ion pumps and glucose transporters) and via channel proteins as AQPs.

The vesicles or caveolae are abundant in the capillary endothelia where they occupy almost 7% of the cell volume. Structurally, they are round or oval shaped with an outer diameter of 50–90 nm and a small neck of 10 nm.[36,37]

The pinocytotic vesicles can cluster together to form a transcellular channel connecting the luminal and the abluminal surface, and higher density of such channels is seen in the venular segment of the capillaries. These vesicular transport systems make continuous capillaries more permeable to large molecules in comparison to the fenestrated capillaries.[38]

Paracellular transport: Junctional Apparatus

Intercellular junctional apparatuses are TJs, AJs, and GJs. Under a normal physiological state, fluids and small molecules having <3 nm radius can diffuse through these junctions. Pathological conditions inciting inflammation loosen these junctions promoting leaking of plasma proteins.

Tight Junctions (Zonula occludens):[39] Tight junctions are composed of several transmembrane adhesive proteins, including occludins, claudins, and junctional adhesion molecules (JAMs), which interact with cytoplasmic scaffolding proteins such as ZO to form the most covalent intercellular junction. These are preferentially distributed in the small artery and arterioles; however, these are also found in capillary distributions where the permeability is limited like the blood–brain barrier or blood–retinal barrier.[39-41]

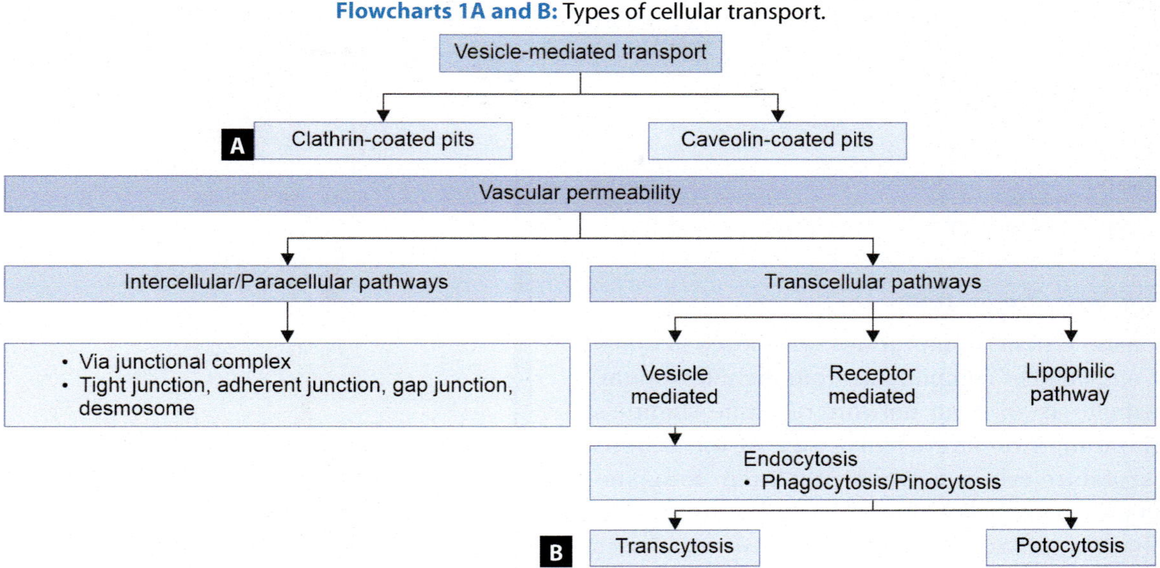

Flowcharts 1A and B: Types of cellular transport.

Adherent junctions (zonula adherence) and desmosomes (macula adherence): These are composed of multiple intercellular adherent molecules and vascular endothelial cadherin-associated α-, β- and p120 catenin adhesion complexes with intracellular anchoring proteins as vimentin, desmin, and cytokeratin. These are localized in the capillaries and PCVs and are thought to be the most important adhesion apparatus that regulates the vascular permeability.[42]

Gap junctions (communicating junctions): Gap junctions are intercellular channels which allow direct passage of ions or molecules from one cell to the other. These facilitate intercellular communication rather than adhesion. It is a cylindrical structure with a diameter of 2.8 nm and consists of two hemichannels which again are formed by circular alignment of six subunits called connexins.[43,44]

These intercellular junctions under the effect of various inflammatory mediators contribute to macromolecular leakage during acute inflammation.

Basement membrane of the endothelium: The basement membrane is a thin sheet which lies at the interface of the endothelial cells and the connective tissue and is primarily composed of glycosaminoglycans as heparan sulfate and chondroitin sulfate which confers it a negative charge.[9]

Glycocalyx of the endothelium: The luminal side of the endothelium is covered with a thin layer which is composed of sialo-conjugates, proteoglycans, and acidic polymers that provide both a fibrous network and a net negative charge to the cell luminal membrane. The thickness is proportionate to the vascular diameter. The proteoglycans contain membrane bound-core proteins as syndecan and glypican attached with a glycosaminoglycan as heparan sulfate. Besides these, several membrane-bound glycoproteins such as integrin and selectin contribute to the formation of the glycocalyx. It maintains blood fluidity and acts as a dynamic barrier that regulates the passage of molecules based on their size, shape, and charge across the microvascular wall. It represents the medium-size pore system of the peritoneal osmotic barrier.[44,45]

Water transport across the endothelium: Initially, it was thought that water transport across continuous capillaries occurs via the paracellular pathway only, but the discovery of the water-specific membrane channel AQP has brough the transcellular pathways to the forefront. There are multiple isoforms, but AQP-1 is the most abundant in the peritoneum. Its present in the endothelial (capillaries, venules, and small veins) as well as mesothelial cells.[46-48]

- Combination of various intracellular and intercellular complexes along with some extracellular matrices governs the vascular permeability.
- The intracellular caveola and the vesicle are the main route for plasma protein transcellular transport at baseline conditions.
- During a pathological condition such as inflammation or malignancy, the paracellular pathways open under the effect of vascular permeability factors as VEGF-A, histamine, and platelet-activating factor (PAF). These also promote the formation of transcellular pores.
- The usual site of occurrence is the PCVs
- Pathological conditions alter the net negative charges on the extracellular matrices reducing their charge-based resistance to anionic plasma proteins.

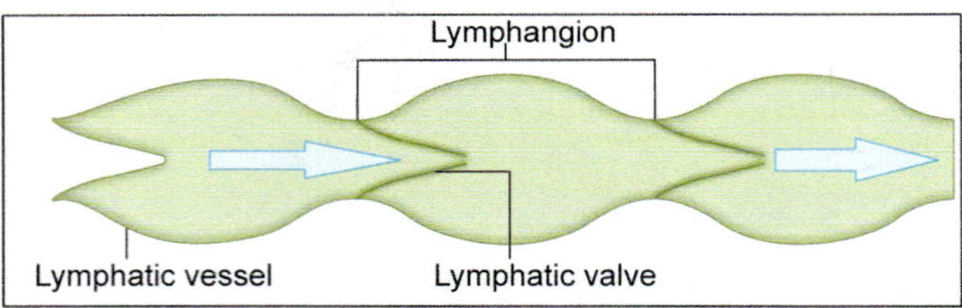

Fig. 4: Schematic representation of the lymphangion units.

Lymphatic Vascular System

The lymphatic systems drain various substances as water, proteins, and cellular components from the interstitium. They originate as an open network of tissue channels that drain along the paravascular area of the venous microvasculature into a network of 0.5 mm long and 20–30 µm wide endothelial tubes called initial lymphatics or lymphatic capillaries. These lymphatic capillaries though mostly devoid of basement membrane have contractile elements in the form of fine actin filaments. These direct the slow downstream movement of the lymph through the collecting channels to the central venous circulation where the directional flow is maintained by peristalsis like rhythmic contraction by consecutive lymphangions. Due to the presence of valves, it requires the generation of sufficient hydrostatic pressure approximately 12 cm of water after which the downstream valves open.[49-51] The contractility is influenced by various mediators as adrenoreceptors, prostaglandins, histamine, etc.[52]

The lymph flows from the collectors to the thoracic duct and the right lymph duct before draining into the subclavian vein **(Figs. 4 and 5)**.

The diaphragmatic lymphatic capillary network is organized as a plexus along the submesothelial surface which communicates with a plexus on the pleural side of the diaphragm.

An important feature of the diaphragmatic lymphatics is the presence of lymphatic lacunae and stomata. Stomata are "pores" formed at the junction of cuboidal mesothelial cells. These cells have cytoplasmic processes that extend to the interior of the pore which may act as "closing doors" for either drainage or inflow to the peritoneal cavity. Lacunae are elongated cisterna-like structures lying beneath the stomata, acting as a drainage system to the precollector small-caliber lymphatic vessels which are devoid of any smooth muscle layer **(Fig. 6)**.[53]

Under typical conditions, lymphatic stomata facilitate the drainage and absorption of fluids from serous cavities,

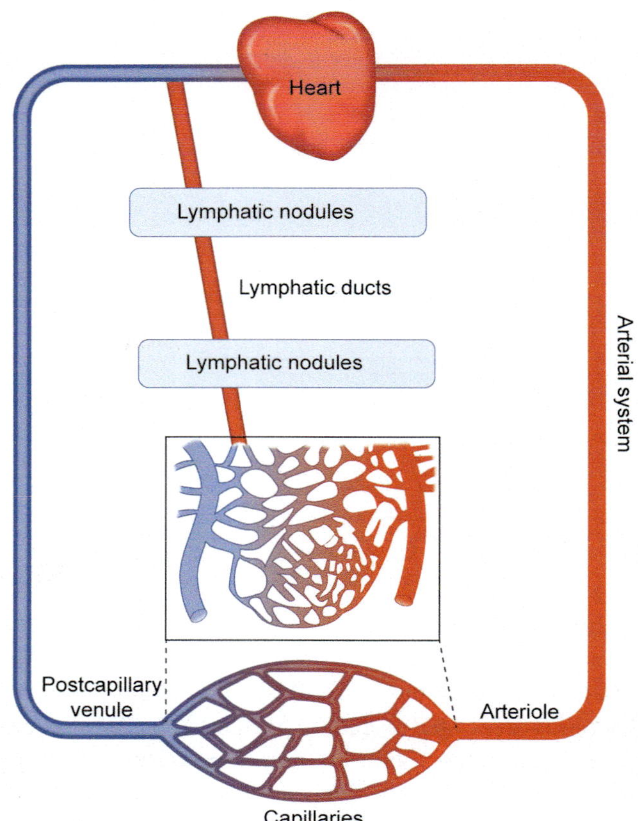

Fig. 5: Schematic representation of the lymphatic system.
Source: Selgas R, Honda K, Lopez-Cabrera M, Hamad C, Gotloib L. Peritoneal structure and changes as a dialysis membrane after peritoneal dialysis. In: Khanna R, Krediet RT (Eds). Nolph and Gokal's Textbook of Peritoneal Dialysis. Cham: Springer.

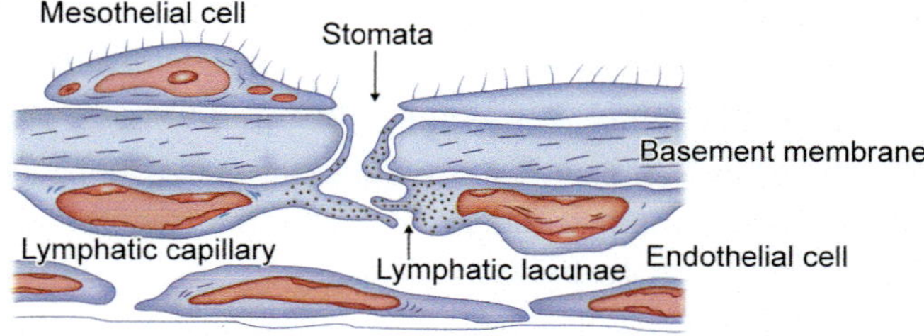

Fig. 6: Relation and structure of lymphatic stomata and lacunae.
Source: Selgas R, Honda K, Lopez-Cabrera M, Hamad C, Gotloib L. Peritoneal structure and changes as a dialysis membrane after peritoneal dialysis. In: Khanna R, Krediet RT (Eds). Nolph and Gokal's Textbook of Peritoneal Dialysis. Cham: Springer.

thereby maintaining homeostasis. Additionally, they enable macrophage migration into these cavities. In pathological states, lymphatic stomata act as the route for ascites, tumor cells, and infections from serous cavities. Clinically, their functions include the absorption of ascites,

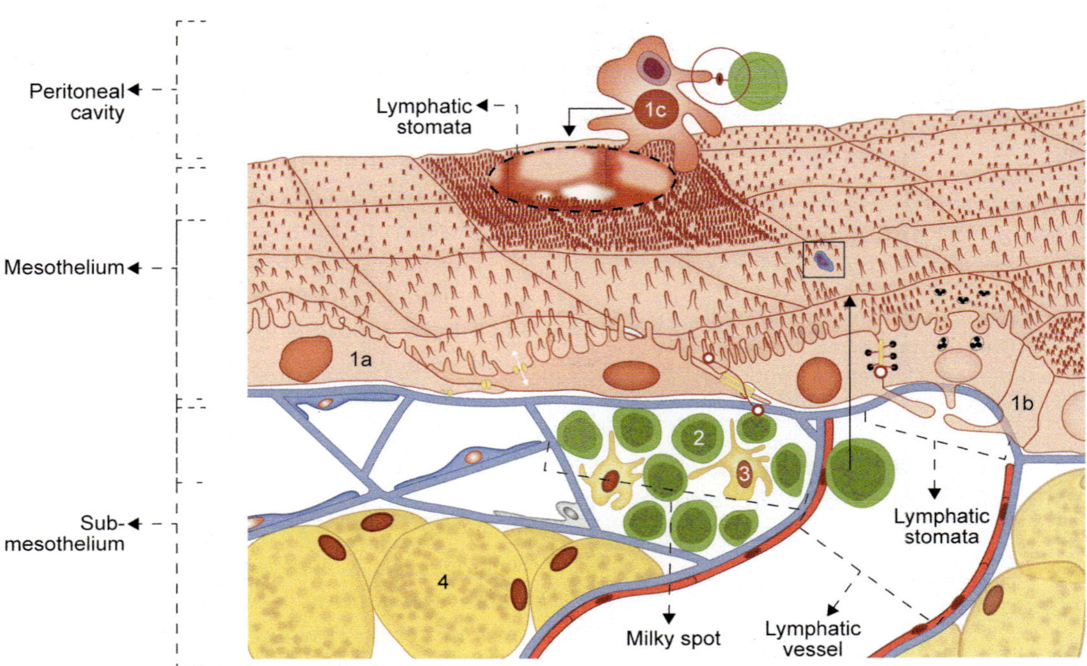

Fig. 7: Cross-sectional schematic image showing the layers as well as the organization of mesothelial cells along with the lymphatic stomata and milky spots.
Source: Isaza-Restrepo A, Martin-Saavedra JS, Velez-Leal JL, Vargas-Barato F, Riveros-Duenas R. The Peritoneum: Beyond the Tissue – A Review. Front Physiol. 2018;9:738.

delivery of intraperitoneal chemotherapy, and transfusion of blood cells for Rh hemolytic fetus treatment.[54]

Another structure seen around the stomata are the milky white spots; although not directly contributing to the lymphatic drainage, these are essentially submesothelial aggregates of macrophages and lymphocytes which are essential for the maturation of resident peritoneal macrophages and are actively involved in peritoneal defense reactions under diverse inflammatory conditions. The cell population of milky spots is made of 400–600 cells, including macrophages (45–70%), lymphocytes (14–29%), and a low number of plasma cells (around 6%). Occasionally, megakaryocytes and adipocytes can also be detected **(Fig. 7)**.[55]

FUNCTIONAL APPLICATION

Models of Transport

Three-pore Model

Postulated by Bengt Rippe, the three-pore model suggests existence of three pores of different sizes in the capillary endothelium. The "large pores" (20–30 nm) formed by the wide interendothelial cleft mainly transport large protein molecules as albumin and account for approximately 5–8% of the total pore area. The "small pores" (4–6 nm) are smaller clefts between endothelial cells which allow movement of water and small solutes as creatinine, sodium, etc. These account for the majority of the porearea (90–93%) The "ultrapores" (0.2–0.4 nm) allow transport of water only and functionally are AQP1. They account for about 2% of the total pore area but can contribute up to 40% of the total capillary ultrafiltrate.[56-58]

Pore-matrix Model

In this model, there are no defined small or large pores, and the permeability is a function of the density of glycoprotein matrix in the cleft.[59]

Distributed Model

In this model, it is assumed that there are uniformly distributed blood vessels in the interstitium present at variable distances from the mesothelial surface and their contribution, although different, collectively determines the effective surface area. Hence, here the degree of vascularity is the main determinant.[59,60]

Anatomical Basis of Ultrafiltration Failure

Changes in the membrane after PD:[9]
- Histological and ultrastructural abnormalities of peritoneum during CAPD
- Mesothelial denudation
- Thickening of mesothelial basement membrane
- Interstitial fibrosis resulting in the thickening of peritoneum
- Diabetiform vascular alterations of postcapillary vessels and small venules
- *Capillaries:* Increased collagen fibers in the media of vasculature, reduplication of basement membrane, degenerate pericytes, proliferation of smooth muscle cells (SMCs) or endothelial cells

The main mediators are advanced glycation end products (AGE) and carbonyl stress-mediated changes **(Flowchart 2)**.

Short-term Changes

The first change after PD initiation is the loss of microvilli of the mesothelial cells followed by the hypertrophy of these cells along with appearance of lipid and crystalline inclusions and reduction in the number of vesicles. In more advanced phases, there are denuded areas with submesothelial fibrosis where there are accumulations of myofibroblasts derived from the epithelial to mesenchymal transformation (EMT) of the mesothelial cell. Apart from the EMT, the mesothelial cells also undergo senescence with cell cycle arrest and alteration in the secretory phenotype.[61-63]

The basement membrane undergoes reduplication in patients treated with PD >6 months; similar findings have been reported in diabetic patients without renal insufficiency.[64]

The submesothelial fibrosis over time intensifies and may develop a peritoneal lining which is fibrous dense and devoid of any mesothelium.[65]

Vascular Changes

Angiogenesis is a neovascularization from preexisting microvasculature as seen in peritoneal biopsies of patients on long-term PD where the number of vessels correlate with the thickness of the peritoneal membrane.[66]

Hyalinizing vasculopathy: It is a vascular change characteristically seen in patients on long-term PD with

Flowchart 2: Pathways leading to alteration in the peritoneal permeability.

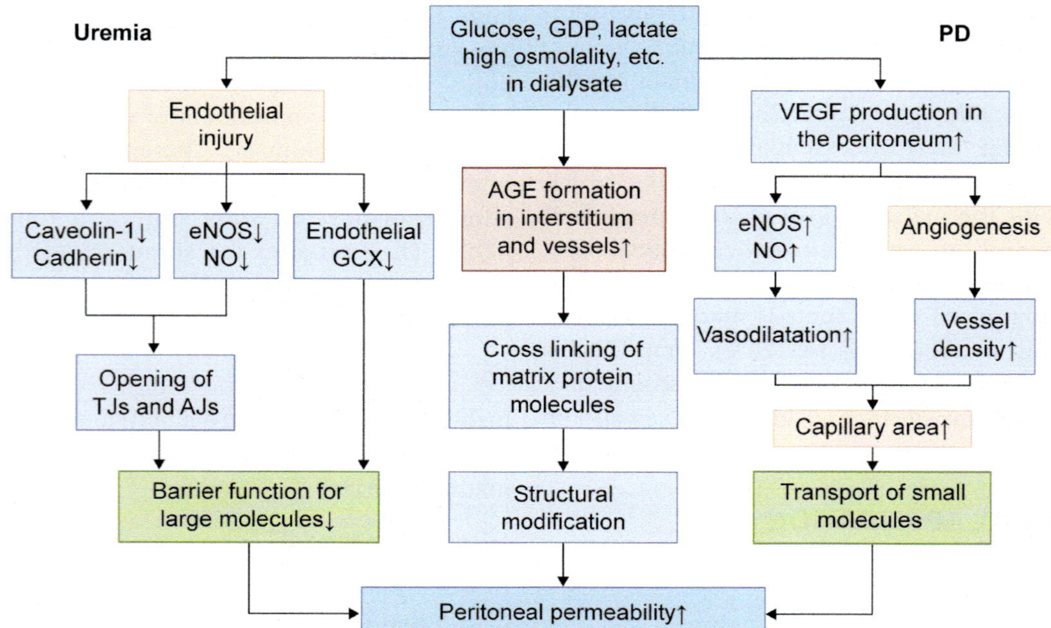

(AGE: advanced glycation end products; AJ: adherent junction; eNOS: endothelial nitric oxide synthase; GCX: glycocalyx; GDP: guanosine diphosphate; NO: nitric oxide; PD: peritoneal dialysis; TJ: tight junction)

Source: Selgas R, Honda K, Lopez-Cabrera M, Hamad C, Gotloib L. Peritoneal structure and changes as a dialysis membrane after peritoneal dialysis. In: Khanna R, Krediet RT (Eds). Nolph and Gokal's Textbook of Peritoneal Dialysis. Cham: Springer.

UFF, with thickening of vascular walls with obstruction of the lumen. Mainly, the capillaries and the PCVs are affected.[31]

Long-term Changes

Encapsulating peritoneal sclerosis: It is a life-threatening devastating complication characterized macroscopically by encapsulation of the intestine within whitish membranes and adhesion of the intestine to each other or the abdominal wall and accumulation of fibrin exudates. Microscopically, it shows various acute and chronic inflammatory changes including inflammatory exudates, neoangiogenesis, and various stages of fibrin deposition and fibrosis.[67]

CONCLUSION

Unlike the hemodialyzer membrane the peritoneal membrane represents a living, dynamic entity which undergoes multitude of modifications in the uremic milieu as well as with the prolonged exposure to the peritoneal dialysis fluid. Clinical observations have paved the way for a deeper understanding of the cell biology. A full discussion of the pathophysiology is beyond the scope of this chapter.

REFERENCES

1. Robinson B. The Peritoneum. Chicago: WT Keener; 1897.
2. Dobbie JW. From philosopher to fish: The comparative anatomy of the peritoneal cavity as an excretory organ and its significance for peritoneal dialysis in man. Perit Dial Int. 1988;8:3-6.
3. Putiloff P. Materials for the study of the laws of growth of the human body in relation to the surface areas of different systems: the trial on Russian subjects of planographic anatomy as a mean of exact anthropometry. In Presented at the Siberian Branch of the Russian Geographic Society, Omsk, 1886.
4. Wegner G. Chirurgische bemerkingen uber die peritoneal Hole, mit Besonderer Berucksichtigung der ovariotomie. Arch Klin Chir. 1877;20:51-9.
5. Esperanca M, Collins DL. Peritoneal dialysis efficiency in relation to body weight. J Pediatr Surg. 1966;1:162-9.
6. Krediet RT, Zemel D, Imholz AL, Struijk DG. Impact of surface area and permeability on solute clearances. Perit Dial Int. 1994;14(Suppl 3):S70-7.
7. Chagnac A, Herskovitz P, Weinstein T, Elyashiv S, Hirsh J, Hammel I, et al. The peritoneal membrane in peritoneal dialysis patients: estimation of its functional surface area by applying stereologic methods to computerized tomography scans. J Am Soc Nephrol. 1999;10(2):342-6.
8. Kastelein AW, Vos LMC, de Jong KH, van Baal JOAM, Nieuwland R, van Noorden CJF, et al. Embryology, anatomy, physiology and pathophysiology of the peritoneum and the peritoneal vasculature. Semin Cell Develop Biol. 2019;92:27-36.
9. Anglani F, Forino M, Del Prete D, Ceol M, Favaro S. Molecular biology of the peritoneal membrane: in between morphology and function. Contrib Nephrol. 2001;(131):61-73.
10. Leak LV. Distribution of cell surface charges on mesothelium and lymphatic endothelium. Microvasc Res. 1986;31(1):18-30.
11. Simionescu M, Simionescu N. Organization of cell junctions in the peritoneal mesothelium. J Cell Biol. 1977;74(1):98-110.
12. Mutsaers SE. Mesothelial cells: their structure, function and role in serosal repair. Respirology. 2002;7:171-91.
13. Remmele W, Richter IE, Wildenhof H. Experimental investigations on cell resorption from the peritoneal cavity by use of the scanning electron microscope. 1975;53(19): 913-22.
14. Ghinea N, Simionescu N. Anionized and cationized hemeundecapeptides as probes for cell surface charge and permeability studies: differentiated labelling of endothelial plasmalemmal vesicles. J Cell Biol. 1985;100(2):606-12.
15. Gotloib L, Shustak A, Jaichenko J. Loss of mesothelial electronegative fixed charges during murine septic peritonitis. Nephron. 1989;51(1):77-83.
16. Gotloib L. Reduplicated skin and peritoneal blood capillaries and mesothelial basement membrane in aged non-diabetic chronic uremic patients. Perit Dial Bull. 1984;4:S28.
17. Di Paolo N, Sacchi G. Atlas of peritoneal histology. Perit Dial Int. 2000;20(Suppl 3):S5–96.
18. Jiménez-Heffernan JA, et al. Peritoneal inflammation and fibrosis in peritoneal dialysis. In: Esbrit P, Alvarez-Arroyo M (Eds). Inflammation and Chronic Disease. Trivandrum: Transworld Research Network; 2006. pp. 89-102.
19. Jiménez-Heffernan JA, Aguilera A, Aroeira LS, Lara Pezzi E, Bajo MA, del Peso G, et al. Immuno-histochemical characterization of fibroblast subpopulations in normal peritoneal tissue and in peritoneal dialysis-induced fibrosis. Virchows Arch. 2004;444(3):247-56.
20. Flessner MF. The importance of the interstitium in peritoneal transport. Perit Dial Int. 1996;16(Suppl 1):S76-9.
21. Lai-Fook SJ, Brown LV. Effects of electric charge on hydraulic conductivity of pulmonary interstitium. J Appl Physiol (1985). 1991;70(5):1928-32.
22. Gilchrist SA, Parker JC. Exclusion of charged macromolecules in the pulmonary interstitium. Microvasc Res. 1985;30(1):88-98.
23. Guyton AC. A concept of negative interstitial pressure based on pressures in implanted perforated capsules. Circ Res. 1963;12:399-414.

24. Scholander PF, Hargens AR, Miller SL. Negative pressure in the interstitial fluid of animals. Fluid tensions are spectacular in plants; in animals they are elusively small, but just as vital. Science. 1968;161(3839):321-8.
25. Rutili G, Arfors KE. Protein concentration in interstitial and lymphatic fluids from the subcutaneous tissue. Acta Physiol Scand. 1977;99(1):1-8.
26. Gotloib L. Hemodynamic effects of increasing intra-abdominal pressure in peritoneal dialysis. Perit Dial Bull. 1981;1:41-2.
27. Flessner MF, Schwab A. Pressure threshold for fluid loss from the peritoneal cavity. Am J Phys. 1996;270(2 Pt 2): F377-90.
28. Ross M, Pawlina W. Cardiovascular system. In: Histology: A Text and Atlas: With Correlated Cell and Molecular Biology, 7th edition. Barcelona: Wolters Kluwer; 2016. pp. 411-27 (Chapter 13).
29. Majno G. Ultrastructure of the vascular membrane. In: Handbook of Physiology, vol. 3. Washington, DC: American Physiological Society; 1965. pp. 2293-375. (Section II-Circulation)
30. Majno G, Palade GE, Schoefl GI. Studies on inflammation. II. The site of action of histamine and serotonin along the vascular tree: a topographic study. J Biophys Biochem Cytol. 1961;11:607-26.
31. Honda K, Nitta K, Horita S, Yumura W, Nihei H. Morphological changes in the peritoneal vasculature of patients on CAPD with ultrafiltration failure. Nephron. 1996;72(2):171-6.
32. Ross M, Pawlina W. Epithelial tissue. In: Histology: A Text and Atlas: With Correlated Cell and Molecular Biology, 7th edition. Barcelona: Wolters Kluwer; 2016. pp. 120-33. (Chapter 5)
33. Gotloib L, Shustak A, Jaichenko J. Fenestrated capillaries in mice sub mesothelial mesenteric microvasculature. Int J Artif Organs. 1989;12(1):20-4.
34. Gotloib L, Shostak A. In search of a role for sub mesothelial fenestrated capillaries. Perit Dial Int. 1993;13(2):98-102.
35. Gotloib L, Shustak A, Bar-Sella P, Eiali V. Fenestrated capillaries in human parietal and rabbit diaphragmatic peritoneum. Nephron. 1985;41(2):2002.
36. Palade GE, Simionescu M, Simionescu N. Structural aspects of the permeability of the microvascular endothelium. Acta Physiol Scand Suppl. 1979;463:11-32.
37. Simionescu M, Simionescu N, Palade GE. Morphometric data on the endothelium of blood capillaries. J Cell Biol. 1974;60(1):128-52.
38. Petersen OW, van Deurs B. Serial-section analysis of coated pits and vesicles involved in adsorptive pinocytosis in cultured fibroblasts. J Cell Biol. 1983;96(1):277-81.
39. Farquhar MG, Palade GE. Junctional complexes in various epithelia. J Cell Biol. 1963;17:375-412.
40. Simionescu M, Simionescu N, Palade GE. Segmental differentiations of cell junctions in the vascular endothelium. The microvasculature. J Cell Biol. 1975; 67(3):863-85.
41. Thorgeirsson G, Robertson AJ. The vascular endothelium. Pathobiologic significance. Am J Pathol. 1978;95:801-48.
42. Dejana E, Orsenigo F, Lampugnani MG. The role of adherens junctions and VE-cadherin in the control of vascular permeability. J Cell Sci. 2008;121 (Pt 13): 2115–22.
43. Komarova YA, Kruse K, Mehta D, Malik AB. Protein interactions at endothelial junctions and signalling mechanisms regulating endothelial permeability. Circ Res. 2017;120(1):179–206.
44. Okamoto T, Suzuki K. The role of gap junction mediated endothelial cell-cell interaction in the crosstalk between inflammation and blood coagulation. Int J Mol Sci. 2017;18(11):2254
45. Reitsma S, Slaaf DW, Vink H, van Zandvoort MA, oude Egbrink MG. The endothelial glycocalyx: composition, functions, and visualization. Pflugers Arch. 2007;454(3):345-59.
46. Agre P, King LS, Yasui M, Guggino WB, Ottersen OP, et al. Aquaporin water channels from atomic structure to clinical medicine. J Physiol. 2002;542(Pt 1):3-16.
47. Devuyst O, Rippe B. Water transport across the peritoneal membrane. Kidney Int. 2013;85(4):750-8.
48. Schoenicke G, Diamant R, Donner A, Roehrborn A, Grabensee B, Plum J. Histochemical distribution and expression of aquaporin 1 in the peritoneum of patients undergoing peritoneal dialysis: relation to peritoneal transport. Am J Kidney Dis. 2004;44(1):146-54.
49. Ohhashi T, Azuma T, Sakaguchi M. Active and passive mechanical characteristics of bovine mesenteric lymphatics. Am J Phys. 1980;239(1):H88-95.
50. Zweifach BW, Prather JW. Micromanipulation of pressure in terminal lymphatics in the mesentery. Am J Phys. 1975;228(5):1326-35.
51. Abu-Hijleh MF, Habbal OA, Moqattash ST. The role of the diaphragm in lymphatic absorption from the peritoneal cavity. J Anat. 1995;186(Pt 3):453-67.
52. Ohhashi T, Kawai Y, Azuma T. The response of lymphatic smooth muscles to vasoactive substances. Pflugers Arch. 1978;375(2):183-8.
53. Leak LV, Rahil K. Permeability of the diaphragmatic mesothelium: the ultrastructural basis for "stomata". Am J Anat. 1978;151(4):557-93.
54. Wang ZB, Li M, Li JC. Recent advances in the research of lymphatic stomata. Anat Rec (Hoboken). 2010;293(5):754-61.
55. Garosi G, Di Paolo N. Recent advances in peritoneal morphology: the milky spots in peritoneal dialysis. Adv Perit Dial. 2001;17:25-8.
56. Rippe B, Stelin G. How does peritoneal dialysis remove small and large molecular weight solutes? Transport pathways: fact and myth. Adv Perit Dial. 1990;6:13-8.

57. Rippe B. A three-pore model of peritoneal transport. Perit Dial Int. 1993;13(Suppl 2):S35-8.
58. Ni J, Verbavatz JM, Rippe A, Boisde I, Moulin P, Rippe B, et al. Aquaporin-1 plays an essential role in water permeability and ultrafiltration during peritoneal dialysis. Kidney Int. 2006;69(9):1518-25.
59. Flessner MF. Peritoneal ultrafiltration: physiology and failure. Contrib Nephrol. 2009;163:7-14.
60. Flessner MF, Dedrick RL. Schultz JS. A distributed model of peritoneal-plasma transport: theoretical considerations. Am J Phys. 1984;246(4 Pt 2):R597-607.
61. Di Paolo N, Sacchi G, De Mia M, Gaggiotti E, Capotondo L, Rossi P, et al. Morphology of the peritoneal membrane during continuous ambulatory peritoneal dialysis. Nephron. 1986;44(3):204-11.
62. Lopez-Cabrera M. Mesenchymal conversion of mesothelial cells is a key event in the pathophysiology of the peritoneum during peritoneal dialysis. Adv Med. 2014;2014: 473134.
63. Aroeira LS, Aguilera A, Sánchez-Tomero JA, Bajo MA, del Peso G, Jiménez-Heffernan JA, et al. Epithelial to mesenchymal transition and peritoneal membrane failure in peritoneal dialysis patients: pathologic significance and potential therapeutic interventions. J Am Soc Nephrol. 2007;18(7):2004-13.
64. Gotloib L, Bar Sella P, Shostak A. Reduplicated basal lamina of small venules and mesothelium of human parietal peritoneum. Perit Dial Bull. 1985;5:212-5.
65. Flessner MF. The effect of fibrosis on peritoneal transport. Contrib Nephrol. 2006; 150:174-80.
66. Honda K, Nitta K, Horita S, Yumura W, Nihei H, Nagai R, et al. Accumulation of advanced glycation end products in the peritoneal vasculature of continuous ambulatory peritoneal dialysis patients with low ultra-filtration. Nephrol Dial Transplant. 1999;14(6):1541-9.
67. Dobbie JW. Pathogenesis of peritoneal fibrosing syndromes (sclerosing peritonitis) in peritoneal dialysis. Perit Dial Int. 1992;12(1):14-27.

CHAPTER

45 Preparing a Patient for Peritoneal Dialysis

Kulwant Singh, Namrata S Rao, Jitendra Kumar

CASE SCENARIO

A 52-year-old lady was diagnosed with end-stage kidney disease (ESKD) 2 years ago, following which she underwent urgent-start hemodialysis (HD) via noncuffed catheter via her right internal jugular vein. Due to primary failure of left radiocephalic arteriovenous fistula and two episodes of catheter-associated infections, she underwent hemodialysis for the next 3 months via noncuffed and later, cuffed dialysis catheters, first in the right and then in the left internal jugular vein.

Four months following her diagnosis of kidney disease, she underwent ABO-compatible renal transplantation, with husband as the kidney donor. Unfortunately, she lost her graft to early graft dysfunction diagnosed as a transplant-associated thrombotic microangiopathy. She was unresponsive to multiple sessions of plasmapheresis, in addition to medication changes. A month after graft nephrectomy, she underwent a computed tomography scan of thoracic veins, which revealed anomalous superior vena cava, attenuated caliber of left brachiocephalic vein, and long segment stenosis of right brachiocephalic vein. The patient and her family was counseled for peritoneal dialysis (PD), at this juncture, by the treating team; however, they refused, and following a failed attempt at balloon dilatation and tunneled dialysis catheter insertion via the right internal jugular vein, she was discharged on the right femoral tunneled catheter. This catheter was salvaged twice over the next 6 months, following episodes of bloodstream infections, but needed removal 9 months later, in view of refractory *Candida glabrata*-associated fungemia.

The patient and her caregivers were again counseled for PD, to which they consented and she was initiated on chronic ambulatory peritoneal dialysis (CAPD) a year back. At 1 year, she is maintaining well, with no residual urine output, four exchanges of 1.5% dextrose a day (including a night dwell), and no episodes of peritonitis during the last year. The case illustrates failed PD counseling at at least two junctures (not being counseled due to urgent-start dialysis initially, and a second time, when she chose right femoral catheter for HD over PD 6 months later).

INTRODUCTION

Renal replacement therapy (RRT) is a term used to encompass all life-supporting treatment options (hemodialysis, peritoneal dialysis, or renal transplant) for end-stage renal disease (ESRD). Thus, it is very important for the primary care provider to understand various indications and contraindications of each modality before preparing the patient for RRT. This chapter details the selection, counseling and preparation for initiating PD among patients requiring longterm RRT.

INDICATIONS AND CONTRAINDICATIONS

In terms of indications for PD, all patients with chronic kidney disease (CKD) must be counseled for PD also as a modality as part of education regarding RRTs.[1,2] However, certain patient characteristics are associated with better suitability for PD such as preserved urine output or residual renal function, sufficient manual dexterity or adequate caregiver support system in place, living in remote areas where in-center HD facilities are unavailable, children (especially school-going, with preserved urine output), and existence of a sterile room to perform PD with adequate sterile precautions **(Box 1)**.[3,4]

Medically, patients with poor tolerance to HD—such as those who have recurrent vascular access failures, intolerant to anticoagulation, poor cardiac reserve [particularly in cases with heart failure with reduced ejection fraction (HFrEF)], or old and bedridden—should be shifted to PD.[5] PD can be a safe and effective treatment

BOX 1: Indications and contraindications for choosing PD.

Favorable characteristics for choosing PD:
- Preserved urine output
- Recurrent vascular access failures
- Intolerant to anticoagulation
- Recurrent hospitalizations for heart failure
- Elderly, bedridden patients with mobility issues
- Chronic heart disease, chronic liver disease with ascites
- *Favorable logistics:* Good manual dexterity/adequate caregiver support
- School-going children, indoor place of work (office job)
- Remote areas far-away from HD units
- Existence of sterile room for PD exchanges

Contraindications for choosing PD:
- Peritoneal pathologies—extensive scarring, adhesions
- Multiple previous abdominal surgeries
- Large abdominal hernias
- Active gastrointestinal inflammation
- Gastrointestinal malignancies with peritoneal spread
- Colostomies such as in patients with congenital anomalies of gastrointestinal and genitourinary tracts

(HD: hemodialysis; PD: peritoneal dialysis)

for patients with chronic liver disease (CLD) and ESKD who have ascites. It helps both in ascites management and in ultrafiltration maintaining hemodynamic stability.[6,7]

Contraindications to PD include those patients with peritoneal pathologies, such as extensive scarring and adhesions, usually in patients with previous abdominal surgeries. In many situations, laparoscopic adhesiolysis has ensured adequate PD.[8,9] Mesh repair of small hernias with simultaneous PD catheter insertion has made PD possible for patients who would otherwise be excluded; however, large hernias can cause uncomfortable distension with PD fluid instillation, and therefore, PD is usually avoided in such settings. Active inflammatory and malignant gastrointestinal pathologies, including peritoneal malignancies and existing colostomies (such as in children with congenital anomalies), may also preclude PD. The benefits and drawbacks of PD are presented in **Figure 1**.

COUNSELING

Counseling should first start with providing education about the modality. The treating nephrologist, trained nurse, or peer counselor can provide initial education depending on institutional protocols. This is a very important step as it lays the foundation for future decision-making. This information can be initially one to one with/without the caregiver, followed by visit/s at home or group discussion/s by PD-trained nurses or educators. In the era of smartphones, informative videos can be easily shared with the patient and caregivers to aid decision-making, and feedback/audio-video calls can be facilitated between prospective PD patients and those successfully performing PD **(Fig. 2)**.

An instructive question-and-answer template (with descriptive answers) that can be used while imparting initial education regarding PD is presented in **Box 2**.

Usually, discussion regarding modalities of RRTs is initiated below an estimated glomerular filtration rate (eGFR) of 20 $mL/min/m^2$. In most scenarios, the treating nephrologist will be the initial educator regarding modalities of RRTs, and also, a vast majority of patients on long-term follow-up with CKD clinics tend to leave modality selection in the hands of their nephrologists. It is imperative that nephrologists (especially when in administration) see PD not just as modality but as a program. If infrastructure permits, every hospital should have a dedicated area for a PD room with a full-time specialized PD nurse on roll, just like HD units. Specialized PD nurses can also positively impact modality selection, so also peer counselors from the PD community.

Survival and Financial Counseling

Patients who are currently deciding about the modality of RRT always want answers on how one modality fares better over the other, in terms of survival and quality of life. In simplistic terms, PD shows better survival at dialysis initiation than HD (first 90 days); PD and HD share similar patient survival at 1 year, but beyond the first few years, PD survival dips faster than HD.[10-12] In terms of quality of life, patients on PD report equal or better quality of life than patients on HD.[13,14] In many low- and middle-income developing countries where government-aided PD programs do not exist, expenditure could be higher for PD than for HD. Accounting for all out-of-pocket expenditure in both modalities is essential when comparing PD and HD financially. While patient and caregiver travel, food expenses, and time-lost on employment need to be factored for choosing HD, transportation of fluids to far-flung areas, especially with increased transport costs in hilly and difficult terrains, schemes available for purchase, or renting of automated peritoneal dialysis (APD) machine (if required) should be taken into consideration. Nephrologists can use the information provided below, to provide optimal survival and financial counseling.

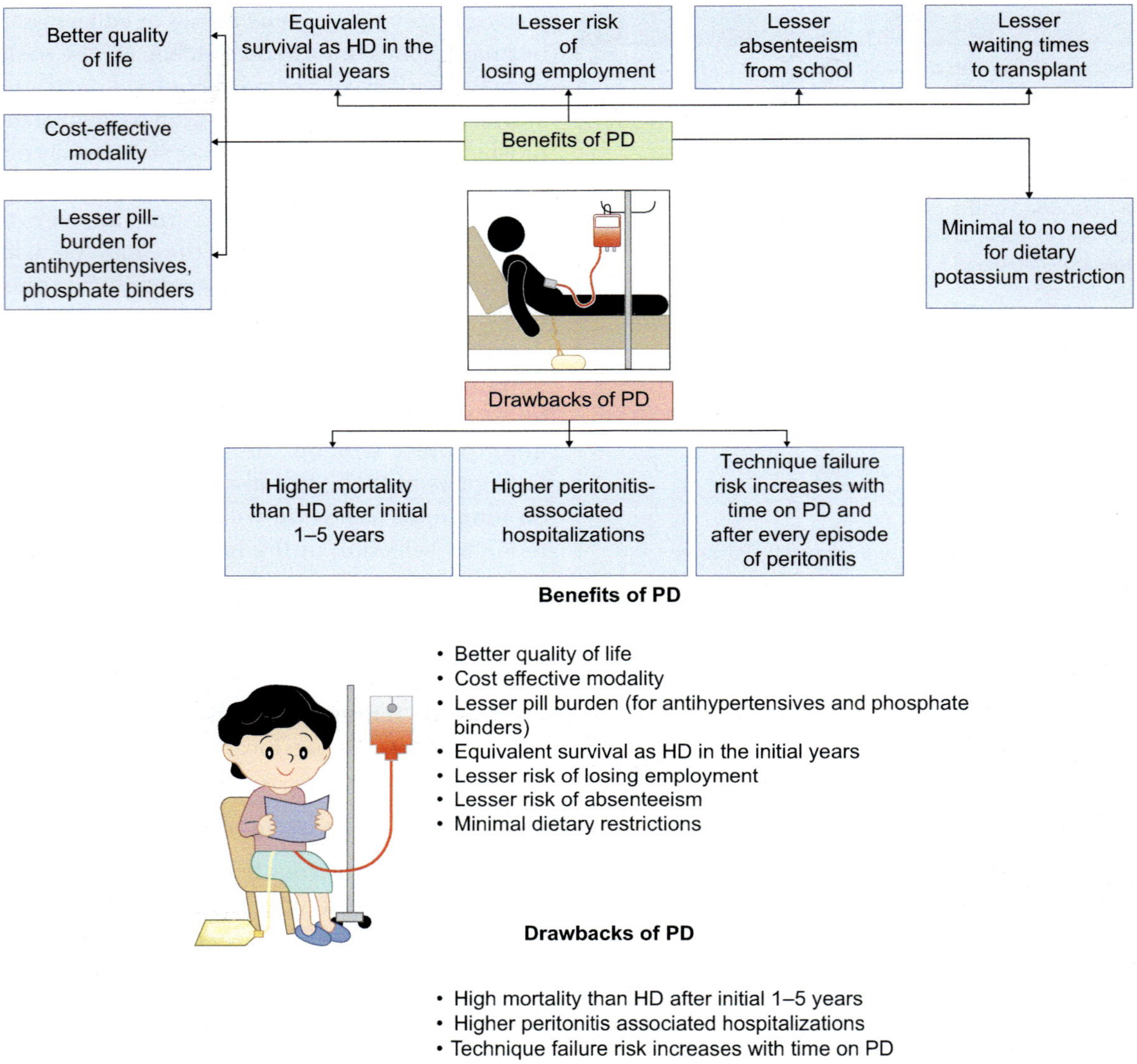

Better quality of life
Equivalent survival as HD in the initial years
Lesser risk of losing employment
Lesser absenteeism from school
Lesser waiting times to transplant
Cost-effective modality
Benefits of PD
Lesser pill-burden for antihypertensives, phosphate binders
Minimal to no need for dietary potassium restriction
Drawbacks of PD
Higher mortality than HD after initial 1–5 years
Higher peritonitis-associated hospitalizations
Technique failure risk increases with time on PD and after every episode of peritonitis
Benefits of PD
• Better quality of life
• Cost effective modality
• Lesser pill burden (for antihypertensives and phosphate binders)
• Equivalent survival as HD in the initial years
• Lesser risk of losing employment
• Lesser risk of absenteeism
• Minimal dietary restrictions
Drawbacks of PD
• High mortality than HD after initial 1–5 years
• Higher peritonitis associated hospitalizations
• Technique failure risk increases with time on PD

Fig. 1: Benefits and drawbacks of peritoneal dialysis (PD). (HD: hemodialysis)

Step 1
Educating about peritoneal dialysis
Sharing audio-visual infographics on Smart Phone or i-Pad
Connecting with other PD patients who can share their experience
PD nurse/counselor
Step 2
Survival counseling
Financial counseling
Helping in decision-making
Nephrologist
PD Nurse/counselor
Initial discussion about RRT

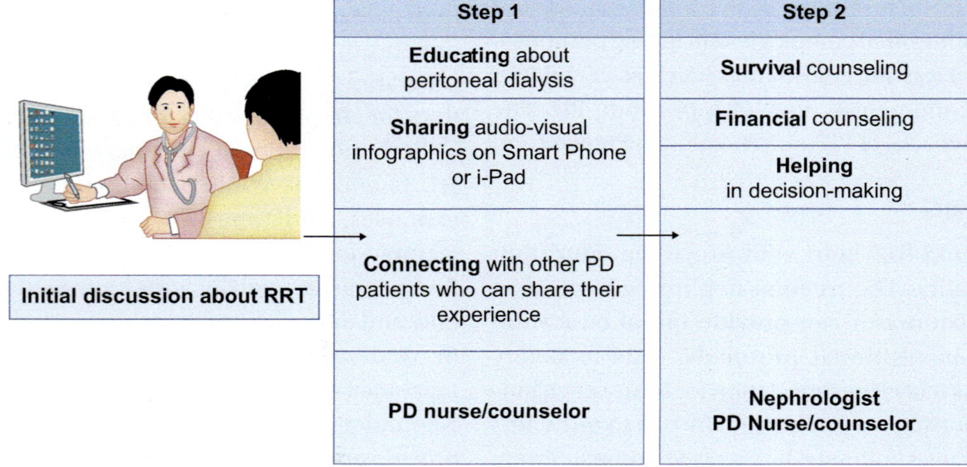

Fig. 2: Stepwise approach for counseling. (PD: peritoneal dialysis; RRT: renal replacement therapy)

BOX 2: Educational questionnaire for preparing a patient for peritoneal dialysis (PD).

- What is PD and how does it work?
- What are the types of PD? (manual vs. automatic) and how does one choose between them?
- Where and how can one set up a sterile room for PD at home?
- How does one prepare for PD—basic preparation for insertion procedure and training?
- What are the problems one could encounter during PD? (early vs. late)

Survival Counseling

Based on evidence from many observational studies and meta-analyses, HD and PD are comparable in terms of overall mortality. However, PD has a survival benefit over HD in the early years of dialysis, in younger patients and in nondiabetic patients. There is evidence to suggest superiority of HD over PD, with longer time on dialysis, though one of the reasons for this may be the shorter waiting time for transplants among those on PD than on HD.[10] In terms of progressing to renal transplantation, patients on PD seem to have a shorter time to receive a transplant than those on HD.[15]

Financial Counseling

It is perceived that PD is an expensive modality as compared to HD. However, globally PD is considered to be the more cost-effective RRT modality, with a strong advocacy for undertaking PD-first or PD-preferred policies.[16] In any RRT modality, there are two types of cost: (1) Direct and (2) indirect. Direct cost includes both hospital system expenses and out-of-pocket expenses. Direct cost which includes cost of consumables may appear higher for PD as these consumables are mostly covered by out-of-pocket expenses only. But indirect cost due to loss of productivity on HD is higher as compared to home-based PD. Both the patients and their caregivers have to visit hospital for HD sessions twice to thrice per week, and on these days they risk incurring complete loss of wages.[17] In addition, studies have shown that patients on PD have less dose requirement of erythropoiesis-stimulating agents (erythropoietins), potassium, and phosphate binders, and these in turn can reduce the monthly medical expenditure for many such patients.[18-20] Better preservation of residual renal function on PD has also been shown to decrease the need for hospitalization for heart failure.[21] Hospitalizations for infection episodes requiring intravenous antibiotics are also higher in HD patients who are on cuffed or noncuffed dialysis catheters. However, infection-related hospitalization risks reduce after the first year in HD (when most patients transition to arteriovenous fistulae) but increase due to greater peritonitis risks in those on PD.[22] Studies from both developed and developing nations (including India) actually have shown PD as a more cost-effective modality as compared to in-center HD.[23,24]

PRACTICES THAT CAN IMPROVE UPTAKE OF PERITONEAL DIALYSIS AS THE INITIAL MODALITY

Urgent-start Peritoneal Dialysis

In patients seen with advanced CKD at first visit, where urgent-start RRT is required, HD is overwhelmingly chosen over PD, such as in emergent situations—refractory hyperkalemia, fluid overload, encephalopathy, uremic seizures, etc. There is a role for choosing PD and initiating PD prior to 2 weeks after catheter placement, in relatively asymptomatic patients with advanced CKD (also referred to as urgent- or early-start PD). This "bridge" practice of early- or urgent-start PD might enhance acceptance of PD as the ultimate RRT modality in a greater number of patients.

Incremental Peritoneal Dialysis

A PD prescription that is less than the standard dose of PD, but fulfills the clinical needs of the patient, based on a good residual renal function, is considered as incremental PD. Incremental PD reduces glucose exposure and financial and time burdens, and is better for the residual renal function, quality of life, and the environment as well. It has also not shown significant differences in patient survival in a single randomized trial.[25] There is a role for discussing incremental PD when counseling a patient with considerable urine output, who is interested in long-term preservation of residual renal function.

CONCLUSION

- Always include peritoneal dialysis as one of the modalities in the initial counseling for renal replacement therapy.
- Every nephrology unit should aim for dedicated PD room with trained PD nurse/counselor.
- Patients with preserved residual renal function, recurrent vascular access failure, poor cardiac reserve. or favorable logistics should be counseled for PD.
- Younger, nondiabetic patients during early years of dialysis can have survival advantage over hemodialysis.
- PD is financially more viable option than HD considering both direct and indirect cost of dialysis.

REFERENCES

1. Porter E, Watson D, Bargman JM. Education for patients with progressive CKD and acute-start dialysis. Adv Chronic Kidney Dis. 2013;20(4):302-10.
2. Prichard SS. Treatment modality selection in 150 consecutive patients starting ESRD therapy. Perit Dial Int. 1996;16(1):69-72.
3. Moist LM, Port FK, Orzol SM, Young EW, Ostbye T, Wolfe RA, et al. Predictors of loss of residual renal function among new dialysis patients. J Am Soc Nephrol. 2000;11(3):556-64.
4. Figueiredo AE, Bernardini J, Bowes E, Hiramatsu M, Price V, Su C, et al. A syllabus for teaching peritoneal dialysis to patients and caregivers. Perit Dial Int. 2016;36(6):592-605.
5. Timóteo AT, Mano TB. Efficacy of peritoneal dialysis in patients with refractory congestive heart failure: a systematic review and meta-analysis. Heart Fail Rev. 2023;28(5):1053-63.
6. Chou CY, Wang SM, Liang CC, Chang CT, Liu JH, Wang IK, et al. Peritoneal dialysis is associated with a better survival in cirrhotic patients with chronic kidney disease. Medicine (Baltimore). 2016;95(4):e2465.
7. Mekraksakit P, Suppadungsuk S, Thongprayoon C, Miao J, Leelaviwat N, Thongpiya J, et al. Outcomes of peritoneal dialysis in cirrhosis: A systematic review and meta-analysis. Perit Dial Int. 2025;45(2):93-105.
8. Kou HW, Yeh CN, Tsai CY, Liu SH, Ho WY, Lee CW, et al. Clinical benefits of laparoscopic adhesiolysis during peritoneal dialysis catheter insertion: A single-center experience. Medicina (Kaunas). 2023;59(6):1014.
9. Haggerty SP, Kumar SS, Collings AT, Alli VV, Miraflor E, Hanna NM, et al. SAGES peritoneal dialysis access guideline update 2023. Surg Endosc. 2024;38(1):1-23.
10. Weinhandl ED, Foley RN, Gilbertson DT, Arneson TJ, Snyder JJ, Collins AJ. Propensity-matched mortality comparison of incident hemodialysis and peritoneal dialysis patients. J Am Soc Nephrol. 2010;21(3):499-506.
11. Termorshuizen F, Korevaar JC, Dekker FW, Van Manen JG, Boeschoten EW, Krediet RT; Netherlands Cooperative Study on the Adequacy of Dialysis Study Group. Hemodialysis and peritoneal dialysis: comparison of adjusted mortality rates according to the duration of dialysis: Analysis of The Netherlands Cooperative Study on the Adequacy of Dialysis 2. J Am Soc Nephrol. 2003;14(11):2851-60.
12. McDonald SP, Marshall MR, Johnson DW, Polkinghorne KR. Relationship between dialysis modality and mortality. J Am Soc Nephrol. 2009;20(1):155-63.
13. Kutner NG, Zhang R, Barnhart H, Collins AJ. Health status and quality of life reported by incident patients after 1 year on haemodialysis or peritoneal dialysis. Nephrol Dial Transplant. 2005;20(10):2159-67.
14. Jung HY, Jeon Y, Park Y, Kim YS, Kang SW, Yang CW, et al. Better quality of life of peritoneal dialysis compared to hemodialysis over a two-year period after dialysis initiation. Sci Rep. 2019;9(1):10266.
15. Snyder JJ, Kasiske BL, Gilbertson DT, Collins AJ. A comparison of transplant outcomes in peritoneal and hemodialysis patients. Kidney Int. 2002;62(4):1423-30.
16. Tonelli M, Nkunu V, Varghese C, Abu-Alfa AK, Alrukhaimi MN, Fox L, et al. Framework for establishing integrated kidney care programs in low- and middle-income countries. Kidney Int Suppl. 2020;10(1):e19-23. Erratum in: Kidney Int Suppl. 2020;10(2):e186.
17. Helanterä I, Haapio M, Koskinen P, Grönhagen-Riska C, Finne P. Employment of patients receiving maintenance dialysis and after kidney transplant: a cross-sectional study from Finland. Am J Kidney Dis. 2012;59(5):700-6.
18. Wetmore JB, Peng Y, Monda KL, Kats AM, Kim DH, Bradbury BD, et al. Trends in anemia management practices in patients receiving hemodialysis and peritoneal dialysis: A retrospective cohort analysis. Am J Nephrol. 2015;41(4-5):354-61.
19. Musso CG. Potassium metabolism in patients with chronic kidney disease. Part II: patients on dialysis (stage 5). Int Urol Nephrol. 2004;36(3):469-72.
20. Kuhlmann MK. Phosphate elimination in modalities of hemodialysis and peritoneal dialysis. Blood Purif. 2010;29(2):137-44.
21. Liu X, Dai C. Advances in understanding and management of residual renal function in patients with chronic kidney disease. Kidney Dis (Basel). 2017;2(4):187-96.
22. van Eck van der Sluijs A, Bonenkamp AA, van Wallene VA, Hoekstra T, Lissenberg-Witte BI, Dekker FW, et al; DOMESTICO study group. Differences in hospitalisation between peritoneal dialysis and haemodialysis patients. Eur J Clin Invest. 2022;52(6):e13758.
23. lomjit N, Kattah AG, Cheungpasitporn W. The cost-effectiveness of peritoneal dialysis is superior to hemodialysis: Updated evidence from a more precise model. Kidney Med. 2020;3(1):15-7.
24. Gupta D, Jyani G, Ramachandran R, Bahuguna P, Ameel M, Dahiya BB, et al. Peritoneal dialysis-first initiative in India: A cost-effectiveness analysis. Clin Kidney J. 2021;15(1):128-35.
25. Yan H, Fang W, Lin A, Cao L, Ni Z, Qian J. Three versus 4 daily exchanges and residual kidney function decline in incident CAPD patients: A randomized controlled trial. Am J Kidney Dis. 2017;69(4):506-13.

CHAPTER 46

Percutaneous Insertion of Peritoneal Dialysis Catheter

Pavitra Manu Dogra, Purva Suhas Bavikar

CASE SCENARIO

History

A 62-year-old female has been suffering from diabetes mellitus and hypertension for the past 15 years. She was diagnosed with chronic kidney disease stage 5 secondary to diabetic kidney disease, approximately 4 months ago when her serum creatinine was 5.8 mg/dL. She was advised for vascular access creation (left brachiocephalic arteriovenous fistula (AVF) which she got constructed 1 month back. She was counseled for dialysis modalities including hemodialysis and peritoneal dialysis but was unsure of either of them. She has now presented with swelling of feet and reduction in urine output for a few days' duration. Urine was frothy. Swelling of feet was associated with periorbital puffiness (early morning predominance) and intermittent breathlessness on exertion. She also had early morning vomiting episodes and nausea (especially, at sight of food). She was brought to a nephrology clinic.

Examination

- *General examination:* The patient had a blood pressure (BP) of 170/100 mm Hg, pulse was 78 beats/min, regular, normal volume and character, respiratory rate (RR) 20 breaths/min and SpO_2 98% at room air. She had pallor, leukonychia, periorbital puffiness and bilateral pitting pedal edema. There was no icterus/clubbing/cyanosis/lymphadenopathy/parotid swelling.
- *Local examination:* Left brachiocephalic AVF is functional with mature venous segment.
- *Systemic examination:* Systemic examination was essentially normal. Lungs revealed vesicular breath sounds. CVS showed LVS4. Fundus examination showed nonproliferative diabetic retinopathy with grade 3 hypertensive retinopathy.

Investigations

Hemoglobin (Hb): 9.2 g/dL, total leukocyte count (TLC): 5,600/mm^3, platelets: 348,000/mm^3; blood urea nitrogen (BUN): 130 mg/dL, serum creatinine: 9.2 mg/dL, serum calcium: 8.6 mg/dL, serum inorganic phosphorus: 7.8 mg/dL, urine RE/ME: Protein-3+, sugar: neg, RBC-2+, WBC: 4–6/HPF, epithelial cells: nil, Casts: nil, crystals: nil. No eosinophils; spot urine protein: Creatinine ratio: Urine Protein: 418.6 mg/dL, urine creatinine: 42 mg/dL, PC ratio: 9966.6 mg/gm of creatinine; 24 hours urinary protein excretion**:** 3.9 gm/day.

Ultrasound KUB (kidney, ureter, and bladder X-ray): Borderline kidney sizes with diffusely increased cortical echogenicity with reduced corticomedullary differentiation (CMD), pelvicalyceal system (PCS) compact; no cyst or calcification or concretion; color Doppler flow imaging (CDFI) renal vessels: no renal artery stenosis; vitamin (25 OH): 23 nmol/L; intact parathyroid hormone (PTH): 569 pg/mL; HBsAg/anti-HCV/anti-HIV: negative; 2D echocardiography: within normal limits.

Final diagnosis: Chronic kidney disease G5A3 (diabetic kidney disease) with uremia.

Plan: The patient was planned for initiation of renal replacement therapy (RRT) in the form of dialysis.

Patient RRT counseling: The patient underwent extensive counseling for RRT and detailed about the pros and cons of hemodialysis and continuous ambulatory peritoneal dialysis (CAPD)/automated peritoneal dialysis (APD).

Patient's decision: She, by virtue of being an educated female, decided on pursuing with a few sessions of hemodialysis via left brachiocephalic AVF, followed by peritoneal dialysis (PD) catheter insertion and initiation of CAPD.

Process ahead: Since the patient has opted for PD as RRT, she shall now be recounseled about the operative procedure by the treating nephrologist and the process of doing daily exchanges of CAPD/APD by the PD technician/nurse.

INTRODUCTION

Peritoneal dialysis is the home therapy option of choice for most patients with kidney failure worldwide. Best-practice PD today provides mortality and quality-of-life outcomes similar to those achieved with in-center hemodialysis (HD) the world over.[1,2] In developing countries such as India, PD is kept as the last option for those with multiple access failures. The major hurdle for PD penetration is the void in insertion technique training amongst young nephrologists.[3,4] Despite extensive promotion of CAPD and APD as a viable kidney replacement therapy (KRT) modality for active young individuals suffering from chronic kidney disease (CKD) stage 5 or end-stage kidney disease (ESKD), much success has not been achieved. The reasons cited for this poor PD penetration amongst the general population are the limited technique survival and high risk of PD peritonitis. With improvement in patient care, fluid dynamics, audiovisual teaching aids, insertion techniques, and microbiological assay techniques for diagnosing culture-positive peritonitis, PD survival has improved tremendously.[5]

Percutaneous PD catheter (PDC) insertion technique has long been under revision to ensure safety and accomplish complication-free outcomes. PD was initially used as the modality for ESKD by Richard Ruben in 1959. This was followed by different insertion methods and development of automated PD machine in Netherlands by Boen et al.[6-8] Henry Tenckhoff developed an indwelling PDC, inserted via a surgical technique in 1968.[9] This was followed by the development of CAPD by Popovich and Monrief.[10] With the advent of the wherewithal for CAPD and APD, insertion techniques underwent further refinement. There was a gradual shift from the ever-popular surgical insertion technique to percutaneous insertion, laparoscopic insertion, and image intensifier-guided percutaneous insertion techniques. There was a gradual shift of PD inserters from surgeons to interventional nephrologists and radiologists.[11-13] In India, PDC insertion is being done by all the three techniques, and the percutaneous technique is being done predominantly by interventional nephrologists with the use of image intensifier[14,15] or without image intensifier.[16-19]

COUNSELING OF PATIENTS FOR PERITONEAL DIALYSIS CATHETER INSERTION

The procedure of counseling of percutaneous PDC insertion is intensive and multi-echeloned. The counseling and clinical examination for patients' feasibility for percutaneous PDC insertion go together. The counseling consists of the following steps:

- *Counseling by PD nurse:* Once a patient has been identified by the nephrology team for percutaneous PDC insertion, the PD nurse should counsel the patient. The patient should be apprised about the procedure in detail including the pros and cons, technique to be followed, self-care during the CAPD/APD, and education about the monitoring of various parameters.
- *Counseling by a nephrologist:* The treating nephrologist counsels the patient about the decision of PD versus HD and the steps of the procedure in brief. The patient is also apprised about the benefits and complications of the procedure. The nephrologist finally assesses the timeline for the procedure in consultation with the patient.
- *Preprocedure counseling:* This is done by the treating nephrologist who is going to do the procedure. It is done on the day prior to the slotted procedure date. The presence of PD nurse is essential during this counseling as the patient shall be in contact of the PD nurse for all pertinent issues.
- *Detailed history:* A detailed preprocedure history should be taken from the patients and should include the following variables:
    - Previous abdominal surgery and complications thereof, e.g., interventions such as laparotomy or laparoscopy or prior solid organ transplants.
    - Previous or current hernias, hernioplasty with or without mesh repair, or complications during the said procedures should be taken.
    - Bowel habits and assessment of risk factors for constipation.
    - Coronary artery disease, arrythmias, any other cardiac disease, vascular disease, and arterial/venous thrombosis.
    - History of antiplatelets such as aspirin, clopidogrel, or anticoagulants. If the patient is on anticoagulants, they are held 5 days before the procedure or converted to unfractionated heparin.

Unfractionated heparin should be withheld 6–8 hours prior to the procedure and restarted 12 hours after the procedure.

INSTRUMENTS REQUIRED FOR PERCUTANEOUS PERITONEAL DIALYSIS CATHETER INSERTION

The procedure of PDC insertion by the percutaneous technique requires a specific set of instruments. These are as follows:

- *PDC catheter kit:* The most common PDC insertion kit used in India is Quinton® PDC insertion kit. It contains a #11 scalpel, 18-G introducer needle, J-shaped guidewire of diameter 0.0035", 16-Fr pull-apart sheath with dilator, two-cuff straight or coiled catheter, a tunneling Stylet, beta-cap adapter, cap, and catheter clamp **(Fig. 1)**.
- *Laparoscopic veress needle:* The laparoscopic veress needle is available in 10 and 12 cm sizes. The ideal length of the veress needle for use in adults is 12 cm. It consists of a 14-G hollow outer cannula with beveled tip and a 16-G spring-loaded inner cannula with soft tip and side eye for passage of fluid or gas. The advantage of this needle is that the outer beveled edge cuts through the stiff tissues and the inner spring-loaded round-tipped needle pops out when the needle enters a hollow cavity or soft, loose tissue area **(Figs. 2A and B)**.
- *Straightening stylet:* This is a 60-cm long solid metal straightening instrument with an external diameter of 3 mm, used to straighten the PDC, and help in effortless slide of the PDC into the pull-apart sheath **(Fig. 3)**.
- *Surgical instruments:* Surgical instruments to be used for percutaneous PDC insertion should include mosquito artery forceps (four), 40 × 10 mm sized Langenbeck retractors (two), 25 × 7 mm sized Langenbeck retractors (two), toothed forceps (one), Allis forceps (two), skin stapler (one), 2-0 vicryl suture (one), and 250 mL collecting bowls (two) **(Figs. 4A and B)**.
- *Monopolar cautery machine with pencil cautery instrument:* This is used for cutting through tissues and coagulating the bleeders, thereby helping to attain a bloodless and clear surgical field.

PERITONEAL DIALYSIS CATHETER (PDC) INSERTION VIA MIDLINE APPROACH (WITH IMAGE INTENSIFIER)

The percutaneous placement of PDC is done using the modified Seldinger technique[20-22] with commercially available PDC kits. It is strongly recommended that this procedure be done under image intensifier, be it C-arm or flat panel detectors. The following steps are followed:

- *Step 1: Bowel preparation and preoperating room preparation*:
  - Hemodialysis should be done a day prior to the procedure.
  - Light dinner should be given, followed by keeping nil orally after 22:00 hours, the night before.
  - Syrup lactulose 30 mL PO at 22:00 hours, the night before

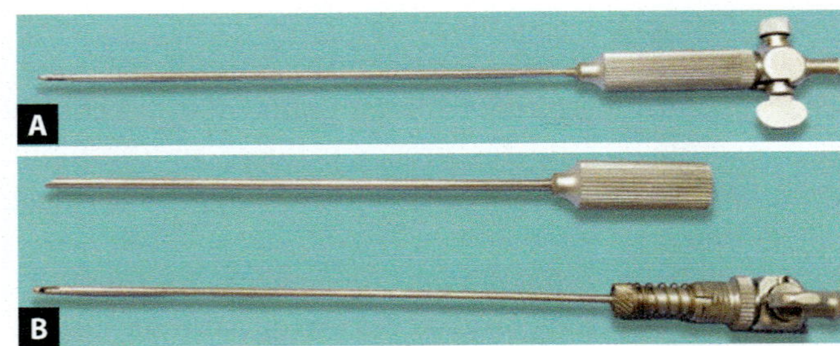

Figs. 2A and B: Laparoscopic veress needle. (A) Assembled (B) unassembled needle with outer sharp bevel edged 14-G needle and inner spring-loaded 16-G round-tipped needle with side eye opening near the tip.

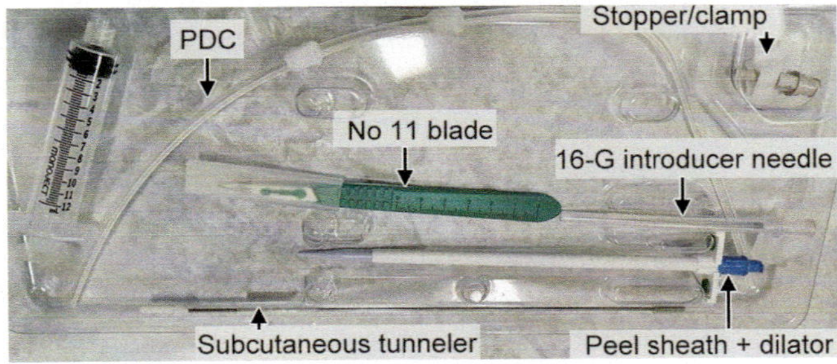

Fig. 1: Peritoneal dialysis catheter (PDC) insertion set with all the contents as described.

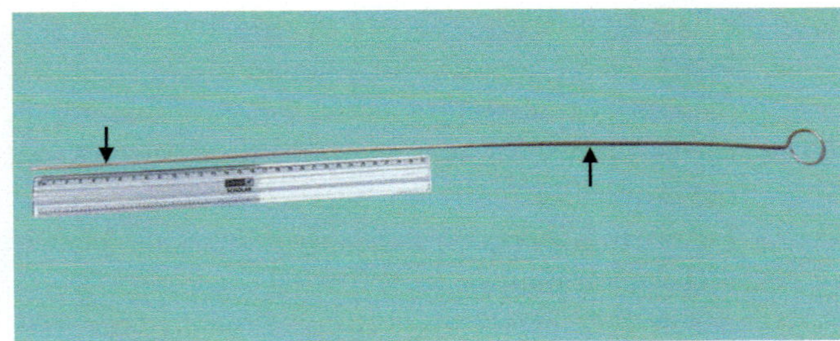

Fig. 3: A 60-cm long straightening stylet, with reference scale kept for size determination.

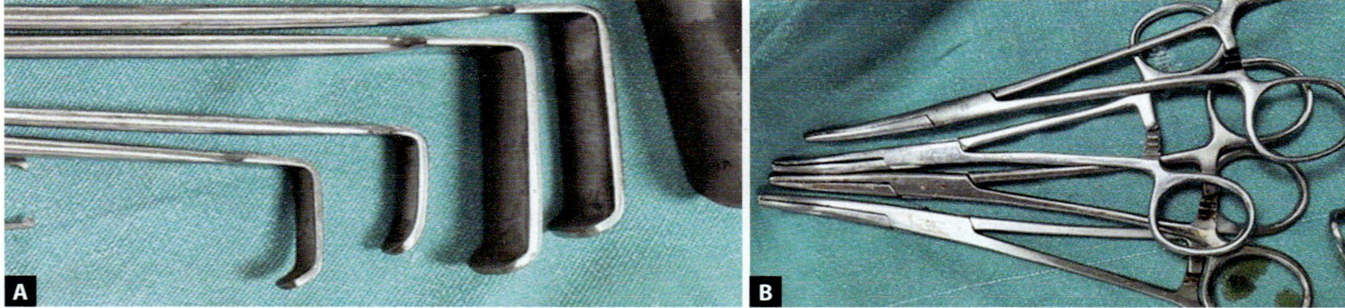

Figs. 4A and B: Set of instruments used for percutaneous peritoneal dialysis catheter insertion. (A) 40 × 10 mm sized Langenbeck retractors; (B) 25 × 7 mm sized Langenbeck retractors mosquito artery forceps.

- Anxiolytic such as tab alprazolam 0.25 mg at 22:00 hours, the night before
- Proctoclysis enema should be given to the patient at 06:00 hours on the day of surgery, followed by clearance of bowels.
- A good soap bath in the morning with cleaning of abdomen and groins
- Injection vancomycin 1,000 mg prior to sending the patient to the operating room
- All the antihypertensive medications should be given to the patient in the morning with a glass of water.
- Take consent for the procedure.
- A fresh set of investigations should be done, including complete hemogram, platelet count, serum electrolytes, urea, creatinine, prothrombin time, and activated partial thromboplastin clotting time.

- *Step 2: Preoperative preparation in operating room*:
  - Secure intravenous access with cannula on the non-AVF forearm.
  - Keep the emergency cardiac resuscitation tray ready with atropine (for vasovagal phenomena) and adrenaline.
  - Patient is given injection fentanyl intravenously @ 0.5 µg/kg over few minutes, to allay anxiety.
  - Preoperative hemodynamics including SpO_2, pulse, BP, and ECG should be taken by a multiparameter cardiac monitor, which should track throughout the procedure.
  - Ensure that two good shadowless lights are focused on the abdomen.
  - Assess the surface anatomy and localize the PDC insertion point at 2 cm below the umbilicus in the midline or paramedian region.
  - Scrub the anterior abdominal wall skin with steriprep solution starting from the point of insertion to peripheral. Umbilicus should be scrubbed last.
  - Apply sterile drapes on to the patient and explain the procedure again to the patient.
- *Step 3: Accessing the rectus sheath*:
  - Local anesthesia is given with injection lignocaine (2%) @ 10 mL until rectus sheath at the operative site
  - A horizontal or vertical midline infra-umbilical skin incision (1–1.5 cm length) is given **(Fig. 5A)**.
  - Blunt dissection is done with curved artery forceps to expose anterior rectus sheath.
  - The point for entry into the peritoneum was locally infiltrated with 2 mL of lignocaine injection.
- *Step 4: Entry into the peritoneal cavity*:
  - *Using laparoscopic veress (pneumoperitoneum) needle:*
    - A veress needle is steadily advanced through the rectus sheath and peritoneum.
    - Veress needle is advanced through rectus sheath vertically at 90° **(Figs. 5B and 6A to D)**. While advancing the veress needle, two clicks will be felt if going in midline. The first click is felt when the needle traverses through the rectus sheath **(Figs. 6B and E)**. Thereafter, the needle should be angled at 45° prior to penetration of parietal peritoneum. Soon, a second click is felt when the needle passes through parietal peritoneum **(Figs. 6D and F)**.
    - Once the second click of veress needle is felt, suggesting the popping out of the inner atraumatic blunt tip needle, a 2.5-mL syringe with saline is used to aspirate **(Fig. 5C)**. If the veress needle is in the peritoneal cavity, there will be a negative suction, and no content shall be aspirated.

- A syringe filled with 10 mL of nonionic radiocontrast media is attached to the veress needle and injected into the peritoneal cavity. Free dissipation of the contrast material outlines the outer surface of the bowel loops, giving a web-like appearance, thus confirming a successful entry into the peritoneal cavity. If the radiocontrast media takes the shape of valvulae conniventes or plicae semilunaris, it refers to small intestine puncture. Similarly, if the bowel haustrations are highlighted by radiocontrast media, it means inadvertent colonic puncture.[23]
- Optionally, then, 1.5 L of CAPD fluid is instilled into the peritoneal cavity through the laparoscopic veress needle, ascertaining a free flow of the fluid **(Fig. 5D)**.
- The veress needle is then gently and slowly advanced by 8–10 cm toward the left iliac fossa at an angulation of 30–45° from the surface. If a resistance is encountered, withdraw the needle slightly and ascertain free flow of fluid into the peritoneal cavity.
- This is followed by removal of the spring-loaded inner needle by gentle unscrewing movement **(Figs. 5E and F)**.
- Keeping the veress needle sturdily held by one hand, the J-tip guidewire is gently progressed into the peritoneal cavity via the outer cannula of the veress needle **(Fig. 5G)** followed by removal of the veress needle.
- A peel-away sheath with plastic dilator is introduced over the guidewire, followed by removal of introducer and guidewire **(Fig. 5H)**.
- PDC (straightened with straightening stylet, keeping the tip of the stylet 0.2 mm short of PDC tip) is slid into the pull-apart sheath, directing toward left iliac fossa or rectovesical pouch, till a gentle resistance is felt.
- Slide the PDC gently over the straightening stylet to allow it to take final position, keeping the deep cuff at the rectus sheath.
- This is followed by gradual withdrawal of straightening stylet keeping a steady tug on the deep cuff, until the stylet is completely withdrawn and removed.
- The pull-apart sheath is then gradually peeled off while keeping a tug on the deep cuff **(Fig. 5I)**.
- The whole procedure is monitored under a fluoroscopic image intensifier **(Figs. 7A to F)**.

- *Using 18-G introducer needle:*
  - An 18-G introducer needle or 16-G FEP-Teflon IV cannula is advanced in midline through the rectus aponeurosis and peritoneum.
  - Once adequate giveaway is felt on breaching the parietal peritoneum, a syringe filled with 10 mL of nonionic radiocontrast media is attached to the veress needle and injected into the peritoneal cavity. Free dissipation of the contrast material outlines the outer surface of the bowel loops, giving a web-like appearance, thus confirming a successful entry into the peritoneal cavity.
  - After confirming the successful peritoneal entry, optionally, 1.5 L of CAPD fluid is instilled into the peritoneal cavity ascertaining free flow.
  - Once the fluid is filled in the peritoneal cavity, a J-tipped guidewire is advanced through the needle.
  - The needle is then removed and the dilator with pull-apart sheath is gently advanced over the guidewire into the peritoneal cavity, with gentle screwing movements.
  - The guidewire is gently removed, followed by removal of the dilator. This is followed by a sudden gush of instilled CAPD fluid through the pull-apart sheath.
  - PDC is loaded on the straightening stylet and advanced through the peel-away sheath into the peritoneal cavity. The PDC is directed toward the left iliac fossa.
  - Keeping a tug on the deep cuff at the rectus sheath, the pull-apart sheath is gradually torn off along with advancement of deep cuff on to the rectus sheath. The deep cuff is either placed on the rectus sheath or pushed into the rectus sheath.
  - Ascertain free flow of CAPD fluid through the PDC by flushing and draining out the fluid.

- *Step 5: Subcutaneous tunnel creation and exit site:*
  - Deep cuff is usually ensured onto the anterior rectus sheath with either a purse string suture on the rectus sheath or by an anchoring suture on the rectus sheath with a bite through the deep cuff material **(Fig. 5J)**. Alternatively, the deep cuff can also be pushed into the space between the rectus sheath and parietal peritoneum with the help of a mosquito artery forceps or a cuff implanter.[24]

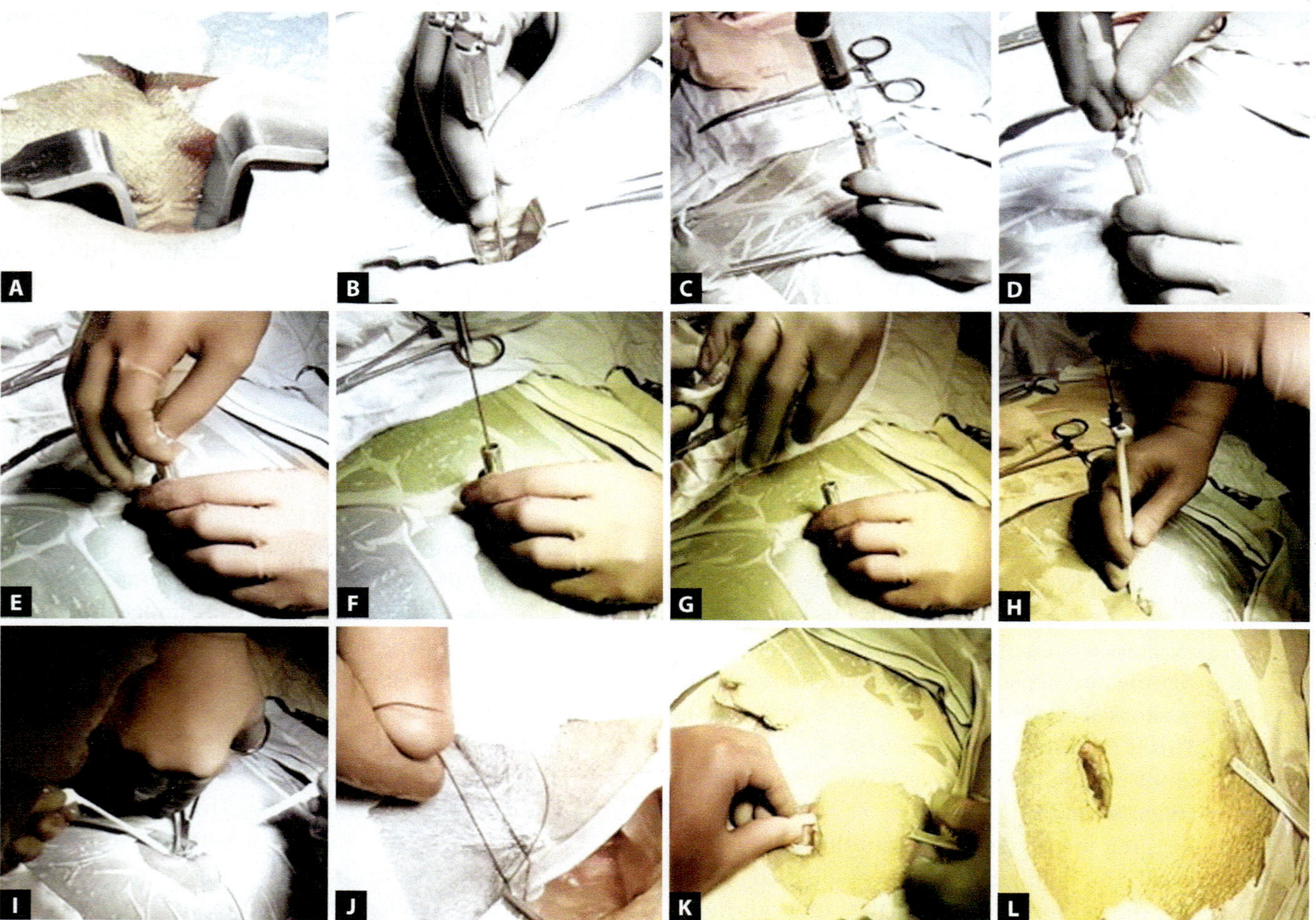

Figs. 5A to L: Procedure steps of percutaneous PDC insertion with the use of laparoscopic veress needle (details are in the text).

- CAPD fluid is quickly drained through the PDC.
- A subcutaneous tunnel with a length of 10–12 cm is made using trocar, ensuring a "n" or inverted parabola configuration of the PDC, with the exit point kept caudolaterally with the outer cuff at least 2–3 cm inside the exit **(Figs. 5K and L)**.
- It is reiterated that a free inflow and draining out of the CAPD fluid through the PDC are ascertained before the closure of incision wound and culmination of the procedure.
- PDC is locked with a heparin lock.
- The final position of the PDC tip is established under image intensifier prior to suturing the entry incision point.
- A check radiogram is usually taken 48 hours after the insertion procedure and prior to first flushing to see the current position of PDC tip **(Fig. 6F)**.

PERITONEAL DIALYSIS CATHETER INSERTION VIA PARAMEDIAN APPROACH (WITH IMAGE INTENSIFIER)

Percutaneous insertion of PDC can also be done using the paramedian incision, usually on the left side; it may be done on the right side too when reinsertion is done. All the steps of the PDC insertion procedure are the same as is done in the midline insertion technique, except for the following variations in the procedure steps:

- Laparoscopic veress needle insertion is associated with three insertion clicks instead of two clicks seen in the midline technique. The first click is felt on traversing the anterior rectus sheath, the second click is felt on traversing the posterior rectus sheath, and the third click is heard on penetration of parietal peritoneum, thus entering the peritoneal cavity.

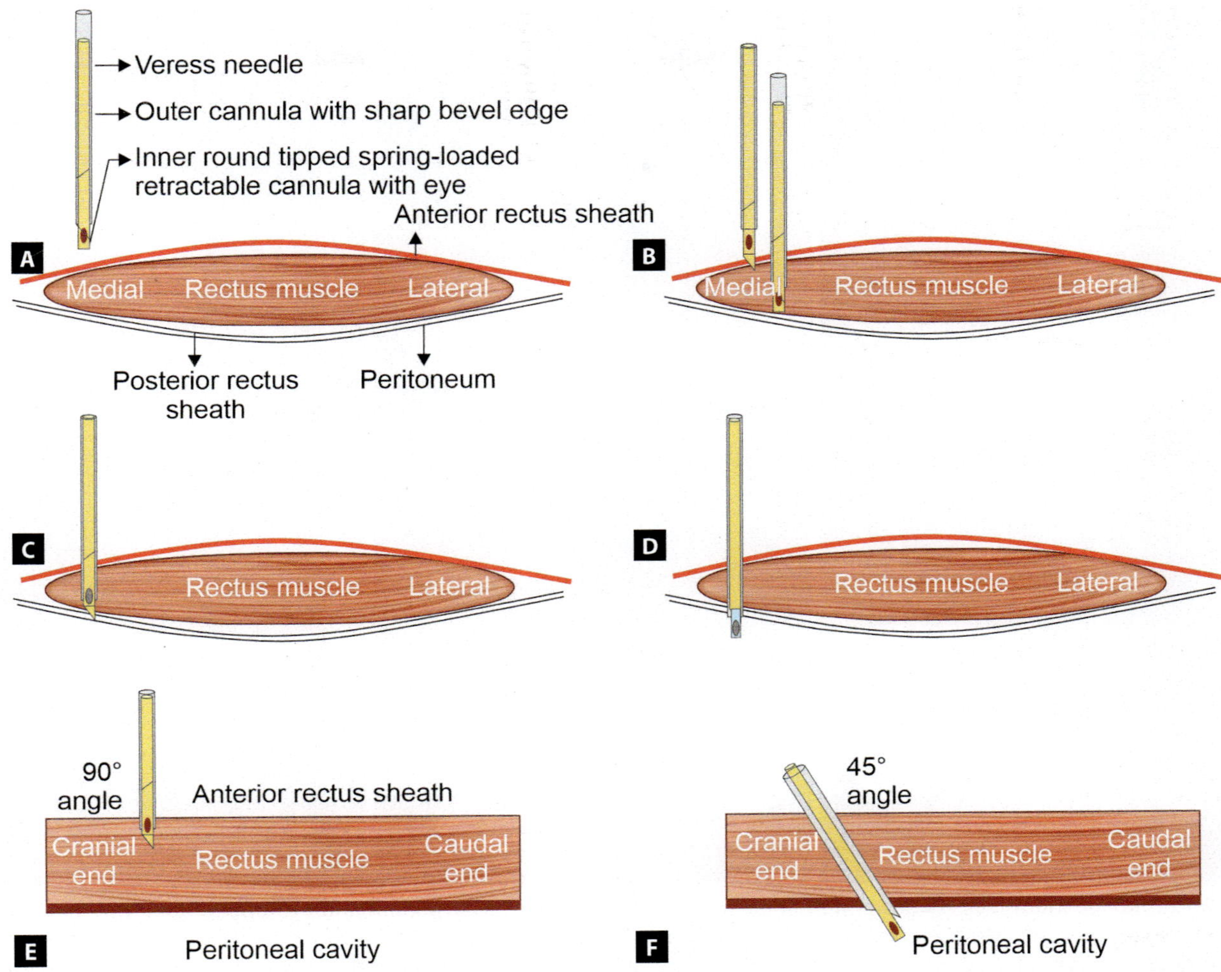

Figs. 6A to F: (A) Relation of rectus apparatus and veress needle prior to insertion in transverse plane; (B and C) The needle traversing through the medial end of the rectus muscle; (D) The needle entering the peritoneal cavity with popping out of the round tipped inner needle; (E and F) Sagittal plane of rectus apparatus showing the angulation of veress needle during insertion.

- Care should be taken while advancing veress needle through the rectus muscle, as to proceed very gently, to avoid injury to vessels or muscle fibers.
- Once the J-tipped guidewire is passed into the peritoneal cavity and the veress needle is withdrawn, a small 0.5-cm incision should be made on the anterior rectus sheath, to aid placement of deep cuff into the rectus muscle body.

COMPLICATIONS OF THIS INSERTION TECHNIQUE AND ITS MANAGEMENT

No surgical procedure is done without its inherent set of complications. The percutaneous technique of PDC insertion has its own share of complications. We should remember that complications are a double-edged sword. On one hand, it gives tremendous experience to the interventional nephrologist, and on the other hand, it might retard the CAPD program by months, if mitigation measures are not taken. These complications and management of specific conditions are as follows:

- *Vasovagal phenomenon:* This usually occurs when the peritoneal cavity is instilled with fluid. It is treated with leg raising, pausing fluid instillation, giving intravenous atropine injection and leaving some residual CAPD fluid in the peritoneal cavity for a tidal effect.
- *Injury to various tissues/structures:*
  - *Bowel and mesenteric perforation:* In such a scenario, there are two approaches. The first is to remove the puncture needle/veress needle immediately and abandon the procedure. In this case the perforation seals itself, being minute in size. The second approach is to keep the needle/

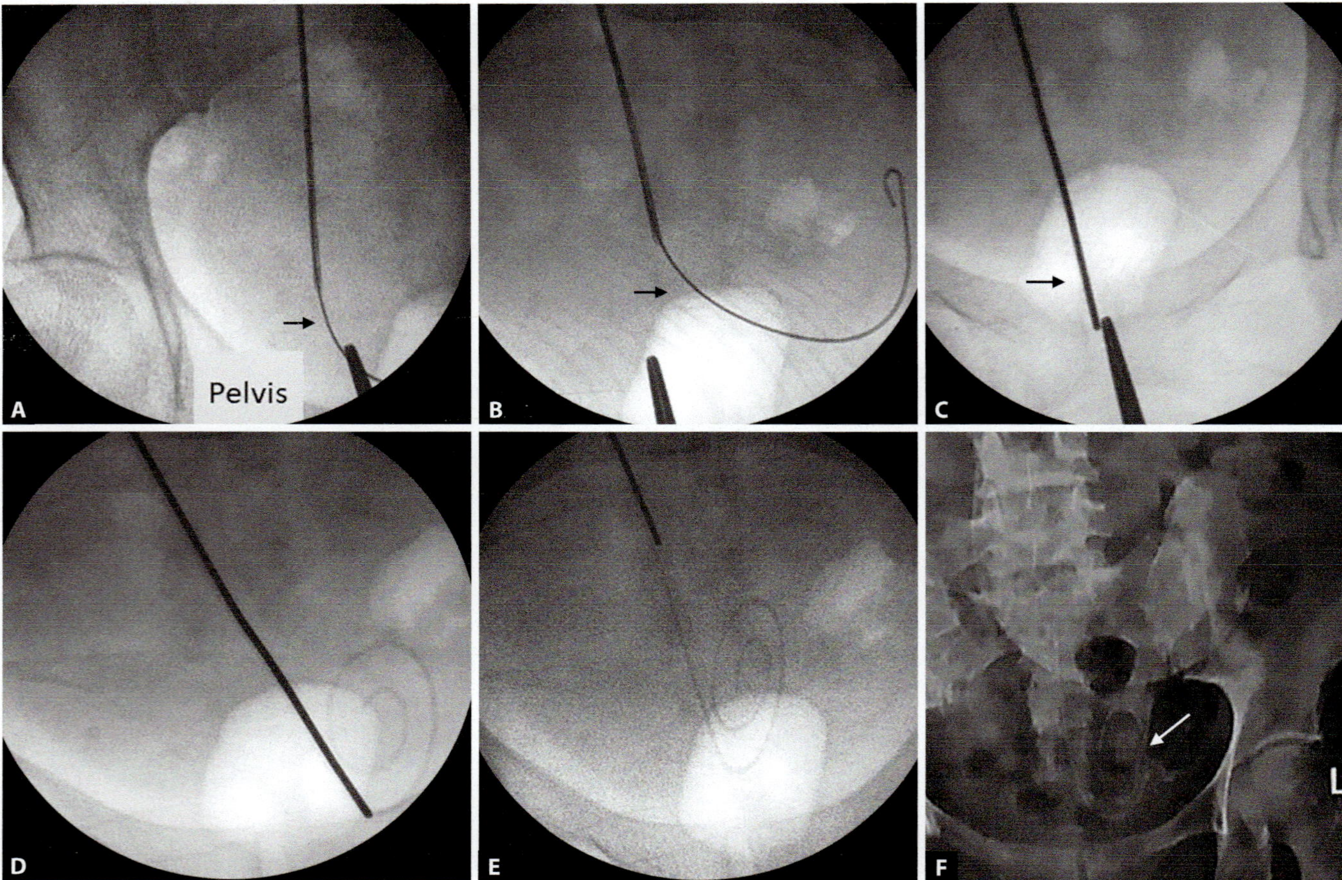

Figs. 7A to F: Image intensifier images of peritoneal dialysis catheter (PDC) insertion. (A and B) J-tipped guidewire being placed through laparoscopic veress needle (black arrows); (C) PDC loaded on straightening stylet being placed deep into the peritoneal cavity (black arrow); (D) Coiled PDC being slid over the straightening stylet; (E) Withdrawal of straightening stylet with placement of PDC; (F) X-ray KUB (kidney, ureter, and bladder X-ray) after 48 hours of insertion showing the coiled PDC tip in pelvis (white arrow).

guidewire in situ at the puncture site and seek immediate surgical intervention. Keeping needle/ guidewire in situ aids the surgeon to identify the puncture site, thus saving on time.

- *Injury to intraabdominal vessels:* This can happen during the initial needle puncture. Vessels such as mesenteric vessels, inferior epigastric vessels, and abdominal aorta can get injured. The best approach is to seek surgical colleagues' intervention, who can proceed with laparotomy and tackle the bleeder.
- *Rectus muscle or abdominal wall hematoma:* These are usually tackled with a conservative approach. Tight abdominal compression bandaging, immobilization, and antifibrinolytic agents such as tranexamic acid, ethamsylate, and epsilon-aminocaproic acid (EACA), etc., are the mitigation measures to prevent further worsening of hematoma. If the hematoma enlarges in size or does not resolve in 48 hours, then re-exploration of the surgical site is recommended to take control of the culprit bleeder.
- *Hemorrhagic PDC outflow:* This is managed by repeated flushing of the PDC with CAPD fluid or saline. It usually settles within a few hours. If hemorrhagic outflow persists and is associated with drop in the hemoglobin of the patient, immediate contrast-enhanced CT abdomen should be done, followed by surgical intervention in form of either laparoscopy or laparotomy to tackle the source of bleeding.
- *Injury to urinary bladder or urinary bladder perforation:* This can occur despite all the standard precautions, if the bladder is distended or the puncture is in the mid lower or lower abdominal

wall. It can be managed with immediate removal of puncture needle/PDC, followed by rest to the urinary bladder by per-urethral catheterization for 48–72 hours, thereby allowing bladder wall to heal.

- *Mechanical complications:*
  - *Preperitoneal placement of the PDC:* This is one of the common complications which can be identified immediately during the contrast instillation or by tremendous abdominal pain during the initial intended filling of peritoneal cavity with CAPD fluid. Treatment is by immediate removal of needle/PDC, followed by either reinsertion in the same sitting or after a rest of 7 days.
  - *Pericatheter dialysate leakage:* This can be identified immediately or in the initial 7 days. It can be managed with PD rest for 14 days or re-exploration of the surgical site, followed by purse-string suture at the site of PDC entry into the rectus sheath.
  - *Incisional hernia:* This is a late and an uncommon manifestation given the size of incision and that the entry into the rectus sheath is very small. This can be managed with surgical intervention, by overlapping the muscular layer or placing a subcutaneous mesh to reinforce the hernial outpouching.
  - *PDC migration out of true pelvis:* This is another common complication. This occurs either due to truncal obesity, right-sided tunnel direction, small-bowel ileus, and constipation or due to omental wrapping. Three patterns of catheter tip migration are described. The first pattern has the catheter tip pointing laterally against the abdominopelvic side wall, the second pattern has the catheter tip point superiorly toward the hypochondrial region, and the third pattern has the catheter tip looping back on itself.[25] The management strategy is to mitigate constipation by using laxatives or cathartics. If this is unsuccessful, then PDC should be replaced either by over-the-guidewire exchange, or surgical reinsertion via a neoincision or a laparoscopic repositioning with omentopexy/omentectomy followed by anterior abdominal wall tugging.[22]
  - *Right-sided hydrothorax:* This occurs due to pleuroperitoneal connections resulting in dialysate leakage into the pleural space. Diagnosis is confirmed by thoracentesis, with recovery of fluid low in protein and high in glucose concentration. Alternatively, the diagnosis can be established by contrast CT peritoneography or technetium-99m peritoneal scintigraphy. Conservative management (peritoneal rest, low-volume dialysis) is rarely successful. Thoracoscopic pleurodesis with talc poudrage or mechanical rub produces 85–100% success rate.[22]
- *Infective complications:*[26] New definitions and management have been published. These include the following:
  - *Pre-PD peritonitis:* This is defined as peritonitis episode occurring after PDC insertion and prior to PD commencement. This is identified within the initial 7 days of PDC insertion during PDC flushing. The treatment is antibiotics including a cover for gram-positive and gram-negative organisms.
  - *PD-related peritonitis:* This is defined as the peritonitis occurring after the commencement of PD. Antibiotics remain the treatment of choice, unless there is refractory peritonitis, which requires PDC removal and reinsertion at a later date (3–4 weeks).
  - *PDC insertion-related peritonitis:* This is defined as PDC insertion-related peritonitis. It is defined as an episode of peritonitis that occurs within 30 days of PDC insertion. Treatment is antibiotics covering both gram-positive and negative organisms.
  - *Dry contamination:* This contamination occurs outside a closed PD system, such as disconnection distal to a closed clamp.
  - *Wet contamination:* This refers to the contamination with an open system, when either dialysis fluid is infused after contamination or the catheter administration set has been left open for an extended period. This includes leaks from dialysate bags, leaks or breaks in tubing proximal to the tubing clamp, breach of aseptic technique, or touch contamination of the connection during a PD exchange. Prophylactic antibiotics are only recommended after wet contamination.

CONCLUSION

Percutaneous technique for PDC insertion for CAPD/APD is a safe procedure and is exclusively being done by the interventional nephrologists and radiologists world over. The use of laparoscopic veress needle and image intensifier during the procedure has added to the safety and surety of PDC tip in the true pelvis, thereby adding to the overall success of the procedure. The complications of this procedure are minimal, if done with caution.

REFERENCES

1. Marshall MR. The benefit of early survival on PD versus HD-why this is (still) very important. Perit Dial Int. 2020;40:405-18.
2. Jung HY, Jeon Y, Park Y, Kim YS, Kang SW, Yang CW, et al. Better quality of life of peritoneal dialysis compared to hemodialysis over a two-year period after dialysis initiation. Sci Rep. 2019;9:10266.
3. Boujelbane L, Fu N, Chapla K, Melnick D, Redfield RR, Waheed S, et al. Percutaneous versus surgical insertion of PD catheters in dialysis patients: a meta-analysis. J Vasc Access. 2015;16(6):498-505.
4. Jha V, Abrahams AC, Al-Hwiesh A, Brown EA, Cullis B, Dor FJMF, et al. Peritoneal catheter insertion: Combating barriers through policy change. Clin Kidney J. 2022;15(12): 2177-85.
5. Nayak KS, Prabhu MV, Sinoj KA, Subhramanyam SV, Sridhar G. Peritoneal dialysis in developing countries. Contrib Nephrol. 2009;163:270-7.
6. Boen ST, Mion CM, Curtis FK, Shilipetar G. Periodic peritoneal dialysis using the repeated puncture technique and an automatic cycling machine. Trans Am Soc Artif Intern Organs. 1964;10:409-14.
7. Peppelenbosch A, van Kuijk WHM, Bouvy ND, van der Sande FM, Tordoir JHM. Peritoneal dialysis catheter placement technique and complications. NDT Plus. 2008;1(Suppl 4):iv23-8.
8. Blagg CR. The early history of dialysis for chronic renal failure in the United States: A view from Seattle. Am J Kidney Dis. 2007;49(3):482-96.
9. Tenckhoff H, Curtis FK. Experience with maintenance peritoneal dialysis in the home. Trans Am Soc Artif Intern Organs. 1970;16:90-5.
10. Popovich RP, Moncrief JW, Nolph KD, Ghods AJ, Twardowski ZJ, Pyle WK, et al. Continuous ambulatory peritoneal dialysis. Ann Intern Med. 1978;88(4):449-56.
11. Allon M, Soucie JM, Macon EJ. Complications with permanent peritoneal dialysis catheters: experience with 154 percutaneously placed catheters. Nephron. 1988;48(1):8-11.
12. Amerling R, Cruz C. A new laparoscopic method for implantation of peritoneal catheters. ASAIO J. 1993;39(3):M787-9.
13. Aal AKA, Guest SS, Moawad S, Mahmoud K, Jackson B, Rageeb PM, et al. Outcomes of fluoroscopic and ultrasound-guided placement versus laparoscopic placement of peritoneal dialysis catheters. Clin Kidney J. 2017;11(4):549-54.
14. Singh V, Mishra SC; Singh P, Rout BB. The influence of peritoneal dialysis catheter tip design on technique survival: A retrospective observational study. Indian J Nephrol. 2023;33(2):119-24.
15. Dogra PM, Nair RK, Sood V, Datt B, Katyal A, Jairam A, et al. Pneumoperitoneum needle vs. introducer needle: Comparison of complications and short-term outcomes in percutaneously inserted peritoneal dialysis catheters in naïve abdomens. Ther Apher Dial. 2022;26(1):212-9.
16. Sampathkumar K, Mahaldar AR, Sooraj YS, Ramkrishnan M, Ajeshkumar, Ravichandran R. Percutaneous CAPD catheter insertion by a nephrologist versus surgical placement: A comparative study. Indian J Nephrol. 2008;18(1):5-8.
17. Varughese S, Sundaram M, Basu G, David VG, Mohapatra A, Alexander S, et al. Percutaneous PD catheter insertion after past abdominal surgeries. Indian J Nephrol. 2012; 22(3):230-1.
18. Dogra PM, Hooda AK, Shanmugraj G, Pramanik SK. Continuous ambulatory peritoneal dialysis catheter insertion technique: a comparative study of percutaneous versus surgical insertion. Indian J Nephrol. 2018;28(4):291-7.
19. Sivaramakrishnan R, Gupta S, Agarwal SK, Bhowmik D, Mahajan S. Comparison of outcomes between surgically placed and percutaneously placed peritoneal dialysis catheters: A retrospective study. Indian J Nephrol. 2016; 26(4):268-74.
20. Tenckhoff H, Schechter H. A bacteriologically safe peritoneal access device. Trans Am Soc Artif Intern Organs. 1968;14:181-7.
21. Crabtree JH, Chow KM. Peritoneal dialysis catheter insertion. Semin Nephrol. 2017;37:17-29.
22. Crabtree JH, Shrestha BM, Chow KM, Figueiredo AE, Povlsen JV, Wilkie M, et al. Creating and maintaining optimal peritoneal dialysis access in the adult patient: 2019 update. Perit Dial Int. 2019;39(5):414-36.
23. Abdel-Aal AK, Dybbro P, Hathaway P, Guest S, Neuwirth M, Krishnamurthy V. Best practices consensus protocol for peritoneal dialysis catheter placement by interventional radiologists. Perit Dial Int. 2014;34(5):481-93.
24. Khudari HE, Abdel-Aal AK, Abaza M, Almehmi SE, Sachdeva B, Almehmi A. Peritoneal dialysis catheter placement: Percutaneous and peritoneoscopic techniques. Semin Intervent Radiol. 2022;39(1):23-31.
25. Reddy YS, Manjusha Y, Kishore CK, Sridhar N, Sriramnaveen P, Sivakumar V. Spontaneous cure of migrated peritoneal catheter. Perit Dial Int. 2012;32(1):107-8.
26. Li PK-T, Chow KM, Cho Y, Fan S, Figueiredo AE, Harris T, et al. ISPD peritonitis guideline recommendations: 2022 update on prevention and treatment. Perit Dial Int. 2022;42(2):110-53.

CHAPTER 47

Surgical Techniques for Peritoneal Dialysis Catheter Insertion

Amrita Dua, Mrinal Pahwa

CASE SCENARIO

A 56-year-old male weighing 70 kg and height 170 cm is known case of diabetes mellitus and hypertension for the last 20 days. He is suffering from end-stage renal disease (ESRD) secondary to diabetic nephropathy for the last 2 years and is on maintenance hemodialysis (HD), thrice weekly, via a permacath access on the right side of his neck. He has suffered from recurrent blood infections and sepsis in the past 4 months. His two-dimensional echocardiogram (2D echo) is suggestive of an ejection fraction of 35%. How can he be further managed?

Continuous ambulatory peritoneal dialysis (CAPD) is a manual, self-care dialysis treatment that uses the patient's peritoneum as a filter to remove waste products from the blood. It is a viable treatment option for patients with ESRD, offering flexibility, autonomy, and cost effectiveness.

INTRODUCTION

End-stage renal disease is a significant global health challenge, with a rapidly growing number of patients requiring renal replacement therapy. Treatment options for ESRD include HD, peritoneal dialysis (PD), and kidney transplantation. The effectiveness of PD as a renal replacement therapy largely depends on establishing long-term, reliable access to the peritoneal cavity using a PD catheter.

In 1959, Richard Ruben was the first to use PD successfully in a patient with ESRD for 6 months.[1] PD is now widely recognized as a cost-effective alternative to HD, offering comparable survival rates, reduced costs, enhanced quality of life, and fewer complications. PD catheters can be placed using various techniques, including open, laparoscopic, and percutaneous methods.[2] Minimally invasive procedures such as percutaneous fluoroscopically guided catheter placement are often performed by interventional radiologists and nephrologists. These methods are typically outpatient procedures, eliminating the need for general anesthesia.

Advantages of these minimally invasive techniques include shorter procedure times, the ability to confirm catheter placement via imaging, and timely placement, particularly in urgent-start PD scenarios. Despite these benefits, interventional radiologists and nephrologists currently place only about 5% of PD catheters.[3]

CATHETER TYPE AND DESIGN

Peritoneal dialysis catheters are available in various designs, including straight, pigtail-curled and swan-neck shapes, with differing lengths and numbers of Dacron cuffs to optimize fixation and tissue ingrowth **(Figs. 1A and B)**. Each catheter consists of a flexible silicone tube with an open-ended port and multiple side holes to enhance drainage and dialysate absorption.

The extraperitoneal segment of the catheter typically features one or two Dacron cuffs. In adult patients, most catheters are double-cuffed, with the proximal cuff

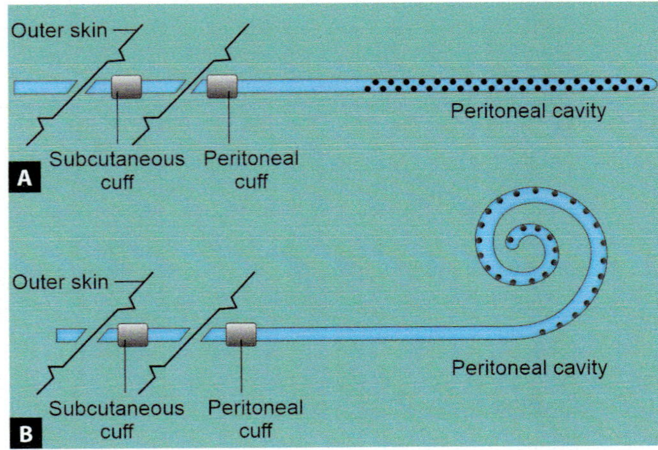

Figs. 1A and B: Two-cuffed straight (A) and curled (B) peritoneal dialysis (PD) catheter types.

implanted in the preperitoneal space and the distal cuff located in the subcutaneous tissue. The proximal cuff secures the catheter in position, while the distal cuff acts as an infection barrier. Selection of the appropriate catheter type and exit site is determined before implantation.

During the preoperative evaluation, patients are examined while fully dressed to identify the belt-line location, which helps guide the choice of exit site. Catheter selection begins with determination of the insertion site. With the patient in a supine position, the insertion site and deep cuff location are identified by aligning the upper border of the catheter coil with the upper border of the pubic symphysis **(Fig. 2)**. The deep cuff's upper border is marked 3 cm lateral to the midline in the paramedian plane. The pubic symphysis is a reliable landmark for positioning the catheter tip in the true pelvis.[4]

Straight and curled catheters perform similarly, and their implantation techniques are straightforward with minimal variation. Curled catheters may offer advantages, such as less pain during fluid inflow and reduced catheter tip dislocation. However, recent research suggests straight catheters might be preferred for better dialysis efficacy. A randomized trial comparing straight and curled catheters in 132 PD patients found no differences in procedure time, catheter-associated infections, or patient survival. However, median patency rate was slightly shorter for curled catheters (1.5 years vs. 2.1 years) due to an increased risk of inadequate dialytic clearance.[5]

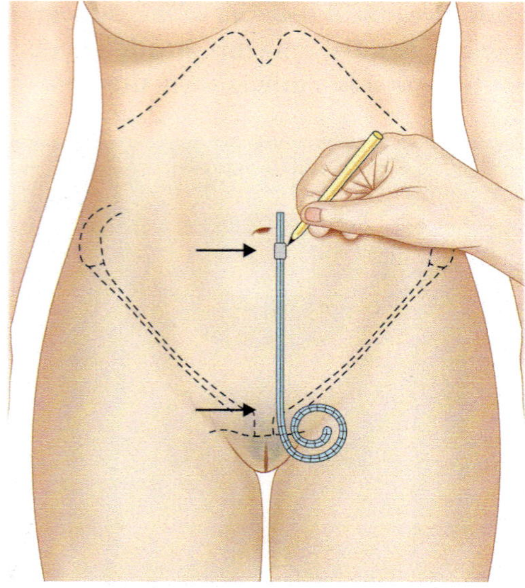

Fig. 2: Schematic illustration indicating the manner in which the catheter-insertion site and deep cuff location are selected, to achieve the proper pelvic position of the curled catheter tip.

Catheter type selection often depends on the surgeon's preference, considering factors such as the insertion method, ease of placement, and local expertise.

PREOPERATIVE EVALUATION AND PREPARATION

The success of PD therapy relies on a thorough preprocedural evaluation to ensure optimal outcomes. This evaluation includes a detailed medical history, physical examination, and assessment for any absolute contraindications to PD catheter placement. Absolute contraindications include active infections, acute diverticulitis, uncontrolled coagulopathy, or recent gastrostomy or enterostomy placement. Additionally, relative contraindications, such as prior abdominal or pelvic surgeries, peritoneal adhesions, chronic constipation, inflammatory bowel disease, abdominal wall hernias or mesh, and morbid obesity, must be carefully considered, with each case evaluated individually.

Proper preparation for PD catheter placement involves a series of systematic steps to ensure success:

- *Patient evaluation:* Assess the patient's preferences, body habitus, and weight to identify the most suitable location for the PD catheter exit site. Options include below the belt line, above the belt line.
- *Preoperative assessment and management:*
  - Conduct a comprehensive evaluation, including:
    - Basic metabolic panel
    - Complete blood count
    - Coagulation profile
  - Address any identified issues such as coagulopathy, electrolyte imbalances, or thrombocytopenia.
  - Manage anticoagulants according to the guidelines provided by the Society of Interventional Radiology.[6]
- *Fasting and sedation:*
  - Since the procedure is performed under moderate sedation, ensure the patient fasts in accordance with institutional protocols.

SURGICAL TECHNIQUES OF CONTINUOUS AMBULATORY PERITONEAL DIALYSIS INSERTION

Open Surgical Technique

The open surgical method is the traditional approach where the catheter is inserted directly through a surgical incision. The key steps of this procedure include marking of skin incision that is a line around 5–10 cm in length perpendicular at a point that is at the junction of medial 1/3rd and lateral 2/3rd on the line joining umbilicus to anterior superior iliac spine. 2% of lignocaine solution is infiltrated in skin and incision is given **(Fig. 3)**. After the skin incision, local anesthesia is instilled in the anterior rectus sheath and the sheath is opened, and the rectus muscle is separated to expose the posterior sheath and peritoneum. Again, local anesthesia is instilled in peritoneum and with a small incision in the peritoneum, the peritoneal cavity is reached **(Fig. 4)**. A Kelly forcep is then passed in pelvis to ensure free space available for placement of catheter **(Fig. 5)**. The catheter is inserted, ensuring the tip lies in the deep pelvis, which facilitates efficient drainage **(Fig. 6)**. A subcutaneous tunnel is created, where the catheter is externalized to prevent infection. The incision is closed in layers with sutures.

Ultrasound-guided Continuous Ambulatory Peritoneal Dialysis Insertion/Percutaneous

Grayscale ultrasonography of the abdominal wall is performed on the planned insertion side to identify the thickest portion of the rectus abdominis muscle for placement of the inner cuff and to ensure there are no underlying bowel loops in the area. Color Doppler imaging is utilized to visualize the epigastric artery, maintaining a puncture site at least 2–3 cm away from the artery. The locations for the deep cuff and the exit site are determined and marked.

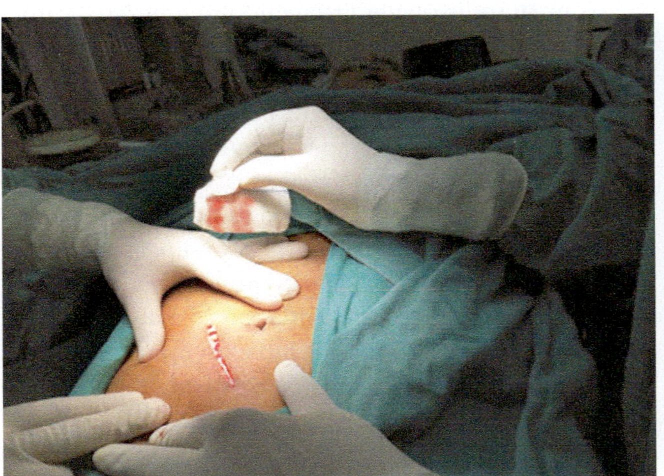

Fig. 3: Incision site.

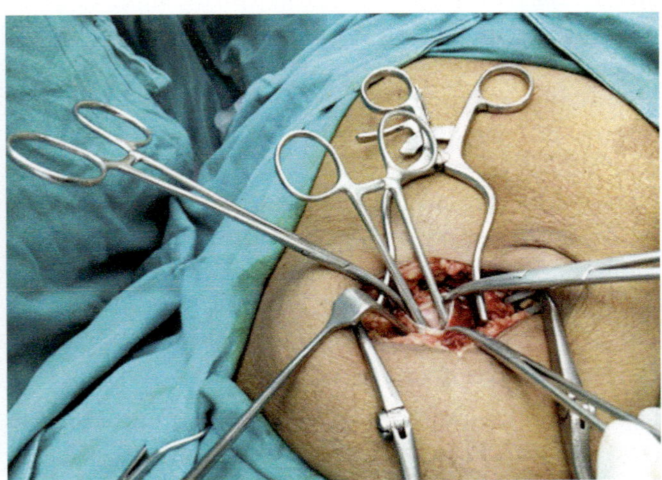

Fig. 5: Passing of long Kelly clamp in pelvis to check for free passage.

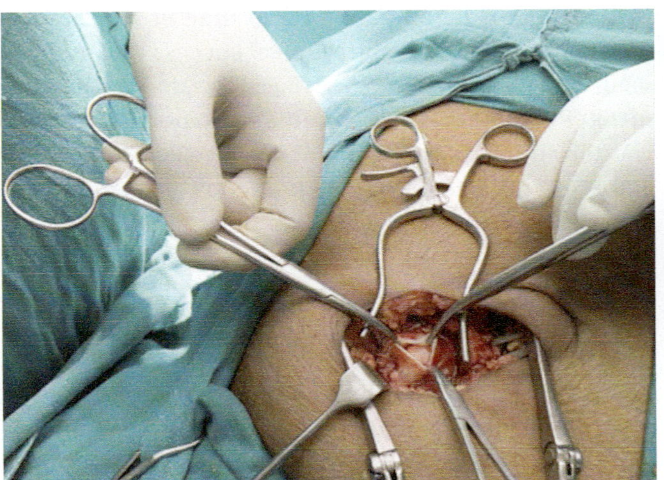

Fig. 4: Application of self-retaining retractors and opening of peritoneum after lifting.

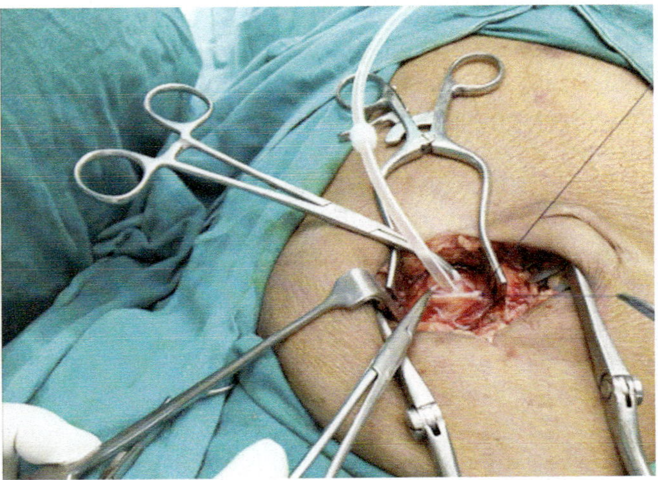

Fig. 6: Introduction of continuous ambulatory peritoneal dialysis (CAPD) catheter.

The entry site is infiltrated with a local anesthetic agent, typically 2% lignocaine. Using the provided introducer needle, insertion is performed at a 45° angle toward the pelvis under ultrasound guidance. The needle tip is positioned just beneath the peritoneum, carefully avoiding bowel loops.

Approximately 1 L of PD fluid is instilled into the peritoneal cavity through the introducer needle, and the free flow of fluid is confirmed using Doppler ultrasound. The guidewire provided in the kit is then advanced through the introducer needle, and with the PD fluid acting as a contrast medium, the guidewire is visualized within the pelvis.

The introducer needle is subsequently removed, and a vertical incision is made at the insertion site. Following dissection, the anterior rectus sheath is exposed, and a 0.5-cm transverse incision is created on the sheath. A peel-away sheath, along with the dilator, is threaded over the guidewire and directed toward the pelvis. The guidewire and dilator are then removed, and the PD catheter is inserted through the peel-away sheath into the peritoneal cavity. The deep cuff is secured to the sheath, and drainage is verified before final tightening **(Figs. 7A to F)**.

Finally, the catheter is placed within a subcutaneous tunnel and externalized through the exit site.

Laparoscopic Continuous Ambulatory Peritoneal Dialysis Insertion

Laparoscopic continuous ambulatory peritoneal dialysis (CAPD) insertion is done under general anesthesia. The patient is positioned supine, and a supraumbilical incision measuring 1–1.5 cm is made. Pneumoperitoneum is established using a Veress needle with carbon dioxide insufflation at a pressure of 12–14 mm Hg. A 10-mm port is inserted, and a laparoscopic camera is introduced for abdominal exploration. A 5-mm port is placed through an incision at the mid-clavicular line, at the umbilical level, and directed laterally toward a point 2 cm from the midline, midway between the umbilicus and pubic symphysis, creating a subcutaneous tunnel. The patient is then tilted to a 30º Trendelenburg position. The PD catheter is passed through the supraumbilical 10-mm port after removing the camera, with its pigtail end directed into the pouch of Douglas (in females) or the rectovesical pouch (in males) using a Maryland forceps introduced through the 5-mm port. The catheter's external end is brought out through the 5-mm port to the inner Teflon cuff under laparoscopic guidance. The 10-mm port site is closed with a purse-string suture using nonabsorbable material such as 0-0 nylon, and the catheter is secured in place with a similar stitch. On-table functionality is confirmed using normal saline. Alternative techniques include Quinton percutaneous catheter placement, the Moncrief-Popovich technique, and extended dialysis catheter methods.

COMPARISON OF IMPLANTATION TECHNIQUES

Randomized prospective studies indicate that outcomes for PD catheters placed surgically via open or laparoscopic techniques are comparable. Although the open surgical method is quicker (14.3 minutes vs. 21.9 minutes; $p < 0.0001$), there is no significant difference in early complication rates.

In one study involving 50 patients randomized to either open surgical or laparoscopic catheter placement with fixation in the pelvis and suture closure of port wounds, fluid leakage occurred in eight patients in the surgical group but in none in the laparoscopic group. Peritonitis rates were similar between the groups, while tip migration occurred in five patients in the open surgical group and in none in the laparoscopic group. These findings suggest that laparoscopic placement results in better catheter function, allowing for the immediate initiation of dialysis without fluid leakage.[7] Additionally, laparoscopic placement facilitates simultaneous performance of other procedures, which is a distinct advantage.[8]

Percutaneous placement of PD catheters, when performed by experienced practitioners, is a well-tolerated procedure that enables rapid initiation of CAPD without requiring operating room time or a peritoneal incision. It boasts a high technical success rate and can often be done on an outpatient basis. A retrospective study of 230 PD catheters—50 placed percutaneously and 180 via conventional surgical methods—revealed comparable catheter survival rates. Percutaneous placement was typically nonelective, reserved for older patients or those unable to undergo general anesthesia or HD. These patients, often with significant underlying conditions, experienced shorter catheter use durations due to early mortality and mechanical failures. Peritonitis rates, however, were similar between the groups.[9]

A recent meta-analysis found no significant differences among the techniques in terms of peritonitis risk, catheter removal or replacement, technical failure, or all-cause mortality.[10]

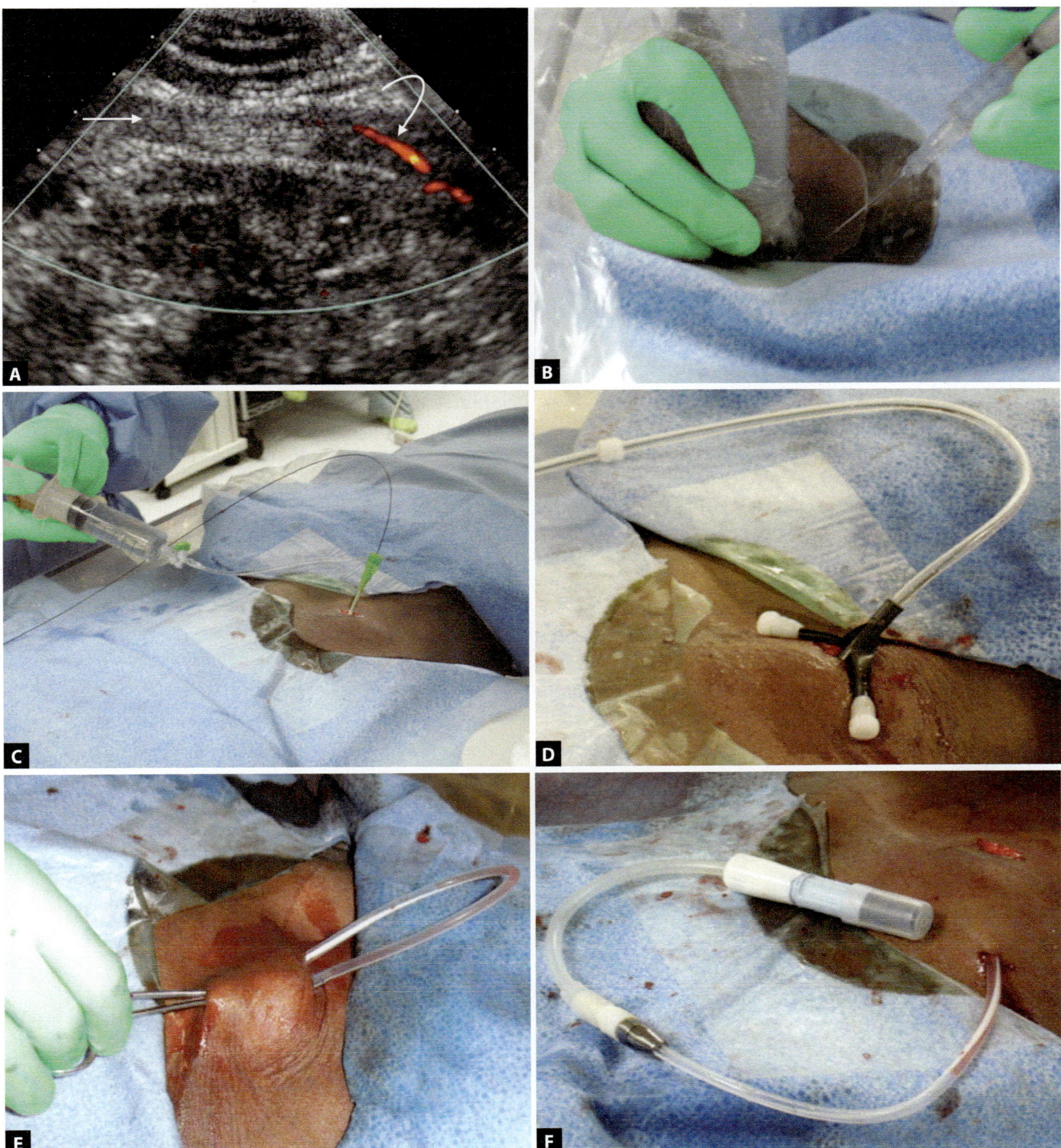

Figs. 7A to F: Various steps in ultrasound guided continuous ambulatory peritoneal dialysis insertion. (A) Color Doppler USG showing epigastric artery (curved arrow) traversing rectus abdominis muscle (straight arrow); (B) Insertion of micro-puncture needle angled 45° caudally; (C) Infusion of normal saline through side arm of introducer sheath; (D) Insertion of catheter over stiff wire, through peel-away sheath; (E) Catheter tunneled through subcutaneous tissue; (F) Extension catheter connected to titanium adaptor.

In our view, both open and laparoscopic techniques are suitable for primary PD catheter placement in patients with no history of prior abdominal surgery. However, in cases involving previous abdominal surgery, the laparoscopic approach is preferred due to its ability to perform adhesiolysis. Additionally, laparoscopic techniques can diagnose and address persistent PD catheter malfunctions, such as those caused by adhesions, omental wrapping, or fibrin clots, during the same procedure. For patients unable to tolerate general anesthesia, percutaneous placement is an appropriate alternative.[11,12]

POST-PERITONEAL DIALYSIS CATHETER INSERTION CARE

The dressing change for the PD catheter should be done by a healthcare provider using sterile technique after a minimum of 7 days following insertion. An earlier dressing change may be necessary if there is visible bleeding or concern about infection. The new dressing should remain in place for another 7 days. Only normal saline should be used to clean the exit site and skin incision. After 2 weeks, prophylactic mupirocin cream or gentamicin can be applied to the exit site. Healing typically takes about 21 days, during which the exit site should be kept dry. Only sponge baths are allowed during this time. Dialysis using the PD catheter usually starts 3–4 weeks after placement. Patients should be advised to avoid heavy lifting for 4 weeks post procedure to prevent dislodging the deep rectus abdominis cuff.

COMPLICATIONS OF CONTINUOUS AMBULATORY PERITONEAL DIALYSIS CATHETER INSERTION

The relative effectiveness of HD and CAPD remains uncertain due to the lack of robust randomized controlled trials.[13] However, CAPD is less expensive than hemodialysis, offers comparable short-term survival, and can be performed at home. CAPD provides additional benefits, including better blood pressure control, improved preservation of residual kidney function, fewer dietary restrictions, and minimal cardiovascular stress.[14,15] As a result, CAPD is often preferred for diabetic patients and those with vascular access challenges or poor cardiac conditions. Many patients opt for CAPD due to the flexibility it offers, allowing them to maintain daily activities and enjoy greater independence and mobility compared to HD.

Despite these advantages, CAPD has notable complications.

The complications of PD catheter are divided into early (within 30 days) and late (within >30 days)[16] **(Table 1)**.

Infectious Complications

Infectious complications are the most common limiting factor to the use of CAPD in long term. Bacterial peritonitis is the most common cause leading to cessation of CAPD, and significantly contributing to morbidity. In order to prevent infections in PD, certain measures are advised and are provided in **Table 2**.

Noninfectious Complications

Noninfectious complications that are clinically important include catheter malfunctions, complications related to increased intra-abdominal pressure (leaks, hernias, and hydrothorax). The presence of dialysate in the peritoneal cavity leads to increased intra-abdominal pressure, which

TABLE 1: Complications of PD catheter are divided into early (within 30 days) and late (within >30 days).

Early complications	*Late complications*
Bleeding	Exit site infection
Bowel perforation	Cuff protrusion
Wound infection	Dialysate leaks
Catheter leakage	Tunnel infection
Outflow failure	Catheter migration
Peritonitis	Hernias

TABLE 2: Measures to prevent infections in peritoneal dialysis (PD).

Timeline	*Intervention*
Pre-PD	• Surgical evaluation, mapping of location of exit site • Patient education on catheter care and healing • Home visit assessment; identifying risk factors for infections (pets, hygiene)
Transition to PD	• Perioperative antibiotics • Selection of double cuff catheter
Post-PD initiation	• Exit site gentamicin/mupirocin • Prophylactic antibiotic use, and antifungal prophylaxis • Prevention of hypokalemia and constipation

increases in proportion to the instilled dialysate volume. Generally, early leaks are thought to be related to catheter insertion techniques, strength of abdominal wall tissues, and time of initiation of dialysis.

The current International Society for Peritoneal Dialysis (ISPD) guidelines recommend a 2-week break in period before starting elective PD. Specific catheter insertion-related interventions to mitigate early complications include utilization of fibrin glue and additional purse-string sutures at the level of deep cuff as well as near the peritoneal membrane. Stopping PD temporarily or employing regimens with minimal impact on intra-abdominal pressure is usually effective in treating early leaks.

Late leaks (>30 days) are often related to mechanical tears in the peritoneum, resulting in extravasation of dialysate into the abdominal wall and external genitalia. CT scans after intraperitoneal contrast and images taken 2–3 hours after dialysate instillation are utilized to visualize these leaks. Abdominal wall leaks necessitate cessation of PD for 1–2 weeks to allow for healing of the leak.

Another late complication of PD is catheter malfunction that can be only outflow or both outflow and inflow. Main causes of obstruction are constipation, catheter tip migration, or omental or bowel wrap.

Flowchart 1: Diagnostic measures for catheter malfunction.

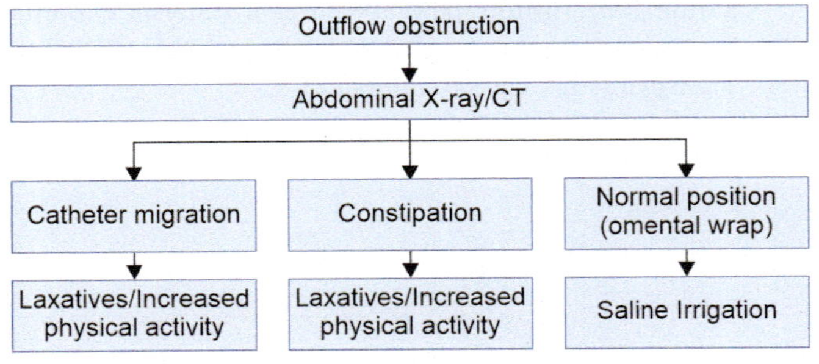

Flowchart 2: Treatment measures for catheter malfunction.

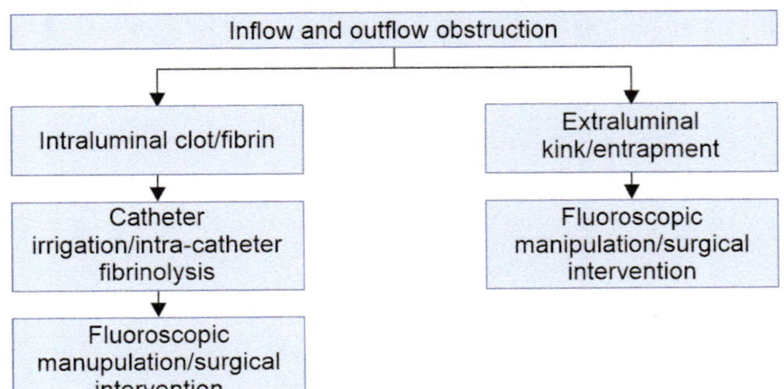

Diagnostic and treatment measures for catheter malfunction are detailed in **Flowcharts 1 and 2**.

If conservative treatments such as laxatives and increased physical activity or saline irrigation of the catheter fails and inflow outflow obstruction still persist, then more invasive management is required as described in **Flowchart 2**.

Surgical intervention can be in form of laparoscopic or open re-exploration under general anesthesia with repositioning of catheter with or without omentectomy.

CONCLUSION

A successful PD program relies heavily on the proper placement of permanent PD catheters, along with a thorough understanding of implantation techniques and potential complications. While the type of catheter used typically does not significantly affect outcomes, the method of placement can offer distinct advantages.

The open surgical technique is favored for its simplicity and accessibility. Surgical residents with experience in abdominal procedures can easily perform this method. Adhesions near the incision site can be dissected with relative ease, and closing the peritoneum and rectus sheath is straightforward, potentially reducing postoperative dialysate leakage.

In contrast, the laparoscopic technique offers advantages such as enhanced visualization of the abdominal cavity, more precise catheter placement with the option of suture fixation, and the ability to perform adhesiolysis, thereby reducing catheter placement failure.

Despite these advancements, PD catheter implantation is associated with complications such as dialysate leakage, exit-site infections, hernias, genital edema, and other discomforts. Catheter malfunction, reported in up to 60% of PD patients, can result from issues such as kinking, displacement, omental wrapping, fibrin coating, or adhesions from prior abdominal infections. Additionally, exit-site and subcutaneous tract infections, along with peritonitis, remain significant concerns. Peritonitis is particularly serious, accounting for 30% of catheter failures and recurring at a rate of approximately 0.5 episodes per patient per year.

A successful PD program also depends on a multidisciplinary approach and a committed healthcare team. Enthusiasm and collaboration among team members are essential to improving catheter outcomes and ensuring long-term success.

REFERENCES

1. Blagg CR. The early history of dialysis for chronic renal failure in the United States: a view from Seattle. Am J Kidney Dis. 2007;3:482-96.
2. Eklund BH. Surgical implantation of CAPD catheters: Presentation of midline incision-lateral placement method and a review of 110 procedures. Nephrol Dial Transpl. 1995;10:386-90.
3. Crabtree JH. Who should place peritoneal dialysis catheters? Perit Dial Int. 2010;30(2):142-50.
4. Crabtree JH. Selected best demonstrated practices in peritoneal dialysis access. Kidney Int Suppl. 2006;103: S27-37.
5. Johnson DW, Wong J, Wiggins KJ, Kirwan R, Griffin A, Preston J, et al. A randomized controlled trial of coiled vs. straight swan-neck Tenckhoff catheters in peritoneal dialysis patients. Am J Kidney Dis. 2006;48:812-21.
6. Davidson JC, Rahim S, Hanks SE, Patel IJ, Tam AL, Walker TG, et al. Society of Interventional Radiology Consensus Guidelines for the Periprocedural Management of Thrombotic and Bleeding Risk in Patients Undergoing Percutaneous Image-Guided Interventions - Part I: Review of anticoagulation agents and clinical considerations: endorsed by the Canadian Association for Interventional Radiology and the Cardiovascular and Interventional Radiological Society of Europe. J Vasc Interv Radiol. 2019;30(8):1155-67.
7. Wright MJ, Bel'eed K, Johnson BF, Eadington DW, Sellars L, Farr MJ. Randomized prospective comparison of laparoscopic and open peritoneal dialysis catheter insertion. Perit Dial Int. 1999;19:372-5.
8. Tsimoyiannis EC, Siakas P, Glantzounis G, Toli C, Sferopoulos G, Pappas M, et al. Laparoscopic placement of the Tenckhoff catheter for peritoneal dialysis. Surg Laparosc Endosc Percutan Tech. 2000;10:218-21.
9. Georgiades CS, Geschwind JF. Percutaneous peritoneal dialysis catheter placement for the management of end-stage renal disease: technique and comparison with the surgical approach. Tech Vasc Interv Radiol. 2002;5:103-7.
10. Strippoli GFM, Tong A, Johnson D, Schena FP, Craig JC. Catheter-related interventions to prevent peritonitis in peritoneal dialysis: a systematic review of randomized, controlled trials. J Am Soc Nephrol. 2004;15:2735-46.
11. Mellotte GJ, Ho CA, Morgan SH, Bending MR, Eisinger AJ. Peritoneal dialysis catheters: a comparison between percutaneous and conventional surgical placement techniques. Nephrol Dial Transplant. 1993;8:626-30.
12. Ozener C, Bihorac A, Akoglu E. Technical survival of CAPD catheters: comparison between percutaneous and conventional surgical placement techniques. Nephrol Dial Transplant. 2001;16:1893-9.
13. Vale L, Cody J, Wallace S, Daly C, Campbell M, Grant A, et al. Continuous ambulatory peritoneal dialysis (CAPD) versus hospital or home haemodialysis for end-stage renal disease in adults. Cochrane Database Syst Rev. 2004;(4):CD003963.
14. Feriani M, Dell'Aquila R, La Greca G. The treatment of diabetic end-stage renal disease with peritoneal dialysis. Nephrol Dial Transplant. 1998;13(suppl 8):53-6.
15. Khalili K, Lan FP, Hanbidge AE, Muradali D, Oreopoulos DG, Wanless IR. Hepatic subcapsular steatosis in response to intraperitoneal insulin delivery: CT findings and prevalence. AJR Am J Roentgenol. 2003;180(6):1601-4.
16. Peppelenbosch A, van Kuijk WHM, Bouvy ND, van der Sande FM, Tordoir JHM. Peritoneal dialysis catheter placement technique and complications. Nephrol Dialysis Transplant Plus. 2008;1(suppl 4):23-8.

CHAPTER

48 Complications Related to Peritoneal Dialysis Catheters

48.1 NON-INFECTIOUS COMPLICATIONS

Santosh Varughese, Manish Lalwani

INTRODUCTION

In 1980, a peritoneal dialysis (PD) patient named Watson became the subject of one of the earliest documented cases of delayed intestinal perforation—a rare but serious noninfectious complication of PD catheter placement. Watson had been on PD for several months without issue when he suddenly developed abdominal pain and dialysate retention. Initial investigations were inconclusive, as free air on imaging was a common finding in PD patients. However, further evaluation revealed a sigmoid colon perforation caused by the catheter, an event so rare at the time that it was first described in the medical literature that same year.

This case underscored the importance of recognizing and managing noninfectious PD complications, which, though often less discussed than infections, can be equally detrimental to catheter function and patient outcomes. Understanding the risk factors, diagnostic approaches, and management strategies for such issues is crucial in ensuring optimal PD catheter function and long-term treatment success.

COMPLICATIONS RELATED TO PERITONEAL DIALYSIS CATHETERS

Complications related to PD catheters are given in **Table 1**.

Classification as per timing of complications is shown in **Flowchart 1**.

TABLE 1: Complications related to peritoneal dialysis catheters.

Complication	*Early complications (n, %)*	*Late complications (n, %)*
Pericatheter bleeding	1 (0.7%)	–
Visceral perforation	0 (0%)	–
Obstruction	1 (0.7%)	0 (0%)
Leakage	4 (2%)	13 (9.8%)
Migration	2 (1.5%)	14 (10.4%)
Omental wrapping	0 (0%)	2 (1.5%)
Exit-site infection	0 (0%)	11 (8.2%)
Tunnel infection	0 (0%)	6 (4.5%)
Peritonitis	3 (2.2%)	1 episode/21.1 patient-months
Hernia	–	2 (1.5%)
External cuff extrusion	–	0 (0%)

Flowchart 1: Classification as per timing of complications.

During insertion	*After insertion*	*While removal*
• Perforation • Bladder perforation • Bleeding • Malposition	• Decreased flow – Malposition • Pericatheter leak • Dialysate leak • Pain – Back pain – Inflow pain – Drain pain • Hemoperitoneum	• Bowel injury • Retained catheter

Intestinal Perforation

Intestinal perforation occurs in approximately 1% or less of all PD catheter placements. The risk is generally independent of the placement technique but may be slightly higher with semirigid, acute PD catheters. The trocar technique carries a higher risk, whereas using a Veress needle could reduce the likelihood of perforation.

Clinical clues to diagnosis: Perforation should be suspected in PD patients presenting with acute abdominal pain after catheter implantation. Key clinical signs include:

- Feculent or bloody dialysate
- Dialysate retention
- Diarrhea after dialysate instillation
- High stool glucose concentration, indicating stool/dialysate admixture
- Gram-negative peritonitis

Rare causes of perforation: A rare but notable cause involves physical injury during percutaneous needle-guidewire catheter insertion. This risk increases if a peritoneal loose body (PLB) is present beneath the bowel. PLBs are solid masses, typically gray or white, that originate from twisted, infarcted, and detached epiploic appendages. These fibrotic masses move freely within the cavity and may serve as a fulcrum, increasing the risk of bowel injury.

Diagnostic approach: Imaging with computed tomography (CT) is the preferred diagnostic tool. Plain radiographs are less effective, as free air is commonly seen in PD patients even without perforation. If not obvious on CT, addition of single-photon emission computed tomography may be helpful in accurate diagnosis and for precise localization of the site of the perforation.

Delayed intestinal perforation is exceedingly rare, with approximately 40 cases reported since Watson's first documentation in 1980. The sigmoid colon is the most commonly affected site, though other areas, such as the small intestine and rectum, have also been implicated.

Risk factors for perforation: Key factors include:

- Diseases of the bowel (e.g., diverticulitis, colon amyloidosis)
- Abdominal wall adhesions
- Use of immunosuppressants
- Increased abdominal pressure from conditions such as polycystic kidney disease
- Prolonged suspension of the catheter without removal
- Nonstandard treatment or prolonged peritonitis

Bladder Perforation

Incidence and Risk Factors

- *Incidence:* Rare, with <1% risk of internal organ perforation during PD catheter placement.
- *Risk factors:*
  - Incomplete bladder emptying (e.g., neurogenic bladder, outlet obstruction)
  - Diabetes, abdominal/pelvic surgery history
  - Intra-abdominal adhesions,
  - Distended bladder preoperatively

Timing and Symptoms

- *Timing:* Usually occurs perioperatively (1 day to 2 weeks postsurgery)
- *Symptoms:* Urgency to void, increased urine output, urinary incontinence, bladder discomfort during PD fills, hematuria, cloudy dialysate, drainage obstruction, or signs mimicking a urinary tract infection (UTI).

Diagnosis

Cystoscopy or cystography; imaging (e.g., CT, ultrasound); indicators include high glucose in urine, dialysate admixture, or clinical symptoms.

We encountered a notable case of bladder perforation in a patient with chronic kidney disease (CKD) caused by long-standing bladder outlet obstruction (BOO). Chronic BOO had led to significant compensatory changes in the bladder wall, characterized by marked hypertrophy and thickening. During corrective surgery, the bladder wall appeared unusually thick and firm, a condition we refer to as a "muskmelon bladder" (unpublished observation), indicative of chronic remodeling and fibrosis due to prolonged obstruction and increased intravesical pressure. Notably, such thick-walled bladders may be at an increased risk for injury.

Bladder perforation is largely preventable by making the patient void to completion prior to the PD catheter insertion and confirmation of the same by ultrasonography. Alternatively, routine preprocedural bladder catheterization, as practiced in some centers, may be beneficial **(Figs. 1A and B)**.

Bleeding

Bleeding that occurs soon after catheter placement is most often due to trauma of small blood vessels located in the abdominal wall and presents as bloody peritoneal dialysate (hemoperitoneum). Mostly, bleeding is mild and can be managed conservatively if the patient's vital signs are stable. The severity of the bleed is gauged by measuring the hematocrit of the effluent whenever there is persistent bleeding. Until the hematocrit decreases beyond 2% from the baseline, conservative treatment will suffice[1] and heparinization of the fluid is enough to prevent clotting of the catheter.

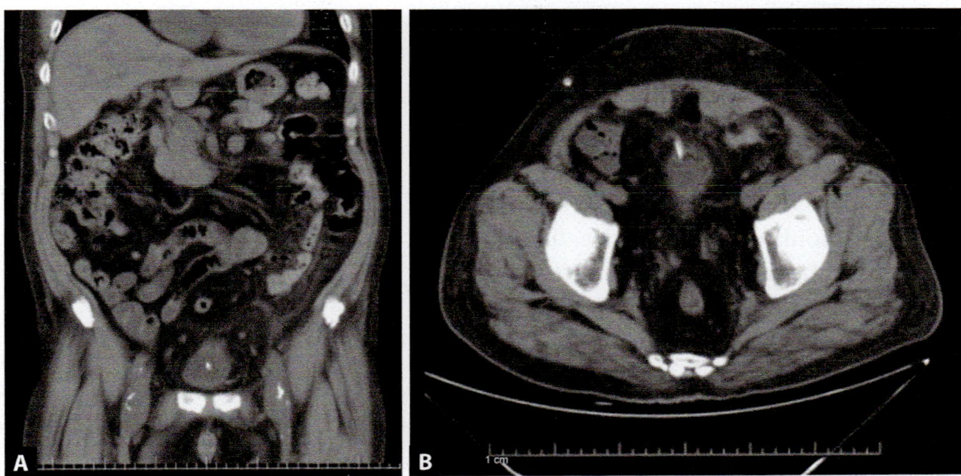

Figs. 1A and B: Peritoneal dialysis (PD) catheter entering bladder wall.
Source: Shi CX, Li ZX, Sun HT, Sun WQ, Ji Y, Jia SJ. Bladder perforation injury after percutaneous peritoneal dialysis catheterization: A case report. World J Clin Cases. 2022;10(20):7054-9.

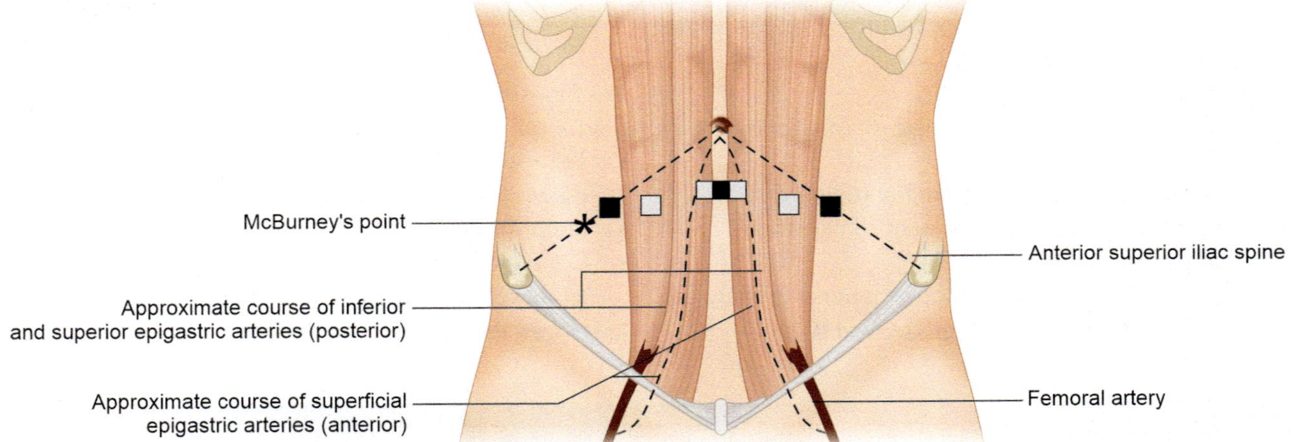

Fig. 2: Operative considerations for peritoneal dialysis catheter insertion.
Source: Ash SR, Narayan R, Agarwal AK. Operative Considerations for Peritoneal Dialysis Catheter. In: Yevzlin AS, Asif A, Salman L, Ramani K, Qaqish SS, Vachharajani TJ (Eds). Interventional Nephrology. Cham: Springer; 2022.

Anticoagulants and clopidogrel should be withheld before percutaneous insertion of PD catheter; however, aspirin need not be withheld. Where urgent-start PD was required, we (SV and ML) have inserted PD catheters percutaneously with minimal dissection and no bleeding. Inferior epigastric artery (IEA) injury is a rare entity that is often iatrogenic in nature following abdominal wall interventions, though occasionally spontaneous, seen more commonly among patients with underlying coagulopathy.[2] IEA injury can be minimized by midline incision and by using ultrasonography to identify the vessel **(Fig. 2)**.

Malposition

When placing the catheter under C-arm guidance, any malposition detected on the table must be corrected before tunneling (described in the next section).

Outflow Failure

Outflow failure occurs when the volume of drained dialysate is significantly less than the inflow volume, without evidence of pericatheter leakage. It often happens soon after catheter placement but may also occur during/after peritonitis or at any time during the catheter's lifespan. Disruption of the shape memory of a PD catheter at the time of insertion may be a factor responsible for tip migration and late catheter dysfunction.

Common causes and management

- *Constipation and urinary retention:*
  - A distended rectosigmoid colon can block catheter side holes or displace the tip. Bladder compression due to urinary retention is less common. It is usually diagnosed by abdominal radiography which shows fecal-filled colon or catheter displacement.
  - *Treatment:*
    - Sorbitol solution (70%), 30 mL every 2 hours until effective
    - Polyethylene glycol (2 L over 4–6 hours) for persistent cases
    - Refractory cases: Stimulant laxatives (bisacodyl) or saline enemas (use cautiously to avoid bacterial migration/peritonitis) or lactulose enemas
- *Tubing kink:*
  - *Cause:* Mechanical kinking leads to two-way obstruction.
  - *Diagnosis:* Flat-plate abdominal radiograph
  - *Treatment:* Catheter revision or replacement
- *Fibrin strands and plug:*
  - It can be prevented by adding heparin to dialysate to prevent fibrin clots **(Figs. 3A and B)**.
  - *Treatment:*
    - Irrigation with heparin (often ineffective if obstruction has occurred) ± thrombolytic therapy with tissue plasminogen activator (tPA) if heparin fails. Recovery of flow with tPA approaches 100% for fibrin clots.
    - tPA is instilled after unsuccessful saline irrigation.
- *Malposition*: Peritoneal dialysis catheter migration is a common complication that can impair dialysate outflow, occurring in *12.7–35%* of patients. Surgical revision is often required in *85–90%* of cases **(Figs. 4A and B)**. Migration typically manifests in three patterns:[3]
  1. *Lateral migration*—catheter tip points against the abdominopelvic sidewall
  2. *Superior migration*—catheter tip points toward the hypochondrial region
  3. *Looping migration*—catheter tip loops back on itself

Predisposing factors: Several factors contribute to catheter migration, including:

- Truncal obesity
- Right-sided or downward tunnel direction
- Small-bowel ileus or absence of peristalsis
- Constipation

However, peritoneal wall anchor techniques (PWAT) have been described to prevent migration of the catheter.

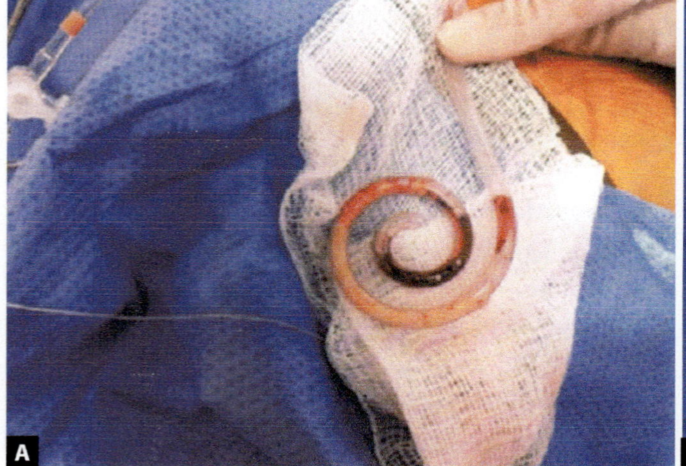

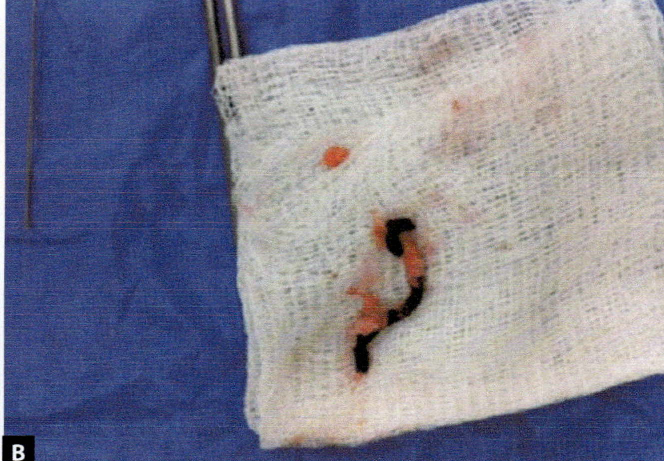

Figs. 3A and B: (A) Fibrin sheath and clots in a coiled peritoneal dialysis (PD) catheter; (B) Debris after being manually removed from the catheter.

Source: Narayan R, Fried T, Chica G, Schaefer M, Mullins D. Minimally invasive fluoroscopic percutaneous peritoneal dialysis catheter salvage. Clin Kidney J. 2014;7(3):264-8.

Management options: Management of PD catheter migration involves conservative, nonoperative, and operative approaches:

- *Conservative measures:*
  - Observation for self-correction is a reasonable initial approach, as spontaneous relocation can occur, though it is rare.

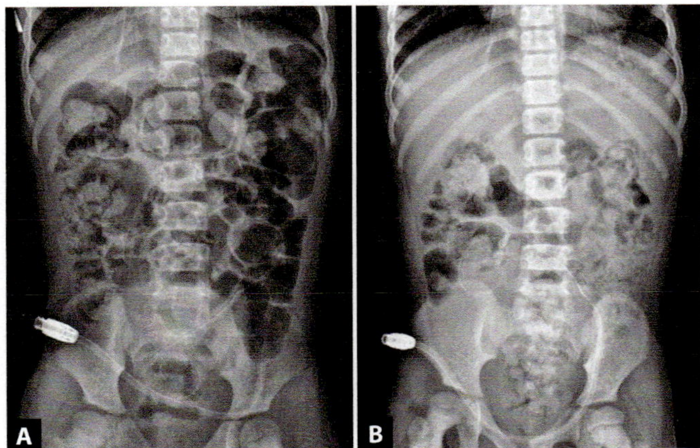

Figs. 4A and B: Normal position of the catheter tip in the pelvic cavity.
Source: Cho MY. Infectious and non-infectious complications of peritoneal dialysis in children. Child Kidney Dis. 2020;24(2):63-8.

- *Nonoperative techniques*:
  - *Fluoroscopy-guidewire manipulation:* This method has a high technical success rate (*85%*) and a clinical success rate of *45–55%*, but it is more complex and costly, with a greater risk of complications.
  - *Fogarty catheter manipulation:* The Fogarty catheter is advanced into the PD catheter, the balloon inflated with sterile saline, and gentle tugging maneuvers performed. Success is confirmed via X-ray and dialysis inflow/outflow. A study of 232 patients reported a *70% success rate* for this method. However, our experience showed success in only *10%* of cases.
  - *Foley catheter stylet or guidewire manipulation* may also be attempted.
- *Operative techniques:*
  - Novel percutaneous catheter repositioning: Using a guidewire through the exit site, percutaneously dissecting the deep cuff free of the surrounding soft tissue, removing and subsequently reinserting the intraperitoneal part of the PD catheter have about 65% success rate at 6 months **(Fig. 5).**[4]
  - *Laparoscopic repositioning:* A minimally invasive option with high success rates but associated with greater cost and complexity

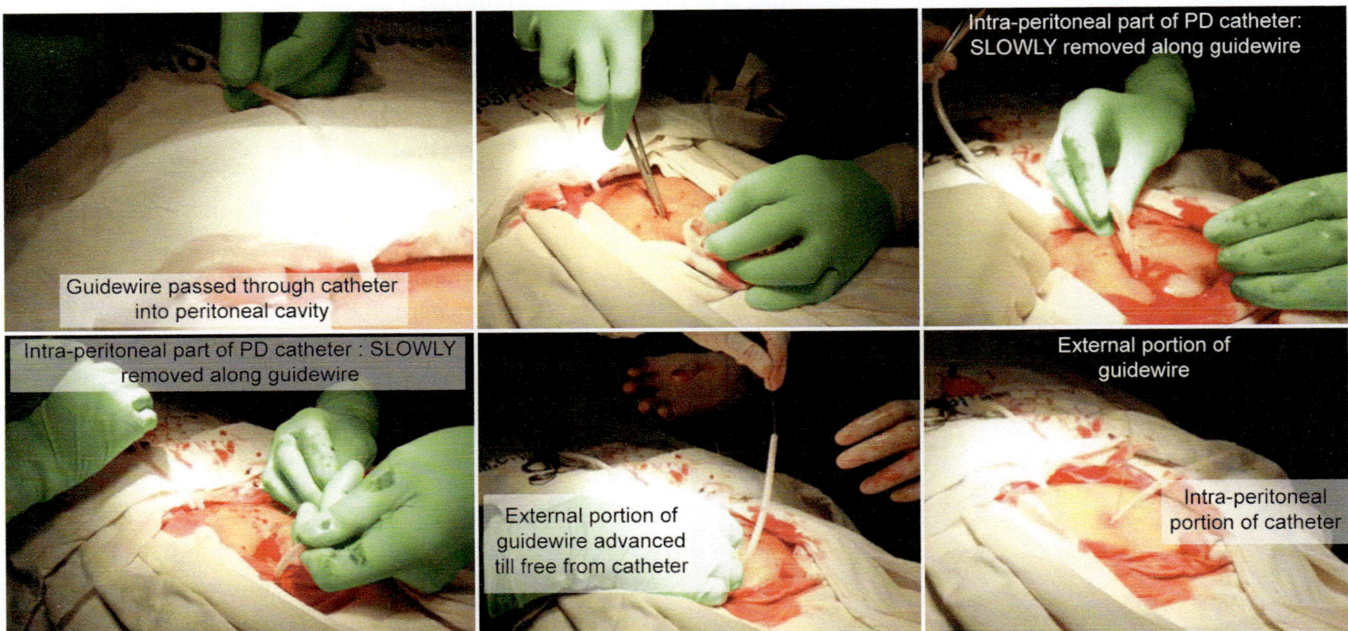

Fig. 5: Novel percutaneous method of peritoneal dialysis (PD) catheter repositioning.
Source: Varughese V, Alexander S, Valson AT, Mohapatra A, David VG, Jacob S, et al. Blind Bedside Peritoneal Dialysis Catheter Repositioning: An Innovative Technique. Indian J Nephrol. 2021;31(3):311-3.

- *Open surgical revision:* This remains the definitive option when all other methods fail. Open surgery has its risks, including *peritonitis, adhesions*, and *dialysis leakage*.

Catheter manipulation for outflow failure: If constipation, urinary retention, tubing kinks, and fibrinolytic therapy fail, obstruction from omentum or adhesions is presumed. Radiologic or laparoscopic interventions are performed. A catheterogram is ideal in this situation **(Fig. 6)**.

- *Radiological intervention*
  - *Procedure:* Fluoroscopic guidewire manipulation redirects displaced or obstructed catheters. Stiff guidewire manipulation can be difficult for catheters with a swan-neck bend. Long-term function is restored in 45–73% of cases. Failure rates are higher (up to 90%) with prior abdominopelvic surgery or peritonitis, likely due to adhesions.
- *Laparoscopic intervention*
  - *Advantages:* Identifies and treats the obstruction reliably
  - *Procedure:*
    - *Omental entrapment:* Strip omentum from the catheter using grasping forceps. Perform omentopexy (suturing omentum to the upper abdomen) to prevent recurrence.
    - *Epiploic appendices/uterine fimbria obstruction:* Laparoscopic resection resolves the issue.
    - *Adhesions:* Laparoscopic adhesiolysis or freeing the catheter. However, adhesiolysis has a 30% failure rate due to adhesion reformation.

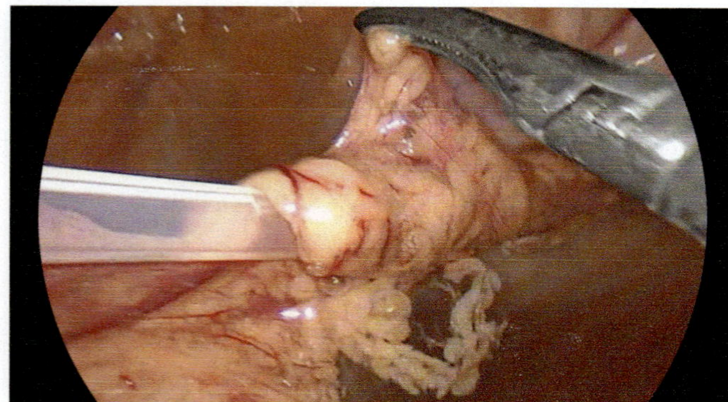

Fig. 6: Omental wrap.
Source: David VL, Mussuto E, Stroescu RF, Gafencu M, Boia ES. Peritoneal Dialysis Catheter Placement in Children: Initial Experience with a "2+1"-Port Laparoscopic-assisted Technique. Medicina. 2023;59(5):961.

- *Catheter tip migration:* Common with straight catheters due to shape-memory forces. Repositioning alone has a high failure rate.
  - *Solution:* Place a laparoscopic suture sling around the catheter and abdominal wall to keep the catheter in position. Sutures to pelvic structures are avoided due to erosion risk.

Pericatheter Leak[5]

The incidence of pericatheter leak is 2–6%.

Risk factors for pericatheter dialysate leaks

- *Early PD initiation:* Starting PD less than 2 weeks after catheter insertion (common in urgent-start PD)
  - *Technical issues during catheter insertion:* Suture failure, inadequate surgical wound closure, improper catheter placement
- Pericatheter hernia development
- Tunnel infections

Clinical manifestations

Swelling in the subcutaneous tissue may precede obvious external fluid leakage. Followed by *visible fluid leakage* around the catheter exit site. Abdominal wall and/or genital edema may occur, even without visible leakage. This can result from peritoneal membrane defects near the catheter tract.

Diagnostic approach

- *Glucose testing:*
  - Perform glucose strip testing on extravasated fluid. *Positive test*: Extremely high glucose concentration indicates *dextrose-containing dialysate*.
- *Imaging*:
  - If leakage is not apparent but suspected (e.g., unexplained outflow failure or abdominal/genital edema), imaging should be performed.
  - *CT peritoneography*:
    - Infusion of contrast-containing dialysate followed by CT imaging is diagnostic.

Management of Pericatheter Leaks[3]

Cuff Extrusion

The incidence is 4–17%.

Cuff extrusion through the exit site can occur due to several factors, including improper positioning, mechanical stress, and infections. An extruded cuff becomes a *bacterial reservoir* near the exit wound. *Daily wetting* of the cuff during routine care exacerbates bacterial contamination, interfering with exit-site hygiene.[6]

Sonographic imaging is critical to evaluate infection in the catheter tunnel or cuffs, as physical examination alone may not optimally assess these areas, particularly at early stages. Evidence of *fluid collection* in the catheter tunnel or near the superficial/deep cuff significantly predicts catheter loss **(Fig. 7)**.[7]

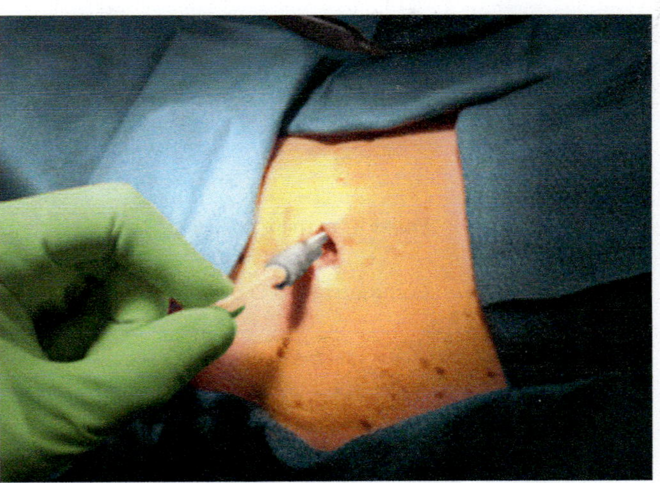

Fig. 7: Cuff extrusion.
Source: Thoracic Key. Mechanical Complications of Peritoneal Dialysis. [online] Available from https://thoracickey.com/mechanical-complications-of-peritoneal-dialysis/ [Last accessed November, 2025].

Pain

Pain as a complication can be back pain, inflow pain, or drain pain. The characteristics of all three are described in **Table 2**.

Pleuroperitoneal Leak

The incidence is 1.6–10%.

The development of a pleural effusion (hydrothorax) in patients on continuous ambulatory peritoneal dialysis (CAPD) may be caused by systemic volume overload, heart failure, or a localized pleural issue. If pleural effusion

TABLE 2: Characteristics of types of pain complications.

Feature	*Back pain*	*Inflow pain*	*Drain pain*
Definition	Pain in the lumbar spine due to mechanical stress, poor posture, or underlying spinal issues	Pain during dialysate infusion into the peritoneal cavity	Pain during the draining phase of peritoneal dialysis
Causes	• Increased intra-abdominal pressure due to CAPD • Lordotic posture • Poor abdominal muscle tone • Degenerative disk disease, osteoporosis	• Acidic pH of conventional dialysate (pH 5.2–5.5) • Poor catheter position • Dialysate temperature Hypertonic glucose solution	• Negative hydraulic pressure during drainage • Catheter abutting bowel, bladder, or peritoneum • Long or malpositioned catheter • Diminished peritoneal space (e.g., polycystic kidneys, uterus)
Risk factors	• CAPD patients • Poor muscle conditioning • Degenerative spine disease	• Use of acidic dialysate • Hypertonic solutions • Poor catheter position	• Use of APD over CAPD • Polycystic kidney disease • Female sex • Constipation
Clinical presentation	• Chronic or acute lower back pain • Possible sciatica	• Abdominal discomfort during infusion • Usually resolves during dwell phase	• Abdominal discomfort (mild to severe) • Referred pain in rectum or perineum
Management/ Treatment	• Decrease dialysate fill volume • Switch to CCPD • Supine position during dialysis *Severe cases:* Switch to hemodialysis	• Raise dialysate pH (use bicarbonate solutions) • Slow infusion rate • Inject local anesthetics into dialysate • Incomplete drainage after dwell • Catheter replacement • Discontinue peritoneal dialysis (severe cases)	• Treat constipation (laxatives) • Switch to tidal PD (TPD) • Evaluate catheter position via radiograph • Catheter repositioning/replacement • Switch to CAPD (gravity-based drainage) • Discontinue peritoneal dialysis (severe cases)

Contd...

Contd...

Feature	*Back pain*	*Inflow pain*	*Drain pain*
Key interventions	• Adjust dialysis modality to CCPD • Posture correction	• Use bicarbonate/lactate dialysate • Local anesthetics in dialysate	• Manage constipation • Use TPD to retain some fluid • Evaluate and correct catheter issues
Severity	Varies from mild to severe	Mild to severe; often transient	Mild to severe; may require modality change
Patient population	Common in CAPD patients	More common in early PD stages	Common in APD patients (25–28% prevalence)

(APD: automated peritoneal dialysis; CAPD: continuous ambulatory peritoneal dialysis; CCPD: continuous cycling peritoneal dialysis; PD: peritoneal dialysis; TPD: tidal peritoneal dialysis)

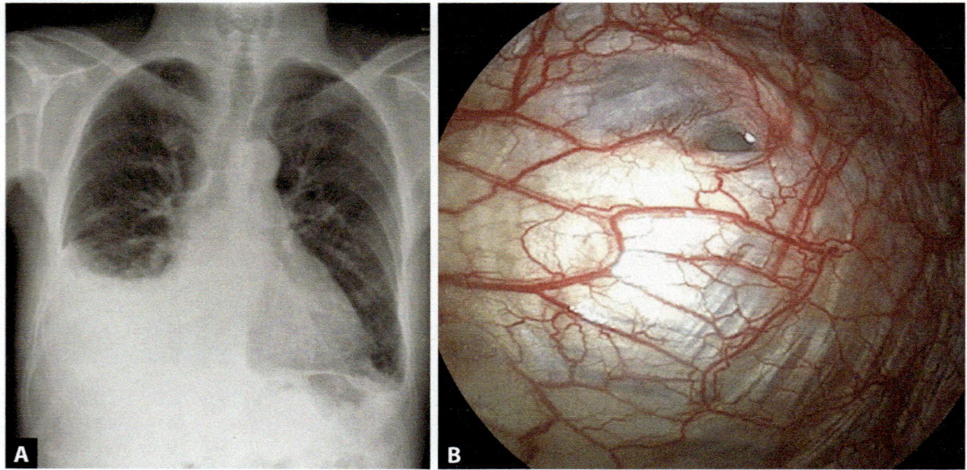

Figs. 8A and B: (A) Chest X-ray showing a right-sided pleural effusion; (B) Pleuroperitoneal leak demonstrated during video-assisted thoracoscopic surgery (VATS).
Source: Nemeth A, Mustafi M, Friedel G, Sayer M, Heyne N, Schlensak, et al. Thoracoscopic mesh implantation as a definitive treatment approach for peritoneal dialysis-associated hydrothorax. Updates Surg. 2022;74:2011-7.

is present without other signs of heart failure or peripheral edema, especially if it is confined to the right side, it should raise suspicion of a pleuroperitoneal communication.

Pleuroperitoneal defects can either be congenital, manifesting at the onset of PD, or be acquired, developing later, often years into the course of dialysis **(Figs. 8A and B)**. Suspecting a pleuroperitoneal communication can be done by keeping the abdomen dry overnight and repeating a chest radiograph in the morning to check if the pleural effusion has decreased.

The diagnosis can be further supported by finding a higher glucose concentration in the pleural fluid compared to plasma or by adding methylene blue dye to the peritoneal fluid. However, to definitively confirm the diagnosis, more advanced imaging techniques such as technetium-99 scintigraphy or MR/CT peritoneography are required.

REMOVAL OF PERITONEAL DIALYSIS CATHETERS

The most commonly used PD catheters have silicon tubing with attached Dacron cuffs. The current standard of care for PD catheter removal is by complete surgical dissection, withdrawing both the tubing and the cuffs. The intention is to avoid infection of any residual part of the catheter. A simple, noninvasive method for removing PD catheters, called the "pull technique,"[8] has become popular in recent years. Physicians still worry, however, about the range of its application and possible complications such as infection of the retained cuff and breakage. Pull technique should not be attempted if the surgeon has put a suture/anchor in deep cuff while inserting the PD catheter. The procedure must always be performed in a sterile environment and a surgical-ready room. It is important to note that catheter-removal techniques vary depending on the type of catheter and its placement method. In general, catheters placed surgically should be removed by a surgeon. An anchored catheter while pulled may cause bowel injury whereas a retained catheter may have to be removed surgically.

REFERENCES

1. Mm F, Ja F. Peritoneal dialysis: an increasingly popular option. Semin Vasc Surg. 1997;10(3):44-50.
2. Dryer EA, Abaza M, Almehmi A. Inferior epigastric artery injury after percutaneous imaging-guided peritoneal dialysis catheter placement. Radiology Case Reports. 2022;17(2):332-5.
3. Reddy YS, Manjusha Y, Kishore CK, Sridhar N, Sriramnaveen P, Sivakumar V. Spontaneous Cure of Migrated Peritoneal Catheter. Perit Dial Int. 2012;32(1):107-8.
4. Varughese S, Alexander S, Valson AT, Mohapatra A, David VG, Jacob S, et al. Blind Bedside Peritoneal Dialysis Catheter Repositioning: An Innovative Technique. Indian J Nephrol. 2021;31(3):311-3.
5. Horowitz L, Ashley J, Brassil M, Marcuzzi D, Peri J. Late Peritoneal Dialysis Exit-Site Leak: A Case Report. Kidney Med. 2023;5(7):100647.
6. Debowski JA, Wærp C, Kjellevold SA, Abedini S. Cuff extrusion in peritoneal dialysis: single-centre experience with the cuff-shaving procedure in five patients over a 4-year period. Clin Kidney J. 2017;10(1):131-4.
7. Plum J, Sudkamp S, Grabensee B. Results of ultrasound-assisted diagnosis of tunnel infections in continuous ambulatory peritoneal dialysis. Am J Kidney Dis. 1994;23(1):99-104.
8. Wang J, Li XS, Zhang FX, Wang RX, Cao F, Tang XH, et al. Minimally invasive 'pull technique' for peritoneal dialysis catheter removal. Perit Dial Int. 2021;41(1):118-21.

48.2 INFECTIOUS COMPLICATIONS

Rajdeb Saha, Saurabh Maruti Thanekar

INTRODUCTION

Peritoneal dialysis is associated with the risk of dreaded complications such as peritoneal dialysis-associated peritonitis (PDAP), exit site, and tunnel infections. Although the rate of infectious complications has drastically reduced with better antimicrobial agents, despite that peritonitis remains the "Achilles heel" for therapy failure, membrane damage, loss of ultrafiltration, and shift to hemodialysis.[1]

CASE 1

A 45-year-old female with end-stage renal disease on continuous ambulatory peritoneal dialysis (CAPD) for 1 year presented with complaints of:

- Abdominal pain, fever, and cloudy dialysate effluent. She reports that the symptoms started 24 hours ago. On examination, there is diffuse abdominal tenderness.
- The white blood cell count in the effluent is 400 cells/mL.
- A sample of the dialysate effluent is sent for Gram stain and culture sensitivity **(Fig. 1)**.
    1. **What is your diagnosis?**
    2. **How will you approach?**

Definition

The recent International Society for Peritoneal Dialysis (ISPD) guidelines published in 2022 provide a clear and comprehensive definition for PDAP.

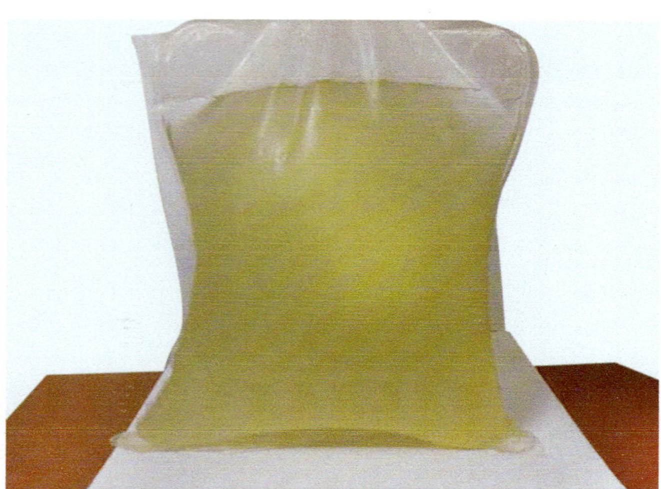

Fig. 1: Dialysate effluent fluid.

Peritonitis

A patient can be labeled as a case of peritonitis if at least two of the following criteria are met:

1. Clinical features consistent with peritonitis, that is, abdominal pain and/or cloudy dialysis effluent
2. Dialysis effluent white cell count >100/mL or >0.1 × 10^9/L (after a dwell time of at least 2 hours), with >50% polymorphonuclear leukocytes (PMN)
3. Positive dialysis effluent culture

Peritonitis is further classified by ***(Flowchart 1)****:*

- *Identification of causative organism:* Bacterial, fungal
- *Simultaneous co-infection* with exit site or tunnel collection having growth similar to effluent fluid
- *Culture-negative peritonitis*
- *Enteric peritonitis:* Peritonitis arising from an intestinal source involving processes such as inflammation, perforation, or ischemia of intra-abdominal organs.

Insertion-related peritonitis **(Fig. 2)**:

- Pre-peritoneal dialysis (PD) peritonitis
- PD catheter insertion-related peritonitis

It is an under-recognized problem, causing under-estimation of peritonitis incidence by 0.03% per patient-year (ppy).[2]

Outcome-specific definitions of peritonitis are given in **Table 1**.

Flowchart 1: Causes of peritonitis based on causative organism and concomitant event.

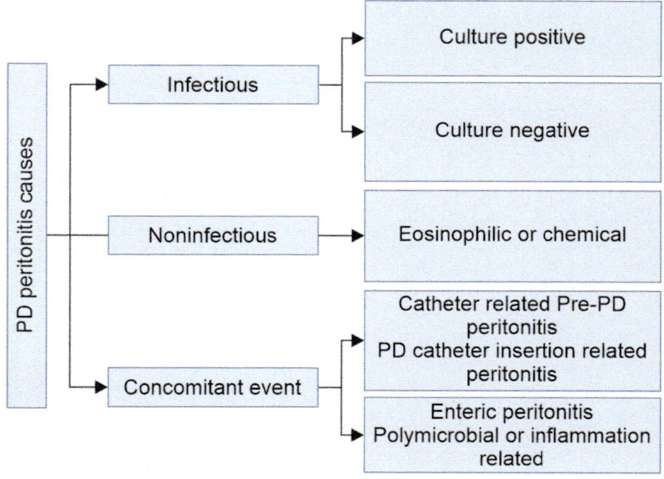

(PD: peritoneal dialysis)

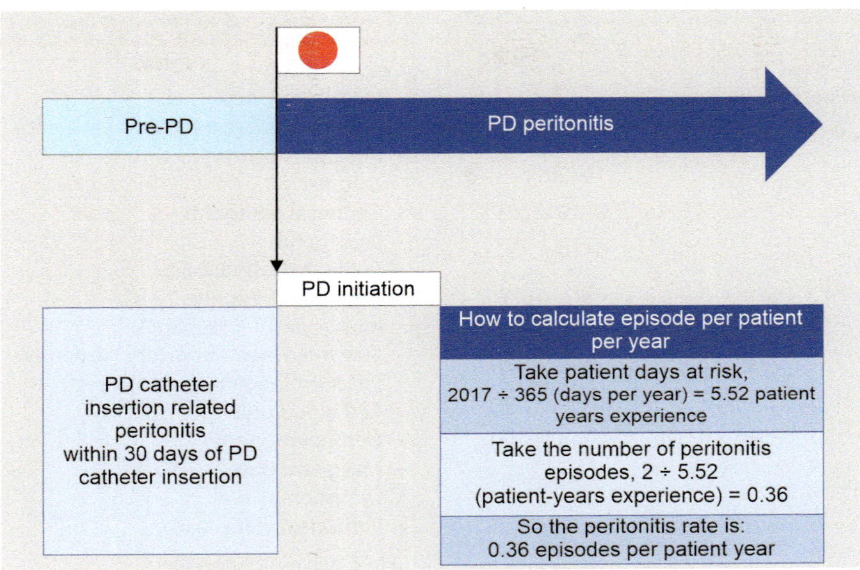

Fig. 2: Peritoneal dialysis (PD) peritonitis timeline.[3]

TABLE 1: Outcome-specific definitions of peritonitis.[2]

Outcome	*Definition*
Medical cure	Complete resolution of peritonitis together with NONE of the following complications: Relapse/recurrent peritonitis, catheter removal, transfer to hemodialysis for 30 days or death
Refractory	Peritonitis episode with persistently cloudy bags or persistent dialysis effluent leukocyte count > 100×10^9/L after 5 days of appropriate antibiotic therapy
Recurrent	Peritonitis episode that occurs within 4 weeks of completion of therapy of a prior episode but with a different organism
Relapsing	Peritonitis episode that occurs within 4 weeks of completion of therapy of a prior episode with the same organism *or* one sterile (culture negative) episode (i.e., specific organism followed by the same organism, culture negative followed by a specific organism, *or* specific organism followed by culture negative).
Repeat	Peritonitis episode that occurs more than 4 weeks after completion of therapy of a prior episode with the same organism

Epidemiology of Peritoneal Dialysis Peritonitis

The global average peritonitis rates decreased from 0.6 episodes ppy in 1992 to 0.3 episodes ppy in 2019; Asia-Pacific countries had the highest peritonitis rates followed by Europe, the Middle East, and Africa.

As per the United States Renal Data System (USRDS) data, the rate of hospitalization for peritonitis decreased from 13.4 per 100 person-years in 2010 to 5.4 per 100 person-years in 2020. The percentage of patients receiving outpatient antibiotics during the year also decreased during this period from 23.6% in 2010 to 15.1% in 2020. Women had higher rates than men, and Black patients had higher rates than members of other race/ethnicity groups.[4]

In western population, Australia and New Zealand, the most common organism was gram-positive bacterium accounting for 50–60% of all peritonitis cases, predominantly coagulase-negative staphylococci (CoNS).

In contrast to the above, in India gram-negative bacteria were more predominant with *Escherichia coli* being the most common bacteria isolated **(Table 2)**.[5]

Pathogenesis of Peritoneal Dialysis Peritonitis

Risk factors

- *Patient-related:*
  - Poor personal hygiene and handwashing techniques
  - Older age, diabetes mellitus (DM), malnutrition
  - Low socioeconomic status
- *Technique-related:*
  - Improper exchange procedures
  - Lack of caregiver support
- *Clinical factors:*
  - Recurrent peritonitis

TABLE 2: Incidence of peritonitis based on microbiological growth.

Microbiological cause of peritonitis	
Staphylococcus epidermidis	30–45%
Staphylococcus aureus	10–20%
Streptococcus species	5–10%
Escherichia coli	5–10%
Other gram-negative species	5%
Pseudomonas species	5%
Others	<5%
Mycobacteria	<1%
Fungus	<1–10%
Culture negative	5–30%

- Polymicrobial infections and structural abnormalities like bowel perforation

Regional variations

- In developed countries, gram-positive organisms dominate due to higher use of antiseptic techniques and improved training.
- In developing countries, gram-negative infections are more prevalent, often linked to suboptimal environmental conditions and healthcare access.

Intraluminal infections occur due to errors in catheter-to-bag or catheter-to-transfer set connections, while *periluminal infections* involve bacteria on the skin surface. *Bowel sources* causing peritonitis are typically seen in diarrheal states or colon instrumentation. *Hematogenous infections* occur when bacteria seed the peritoneum through the bloodstream. *Transvaginal infections* are also reported.[1]

Diagnosis of Peritoneal Dialysis Peritonitis

How to collect a specimen

Whole bag or minimum 100 mL effluent fluid after a dwell time of at least 2 hours should be sent immediately to the laboratory (within 6 hours). In 75% cases, microbiological diagnosis is established in <3 days.

Investigations

Dialysate culture methods

When a fluid sample is sent for examination, it is recommended to send for peritoneal dialysis fluid to examine cell count, differential count, Gram stain, and culture sensitivity.

TABLE 3: Causes differential diagnosis of cloudy effluent fluid.

Cellular causes:	*Noncellular causes:*
• PMN leukocytes	• Fibrin
• Culture-positive infectious peritonitis	• Triglycerides (milky white appearance of effluent)
• Infectious peritonitis with sterile cultures	• Calcium channel blockers
• Chemical peritonitis	• Lymphatic obstruction
• Eosinophils	• Acute pancreatitis
• Dialysate eosinophilia	
• Chemical peritonitis	
• Monocyte/macrophages	
• Specimen taken from "dry" abdomen (after prolonged peritoneal rest)	
• Red blood cells	
• Hemoperitoneum	
• Malignant cells	
• Lymphoma	
• Peritoneal metastasis	

(PMN: polymorphonuclear)

Fifty milliliters of peritoneal fluid is collected in sterile containers, while 10 mL is injected into aerobic and anaerobic blood culture bottles to be processed by the BACTEC method and a loop full of sediment from centrifuged PD fluid is plated into various culture medias.

If cultures remain negative after 3–5 days of incubation, then PD fluid should be sent for repeat cell count, differential count, fungal, and Mycobacteria culture **(Table 3)**.

Prevention of Peritoneal Dialysis Peritonitis

Catheter placement: Administration of systemic antibiotics is recommended as per recent ISPD 2022 guidelines prior to the procedure. Single-dose intravenous cefuroxime or vancomycin prophylaxis is often employed, guided by local resistance pattern.

Exit-site care: Topical application of antibiotic cream or ointment to the exit site is recommended although such practice varies among various centers.[6-8]

Contamination of peritoneal dialysis: "Dry contamination" is contamination that occurs outside a closed PD system, such as disconnection distal to a closed clamp, while "*wet contamination*" occurs within an open system, when either dialysis fluid is infused after contamination or the catheter administration set is left open for an extended period.

Yap et al. revealed that 548 episodes of touch contamination had a relatively low rate of peritonitis (3.1%), while peritonitis occurred only after wet contamination (5.6%).[9]

In case of suspected contamination, cell count and culture should be monitored and a single dose of intraperitoneal (IP) cefazolin is a reasonable option.

Invasive gastrointestinal and gynecological procedures: All PD patients undergoing gastrointestinal (GI) procedure and invasive gynecological procedure require antibiotic prophylaxis and are required to drain their PD fluid prior to any procedures. Most commonly reported bacterial pathogens are *Streptococcus*, followed by *E. coli*, *Enterococcus*, *Staphylococcus*, and infrequently *Candida*.

The highest peritonitis complication rate after endoscopic or instrumental procedures is reported after invasive gynecological procedures, ranging from 26.9 to 38.5%.[10-12]

Domestic pet and zoonotic infection: Around one-fifth of PD patients surveyed in a single PD center were keeping pets.

"*Cat-bite peritonitis*", the aerobic gram-negative coccobacillus *Pasteurella multocida* is found in the upper respiratory tract and oral cavity of many domestic and wild animals including dogs and hamsters.

Pet-related damages include PD tubing cut, scratches, or chewing, ultimately leading to leaks. The patient should be advised to follow hand washing before and after PD exchanges as well as after handling pets.[13-18]

Peritoneal Dialysis Equipment and Training program: Comprehensive and tailored PD training, adherence to standardized exchange techniques, and periodic retraining **(Box 1)** have been shown to reduce peritonitis.

The Peritoneal Dialysis Outcomes and Practice Patterns Study (PDOPPS) noted marked variation in training practices across 120 facilities across 7 countries; timing of commencement, duration of training, and location or use of competency assessments were not predictive of peritonitis risk.[19-21]

BOX 1: Indications of retaining peritoneal dialysis (PD) catheter in case of peritonitis.

- Following prolonged hospitalization
- Following peritonitis and/or catheter infection
- Following change in dexterity, vision, or mental acuity
- Following change to another supplier or a different type of connection
- Following change in caregiver for PD exchange
- Following other interruptions in PD (e.g., period of time on hemodialysis)

Modifiable risk factors: To promote use of disconnect system with "flush before fill" design: During this process, the remaining fluid from the previous dwell is drained out (flush) prior to infusing the fluid (fill) for the current dwell period, hence avoiding stagnation of fluid within the peritoneal cavity.

Avoid hypokalemia: Under PDOPPS study, hypokalemia persistent for 4 months was associated with 80% higher subsequent peritonitis rates after adjustment for confounders.[22]

Avoid GI problems: Constipation and enteritis have been reported to be associated with peritonitis due to enteric organisms.

Avoid histamine 2 antagonist: Suppression of gastric acid is an emerging risk factor for peritonitis.

Secondary prevention: For each peritonitis episode, a root-cause analysis should be performed to determine the etiology to prevent another episode.[2]

To prevent fungal peritonitis, it is recommended to coprescribe antifungal prophylaxis whenever a course of antibiotics is advised **(Fig. 3)**.

Treatment of Peritonitis

All fluid presenting as cloudy fluid should be assumed as peritonitis unless proven otherwise and the patient should be put on empirical antibiotics intraperitonially. The systemic route is preferred only in case of suspected systemic sepsis. A delay in administration of antibiotics has shown to increase the risk of PD failure or sometimes even death by as high as 5.5%.

The decision to hospitalize should depend on:

- Hemodynamic status of the patient
- Severity of signs and symptoms
- Social support

The algorithm for initiation of empirical therapy in suspected peritonitis is explained in **Flowchart 2.**

Fourth-generation cephalosporins and imipenem/cilastatin monotherapy have shown to be noninferior and could be used as an alternative to dual therapy. Empirical aminoglycoside demonstrated a higher likelihood of medical cure than ceftazidime, as reported in PDOPPS.[23,24]

The antibiotic regimen should always be initialized based on the local antibiotic stewardship. The antibiotic should be de-escalated once the antibiotic sensitivity pattern is available **(Tables 4 to 6)**.

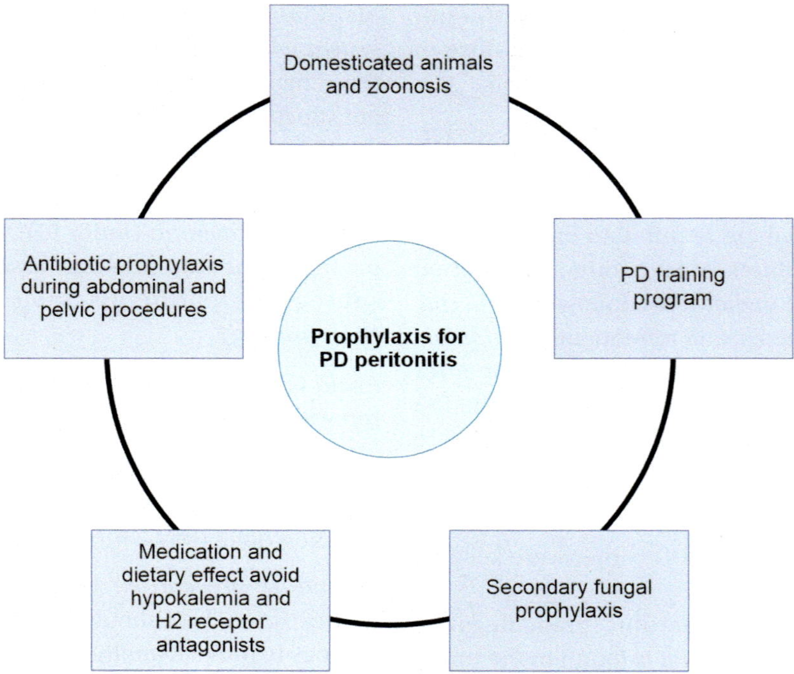

Fig. 3: Prophylaxis of peritoneal dialysis (PD) peritonitis.

Flowchart 2: Initial management algorithm of suspected cases of peritoneal dialysis (PD) prophylaxis.

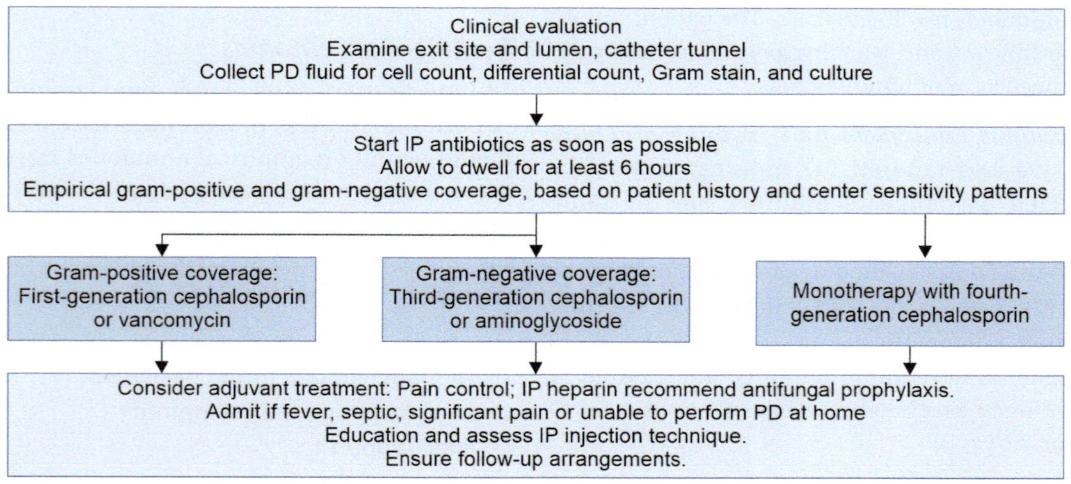

TABLE 4: Antibiotics recommended in peritonitis, IP dosing.

	Intermittent (one exchange daily)	*Continuous (all exchanges)*
Aminoglycosides		
Amikacin	2 mg/kg daily	LD 25 mg/L, MD 12 mg/L
Gentamicin	0.6 mg/kg daily	LD 8 mg/L, MD 4 mg/L
Netilmicin	0.6 mg/kg daily	MD 10 mg/L
Tobramycin	0.6 mg/kg daily	LD 3 mg/kg, MD 0.3 mg/kg

Contd...

Contd...

	Intermittent (one exchange daily)	*Continuous (all exchanges)*
Cephalosporins		
Cefazolin	15–20 mg/kg daily	LD 500 mg/L, MD 125 mg/L
Cefepime	1,000 mg daily	LD 250–500 mg/L, MD 100–125 mg/L
Cefoperazone	No data	LD 500 mg/L, MD 62.5–125 mg/L
Cefotaxime	500–1,000 mg daily	No data
Ceftazidime	1,000–1,500 mg daily	LD 500 mg/L, MD 125 mg/L
Ceftriaxone	1,000 mg daily	No data
Penicillins		
Penicillin G	No data	LD 50,000 unit/L, MD 25,000 unit/L
Amoxicillin	No data	MD 150 mg/L
Ampicillin	No data	MD 125 mg/L
Ampicillin/Sulbactam	2 g/l g every 12 hours	LD 750–100 mg/L, MD 100 mg/L
Piperacillin/Tazobactam	No data	LD 4 g/0.5 g, MD 1 g/0.125 g
Others		
Aztreonam	2 g daily	LD 1,000 mg/L, MD 250 mg/L
Ciprofloxacin	No data	MD 50 mg/L
Clindamycin	No data	MD 600 mg/bag
Daptomycin	No data	LD 100 mg/L, MD 20 mg/L
Imipenem/Cilastatin	500 mg in alternate exchange	LD 250 mg/L, MD 50 mg/L
Ofloxacin	No data	LD 200 mg, MD 25 mg/L
Polymyxin B	No data	MD 300,000 unit (30 mg)/bag
Meropenem	1 g dally	125 mg/L (case report)
Teicoplanin	15 mg/kg every 5 days	LD 400 mg/bag, MD 20 mg/bag
Vancomycin	15–30 mg/kg every 5–7 days (Supplement doses for APD patients)	LD 30 mg/kg, MD 1.5 mg/kg/bag
Antifungals		
Fluconazole	IP 200 mg every 24–48 hours	No data
Voriconazole	IP 2.5 mg/kg daily	No data

(APD: automated peritoneal dialysis; IP: intraperitoneal; LD: loading dose in mg; MD: maintenance dose in mg)
Source: Adapted and modified from Li PKT, Szeto CC, Piraino B, de Arteaga J, Fan S, Figueiredo AE, et al. ISPD Peritonitis Recommendations: 2016 Update on Prevention and Treatment. Perit Dial Int. 2016;36(5):481-508.

TABLE 5: Systemic antibiotics recommended for treatment of PD peritonitis.

Drug	*Dosing*
Antibacterials	
Ciprofloxacin	Oral 250 mg BD (500 mg BD, if residual renal function >5 mL/min)
Colistin	IV 300 mg loading, then 150–200 mg daily (expressed as CBA)
Ertapenem	IV 500 mg daily
Levofloxacin	Oral 250 mg daily
Linezolid	IV or oral 600 mg BD
Moxifloxacin	Oral 400 mg daily
Rifampicin	450 mg daily for BW <50 kg; 600 mg daily for BW ≥50 kg
Trimethoprim/sulfamethoxazole	Oral 160 mg/800 mg BD

Contd...

Contd...

Drug	*Dosing*
Antifungals	
Amphotericin	IV test dose 1 mg; starting dose 0.1 mg/kg/day over 6 hours; increased to target dose 0.75 mg/kg/day over 4 days
Caspofungin	IV 70 mg loading, then 50 mg daily
Fluconazole	Oral 200 mg loading, then 50–100 mg daily
Posaconazole	IV 400 mg every 12 hours
Voriconazole	Oral 200 mg every 12 hours

(BD: twice a day; BW: body weight; CBA: colistin base activity; IV: intravenous)

Source: Adapted and modified from Li PKT, Szeto CC, Piraino B, de Arteaga J, Fan S, Figueiredo AE, et al. ISPD Peritonitis Recommendations: 2016 Update on Prevention and Treatment. Perit Dial Int. 2016;36(5):481-508.

TABLE 6: Treatment of bacterial peritoneal dialysis (PD) peritonitis.

Organism-specific therapy		
Organism	***Antibiotics of choice (dosage)***	***Comments***
Methicillin-susceptible *Staphylococcus aureus* (MSSA)	First-generation cephalosporin	Associated with exit-site or tunnel infection, likely touch contamination
Methicillin-resistant *Staphylococcus aureus* (MRSA)	Vancomycin (15–30 mg/kg) q5 days for continuous ambulatory peritoneal dialysis (CAPD) and 15 mg/kg every 4 days for automated peritoneal dialysis (APD)	
Streptococcus group	• Cefazolin 15 mg/kg q24 hours for long dwell and 20 mg/kg q24 hours for short dwell • If allergic/resistant change to vancomycin IP • Treat for 14 days	• Most common organisms were viridans groups (including *Streptococcus oralis*, *Streptococcus sanguinis*, and *Streptococcus gordonii*) • Viridans peritonitis indicates dental problems
Corynebacterium	IP vancomycin for 3 weeks	Found as skin commensal
Enterococcus	Oral amoxicillin for 2–3 weeks	Mostly associated with polymicrobial peritonitis (PMP)
Vancomycin-resistant enterococcus (VRE)	• Oral or intravenous linezolid or IP daptomycin, or teicoplanin • Treat for 21 days	Newer agents like dalbavancin or combination treatment strategies (including tigecycline and fosfomycin) can be used
Pseudomonas	• IP ceftazidime or cefepime + IP gentamycin/tobramycin/amikacin • Or oral ciprofloxacin • Duration of treatment 21 days	For nonfermenting gram-negative bacteria even if peritonitis resolves but persistent exit site or tunnel infection consider for catheter and reinsertion
Acinetobacter ± CRAB (carbapenem-resistant *Acinetobacter baumannii*)	• IP ciprofloxacin, broad-spectrum cephalosporin, a combination of beta-lactam/beta-lactamase inhibitor or a carbapenem • To treat for 21 days	*In case of CRAB:* Use IP aminoglycoside or LP colistin ± a sulbactam-containing agent
Enterobacterales	• Fourth-generation cephalosporin (cefepime), quinolones, or carbapenem • Treat for 21 days	Commonly associated with high resistance to antibiotics, treatment failure rates, worse clinical outcomes
Polymicrobial peritonitis	• Metronidazole plus Vancomycin, in combination with ceftazidime or an aminoglycoside • Monotherapy with a carbapenem or piperacillin/tazobactam may be considered.	• Suspicion of possibility of intra-abdominal pathology • Computed tomographic (CT) scan may help to identify the pathology, especially in the presence of hemodynamic instability

Notes: For all bacterial infections: If no improvement after 5 days on appropriate antibiotics, remove catheter and treat with appropriate antibiotics for 14–21 days.

It is not necessary to switch patients on automated peritoneal dialysis (APD) to CAPD temporarily during peritonitis episodes.[25]

Vancomycin remains the drug of choice in centers with a high prevalence of methicillin-resistant *Staphylococcus aureus* (MRSA) and other relevant organisms with IP being the preferred route as 90% of the drug is absorbed in the presence of peritonitis. Aminoglycosides have a concentration-dependent activity, making it favorable for intermittent daily dosing.[23]

CASE 2

Patient X, a 67-year-old patient, diagnosed as end-stage kidney disease (ESKD) secondary to lupus nephritis arrives at the emergency department with complaints of abdominal pain, nausea, and vomiting over the past 3 days. She also reports a fever and a general feeling of malaise. She notes that her abdominal pain is diffuse and worsens with movement.

Clinical Findings

- *Vital signs:* Temperature 100.9°F (38.3°C), blood pressure 130/85 mm Hg, heart rate 88 bpm
- *Abdominal examination:* Diffuse abdominal tenderness with rebound tenderness and guarding. Bowel sounds are decreased. The exit site appears normal with no visible signs of infection.
- *Peritoneal dialysis effluent analysis:*
  - *Cell count:* Elevated white blood cells (>100 cells/μL, predominantly neutrophils)
  - *Gram stain:* No organisms visualized
  - *Culture results:* Negative (no growth after 48 hours)
  - *Peritoneal fluid lactate:* Elevated

What is the probable diagnosis?

Culture-negative Peritonitis

The ISPD recommends that culture-negative peritonitis rates should be kept <15%. If fluid yields no growth, repeat WBC count with differential should be obtained, together with special culture request to exclude unusual organisms such as mycobacteria, nocardia, filamentous fungus, and other fastidious bacteria **(Box 2; Flowchart 3)**.

BOX 2: Causes of culture-negative peritoneal dialysis peritonitis.

Infectious causes:
- Recent antibiotic exposure,
- Suboptimal sample collection
- Culture methods
- Slowly growing atypical organisms (e.g., mycobacteria, fungus)

Noninfectious cause:
- Eosinophilic or chemical (e.g., icodextrin) peritonitis

Tuberculosis Peritonitis

Tuberculosis peritonitis typically presents as part of disseminated tuberculosis (TB) but can also occur in isolation. The disease manifests through inflammation of the peritoneal cavity, leading to symptoms such as abdominal pain, cloudy effluent, and fever.

Reports indicate that TB peritonitis accounts for 1–3% of all PD-related peritonitis cases in endemic regions.

Risk factors include DM, HIV infection, and immunosuppressive therapy.

Although rare, nontuberculous mycobacteria (NTM) may also cause peritoneal infections, but these cases are relatively rare in PD.

Diagnosis

- *Mycobacterial culture:* The gold standard for diagnosis
- *Polymerase chain reaction (PCR) and GeneXpert:* These offer faster and more reliable detection of *Mycobacterium tuberculosis*, with better sensitivity than conventional culture methods.
- *Imaging:* Abdominal ultrasound or CT scans can reveal signs of peritoneal thickening or abscess formation.
- *Peritoneal biopsy:* Laparoscopic peritoneal or omental biopsies can yield better results.

Treatment

The treatment of TB peritonitis is based on the standard anti-TB regimen as per the recent national guidelines.

The total treatment duration is typically 9 months, but it may be extended in immunocompromised patients or those with complications.[2]

Corticosteroids may be added as an adjuvant therapy in certain cases to reduce inflammation and prevent peritoneal fibrosis.

Complications

Include significant peritoneal fibrosis, bowel perforation, or abscess formation.

According to the Indian guidelines for CAPD-related TB peritonitis, PD catheter removal is indicated in the following cases:

- Failure to respond to anti-TB therapy
- Refractory or relapsing infections

Flowchart 3: Management algorithm of culture-negative peritonitis.

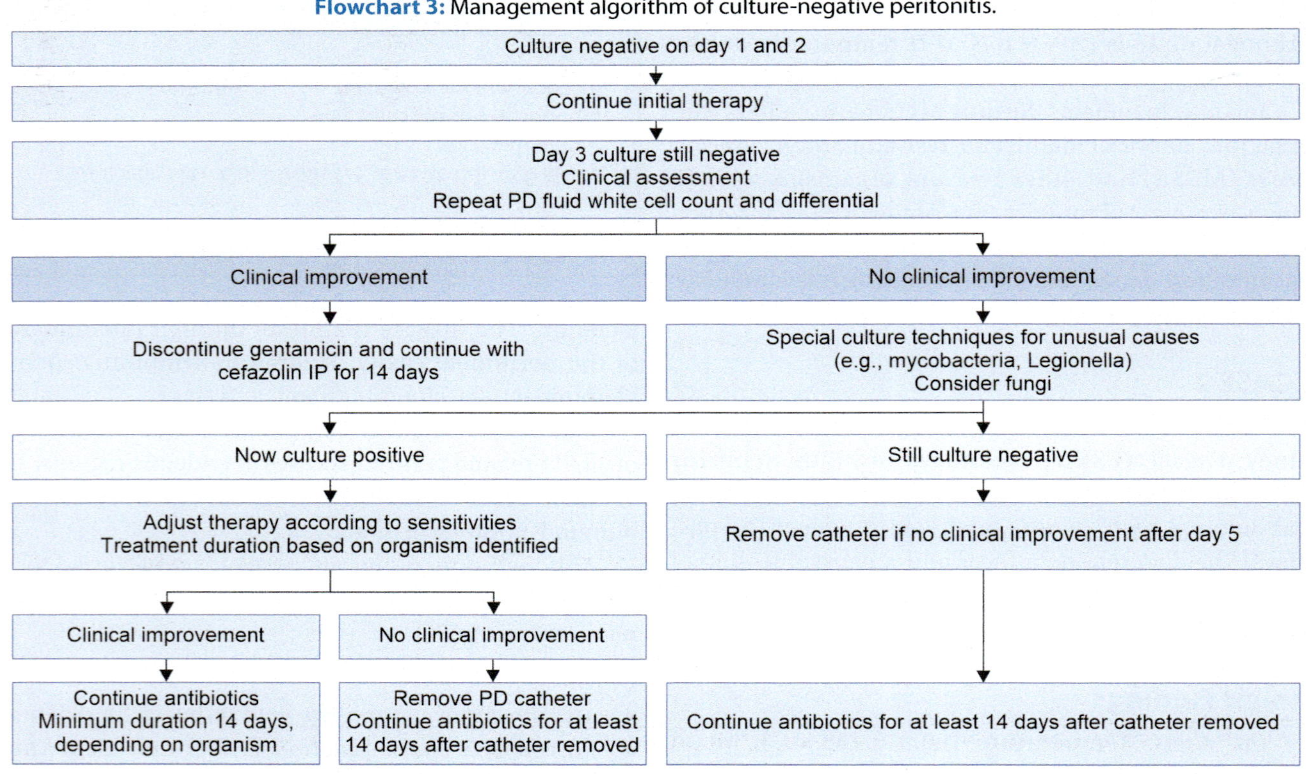

(PD: peritoneal dialysis)

Screening and treatment of latent TB along with TB prophylaxis for high-risk individuals may help prevent TB peritonitis.

CASE 3

Mr A, a 55-year-old male farmer, diagnosed as chronic kidney disease (CKD) on PD for 3 years, DM, hypertension (HTN), presents with complaints of severe and progressive abdominal pain, fever, and cloudy PD effluent since 4 days. *Clinical examination* revealed temperature 38.5°C, blood pressure 140/90 mm Hg, and heart rate 100 bpm. *Abdominal examination* showed diffuse tenderness, guarding, and rebound tenderness.

Investigations:

- *Complete blood count (CBC):* 18,000 cell/mL
- *Peritoneal dialysis effluent analysis:* Elevated white blood cell count with a predominance of neutrophils
- *Gram stain:* Negative
- *Culture:* Growth of *Candida* species

How will you manage?

Fungal Peritonitis

Fungal infections are often insidious in onset and are associated with prolonged inflammation and higher mortality rates if not addressed promptly.

Studies suggest approximately 2–15% incidence of fungal peritonitis among all cases of PD-related peritonitis. The incidence is higher in immunocompromised patients.

Clinical Features of Fungal Peritoneal Dialysis Peritonitis

The clinical presentation may overlap with bacterial peritonitis. Key features include:

- Abdominal pain and tenderness
- Cloudy dialysis effluent
- Systemic symptoms like fever point toward the systemic spread of the infection
- Delayed response to antibiotics
- In severe cases, the patient may present with sepsis, bowel perforation, and peritoneal abscess formation.

Diagnosis of Fungal Peritoneal Dialysis Peritonitis

Microbiological testing: Peritoneal fluid culture is the gold standard for diagnosis.

Common Organisms Causing Fungal Peritonitis

Fungal peritonitis is classically seen with opportunistic pathogens like:

- *Candida* species: *Candida albicans* is the most frequently encountered organism, although *Candida tropicalis* and other nonalbicans species are also involved.
- *Aspergillus* species are a rare cause of fungal peritonitis in PD patients.
- Other rare fungi reported to cause fungal peritonitis include *Fusarium*, *Histoplasma*, and *Rhizopus* species.

Management

- *Candida*- or *Aspergillus*-related peritonitis warrants catheter removal due to the high relapse rate and complications.
- Empiric antifungal therapy should be promptly initiated after collecting peritoneal effluent samples.
- Fluconazole (for *Candida*) and amphotericin B (for molds) are commonly used as initial agents.
- Treatment should be continued for a minimum of 2–4 weeks, with adjustments based on clinical response and microbiological clearance.

Adjunctive therapy

- *Heparin:* 500 units/L IP may help prevent occlusion of the catheter by fibrin.
- *Analgesic* may help in symptomatic improvement.
- *Augmented peritoneal lavage* with one or two rapid PD exchanges is often performed for pain relief although not enough supportive data is available.
- *Switch to icodextrin:* PDOPPS suggests that temporary switching to icodextrin may improve ultrafiltration and alleviates signs of volume overload.
- *Urokinase* and *oral rifampicin* showed catheter salvage in 64% cases of persisting CoNS.

Response monitoring and catheter removal

The effluent fluid, catheter lumen, exit site, and tunnel should be re-examined regularly.

If no response is seen after 48 hours, fluid cell counts and cultures should be repeated.

Monitoring of WBC count in PD effluent may also predict treatment response.[25]

Indications of catheter removal are:

- Refractory peritonitis
- Relapsing, recurrent, or repeat peritonitis episodes
- Fungal peritonitis
- Treatment failure in individualized cases of tuberculous and nontuberculous mycobacterial infection

Timing for reinsertion: Reinsertion can be considered after culture of the PD effluent has become negative and the PD effluent white cell count is below 100/mL, in the absence of concomitant exit site or tunnel infection.

Reinsertion of catheter can be considered after 2–4 weeks of bacterial and 4–6 weeks of fungal peritonitis along with complete resolution of peritoneal symptoms.

Alternative dialysis modes

Hemodialysis (HD) should be considered, particularly if the infection requires PD catheter removal, to allow peritoneum healing.

The clinical status of the patient should be reassessed for disease remission and reinsertion of the PD catheter may be considered after 4–6 weeks.[2,23,26,27]

CONCLUSION

Peritonitis remains a critical concern in patients undergoing PD. Advances in PD technique, prophylaxis, patient education, and prompt treatment have improved outcomes but have not eliminated the risk of infection-related complications.

Efforts to identify modifiable risk factors, improvement in training programs, and tailored antibiotic regimens based on local resistance patterns are essential. Ensuring adherence to ISPD guidelines, conducting thorough root-cause analyses following each episode, and implementing secondary prevention measures can help maintain membrane integrity, prolong technique survival, and enhance a patient's quality of life.

REFERENCES

1. KV Dakshinamurthy, Siva Kumar V, Ram R, Sangeetha Lakshmi B. Peritoneal Dialysis Primer, 1st edition. Tirupati: SVIMS; 2017. pp. 316-76.
2. Li PKT, Chow KM, Cho Y, Fan S, Figueiredo AE, Harris T, et al. ISPD peritonitis guideline recommendations: 2022 update on prevention and treatment. Perit Dial Int. 2022;42(2):110-53.
3. Cristina Popa (@NephroSeeker)/X. [online] Available from https://x.com/NephroSeeker [Last accessed July, 2025].

4. USRDS. (2024). Annual data report. [online] Available from https://usrds-adr.niddk.nih.gov/ [Last accessed July, 2025].
5. Vikrant S, Guleria RC, Kanga A, Verma BS, Singh D, Dheer SK. Microbiological aspects of peritonitis in patients on continuous ambulatory peritoneal dialysis. Indian J Nephrol. 2013;23(1):12-7.
6. Wikdahl AM, Engman U, Stegmayr BG, Sörenssen JG. One-dose cefuroxime i.v. and i.p. reduces microbial growth in PD patients after catheter insertion. Nephrol Dial Transplant. 1997;12(1):157-60.
7. Lye WC, Lee EJ, Tan CC. Prophylactic antibiotics in the insertion of Tenckhoff catheters. Scand J Urol Nephrol. 1992;26(2):177-80.
8. Gadallah MF, Ramdeen G, Mignone J, Patel D, Mitchell L, Tatro S. Role of preoperative antibiotic prophylaxis in preventing postoperative peritonitis in newly placed peritoneal dialysis catheters. Am J Kidney Dis. 2000;36(5):1014-9.
9. Yap DYH, Chu WL, Ng F, Yip TPS, Lui SL, Lo WK. Risk Factors and Outcome of Contamination in Patients on Peritoneal Dialysis—A Single-Center Experience of 15 Years. Perit Dial Int. 2012;32(6):612-6.
10. Gweon TG, Jung SH, Kim SW, Lee KM, Cheung DY, Lee BI, et al. Risk factors for peritonitis in patients on continuous ambulatory peritoneal dialysis who undergo colonoscopy: a retrospective multicentre study. BMC Gastroenterol. 2019;19(1):175.
11. Al-Hwiesh AK, Abdul-Rahman IS, Hussameldeen MA, Al-Audah N, Abdelrahman A, Moaigel HM, et al. Colonoscopy in Automated Peritoneal Dialysis Patients: Value of Prophylactic Antibiotics: A Prospective Study on a Single Antibiotic. Int J Artif Organs. 2017;40(10):550-7.
12. Wu HH, Li IJ, Weng CH, Lee CC, Chen YC, Chang MY, et al. Prophylactic Antibiotics for Endoscopy-Associated Peritonitis in Peritoneal Dialysis Patients. PLoS One. 2013;8(8):e71532.
13. Makin AJ, Cartwright KA, Banks RA. Keeping the cat out of the bag: a hazard in continuous ambulatory peritoneal dialysis. BMJ. 1991;303(6817):1610-1.
14. Sedlacek M, Cotter JG, Suriawinata AA, Kaneko TM, Zuckerman RA, Parsonnet J, et al. Mucormycosis Peritonitis: More Than 2 Years of Disease-Free Follow-up After Posaconazole Salvage Therapy After Failure of Liposomal Amphotericin B. Am J Kidney Dis. 2008;51(2):302-6.
15. Campos A, Taylor JH, Campbell M. Hamster bite peritonitis: Pasteurella pneumotropica peritonitis in a dialysis patient. Pediatr Nephrol. 2000;15(1-2):31-2.
16. Freeman AF, Zheng XT, Lane JC, Shulman ST. Pasteurella aerogenes hamster bite peritonitis. Pediatr Infect Dis J. 2004;23(4):368.
17. Paul RV, Rostand SG. Cat-bite peritonitis: Pasteurella multocida peritonitis following feline contamination of peritoneal dialysis tubing. Am J Kidney Dis. 1987; 10(4):318-9.
18. Shanmuganathan M, Goh B, Lim CTS. *Streptococcus gallolyticus* subsp. *pasteurianus* peritonitis in a patient on continuous ambulatory peritoneal dialysis. Indian J Nephrol. 2017;27(6):488.
19. Rope R, Nanayakkara N, Wazil A, Dickowita S, Abeyeskera R, Gunerathne L, et al. Expanding CAPD in low-resource settings: A distance learning approach. Perit Dial Int. 2018;38(5):343--8.
20. Yi C, Guo Q, Lin J, Li J, Yu X, Yang X. Patient-Doctor Contact Interval and Clinical Outcomes in Continuous Ambulatory Peritoneal Dialysis Patients. Am J Nephrol. 2017;45(4):346-52.
21. Russo R, Manili L, Tiraboschi G, Amar K, De Luca M, Alberghini E, et al. Patient re-training in peritoneal dialysis: why and when it is needed. Kidney Int Suppl. 2006;(103):S127-132.
22. Ribeiro SC, Figueiredo AE, Barretti P, Pecoits-Filho R, de Moraes TP; all centers that contributed to the BRAZPD II study. Low Serum Potassium Levels Increase the Infectious-Caused Mortality in Peritoneal Dialysis Patients: A Propensity-Matched Score Study. PLoS One. 2015;10(6):e0127453.
23. Jeloka T, Abraham G, Bhalla A, Balasubramaniam J, Dutta A, Gokulnath, et al. Continuous ambulatory peritoneal dialysis peritonitis guidelines – Consensus statement of peritoneal dialysis society of India - 2020. Indian J Nephrol. 2021;31(5):425.
24. Kitrungphaiboon T, Puapatanakul P, Chuengsaman P, Tiskajornsiri K, Halue G, Siribamrungwong M, et al. Intraperitoneal Cefepime Monotherapy Versus Combination Therapy of Cefazolin Plus Ceftazidime for Empirical Treatment of CAPD-Associated Peritonitis: A Multicenter, Open-Label, Noninferiority, Randomized, Controlled Trial. Am J Kidney Dis. 2019;74(5):601-9.
25. Whitty R, Bargman JM, Kiss A, Dresser L, Lui P. Residual Kidney Function and Peritoneal Dialysis-Associated Peritonitis Treatment Outcomes. Clin J Am Soc Nephrol. 2017;12(12):2016.
26. Al Sahlawi M, Bargman JM, Perl J. Peritoneal Dialysis-Associated Peritonitis: Suggestions for Management and Mistakes to Avoid. Kidney Med. 2020;2(4):467-75.
27. Nochaiwong S, Ruengorn C, Koyratkoson K, Thavorn K, Awiphan R, Chaisai C, et al. A Clinical Risk Prediction Tool for Peritonitis-Associated Treatment Failure in Peritoneal Dialysis Patients. Sci Rep. 2018;8(1):14797.

CHAPTER 49

Peritoneal Dialysis Catheter Insertion in Pediatric Patients

Sowrabha Rajanna, Kanav Anand, Rekulapally Praneetha

CASE SCENARIO

A 6-month-old infant weighing 5 kg presented with acute decompensation characterized by lethargy, refusal to feed, and irritability. The child had diarrhea and septic shock that was not responsive to fluid resuscitation and required inotropic support. Despite 3 days of treatment, the patient remained anuric and did not respond to fluid boluses or diuretics. Examination revealed fluid overload. Laboratory results showed:

- *Serum sodium:* 130 mEq/L
- *Serum potassium:* 7 mEq/L
- *Blood urea nitrogen:* 75 mg/dL
- *Serum creatinine:* 4 mg/dL
- *Arterial blood gas (ABG):* pH 6.9
- *Serum bicarbonate:* 10

Given the poor response to conservative management, peritoneal dialysis (PD) was initiated using a 1.5% dextrose solution via a catheter inserted by the Seldinger technique at the bedside. The dialysis prescription consisted of:

- *Dwell volume:* 20 mL/kg (100 mL per cycle)
- *Fill time:* 5 minutes
- *Dwell time:* 30 minutes
- *Drain time:* 20 minutes

Over the course of 3 days, the infant showed improvement, with the resolution of hyperkalemia, acidosis, and reduced fluid overload. The infant began passing urine, and PD was subsequently discontinued.

INTRODUCTION

"Children are not just small adults."

Peritoneal dialysis initiation is a practical skill of great value in caring for pediatric patients. It can be taken up in sick neonates and hemodynamically unstable children with minimal resources. Vascular access is challenging in children and initiation of hemodialysis requires specific consumables which may not be readily available at all centers. In comparison, peritoneal dialysis catheter insertion is a life-saving skill and has a short learning curve. Methods to prepare modified catheters and locally prepare peritoneal fluid are also discussed in this chapter.

INDICATIONS FOR RENAL REPLACEMENT THERAPY[1]

Renal indications:

- *Oliguria* unresponsive to diuretics or fluid challenge
- *Pulmonary edema* with acute kidney injury (AKI)
- *Severe metabolic acidosis* (pH <7.2 despite bicarbonate therapy)
- *Severe or persistent hyperkalemia* (K^+ > 6.5 mEq/L, or 5.5–6.5 mEq/L with ECG changes)
- *Uremic symptoms* (encephalopathy, seizures, myopathy, pericarditis, bleeding)
- *Symptomatic hyponatremia*
- *Need for large volume* of medications, blood products, or total parenteral nutrition (TPN) in an oligoanuric patient

Nonrenal indications:

- *Fluid overload* >20% it is associated with increased mortality (3% increase per 1% increase in fluid overload)
- *Large transfusions* in trauma or coagulopathy
- *Inborn errors of metabolism*
- *Sepsis*
- *Postcardiopulmonary bypass* systemic inflammatory response syndrome
- *Drug overdose* or poisonings

PERITONEAL DIALYSIS HARDWARE

Catheter Types

- *Rigid catheters* **(Fig. 1)**:
  - *Description:* Suitable for short-term use (up to 72 hours) and cost-effective
  - Available in two sizes:
    1. *20 cm* for infants
    2. *30 cm* for older children
  - *Advantages:* Low-cost, easy to insert
  - *Disadvantages:* Higher risk of complications, less comfortable
- *Tenckhoff catheters (soft PD catheters)* **(Fig. 2)**:
  - *Description:* Flexible, can be inserted percutaneously or via open surgery. Available in sizes:
    - *31 cm* for neonates and infants
    - *37 cm* for small children
    - *41 cm* for adolescents

    All sizes are available in various shapes (straight tip, coiled tip, and swan neck).
  - *Advantages:* Long-term use; fewer complications
  - *Disadvantages:* Requires surgical or bedside insertion by trained personnel; more expensive
- *Improvised catheters* **(Figs. 3 and 4)**:
  - *Description:* Alternative catheters used when standard PD catheters are unavailable (e.g., infant feeding tubes, pig-tail drainage catheters)
  - *Advantages:* Useful in resource-limited settings
  - *Disadvantages:* Higher risk of infection and complications

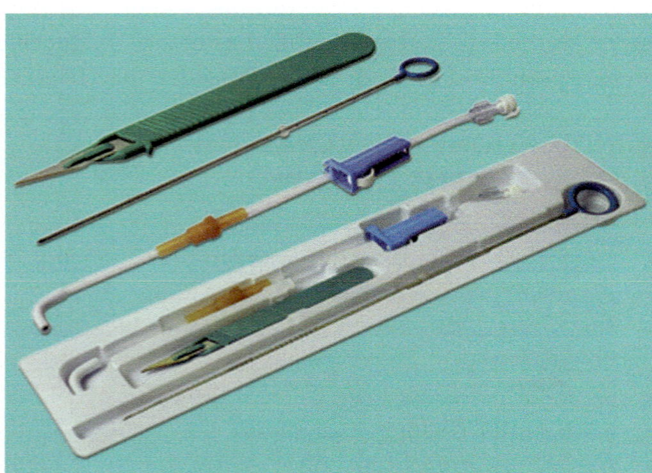

Fig. 1: Rigid peritoneal dialysis (PD) catheter.

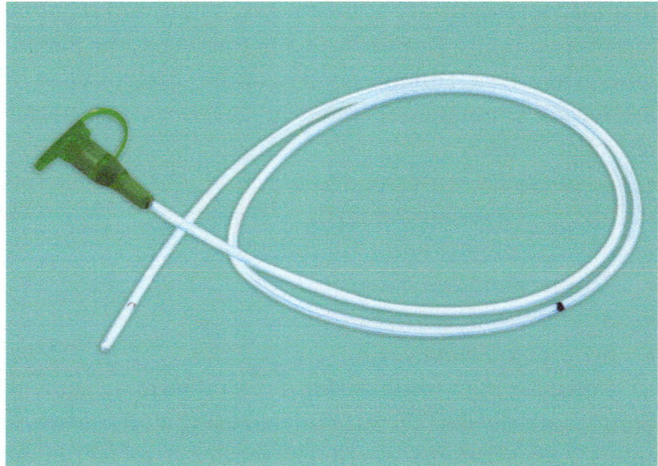

Fig. 3: Infant feeding tube.

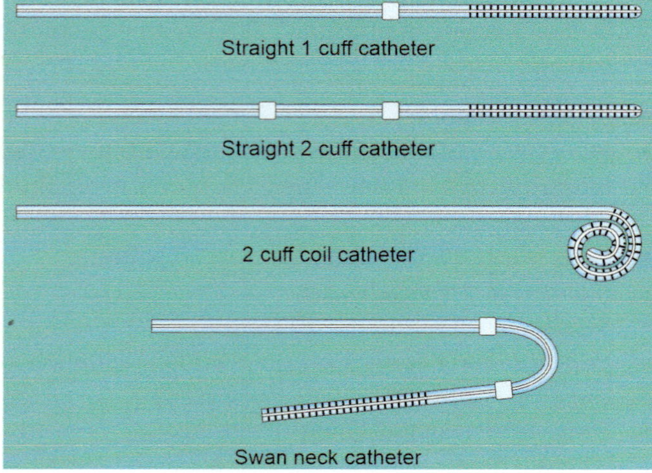

Fig. 2: Tenckhoff catheter.

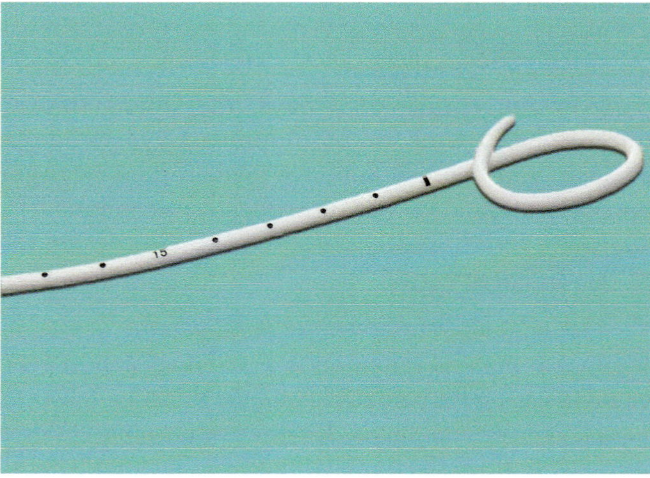

Fig. 4: Pigtail drainage catheter.

Dialysis Fluids

- *Commercially available PD fluids*
  Acute PD solution contents:
  Each 100 mL contains (values in mmol/L):
  - Sodium: 130
  - Potassium: 2
  - Calcium: 1.5
  - Chloride: 100
  - Magnesium: 0.75
  - Acetate: 35
  - Dextrose: 95 (1.7 g/100 mL)

  Continuous ambulatory peritoneal dialysis (CAPD) solutions vary by dextrose concentration and osmolality. These solutions are selected based on the patient's needs, including electrolyte balance, osmolality, and glucose control **(Table 1)**.
- *Customized PD fluids:* Tailored solutions may be prepared for patients with specific metabolic needs, such as those with hepatic dysfunction or severe electrolyte imbalances **(Table 2)**.
  Table 2 can be used to guide the preparation of customised PD fluids as recommended by the ISPD.

PATIENT PREPARATION FOR PERITONEAL DIALYSIS CATHETER INSERTION

Proper patient preparation is crucial to ensure a successful PD catheter insertion and minimize complications.

Preoperative Assessment[3]

- *Medical history:* Review comorbidities such as diabetes, prior abdominal surgeries, or peritonitis.
- *Physical examination:* Assess for infection, hernias, or abdominal scars.
- *Laboratory tests*:
  - *Baseline tests:* Complete blood count, coagulation profile, and kidney function

TABLE 1: Types of continuous ambulatory peritoneal dialysis (CAPD) solutions with different dextrose concentration and osmolality.

Type	*Na (mEq/L)*	*Lactate (mmol/L)*	*K (mEq/L)*	*Cl (mEq/L)*	*Dextrose (mg/dL)*	*Osmolality (mOsm/L)*
1.7%	130	35	3	108	1,700	363
1.5%	132	40	3.5	96	1,360	346
2.5%	132	40	3.5	96	2,270	396
4.5%	132	40	3.5	96	3,860	485

TABLE 2: Local preparation of customized peritoneal dialysis (PD) fluids (ISPD guidelines).[2]

Local preparation of solutions									
Type of fluid	NA^+	K^+	Ca^{2+}	Mg	Cl^-	HCO_3^-	Lactate	pH	Osm.
Hartmann's solution	131	5	2.0		111		29	7.0	278
Ringer's lactate	131	5	1.8		112		28	6.5	279
Plasmalyte B	130	4	0	1.5	110	27		7.4	273
½ Normal saline	77				77			5.0	154

(Ca: calcium; Cl: chlorine; HCO_3^-: bicarbonate; K: potassium; Mg: magnesium; Na: sodium; Osm: osmolarity)

Preparation of dialysis solutions using the above intravenous solutions:

1 L Plasmalyte + 30 mL 50% dextrose (15 g) will generate a solution with the following concentrations: Glucose 1.45%, Na 126 mmol/L, HCO_3^- 27 mmol/L, K 3.8 mmol/L, Mg 1.45 mmol/L, Osm 342. This is very similar to some of the bicarbonate-based solutions sold by industry.

1 L Ringer's lactate + 30 mL 50% dextrose (15 g) will generate a solution with the following concentrations: Na 127 mmol/L, lactate 27 mmol/L, Ca 1.36 mmol/L, K 3.8 mmol/L, glucose 1.45%, Osm 346.
This is similar to lactate-based PD solutions.

Note: Both above solutions contain potassium.

1 L 1/2 normal saline + 40 mL 8.5% Na Bic (40 mmol) + 40 mL 50% dextrose (20 g) + 60 mL 3% NaCl (30 mmol) will generate a solution with approximately the following concentrations: Na ± 130 mmol/L, Bicarb 35 mmol/L, glucose 1.7%, Osm: 340

Source: Cullis B, Abdelraheem M, Abrahams G, Balbi A, Cruz DN, Frishberg Y, et al. Peritoneal dialysis for acute kidney injury. Perit Dial Int. 2014;34(5):494-517.

- *Infection markers:* Screen for Methicillin-resistant *Staphylococcus aureus* (MRSA), treat if needed.
- *Blood glucose:* Ensure optimal control.
- *Imaging:* Abdominal ultrasound or CT scan to check for adhesions, ascites, or anatomical issues.

Patient Education

- *Procedure explanation:* Discuss the steps, risks, and benefits of PD catheter insertion.
- *Postprocedure care:* Teach the family about catheter care and infection prevention.

Skin and Site Preparation

- *Skin cleaning:* Bathe with antiseptic soap and shave the abdominal area.
- *Bowel preparation:* Use a laxative (polyethylene glycol) to reduce the risk of bowel injury.

Infection Prophylaxis

- *Antibiotics:* Administer prophylactic antibiotics (e.g., cefazolin or vancomycin) 30–60 minutes before the procedure.
- *Skin antisepsis:* Use chlorhexidine or iodine-based antiseptic.

Anesthesia and Sedation

- *Local anesthesia:* For percutaneous techniques
- *General anesthesia:* For laparoscopic or open surgical approaches
- *Sedation:* Mild sedation may be given to ease anxiety.

Positioning

Supine position: With slight elevation of the head to optimize access to the peritoneal cavity.

The above-mentioned steps are mandatory for CAPD catheter insertion in children. However, in acute PD catheter insertion by the percutaneous technique (described in the following text), MRSA screening may be skipped.

TECHNIQUES FOR PD CATHETER INSERTION IN PEDIATRICS[4-6]

Open Surgical Technique

- *Procedure:* Performed under general anesthesia, with an infraumbilical or paraumbilical incision. A purse-string suture secures the peritoneal lining around the catheter.
- *Advantages:* High success rate with direct visualization
- *Disadvantages:* Requires operating room facilities and longer recovery

Percutaneous Technique (Rigid Catheters)

- *Procedure:*
  - Site of insertion **(Fig. 5)**
    - Midpoint of line joining the umbilicus to pubic symphysis
    - Paramedian line just lateral to rectus sheath, preferably left side
  - Give local anesthesia till the peritoneum. Insert 16- or 18-gauze cannula at the planned site of catheter insertion and infuse 30 mL/kg of dialysate fluid to create artificial ascites, ensuring full flanks.
  - Make small skin incision (stab wound) with an 11 number surgical blade and insert the catheter with the stylet through abdominal wall in a screwing motion. On penetration of the peritoneum a sudden "give way" feeling is appreciated and gush of dialysate fluid is seen into the catheter.
  - Once peritoneal cavity is entered, withdraw stylet by 1 cm. Advance the catheter toward right anterior superior iliac spine with simultaneously withdrawal of stylet. Attach the connecting set to the catheter and run in dialysate fluid to confirm free flow. Allow about half of dialysate fluid to drain out by gravity and then start next inflow. Initially four to five rapid cycles (in followed by out, with no dwell) are done prior to initiating dwell.

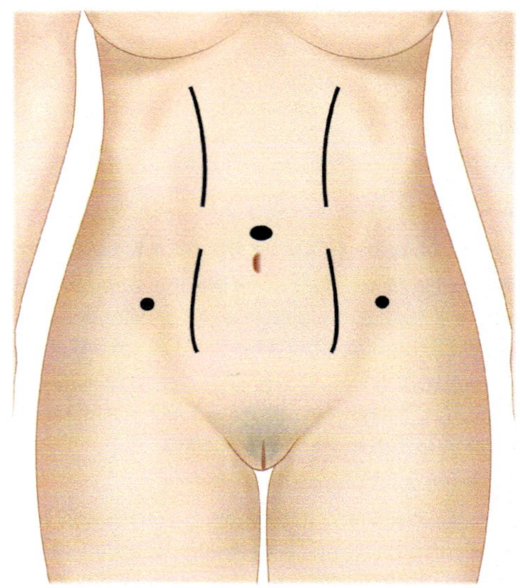

Fig. 5: Site of insertion.

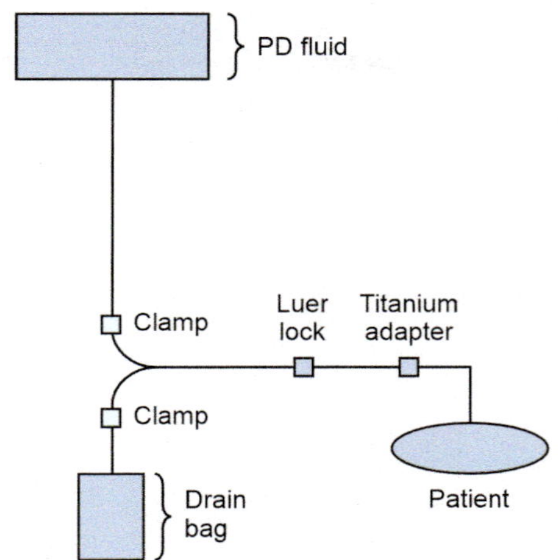

Fig. 6: Flow diagram of peritoneal dialysis (PD) set.

- Purse string suture may be put in order to fix the catheter so as to prevent pericatheter leak.
- When "Y"-shaped connector is not available, a "three way" with two IV sets (one for inlet and other for outlet) may be used **(Fig. 6)**. If neonatal size PD catheter is not available, pediatric size PD catheter can be trimmed and used.

- *Advantages:* Minimal invasion, bedside procedure
- *Disadvantages:* Higher risk of complications such as bowel perforation or catheter blockage

Laparoscopic-assisted Technique[7-9]

- *Procedure:* Pneumoperitoneum is established, and a laparoscope is used for visual guidance. The catheter is tunneled subcutaneously.
- *Advantages:* Direct visualization and ideal for complex cases
- *Disadvantages:* Requires specialized equipment and expertise

Seldinger Technique for Tenckhoff Catheters

- *Procedure:* A needle is inserted into the peritoneal cavity, followed by catheter insertion over a guidewire.
- *Advantages:* Minimally invasive and suitable for bedside placement
- *Disadvantages:* Technical challenges in small children

PERITONEAL DIALYSIS PRESCRIPTION

- *Volume of fluid (fill volume):* The range is 20–40 mL/kg (800–1,100 mL/m^2). We may start from a lower volume and gradually increase depending upon the tolerance of the child. Patients with pulmonary compromise may worsen with increased abdominal dialysate volumes; hence, lower dwell volumes are preferred in such patients.
- *Length of time in abdomen (dwell time):* Usually 30 minutes
- *Total duration of a cycle:* Run-in time 5–10 minutes, dwell time 30 minutes and outflow time 20–25 minutes; thus, each cycle usually lasts for 1 hour.
- Total number of cycles
- *Additives to dialysis solution:*
  - Addition of potassium to the dialysis fluid may be withheld for initial 8–10 cycles. Subsequently once the serum potassium levels fall below 4 mEq/L, 2–4 mEq/L of KCl can be added depending on the serum potassium level.
  - Heparin (250–500 IU/L) may be added to prevent clot formation particularly to first liter of fluid and when outflow contains blood and fibrinous material.

Modifications

- Dwell time should be shorter (20 minutes) in an infant and when doing PD for hypercatabolic states. In older children, the dwell time can be increased up to 1 hour.
- In pulmonary edema, the dwell time can be shortened to 15–20 minutes and concentrated dialysate fluid (2.5%) can be used to remove fluid rapidly.
- In severe metabolic acidosis, "bicarbonate-based PD" can be done with shorter dwell time.
- *Continuous flow peritoneal dialysis (CFPD):* It can be considered as a PD treatment option when an increase in solute clearance and ultrafiltration is desired but cannot be achieved with standard acute PD. Therapy with this technique should be considered experimental since experience with the therapy is limited. It can also be considered for dialysis therapy in children with AKI when the use of only very small fill volumes is preferred (e.g., children with high ventilator pressures).

Monitoring

- Vitals along with accurate input output and weight records
- Color of peritoneal fluid and fibrin threads in PD drain fluid
- Serum electrolytes and blood sugar every 12 hours
- Blood urea and creatinine once a day
- PD fluid should be sent for analysis if the patient is febrile or PD drain fluid is altered in color.

Cycle number	*Inflow time*	*Inflow volume*	*Dwell time*	*Outflow time*	*Outflow volume*	*Cycle balance*	*Cumulative balance*	*BP*	*RBS*

Complications

- *During insertion:*
  - *Bleeding:* It usually diminishes with subsequent cycles. Add heparin to dialysate fluid to prevent catheter blockage.
  - *Bowel perforation:* Uncommon when artificial ascites is created prior to procedure. It manifests with watery diarrhea and fecal material in dialysate effluent.
  - *Bladder perforation:* Rare if bladder is catheterized prior to procedure
- *Poor drainage:* Catheter may be blocked with fibrin or omental plug, and managed by flushing, repositioning or removal and reinsertion of catheter.
- *Leakage:* Purse string suture at base prevents it. Use smaller fill volumes if leak is detected. Ensure all holes are intraperitoneal while inserting the catheter.
- *Abdominal pain:* Pain during inflow is usually because of peritonitis, cold dialysate fluid, hypertonic solution, or excessive abdominal distention.
- Electrolyte disturbances (hypokalemia and hypernatremia) and hyperglycemia
- Dehydration
- *Peritonitis:* It manifests by abdominal pain, cloudy peritoneal fluid containing >100 cells/mm^3 or any number of cells with >50% neutrophils. Usual organisms are gram positive bacteria (*Staphylococcus epidermidis*, *S. aureus*). Initial treatment started with intraperitoneal antibiotics covering for both gram-positive and gram-negative organisms till availability of gram stain or culture.
- Respiratory embarrassment (abdominal compartment syndrome) because of over distention of abdomen, pleural effusion

CONTRAINDICATIONS

Peritoneal dialysis is absolutely contraindicated in patients with diaphragmatic defects. It is generally not recommended in patients with recent abdominal surgery or trauma, ventriculoperitoneal shunts, prune belly syndrome, and ventilation via the high-frequency oscillator because of the high risk of catheter leak due to abdominal movement.

CONCLUSION

Peritoneal dialysis remains an essential treatment option for pediatric patients with AKI. Successful catheter insertion and the choice of PD technique depend on the patient's condition and available resources. Proper preoperative preparation, careful technique during insertion, and vigilant postoperative care are crucial to minimize complications and ensure the effectiveness of PD in managing renal failure in young patients.

REFERENCES

1. Khwaja A. KDIGO clinical practice guidelines for acute kidney injury. Nephron Clin Pract. 2012;120(4):c179-84.
2. ISPD guidelines for peritoneal dialysis in acute kidney injury: 2020 Update (paediatrics). Perit Dial Int. 2021;41(2):139-57.
3. Peritoneal dialysis in the pediatric intensive care unit setting: techniques, quantifications, and outcomes. Blood Purif. 2013;35(1-3):77-80.

4. Szeto CC, Li PK, Johnson DW, Bernardini J, Dong J, Figueiredo AE, et al. ISPD Catheter-Related Infection Recommendations: 2017 Update. Perit Dial Int. 2017;37(2): 141-54.
5. Chow KM, Szeto CC, Leung CB, Kwan BC, Pang WF, Li PK. Tenckhoff catheter insertion by nephrologists: open dissection technique. Perit Dial Int. 2010;30:524-7.
6. Wright MJ, Bel'eed K, Johnson BF, Eadington DW, Sellars L, Farr MJ. Randomized prospective comparison of laparoscopic and open peritoneal dialysis catheter insertion. Perit Dial. 1999;19:372-5.
7. Crabtree JH. Selected best demonstrated practices in peritoneal dialysis access. Kidney Int. 2006;70:S27-37.
8. Attaluri V, Lebeis C, Brethauer S, Rosenblatt S. Advanced laparoscopic techniques significantly improve function of peritoneal dialysis catheters. J Am Coll Surg. 2010;211: 699-704.
9. Medani S, Hussein W, Shantier M, Flynn R, Wall C, Mellotte G. Comparison of percutaneous and open surgical techniques for first-time peritoneal dialysis catheter placement in the unbreached peritoneum. Perit Dial Int. 2015;35(5):576-85.

Index

Page numbers followed by *b* refer to box, *f* refer to figure, *fc* refer to flowchart, and *t* refer to table.

A

B

C

I

J

K

T

W

X

Z